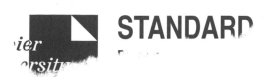
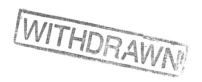
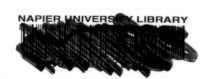

GERONTOLOGICAL REHABILITATION NURSING

GERONTOLOGICAL REHABILITATION NURSING

Kristen L. Easton, MS, RN, CRRN-A

Assistant Professor of Nursing
Valparaiso University
Community Health Education Director
Porter Memorial Hospital
Valparaiso, Indiana
Doctoral Candidate
Wayne State University
Detroit, Michigan

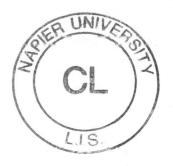

W.B. SAUNDERS COMPANY
A Division of Harcourt Brace & Company
Philadelphia   London   Toronto   Montreal   Sydney   Tokyo

W.B. SAUNDERS COMPANY
A Division of Harcourt Brace & Company

The Curtis Center
Independence Square West
Philadelphia, Pennsylvania 19106

Library of Congress Cataloging-in-Publication Data

Easton, Kristen L.

Gerontological rehabilitation nursing / Kristen L. Easton.

p.   cm.

ISBN 0–7216–6344–3

1. Geriatric nursing.   2. Rehabilitation nursing.   3. Aged—Rehabilitation.
   4. Aged—Nursing home care.   I. Title. [DNLM: 1. Geriatric Nursing.
   2. Rehabilitation Nursing.   WY 152 E13g 1999]

RC954.E226 1999   610.73′65—dc21

DNLM/DLC   98–37373

GERONTOLOGICAL REHABILITATION NURSING   ISBN 0–7216–6344–3

Printed in the United States of America.

Last digit is the print number: 9   8   7   6   5   4   3   2   1

Dedication

To my father, Peter Gibson, M.D.,
upon his retirement from a lifetime of service
to medicine in the specialty of pediatric surgery.

For the thousands of lives that you helped to save
and improve, Dad, that so many children could grow
to know the joys of old age,
and for the excellent example of a life well lived
that you set for all of us.

■

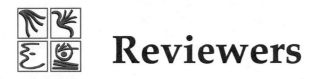

Reviewers

Carolyn K. Braudaway, MS, RN
Columbia Union College
Takoma Park, Maryland

Bonnie L. Closson, RN, CRRN*
Clinical Nurse Specialist
Mayo Clinic
Rochester, Minnesota

Sue Cohen, MA, OTR/L
MossRehab Hospital
Philadelphia, Pennsylvania

Patricia A. Dalleske, MSN
Formerly Instructor, Department of Nursing
Youngstown State University
Youngstown, Ohio

Bonnie A. Hall, MScN, RN
Clinical Nurse Specialist, Geriatrics
Queensway-Carleton Hospital
Nepean, Ontario
Clinical Assistant and Faculty of Health
  Science
University of Ottawa School of Nursing
Ottawa, Ontario
Canada

Geri Richards Hall, ARNP, CNS
Gerontology Clinical Nurse Specialist
Mayo Clinic, Scottsdale
Scottsdale, Arizona

Sandra P. Hirst, MSc(NEd), RN
Associate Professor
University of Calgary
Calgary, Alberta
Canada

Patricia McLean Hoyson, MSN, RN, CDE
Assistant Professor of Nursing
Youngstown State University
Youngstown, Ohio

Sharon E. Melberg, RN, MPA
University of California, Davis,
  Medical Center
Sacramento, California

Jeanne Mervine, RN, MS, CRRN
Rehabilitation Institute of Chicago
Chicago, Illinois

Henry M. Plawecki, PhD, RN
Professor
Purdue University Calumet
Hammond, Indiana

Susan M. Rawl, PhD, RN
Assistant Research Scientist
Indiana University School of Nursing
Indianapolis, Indiana

Barbara Resnick, PhD, CRNP
University of Maryland School of Nursing
Baltimore, Maryland

---

*Deceased

Preface

This book was written as a reference for long-term caregivers and emphasizes the application of rehabilitation and gerontological principles in post-acute care settings. In my years of nursing practice in long-term care, I came to realize that there was a need for a gerontological nursing text based on rehabilitation principles and concepts. I first felt the frustration experienced by many long-term caregivers many years ago when I worked as a nursing assistant in a nursing home. I recall thinking: Is this all there is? Isn't there any way to improve the quality of life for elderly residents in long-term care? What is the key to quality care for these older patients? I have spent the rest of my professional career pursuing the answer to those questions. The answer lies in a new specialty called gerontological rehabilitation nursing.

The field of gerontological nursing is quickly expanding. Care of the older adult with long-term illnesses cannot be adequately given apart from the principles and concepts of rehabilitation. A nurse educated in the principles of rehabilitation, with sufficient knowledge of the aging process, will be able to meet the future challenges of the complex elderly population. New roles for health professionals may emerge, and families will likely play a more crucial part in care of the aged than ever before. More aged adults will be cared for in the home. But how can health care professionals teach families and patients things that they themselves never learned? What is the key to quality care for our elderly patients? The answer lies in the marriage between rehabilitation concepts and gerontological nursing.

Gerontological nursing apart from rehabilitation concepts and practice is nothing more than medical-surgical nursing applied to older adults. That is why I felt a text based on rehabilitation was needed by practitioners. However, by introducing such a reference into the literature, I felt compelled to provide some explanations as to its origins, as Part I suggests. Understanding this background is essential to defining gerontological rehabilitation as a specialty in nursing.

This text is not designed to be a comprehensive gerontological nursing book and a rehabilitation text. It is assumed that the reader has basic knowledge of the nursing process and the aging process. This text presents holistic nursing care (based on rehabilitation principles) for older clients with chronic health alterations. The emphasis is on post-acute, tertiary care of older adults who have long-term health alterations. The content focuses on the application of rehabilitation practices to care of long-lived adults who have chronic health problems. The reader is encouraged to value the adult with a long-term health alteration as a holistic being who perpetually interacts with and is influenced by the internal and external environment. Rehabilitation concepts are explained, and gerontological nursing is discussed, with an emphasis on health maintenance, promotion of self-care, and prevention of secondary complications.

The information is organized into four units. Part I provides an introduction to rehabilitation and long-term care, discussing concepts, principles, definitions, holistic care, the interdisciplinary team, roles of the nurse, and a brief discussion of related theories. This forms the framework for gerontological rehabilitation nursing practice.

Part II deals with assisting the person toward self-care through application of rehabilitation principles and knowledge of the aging process. Part II focuses on practical, clinical information on improving nutritional status, maintaining and promoting skin integrity, mobility, establishing bowel and bladder patterns, and enhancing sensory perception. For example, in the chapter on mobility, different types of transfers (including proper positioning of the wheelchair, the patient, and the caregiver during various transfers) are discussed, as is proper use of transfer belts and gait belts, promoting back safety when lifting, and how to teach patients to maximize self-care related to mobility and transfers.

Part III presents nursing implications related to selected common diagnoses in the older adult. This includes a practical discussion of rehabilitative, long-term care of the adult who has experienced such problems as stroke, spinal cord injury, various other neurological disorders, and orthopedic problems such as arthritis, hip and knee replacements, and amputation. Those conditions that were discussed generally in terms of systems in Part II are explained more fully in Part III. This is one of the most distinguishing characteristics of the book. Case studies are included to enhance critical thinking.

Part IV presents additional considerations in long-term care. Cultural competence; psychosocial issues; ethical, legal, and moral considerations; and trends in gerontological rehabilitation nursing are discussed. Topics such as the right to die, death with dignity, assisted suicide, polypharmacy, abuse of the aged, and support for the family and caregiver are addressed. Case studies and suggested resources are included.

As with any endeavor, this work represents only a beginning. The author hopes that others will continue to explore and expand this body of knowledge to further nursing science and to more fully define the specialty of gerontological rehabilitation nursing.

KRISTEN L. EASTON

Acknowledgments

Many friends, family members, and colleagues contributed to the writing of this book through their encouragement, enthusiasm, and support. I would particularly like to thank the nursing staff who worked with me on 1 East, Rehabilitation, at St. Margaret Mercy Healthcare Centers in Hammond, Indiana—their commitment to quality patient care inspired me to write this book. I am equally indebted to the nursing faculty at Valparaiso University, whose high standards for nursing education keep me constantly challenged to strive for excellence. A sincere thanks to some special friends who provided constant encouragement and support, as well as listening ears: Nola, Jenecia, and Susan (my fellow doctoral students at Wayne State), Phyllis, Freda, Linda, Roberta, Michelle, and Pat. Thank you to Donna, Mary, and Madonna for help with pictures. A special thanks to Greg, and to my children, Rachel, Kenny, and Daniel, for all the hours you sacrificed "mom" to her writing. Thanks to my brother, Don, sisters, Kathy and Valeri, and my parents, Pete and Kay Gibson, for staying in touch even when I didn't.

KRIS

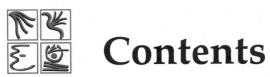

Contents

Part I

Introduction to Rehabilitation and Long-Term Care

■

Chapter 1

Aging, Disability, and Chronic Illness

■

THE AGING POPULATION

The face of America is showing its age. Never before have so many lived for so long. As of 1990, people older than 65 years old accounted for 12.7% of the United States population, or about 32.8 million individuals (Fowles, 1994). At present, one in every eight Americans is elderly (U.S. Department of Commerce & U.S. Department of Health and Human Services, 1991). As the "baby boomers" (those born after World War II, 1946–1964) reach the age of 65, the nation will see a surge in the growth of the elderly population (Fig. 1–1).

The U.S. Bureau of the Census projects that the number of elderly will peak by the year 2050, accounting for about 79 million people, or about one of every five Americans (Goldstein & Damon, 1993). As the number of elderly in the population has increased, researchers have designated classifications to help distinguish differences in this diverse group. The most commonly used terms are the *young-old* (age 65–74 years), *middle-old* (age 75–84 years), and *old-old* (age 85 and older). The young-old group is made up of individuals who have most recently been labeled "seniors," but many of them do not present with the problems seen in later life. For example, in 1990, only 1.4% of the young-old population lived in nursing homes, compared with 6% of the middle-old and 25% of the old-old (Goldstein & Damon, 1993). Changes in living arrangements, marital status, and functional ability also occur with age (U.S. Department of Commerce & U.S. Department of Health and Human Services,

1993), further emphasizing the diversity within this elderly group.

The old-old population, sometimes referred to as the frail elderly, has experienced a growth of 35% from 1980 to 1990 and is only expected to continue to grow (U.S. Department of Commerce & U.S. Department of Health and Human Services, 1993). This group represents 10% of the elderly population (U.S. Department of Commerce & U.S. Department of Health and Human Services, 1991). It should be noted that although the growth rate appears high, the people 85 years

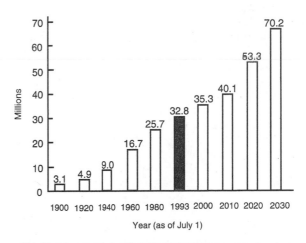

Figure 1–1 Number of persons 65 years and older: 1900 to 2030. (From the American Association of Retired Persons (AARP). (1994). *A profile of older Americans*. [Based on data from the U.S. Bureau of the Census]. Washington, DC: Author. Copyright 1995, American Association of Retired Persons. Reprinted with permission.)

and older accounted for just over 1% of the U.S. population in 1990 (U.S. Department of Commerce & U.S. Department of Health and Human Services, 1992). In 2050, at the peak of the elderly population growth, it is projected that nearly 20% of the U.S. population will be 85 years and older, making this the fastest growing age group in the country. In addition, the 1990 census revealed nearly 1 million people reporting their age as 90 years or older, with centenarians (those 100 years or older) numbering 36,000 (U.S. Department of Commerce & U.S. Department of Health and Human Services, 1991), a figure also expected to increase.

But the United States is not the only country whose elderly population is growing. While life expectancy in the United States has increased significantly in the past century, from 47 years in 1900 to over 75 years in 1990 (Goldstein & Damon, 1993), other nations have experienced similar trends. During the past several decades, most developing countries have experienced significant reductions in mortality rates and subsequent increases in longevity. With the increase in availability of advanced medical treatment, life expectancy—perhaps as a result of both a reduction of mortality and a decreased birth rate—is predicted to continue to increase. Between 1950 and 2025, the total number of persons worldwide age 60 and older is expected to increase to about 1.1 billion (United Nations, 1991). If these projections are correct, many countries are experiencing a demographic transition to an older population structure. In 1980, the countries that had the most aged populations, with 10% or more at age 65 and older, included Poland, Romania, Australia, United States, Portugal, Spain, Netherlands, Bulgaria, Czechoslovakia, France, Hungary, Greece, Belgium, West Germany, Switzerland, Italy, Denmark, United Kingdom, Austria, East Germany, and Sweden (Cowgill, 1986; Sokolovsky, 1987). According to the United Nations International Conference on Ageing Populations in the Context of Urbanization, by the year 2025, the proportion of elderly in more developed regions will exceed 25%, and the populations of less developed areas would still have at least 12% of the population older than 60 years of age (United Nations, 1991).

Thus, the experience of aging is not limited to one particular country or continent, but is a universal phenomenon. This process is one that occurs to all human beings regardless of racial, cultural, religious, or ethnic differences. However, many factors affect the aging process, just as growing old has certain predictable effects.

AGING AND DISABILITY

As the body ages, individuals experience a wide variety of changes in bodily systems and their functions. Some of these result from "normal" aging and are generally expected. Other changes are considered abnormal and may require the elderly person to use the health care system more frequently than before. In fact, most elderly suffer from at least one chronic illness (Eliopoulos, 1997). Many such long-term health problems may lead to disability.

Caring for aged patients accounts for a large portion of health care dollars spent each year. However, many federal programs that provide assistance to the disabled elderly are inadequately funded, understaffed, and overwhelmed. For example, The Social Security Disability Insurance (SSDI) program was originally designed to provide partial replacement of earnings for those older than 50 years of age who experienced a disability. Since its inception, the SSDI has grown to tackle more diverse purposes, often to the unintentional exclusion of those whom it was intended to serve. In fact, defining who is classified as disabled has become one of the more difficult tasks of the federal government.

The probability of having multiple chronic conditions increases with chronological age. More than 80% of the elderly report having at least one chronic problem (Zarle, 1989). Table 1–1 lists some of the most frequently reported chronic illnesses. Arthritis is the most common, with more than half of those age 65 and older reporting this problem. The second most common condition is hypertension, especially prevalent among African-Americans. Approximately half of the old-old population complain of hearing loss. Heart

Table 1–1   COMMON CHRONIC HEALTH COMPLAINTS OF OLDER ADULTS

Arthritis	Visual disturbances
Hypertension	Cancer
Hearing impairments	Diabetes
Heart conditions	Varicose veins
Orthopedic problems	Hemorrhoids
Sinusitis	Depression
Respiratory disorders	Skin disorders
Stroke	

conditions, chronic sinusitis, visual disturbances, orthopedic problems, and respiratory conditions are also frequently reported conditions.

Arthritis, the number one chronic condition among the elderly, can have severe negative effects on mobility and functional capacity (Lyngberg, Harreby, Bentzen, Frost, & Danneskiold-Samsoe, 1994; Montgomery Orr & Bratton, 1992; Mulrow et al., 1994). Arthritis affects such a large portion of the elderly population that it is considered by some to be a normal part of aging. Even the aging process itself, apart from disease or illness, tends to be accompanied by increased frailty and a decrease in self-care capacity (Boult et al., 1994; Hasselkus, 1989; Jopp, Carroll, & Waters, 1993; Mulrow et al., 1994). Many elderly individuals who are unable to care for themselves will require some type of nursing care as they age, owing largely to factors related to mobility. According to a study by Ettinger et al. (1994), the most common diseases reported by the elderly to cause difficulty with physical tasks included arthritis, heart disease, lung disease, and stroke, along with old age and injury.

Hypertension significantly increases the chance of heart attack, heart failure, kidney damage, and eye problems (American Heart Association, 1990). High blood pressure is also the number one risk factor for stroke. According to the National Stroke Association (1994), every year nearly 500,000 Americans experience a stroke. Of the approximately 350,000 who survive, many will have residual disabilities, and all will experience some kind of change in their lives, whether temporary or permanent. Although not exclusively a disease of old age, the majority of strokes do occur in those age 65 and older. Even modifiable risk factors of stroke, such as hypertension and cardiovascular diseases, are often associated with aging.

Approximately 13% of the United States and world population is disabled (Rehabilitation Institute of Chicago, 1993). Many of the disabled are also elderly. These two groups, the aged and the disabled, comprise people from all racial, cultural, religious, and socioeconomic backgrounds. The disabled elderly, then, could be considered a double minority. However, as life expectancy increases, so do the number of elderly and the number of aged people living with disabilities.

In fact, as the number of elderly in the general population increases, so does the percentage of persons needing assistance with everyday activities. Approximately 45% of noninstitutionalized persons older than the age of 85 years require such assistance (Goldstein & Damon, 1993; U.S. Department of Commerce & U.S. Department of Health and Human Services, 1991), compared with only 2.4% of those younger than 65. Indeed, there appears to be a strong relationship between age and the need for assistance. Depending on the definitions of activities of daily living (ADLs), studies estimate a range of between 4.4 million and 6.7 million of the noninstitutionalized elderly with functional dependencies (Taeuber, 1993). By the year 2000, it is expected that 7.3 million elderly will require some type of assistance to remain independent. This figure may increase to about 14.4 million by the year 2050 (Zarle, 1989).

Unfortunately, the funds available to care for these individuals do not match the increased need. Because it is well documented that the elderly experience many common chronic health problems that often result in disability, the health system must prepare itself to use creative methods for providing long-term care.

IMPLICATIONS FOR HEALTH CARE

Research has shown that rehabilitation of the elderly can increase their ability to perform self-care (Gill & Balsano, 1994; Gregor, McCarthy, Chwirchak, Meluch, & Mion, 1986; Heacock, Walton, Beck, & Mercer, 1991; Kalra, 1994). Numerous studies have been conducted that demonstrate correlations between exercise or activity programs and functional capacity (Bohannon & Cooper, 1993; Gregor et al., 1986; Judge, Underwood, & Gennosa, 1993; Lyngberg et al., 1994; Mills, 1994; Nugent, Schurr, & Adams, 1994). Many studies examine the elderly population with orthopedic problems such as hip fracture, arthritis, and amputation, as well as combinations of these disorders. These groups have also been shown to improve function with rehabilitation (Bohannon & Cooper, 1993; Fisher et al., 1993; Montgomery Orr & Bratton, 1992). Mehta and Nastasi stated that although reduction and immobilization of fractures in the elderly may often be unnecessary, "rehabilitation is always essential" (1993, p. 717).

Rehabilitation after a stroke also significantly affects functional recovery (Dobkin, 1991; Kalra, 1994; Khader & Tomlin, 1994; Nakayama, Jorgensen, Raaschou, & Skyhoj

Olsen, 1994). Most stroke patients participating in an inpatient rehabilitation program maintain gains achieved and even continue to improve after discharge home (Davidoff, Keren, Ring, & Solzi, 1991; Rawl, Easton, Zemen, Kwiatkowski, & Burczyk, 1998). Even cognitively impaired elderly benefit from a rehabilitative focus to care (Heacock et al., 1991). Despite differences in diagnoses, rehabilitation plays a significant role in the outcomes and hence the discharge and health maintenance status of elderly patients.

Yet rehabilitation does not only affect physical outcomes. Rawl et al. (1998) found that elderly rehabilitation patients who received follow-up from a rehabilitation nurse after discharge used more positive coping strategies than those receiving less specialized follow-up care. Other researchers have examined the connection between such variables as self-care, decision-making, coping, health-promoting lifestyles, quality of life, and the like (Aller & Van Ess Coeling, 1995; Stuifbergen & Becker, 1994). These findings generally indicate that a person's self-perception and coping ability improve throughout the rehabilitation process and can be linked to the capacity to perform or direct self-care.

The role of the spouse, caregiver, and/or significant other has also been shown to have a positive effect on outcomes, both functional and psychological, of the elderly rehabilitation patient (Baker, 1993; Folden, 1993; Watson, 1986). Cummings et al. (1988) found that patients, particularly those 60 years and older, who had a greater number of social supports recovered more completely (closer to prefracture level of function) after a hip fracture. Conversely, however, caregiver-related problems can also negatively affect the long-term care situation (Evans, Bishop, & Haselkorn, 1991; Periard & Ames, 1993). In addition, coping strategies of patients with long-term disabilities, as well as their caregivers, have also been shown to be positively influenced by the rehabilitation process (White, Richter, & Fry, 1992).

The effectiveness of nursing interventions in long-term care and rehabilitation is an area where further research is needed. Much of the literature is focused on discharge planning, indicating that this is a critical component to the nursing role (Haddock, 1991; Shiell, Kenny, & Farnworth, 1993). Supportive-educative nursing interventions have also been largely influential in helping patients and family members to cope with long-term health alterations. Outcomes that may be af-

fected by nursing interventions include, but are not limited to, a decreased length of stay, improvement in functional status including mobility skills, increase in use of positive coping mechanisms, and the increased likelihood of a home discharge destination (Folden, 1993; Gill & Ursic, 1994; Heafey, Golden-Baker, & Mahoney, 1994; Lichtenstein, Semaan, & Marmar, 1993; Miller, Wikoff, McMahon, Garrett, & Ringel, 1988).

COMMONLY USED TERMS

Defining who is disabled for the purpose of dispersing federal funds is one of the most challenging tasks assigned to the government. However, for the layperson and the health care professional, certain commonly used terms should be recognized. The following sections define and discuss words often used in long-term care of the elderly.

Elderly/Aged

Society typically has defined the *elderly* or *senior citizen* as any person age 65 or older; however, this restriction is largely a result of the need for a chronological age to determine eligibility for social security, retirement benefits, and pension. Many so-called older adults lead very active lives, participating in such vigorous activities as scuba diving, water-skiing, marathon running, and the like. Others in this age group become more sedentary and thus are likely to sooner experience the normal effects of aging. Yet, aging is a highly individualized experience influenced by a variety of factors. Such variables include cultural, racial, ethnic, and religious differences. The attitudes that people hold toward growing old also influence perceptions of the aging process. Others define aging in terms of functional capacity or biological changes.

For the purposes of this text, a traditional definition of elderly or the aged (those 65 years of age and older) is used. Most of the research done with older adults defines this age group similarly, but it should be noted that significant differences in many areas such as lifestyle, living arrangements, and functional capacity are found even within this population. Thus, as stated earlier in this chapter, the elderly are often classified into the *young-old, middle-old*, and *old-old* (or frail elderly) categories. In general, the American elderly are described as a diverse and growing population.

Disability

Disability is an appropriate term to use in reference to the limitations an individual may experience as the result of an impairment due to illness, injury, or birth defect. Disability has also been defined as the "inability to perform some key life functions" (Dittmar, 1989). *Functional limitations* is a closely related term, often used interchangeably, and refers to difficulties persons may experience in carrying out ADLs.

Disabilities can take many forms: physical, communicative, developmental, sensory, or cognitive. Many older adults have a combination of disabilities. Although a disability may limit a person's functional status, there are still many different ways individuals adapt to these changes, making them "able" in other capacities.

Many people labeled as "disabled" do not consider themselves as such. They acknowledge their limitations and take the necessary steps to adjust to them. In their eyes, this makes them "able." In order to avoid judgmental verbiage, health care professionals need to examine their use of language in discussing persons with disabilities.

Impairment

Impairment, also an appropriate rehabilitation term, refers to residual limitation that results from disease, injury, or birth defect. Impairment implies a decrease in an ability, but not total loss. This term can be linked with other descriptors to further describe an individual's status without verbal bias. For example, hearing impairment is a broad term that could be used to describe a range of disabilities from "slightly hard of hearing" to deafness. *Functional impairment* is used to describe difficulties performing routine activities such as ADLs. This term is akin to *functional limitations*.

Handicap

The word *handicap* is considered by some to be an inappropriate term that applies to bowling, golf, and horse racing but not people. More recent models for rehabilitative care do not use this term. The World Health Organization (WHO), however, makes a distinction between the definitions for *impairment, disability,* and *handicap*. The WHO states that an impairment occurs at the organ level, a disability occurs at the personal level, and a handicap occurs at the societal level (Storck & Thompson-Hoffman, 1991). The word *handicap* suggests interaction between the person with a disability and the environment. A handicap is the disadvantage a person may experience (as a result of impairment or disability) that limits or prevents usual function for that individual.

Chronic Illness

The word *chronic* is difficult to define, much less comprehend, unless one has experienced a long-term illness. Discussion must arise as to what is considered chronic and what is called acute. There is no precise dividing line between the two. Does a patient who has experienced a headache for more than 2 weeks still consider it a temporary problem? When does the individual with a back injury resulting in pain and spasms call it a chronic problem? The definition of chronic illness may well vary from person to person. Nonetheless, it is helpful to attempt to use some guidelines by which to measure chronicity.

According to the Commission on Chronic Illness, chronic illness is defined as "all impairments or deviations from normal which have one or more of the following characteristics: are permanent, leave residual disability, are caused by a nonreversible pathological condition, require special training of the patient for rehabilitation, may be expected to require a long period of supervision, observation or care" (Strauss, 1975, p. 1).

This definition encompasses a myriad of long-term health alterations. Those diseases that in the past were considered chronic do not always fit within this framework. For example, cancer, once considered the prime example of chronic illness, is no longer always irreversible, results in impairments or disability, or necessitates a long period of supportive care. Other conditions may be chronic depending on their severity, such as an incomplete spinal cord injury, mild stroke, or Guillain-Barré syndrome, which may for a time require extensive care, but can result in complete recovery with no residual effects, and thus may not always be considered a "chronic illness."

Based on this definition, several chronic illnesses can be identified, as shown in Table 1–2. These would include conditions that may result in some form of disability, and usually require long-term supervision. Chronicity is a concept involving a wide variety of variables, requiring the health care professional to care-

Table 1–2 EXAMPLES OF COMMON CHRONIC ILLNESSES

AIDS
Diabetes
Multiple sclerosis
Muscular dystrophy
Cerebral palsy
Polio
Disfiguring burns
Amputation
Parkinson's disease
Rheumatoid arthritis
Many types of cancer
Schizophrenia
Alzheimer's disease and other forms of dementia
Complete spinal cord injury, and some
    incomplete injuries
Cerebrovascular accident with residual limitations
Chronic obstructive pulmonary disease (COPD)

Based on the definition from the Commission on Chronic Illness (1956).

fully examine an individual's situation in a holistic manner for successful treatment.

GERONTOLOGY AND GERIATRICS

Gerontology refers to the study of aging and/ or the elderly. *Geriatrics* is one subspecialty of gerontology and is defined as the medical care of the aged. Both are rapidly growing fields, but ones in which there is still a severe shortage of health care professionals. According to the Alliance for Aging Research, the nation's academic health centers are not well prepared to teach geriatrics, with an inadequate number of physicians educated in this specialty. Likewise, the need for nurses caring for the elderly will increase dramatically by the year 2020, with an estimated need for 600,000 additional full-time equivalent registered nurses (RNs). Data from the Division of Nursing, Bureau of Health Professions predict that more than half of the total supply of RNs will be caring for persons in the older age category (*Shortage of Health Care Professions*, 1993).

GERONTOLOGICAL NURSING

The specialty of gerontological nursing, or nursing care of the elderly, was first suggested in 1925 in an editorial published by the *American Journal of Nursing*, although an article in the same journal was published in 1904 on care of the aged. The first textbook on this specialty was published in 1950. To-

day there are many fine resource books on this subject.

Gerontological nursing, sometimes mistakenly referred to as geriatric nursing (a misnomer), has only recently been welcomed into the curriculum of some nursing programs. Although the concept of gerontological nursing has been well represented in the literature for decades, the educational arena has been slower to adopt it. Many baccalaureate programs now include a course on care of the older adult, but few associate degree programs have such a single required course. The challenging task of integrating these principles throughout the curriculum (although this should occur regardless of the existence of a concentrated class in this area) then becomes the work of the faculty and is often underemphasized.

The importance of educating nursing students in the area of elderly care cannot be overemphasized. Recent strides have been taken to ensure that every gerontological nurse, regardless of educational background, shares a similar goal: "health care for elderly Americans should be affordable, and should foster autonomy, promote health, provide excellent illness care, and support a death with dignity" (Burke & Sherman, 1993, pp. 60–61). This statement truly represents a step in the right direction.

REHABILITATION AND REHABILITATION NURSING

Rehabilitation is a lifelong process in which the client with a long-term health alteration works together with the family, the rehabilitation team, and society to achieve his or her optimum level of functioning as a holistic person, with the goals of preventing secondary complications, fostering maximal independence, maintaining dignity, and promoting quality of life. The process of rehabilitation is complex and involves the coordinated efforts of a variety of professionals. The members of the interdisciplinary health care team collaborate with the client, formulating mutually established goals and adapting an individualized plan of care to assist the client toward maximal independence. Members of the rehabilitation team support one other, sharing expertise in their respective areas to provide a holistic approach to comprehensive care planning, with the common goal of assisting the client to achieve optimal outcomes.

Although rehabilitation demands the coordinated efforts of many health care professionals, the client is considered the most important member of the team. Many clients describe the rehabilitation program as the place where they learn to live again. The word *rehabilitate* comes from the Latin *re-* and *habilitare*, or *habilis*, meaning to "again fit" or "suit." The term denotes restoration to a former or better state.

Rehabilitation nursing has distinguished itself as an emerging and rapidly growing specialty. As of 1994, there were approximately 60,000 rehabilitation nurses in the United States. A large portion of this number have earned the distinction of rehabilitation nursing certification (CRRN, or certified rehabilitation registered nurse), further validating their expertise. Rehabilitation nurses work in a variety of settings, from hospitals to subacute facilities, long-term care, home health care, and community and governmental agencies, and for private companies such as insurance or consulting firms. They care for individuals and their families who have experienced a disabling injury or chronic illness, helping them to cope and adapt to their changing situation.

Nurses working in the field of rehabilitation must have a broad knowledge base, be able to work cooperatively with the interdisciplinary team, and be optimistic and creative. The rehabilitation nurse assumes many roles, including those of caregiver, teacher, researcher, manager, advocate, counselor, consultant, leader, and lifelong learner. Good communication and assessment skills are essential to promote quality patient outcomes.

GERONTOLOGICAL REHABILITATION NURSING

This is a subspecialty that has yet to be adequately defined. The Association of Rehabilitation Nurses (ARN) describes this field thus: "gerontological rehabilitation nursing practice provides care and expertise to promote health, maintain and restore function, and provides education and counseling to older clients and their families. Gerontological rehabilitation nurses combine rehabilitation knowledge and skills with gerontological principles to focus on individuals who are 65 years of age and older" (Association of Rehabilitation Nurses, 1994). The ARN first formed a special interest group in 1991 for rehabilitation nurses working with the elderly. Since that time, this group within the organization has continued to grow and is currently working on more thoroughly defining this field of practice. Most nurses considering themselves gerontological rehabilitation nurses have a strong background in rehabilitation and specific expertise in the area of older adults. Usually these practitioners are first rehabilitation nurses, but they may have had prior experience in long-term care. Their focus combines knowledge of both the aging process and rehabilitation concepts and practice to specialize in caring for the aging adult with a disability or long-term health problem. However, nurses who have training in gerontological nursing cannot automatically deem themselves gerontological rehabilitation nurses, for the principles of rehabilitation are not typically taught in depth in nursing school, neither are they learned overnight. The practice of this type of nursing continues to evolve and define itself. There are currently no nursing journals exclusively for gerontological rehabilitation nursing, but their development may not be far off.

Given the great patient/client numbers that will be included in this group in the coming years, gerontological rehabilitation is a specialty that demands particular attention. The purpose of this reference book is to provide definition and scope to the practice of gerontological rehabilitation nursing. The role of the gerontological rehabilitation nurse is further discussed in Chapter 4.

REFERENCES

Aller, L. J., & Van Ess Coeling, H. (1995). Quality of life: Its meaning to the long-term care resident. *Journal of Gerontological Nursing, 21*(2), 20–25.

American Heart Association. (1990). *About high blood pressure in African Americans* [Brochure]. Dallas, TX: Author.

Association of Rehabilitation Nurses. (1994). *Rehabilitation nurses make the difference* [Brochure]. Skokie, IL: Author.

Baker, A. (1993). The spouse's positive effect on the stroke patient's recovery. *Rehabilitation Nursing, 18*(1), 30–33.

Bohannon, R. W., & Cooper, J. (1993). Total knee arthroplasty: Evaluation of an acute care rehabilitation program. *Archives of Physical Medicine and Rehabilitation, 74*, 1091–1094.

Boult, C., Boult, L., Murphy, C., Ebbitt, B., Luptak, M., & Kane, R. L. (1994). A controlled trial of outpatient geriatric evaluation and management. *Journal of the American Geriatrics Society, 42*(5), 465–470.

Burke, M., & Sherman, S. (Eds.). (1993). *Gerontological nursing: Issues and opportunities for the twenty-first century.* New York: National League for Nursing Press.

Cowgill, D. O. (1986). *Aging around the world*. Belmont, CA: Wadsworth Publishing.

Cummings, S. R., Phillips, S. L., Wheat, M. E., Black, D., Gossby, E., Wlodarczyk, D., Trafton, P., Jergesen, H., Hunter Winograd, C., & Hulley, S. B. (1988). Recovery of function after hip fractures: The role of social supports. *Journal of the American Geriatrics Society, 36*, 801–806.

Davidoff, G. N., Keren, O., Ring, H., & Solzi, P. (1991). Acute stroke patients: Long-term effects of rehabilitation and maintenance of gains. *Archives of Physical Medicine and Rehabilitation, 72*, 869–873.

Dittmar, S. (1989). *Rehabilitation nursing: Process and application*. St. Louis, MO: C. V. Mosby.

Dobkin, B. H. (1991). The rehabilitation of elderly stroke patients. *Clinics in Geriatric Medicine, 7*(3), 507–523.

Eliopoulos, C. (1997). *Gerontological nursing*. Philadelphia: Lippincott-Raven.

Ettinger, W. H., Fried, L. P., Harris, T., Shemanski, L., Schulz, R., & Robbins, J. (1994). Self-reported causes of physical disability in older people: The cardiovascular health study. *Journal of the American Geriatrics Society, 42*(10), 1035–1044.

Evans, R. L., Bishop, D. S., & Haselkorn, J. K. (1991). Factors predicting satisfactory home care after stroke. *Archives of Physical Medicine and Rehabilitation, 72*, 144–147.

Fisher, N. W., Gresham, G. E., Abrams, M., Hicks, J., Horrigan, D., & Pendergast, D. R. (1993). Quantitative effects of physical therapy on muscular and functional performance in subjects with osteoarthritis of the knees. *Archives of Physical Medicine and Rehabilitation, 74*, 840–847.

Folden, S. L. (1993). Effect of a supportive-educative nursing intervention on older adults' perceptions of self-care after a stroke. *Rehabilitation Nursing, 18*(3), 162–166.

Fowles, D. G. (1994). *A profile of older Americans*. Washington, DC: American Association of Retired Persons and Administration on Aging, U.S. Department of Health and Human Services.

Gill, H. S., & Balsano, A. E. (1994). The move toward subacute care. *Nursing Homes, 43*(4), 6–7, 9–11.

Gill, K. P., & Ursic, P. (1994). The impact of continuing education on patient outcomes in the elderly hip fracture population. *Journal of Continuing Education in Nursing, 25*(4), 181–185.

Goldstein, A., Damon, B., & U.S. Department of Commerce, Economics and Statistics Administration, Bureau of the Census. (1993). *We the American elderly*. Washington, DC: U.S. Government Printing Office.

Gregor, S., McCarthy, K., Chwirchak, D., Meluch, M., & Mion, L. C. (1986). Characteristics and functional outcomes of elderly rehabilitation patients. *Rehabilitation Nursing, 11*(3), 10–14.

Haddock, K. S. (1991). Characteristics of effective discharge planning programs for the frail elderly. *Journal of Gerontological Nursing, 17*(7), 10–13.

Hasselkus, B. R. (1989). Occupational and physical therapy in geriatric rehabilitation. *Physical & Occupational Therapy in Geriatrics, 7*(3), 3–20.

Heacock, P., Walton, C., Beck, C., & Mercer, S. (1991). Caring for the cognitively impaired: Reconceptualizing disability and rehabilitation. *Journal of Gerontological Nursing, 17*(3), 23–25.

Heafey, M. L., Golden-Baker, S. B., & Mahoney, D. W. (1994). Using nursing diagnoses and intervention in an inpatient amputee program. *Rehabilitation Nursing, 19*(3), 163–168.

Jopp, M., Carroll, M. C., & Waters, L. (1993). Using self-care theory to guide nursing management of the older adult after hospitalization. *Rehabilitation Nursing, 18*(2), 91–94.

Judge, J. O., Underwood, M., & Gennosa, T. (1993). Exercise to improve gait velocity in older persons. *Archives of Physical Medicine and Rehabilitation, 74*, 400–406.

Kalra, L. (1994). The influence of stroke unit rehabilitation on functional recovery from stroke. *Stroke, 25*, 821–825.

Khader, M. S., & Tomlin, G. S. (1994). Change in wheelchair transfer performance during rehabilitation of men with cerebrovascular accident. *The American Journal of Occupational Therapy, 48*(10), 899–905.

Lichtenstein, R., Semaan, S., & Marmar, E. C. (1993). Development and impact of a hospital-based perioperative patient education program in a joint replacement center. *Orthopaedic Nursing, 12*(6), 17–23.

Lyngberg, K. K., Harreby, M., Bentzen, H., Frost, B., & Danneskiold-Samsoe, B. (1994). Elderly rheumatoid arthritis patients on steroid treatment tolerate physical training without an increase in disease activity. *Archives of Physical Medicine and Rehabilitation, 75*, 1189–1195.

Mehta, A. J., & Nastasi, A. E. (1993). Rehabilitation of fractures in the elderly. *Clinics in Geriatric Medicine, 9*(4), 717–727.

Miller, P., Wikoff, R., McMahon, M., Garrett, M. J., & Ringel, K. (1988). Influence of a nursing intervention of regimen adherence and societal adjustments postmyocardial infarction. *Nursing Research, 37*(5), 297–302.

Mills, E. M. (1994). The effect of low-intensity aerobic exercise on muscle strength, flexibility, and balance among sedentary elderly persons. *Nursing Research, 43*(4), 207–211.

Montgomery Orr, P., & Bratton, G. N. (1992). The effect of an inpatient arthritis rehabilitation program on self-assessed functional ability. *Rehabilitation Nursing, 17*(6), 306–310.

Mulrow, C. D., Gerety, M. B., Kanten, D., Cornell, J. E., DeNino, L. A. Chiodo, L., Aguilar, C., O'Neil, M. B., Rosenberg, J., & Solis, R. M. (1994). A randomized trial of physical rehabilitation for very frail nursing home residents. *Journal of the American Medical Association, 271*(7), 519–524.

Nakayama, H., Jorgensen, H. S., Raaschou, H. O., & Skyhoj Olsen, T. (1994). Recovery of upper extremity function in stroke patients: The Copenhagen Stroke Study. *Archives of Physical Medicine and Rehabilitation, 75,* 394–398.

National Stroke Association. (1994). *Stroke prevention: Reducing risk & recognizing symptoms* [Brochure]. Englewood, CO: Author.

Nugent, J. A., Schurr, K. A., & Adams, R. D. (1994). A dose response relationship between amount of weight bearing exercise and walking outcome following cerebrovascular accident. *Archives of Physical Medicine and Rehabilitation, 75,* 399–402.

Periard, M. E., & Ames, B. (1993). Lifestyle changes and coping patterns among caregivers of stroke survivors. *Public Health Nursing, 10*(4), 252–256.

Rawl, S., Easton, K. L., Zemen, D., Kwiatkowski, S., & Burczyk, B. (1998). Effectiveness of a nurse-managed follow-up program for rehabilitation patients after discharge. *Rehabilitation Nursing, 23*(4), 204–209.

Rehabilitation Institute of Chicago. (1993). *What do you say after you see they're disabled?* [Brochure]. Chicago, IL: Author.

Shiell, A., Kenny, P., & Farnworth, M. S. (1993). The role of the clinical nurse co-ordinator in the provision of cost-effective orthopaedic services for elderly people. *Journal of Advanced Nursing, 18,* 1424–1428.

Shortage of health care professions caring for the elderly: Recommendations for change: A report by the Chairman of the Select Committee on Aging, House of Representatives, One Hundred Second Congress, second session (1993). Washington, DC: U.S. Government Printing Office.

Sokolovsky, J. (1987) *Growing old in different societies: Cross-cultural perspectives.* Littleton, MA: Copley Publishing Group.

Storck, I. F., & Thompson-Hoffman, S. (1991). Demographic characteristics of the disabled population. In S. Thompson-Hoffman & I. F. Storck (Eds.), *Disability in the United States: A portrait from national data* (pp. 1–12). New York: Springer Publishing.

Strauss, A. L. (1975). *Chronic illness and the quality of life.* St. Louis, MO: C. V. Mosby.

Stuifbergen, A. K., & Becker, H. A. (1994). Pre-dictors of health-promoting lifestyles in persons with disabilities. *Research in Nursing and Health, 17,* 3–13.

Taeuber, C. (1993). *Sixty-five plus in America* (pp. 3, 11–16) [Brochure]. Washington, DC: U.S. Department of Commerce, Economics and Statistics Administration, Bureau of the Census.

United Nations, Department of International Economic and Social Affairs. (1991). *Ageing and urbanization.* Proceedings of the United Nations International Conference on Ageing Population in the Context of Urbanization. New York: United Nations.

U.S. Department of Commerce, Economics and Statistics Administration, Bureau of the Census, & U.S. Department of Health and Human Services, National Institutes of Health, National Institute on Aging. (1991). *Profiles of America's elderly: Growth of America's elderly in the 1980's.* Washington, DC: U.S. Government Printing Office.

U.S. Department of Commerce, Economics and Statistics Administration, Bureau of the Census, & U.S. Department of Health and Human Services, National Institutes of Health, National Institute on Aging. (1992). *Profiles of America's elderly: Growth of America's oldest-old population.* Washington, DC: U.S. Government Printing Office.

U.S. Department of Commerce, Economics and Statistics Administration, Bureau of the Census, & U.S. Department of Health and Human Services, National Institutes of Health, National Institute on Aging. (1993). *Profiles of America's elderly: Living arrangements of the elderly.* Washington, DC: U.S. Government Printing Office.

Watson, P. G. (1986). Stroke in the family: Theoretical considerations. *Rehabilitation Nursing, 11*(5), 15–17.

White, N. W., Richter, J. M., & Fry, C. (1992). Coping, social support, and adaptation to chronic illness. *Western Journal of Nursing Research, 14*(2), 211–224.

Zarle, N. S. (1989). Continuity of care: Balancing care of elders between health care settings. *Nursing Clinics of North America, 24*(3), 697–705.

Chapter 2

The Nature of Long-Term Care: Practice Settings for the Gerontological Rehabilitation Nurse

■

An understanding of the numerous settings in which gerontological rehabilitation nurses (GRNs) may practice and the various levels of care often required by the elderly will assist in planning quality care. Although GRNs will need to integrate the various roles (as described in Chapter 4) to different extents depending on the individual needs of patients in each setting, some general comments about each practice environment may be helpful.

ACUTE CARE HOSPITAL

The term *acute care* in reference to health services for the elderly is rather vague. This phrase has come to mean services rendered to an individual within an acute care setting or hospital. With the development of terms such as *subacute care*, *subacute rehabilitation*, and *acute rehabilitation*, acute care usually refers to the point at which most elderly individuals enter the health care system for initial treatment of an illness of sudden, severe onset and limited duration. However, for many aged patients, an acute problem is complicated by other factors such as the presence of chronic illnesses and the normal changes associated with aging.

The GRN working in the acute care setting still uses the principles of rehabilitation, although the focus of care may be to return the patient to a state of medical stability. In the acute care hospital, the aged person needs assistance with surviving the initial bodily insult that caused admission, stabilizing his or her medical status, and regaining of

strength. The role of the GRN as caregiver takes precedence. Although therapy may be instituted relatively quickly within the hospital setting, it is not the primary focus of this care environment and thus lacks the duration and intensity of a rehabilitation unit. Yet it is essential that prevention of secondary complications be foremost in the GRN's mind so that the potential for rehabilitation when the person is physically able is maximized. As teachers and leaders, GRNs can help direct other health care professionals, as well as the patient and family, to look at the long-range picture during the acute care phase.

What may have been a short-term illness for a younger person can become a life-altering event for an older adult. When routine treatment does not result in the elderly patient's ability to return to the premorbid living situation, several options are available. These are discussed in the following sections.

POST-ACUTE CARE OPTIONS

There are many long-term care options for the elderly adult after discharge from the acute care hospital. Many facilities, such as nursing homes or transitional care units, are utilized by the aged with the hopes of continued strengthening and eventual discharge home. The older adult may enter the post-acute care web directly from the inpatient hospital or from the community. This maze of care options has only continued to grow in the past decade, causing a great deal of confusion for consumers, health care providers, and insurance companies.

To understand the complexities of the multiple levels of care available, the nurse must be aware of both the similarities and differences between options. The somewhat overlapping sources of services for the elderly have been primarily motivated by cost effectiveness, cost containment, and a need to fill gaps in the health care system. Because the GRN is often in a position to make referrals or suggestions as to the level of care most appropriate for each patient, knowledge in this area is essential.

Generally, post-acute care units or facilities vary in several ways. Each level of care defines itself differently, has distinct goals, services a specific patient population, has unique facility requirements and criteria for admission, has certain nursing hours per patient day (NHPPD), has separate reimbursement rules, and has a range for average length of stay (LOS). The major options for elderly adults available today include rehabilitation (inpatient/outpatient), subacute care (also sometimes called transitional or skilled care), adult day care, assisted living, group homes, extended or long-term care (such as nursing homes), hospice (in home or on a special unit), home health care (ranging from professional paid caregivers to nonprofessional, family support), and outpatient therapy. Older adults often move from one level of care to another and back again (Fig. 2–1). Much of this use of the health care system is a result of the number of chronic illnesses experienced by adults as they reach the old-old age group.

The objective of most post-acute care units is that the patient return home as soon as possible; however, this is not always a feasible option. For example, a frail elderly widow living alone who falls and fractures her hip may, after replacement surgery, go to inpatient rehabilitation for intensive therapy with the goal of home discharge to her premorbid living habits. However, while in rehabilitation, she develops a deep vein thrombosis and is transferred back to the acute care hospital for treatment. A week or so later, having been on bedrest, she is now unable to tolerate the rigorous therapy schedule of the rehabilitation program and is sent to subacute care, which may be less demanding but still provides her needed therapy. From there she may be discharged home, or, if further complications arise, could return to the acute care setting or be placed in a long-term care facility if unable to care for herself. The use of multiple levels of post-acute care by the older

adult during even one episode of illness or injury is not unusual. Figure 2–1 illustrates the "web" of health care for the elderly.

REHABILITATION UNIT

Brody and Morrison captured the essence of rehabilitation by stating "rehabilitation intervention is often the 'glue' that links acute, transitional, and long-term-care systems, so that continuity of care may maximize the functioning of the elderly disabled" (1992, p. 44). Rehabilitation units set the standard by which all other post-acute treatment should be measured. Before the acceptance of subacute units, most patients who had experienced a long-term health crisis or chronic illness, and met admission standards, were sent to the rehabilitation unit to receive intensive therapy, with the goal of home discharge. The types of individuals benefiting from rehabilitation included those with diagnoses of stroke, traumatic brain injury, spinal cord injury, musculoskeletal and orthopedic disorders such as hip fracture and amputation, and neurological disorders such as multiple sclerosis and Guillain-Barré syndrome. Not all individuals experiencing these problems require post-acute rehabilitation. Some individuals recover fully with traditional therapy in the hospital setting or with outpatient therapy. Others, with greater functional deficits, are transferred to rehabilitation (now often referred to as acute rehabilitation).

Rehabilitation care is holistic and involves the cooperative efforts of an interdisciplinary team. Support available to rehabilitation patients includes physical, occupational, speech, and recreational therapy; social services; and around-the-clock nursing care. Other assistance provided on the rehabilitation unit may include nutritional counseling, vocational counseling, pastoral care, and community reintegration training, to name a few. All team members work together to provide a comprehensive program for each patient. The patient is considered part of the team and helps develop a plan of care to suit his or her particular needs. Despite the obvious benefits of such individualized and multifaceted care, many patients will not receive rehabilitation because it is a costly service. A more thorough discussion of rehabilitation is provided in Chapter 3.

The acute rehabilitation unit that cares for a large population of elderly, often called a general rehabilitation unit, is an ideal place for GRNs to use their skills. Nurses with ex-

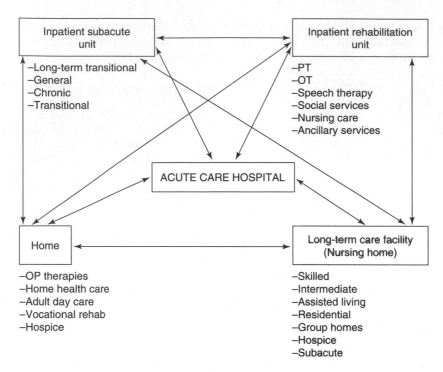

Figure 2–1 The "web" of health care for the elderly. OP, outpatient; OT, occupational therapy; PT, physical therapy.

pertise in care of older adults will find that working in rehabilitation requires excellent assessment and communication skills. Working with the interdisciplinary team is a challenging and rewarding venture. Developing expertise in the roles of teacher, leader, consultant, and mediator will be increasingly essential for GRNs in the rehabilitation setting. Instead of the heavy emphasis on the role of caregiver (as in the acute hospital), GRNs focus on assisting older adults to perform self-care. Nurses can use a variety of talents to devise quality care plans for this diverse group of patients.

General requirements for admission to a rehabilitation unit include the ability to tolerate at least 3 hours of therapy per day, presence of family or social support, goal of home discharge, and adequate insurance coverage. Unfortunately, some patients who would otherwise qualify for inpatient rehabilitation admission are denied because of reimbursement issues. The cost of multiple therapeutic services provided on an inpatient basis by licensed professionals is high. Subacute care has emerged as an option for those individuals requiring a level of care less than the acute care hospital provides but more than a skilled nursing facility (SNF) or extended care facility (ECF) provides. Those who do not qualify for inpatient acute rehabilitation or do not re-

quire as intense a rehabilitative program now have the additional option of subacute care.

SUBACUTE CARE

Subacute care, also called transitional or continual care, is considered by many to be the future of health care. This concept has emerged as an alternative level of care to fill the treatment gap. The acceptance of subacute care has grown recently and has been the subject of much controversy. In an effort to define this type of care, the Joint Commission on Accreditation of Healthcare Organizations (JCAHO) stated that subacute care is "generally more intensive than traditional nursing facility care and less than acute care. It requires frequent (daily to weekly) recurrent patient assessment and review of the clinical course and treatment plan for a limited (several days to several months) time period, until a condition is stabilized or a predetermined treatment course is completed" (Stahl, 1994, p. 34). Such wide variation in length of stay and depth of treatment plans has allowed for a varied interpretation of this level of care.

There are four levels of subacute care as depicted in Table 2–1, and they vary according to population focus, admission criteria, facility requirements and goals, nursing hours per patient day (NHPPD), and average length of stay (LOS). Typical individuals seen in subacute care are those needing assistance as a result of non-healing wounds, chronic ventilator dependence, renal problems, intravenous therapy, and coma management and those with complex medical and/or rehabilitative needs, including pediatrics, orthopedics, and neurological. These units are designed to promote optimum outcomes in the least expensive cost setting. Subacute units can be composed of a single type of patients, such as a chronic ventilator unit, or a mixture of them. Because the regulations for reimbursement are currently broad and ill-defined, patients in subacute care may receive less than the needed therapy, depending on the individual goals of the unit's administration. Competition has also arisen among rehabilitation units and subacute care, because there is some overlap between the types of patients each services.

The driving force behind the subacute movement is managed care. Alliances between acute care, rehabilitation, and extended care are a benefit to all. Subacute care was developed to bridge the gap between these levels of care (Gill & Balsano, 1994). In addition to long-term care facilities or nursing homes, many acute care hospitals are opening subacute units. As of 1995, about 25% of subacute capacity was in the hospital setting (Peck, 1995). While subacute may be the new buzzword, gerontological nurses will recognize that subacute care has been practiced in many skilled nursing facilities for years. Some units that call themselves transitional care units (TCUs) also fall under the category of subacute nursing.

Indeed, experts have a variety of opinions as to which type of nurse is best suited for work in subacute care. There are those who feel that a nurse with a critical care background would function optimally (Glosner Walsh, 1995). Because the subacute nurse may be called on to provide intravenous therapy, ventilator and tracheostomy care, cardiac monitoring, peritoneal dialysis, pain management, and wound care, it may be seen as a viable option for those nurses interested in caring for patients with complex needs through a longer course of stay than the acute care setting. Thus, the role of the GRN as caregiver is maximized. Others feel that a diverse staff is necessary because of the broader knowledge base used (Dewease, 1994). Garfinkle (1994) suggested that the unit manager have a strong background in critical care nursing or be a certified rehabilitation

nurse. Because critical care and rehabilitation represent opposite ends of a nursing mindset (acute care versus chronic care), this is a controversial subject. Yet these varying opinions represent the problem with management of subacute care units. So much has been left to individual interpretation that there may be vast discrepancies in the quality of care provided from institution to institution. However, recent legislative changes have tightened the rules, regulations, and reimbursement policies related to subacute care, so future changes are inevitable.

The dilemma of maintaining consistent quality of care is the subject of a study conducted by Mayer, Buckley, and White (1990). These authors suggested that nursing assistants can and do appropriately provide the majority of direct care in subacute facilities. Licensed vocational nurses performed the technical aspects of care, and the registered nurse acted mainly as planner, coordinator, and evaluator of outcomes and assumed some responsibility for psychosocial interventions, respiratory care, and some medications. According to this study, the registered nurse provided only 2.6% of all direct care, whereas the nursing assistant provided 68.4% of direct care. These caregiving patterns are much more consistent with nursing home ratios than acute rehabilitation within a hospital setting.

An additional concern is the development of subacute units within nursing homes. Although many extended care facilities have provided skilled nursing services for quite some time, this type of care will probably expand as a result of the subacute movement. This will require long-term care nurses to be more knowledgeable of acute care diagnoses, interventions, and technology (Patterson, 1994). Many nurses and assistants working in nursing homes are ill prepared to meet this challenge.

Those subacute units with a rehabilitative focus represent the model or ideal for this type of cost-effective care. Individuals still receive therapy, but at a substantially lower and reimbursable cost than acute rehabilitation. Because reimbursement for ancillary services is at a premium in subacute care, and most of these types of units should be inherently rehabilitation-focused, this is an excellent place for the GRN to practice.

The subacute movement has provided a missing link from the ECF to the acute care system. Nursing homes and long-term care facilities have been encouraged to develop

Table 2-1   STANDARDS OF CARE FOR SUBACUTE PATIENTS

Type of Subacute Patient	Clinical Criteria for Admission	Nursing Hours PPD	Average Length of Stay

I. Transitional Subacute:
 	
A. Definition: Serves as substitute for continued hospital stay rather than alternate hospital discharge placement.
B. Facility Requirements:
   1. Physician program director or consultant
   2. Dedicated RN staff of acute or CCRN with ACLS certification
   3. 24-hour respiratory therapy
   4. 7 days/week rehabilitation therapies
   5. Nutritional therapist
C. Goals:
   1. Manage patient's care and therapy in a less expensive setting for cost effectiveness
   2. Discharge patient to home or in other alternative less expensive setting such as assisted living or long-term care
	1. Wound management for burns
	2. Stroke patients by 5th day of hospitalization
	3. Coronary bypass patients, not off ventilator within 4–5 days for weaning
	4. Pulmonary management of tracheostomies
	5. Multiple stage III and IV decubitus
	6. Cardiac patients recovering from heart attack or cardiac surgery
	7. Oncology surgery, including chemotherapy
	8. Rehabilitation for CVAs or for complications following orthopedic surgery
	9. Medically complex patients with diabetes, digestive disorders, or renal disorders/failure
	10. Following vascular or other surgeries
		5–8 hours	5–40 days

II. General Medical-Surgical Subacute
 	
A. Definition: Provides care for patients who require medical care and monitoring at least weekly, certain rehabilitation therapies, and moderate nursing care services.
B. Facility Requirements:
   1. Physician consultant
   2. RN staff with acute or CCRN background
   3. 6 days/week rehabilitation therapies
   4. Respiratory therapy consultant
   5. Nutritional therapist/dietitian
   6. Medicare certified beds
C. Goals:
   1. Manage patient's care in a cost-effective manner
   2. Discharge patient to home or assisted living facility
	1. Patients requiring I.V. therapy for septic conditions without other significant medical complications
	2. Patients with tracheostomy who require monitoring and tending or tracheostomy care
	3. Stabilized medical patients with cardiac problems, diabetes, digestive disorders, or renal disorders
	4. Stroke, CVAs requiring continued rehabilitation therapies, e.g., PT, OT, ST (1–3 hr PPD)
	5. Orthopedic patients requiring physical rehabilitation therapies of 1–3 hr PPD
	6. HIV patients
		3–5 hours	7–21 days

III. Chronic Subacute

3–5 hours   60–90 days

A. Definition: Provides care for patients with little hope of ultimate recovery and functional independence.
B. Facility Requirements:
1. Physician consultant
2. RN and LPN with medication certification
3. Restorative nursing
4. PT, OT, ST consultants

1. Ventilator-dependent patients
2. Long-term comatose patients
3. Patients with progressive neurological disease
4. Patients in need of restorative care provided by RN/LPN with assistance from PT, OT, ST

IV. Long-Term Transitional Subacute

6.5–9 hours   25 days or more

A. Definition: Provides care for medically complex patients or acute ventilator-dependent patients, e.g., Vencor Hospital.
B. Facility Requirements:
1. Physician director
2. Pulmonologist, physiatrist, cardiologist, endocrinologist, cardiovascular surgeon, gastroenterologist consultant
3. Nutritional therapist/dietitian
4. Respiratory therapist
5. RN with acute care experience, CCRN certification preferred

1. Acute ventilator-dependent patients requiring intensive daily care and management
2. Medically complex patients with at least two medical or surgical concurrent diagnoses requiring medical specialists and primarily RN interventions

ACLS, advanced cardiac life support; CCRN, critical care registered nurse; CVAs, cerebrovascular accidents; LPN, licensed practical nurse; OT, occupational therapist; PPD, per patient day; PT, physical therapist; RN, registered nurse; ST, speech therapist.
Reproduced with permission from the article "Subacute Care: The Future of Health Care," from the October, 1994 issue of *Nursing Management*, © Springhouse Corporation.

alliances and partnerships to take full advantage of this new level of care. This includes the development of managed care contracts (Gill & Balsano, 1994). In addition to enhanced continuous quality improvement, elderly patients benefit from a smooth transition as they move throughout the health care system (Singleton, 1994).

Hillary Rodham Clinton's idea was to provide subacute care in nursing homes rather than in the more expensive setting of hospitals. However, there are many facilities jumping on the "subacute bandwagon" that have less than the patients' best interests in mind. In fact, some refer to subacute care as "the last great government giveaway." Until more definitive standards for treatment and reimbursement are delineated, subacute care units cannot guarantee the quality of service offered by inpatient rehabilitation, but they are a cost-effective option for care.

NURSING HOMES AND EXTENDED CARE

Extended care facility (ECF) is the term most often used in reference to nursing homes; it is used interchangeably with *long-term care* (LTC) *facility.* The distinctions between skilled nursing care, transitional care, extended care, and long-term care are often blurred. But regardless of the name, LTC facilities are cost-effective compared with acute care facilities, resulting in savings of 70% to 80% over hospitals (Curry-Baggett, 1994). Nursing homes can provide a variety of levels of care, including skilled (which may or may not be renamed or restructured to conform to subacute standards), intermediate, assisted living, and residential. The GRN working in long-term care utilizes all the roles described in Chapter 4 to provide comprehensive quality care to the elderly in these settings.

Skilled Nursing

Skilled nursing care has a wide range of interpretations. Many nursing homes provide this type of care on a designated unit with a specific number of licensed beds. Some subacute care units began as skilled nursing units. Despite the title, skilled nursing care is practiced at many levels. Patients within the nursing home setting who are placed on the skilled unit are those who require more intense, direct care. These patients or residents often have complex needs involving several body systems. Nurses working in skilled care per-

form a variety of tasks such as tube feedings, intravenous therapy (including hyperalimentation therapy and maintenance of Infuse-A-Ports or Port-A-Caths), extensive wound care and dressing changes, medication management, rehabilitation, hospice care, and care of the patient on a ventilator.

Intermediate

This level of care within the nursing home setting is for those who require less assistance than skilled nursing but who are unable to perform all activities of daily living (ADLs) independently. Most long-term care facilities provide intermediate level beds for a variety of patients. An example of this type of patient would be an elderly, insulin-dependent diabetic who may be unable to manage his own injections because of severe arthritis combined with retinopathy. Residents on this kind of unit vary as to their functional capabilities but share a lack of total independence. Some of them might be able to live at home with assistance but lack sufficient family support or financial resources.

Residential

Some elderly individuals need only occasional supervision with day-to-day activities. They may not need nursing home care but do not desire to live alone any longer in an isolated environment. Some nursing homes make a distinction between assisted living and residential care, whereas others consider these the same level. The concept of assisted living outside of the long-term care setting is discussed later in this chapter.

Many extended care facilities have separate living quarters on the premises. These may be private apartments or clusters of small homes, sometimes referred to as a village. Other nursing homes have a special unit designated as residential. This type of care provides the elderly with a more home-like community environment, while keeping health professionals close to them. The services provided in residential care may vary slightly between facilities. Assistance may range from none (total independent living) to telephone calls or daily house checks by the staff, emergency call systems, or availability for group dining and camaraderie. Some senior housing is similar to residential living as a part of the long-term care facility.

Implications for Gerontological Rehabilitation Nursing

Long-term care placement for the elderly may mean that this facility becomes their home. Although a few individuals will enter a nursing home to regain strength as a transition to home, this will become less true with the increased use of subacute care units. The long-term care facility will be increasingly viewed as an end point for seniors unable to live alone or assisted at home. This has enormous implications for the already often negatively viewed nursing home. Issues such as quality of life, death with dignity, and the importance of self-care are certain to receive more attention.

Nursing homes or extended care facilities offer challenging places for GRNs to practice. The vast diversity in levels of care allows nurses to choose between working with patients requiring skilled assistance or with the more healthy elderly. Some professionals float between such units, gain experience, and enjoy variety by working across the spectrum of tertiary care.

For many years, the prevailing attitude within the nursing profession suggested that nurses working in long-term care were inferior practitioners with no other options, or were just plain lazy. This negative stereotype has deterred many graduate nurses from gerontological practice. Some current proponents of gerontological nursing, particularly educators in the academic setting, have praised the value of this type of practice environment for the nurse in training. Others believe that long-term care experiences for students are less helpful than other types of experiences and should be limited to upper class students only. Current trends are toward collaborative projects between educators, practitioners, and the community. Experts agree that the education of student nurses in the principles of gerontology should occur throughout the curriculum and is critical to prepare nurses to meet the future needs of the growing elderly population (Bahr, 1993; Burke & Sherman, 1993; Heine, 1993; Waters, 1994). However, gerontological nursing apart from the concepts of rehabilitation is much like medical-surgical nursing applied to older adults. One can easily see this trend by examining the gerontological books currently on the market. Most of these references contain a scant chapter on rehabilitation of the elderly, apparently minimizing its usefulness. Nonetheless, the future of care for the elderly is in rehabilitative practice. Primary prevention is no longer enough, because most elderly are living with at least one chronic disease, some occurring as a normal part of aging as a result of extended life span. Nursing professionals cannot sufficiently practice in the tertiary gerontological setting without knowledge and skill in rehabilitation principles. With the marriage of these two specialties, new potential emerges for improved quality of care for the older population.

The use of rehabilitation principles and promotion of self-care have been shown to enhance the quality of life of nursing home residents (Aller & Van Ess Coeling, 1995). The hazards of immobility and/or institutionalization, combined with the usual effects of aging, put the elderly at substantial risk of harm. The GRN can make a difference in the lives of older adults not only by preventing secondary complications, but by improving function, self-esteem, and the quality of life experienced by the aged.

Long-term care offers enormous benefits in terms of professional satisfaction. The gerontological rehabilitation nurse is able to build rapport with residents and their family members, helping to promote a positive self-image through goal achievement. Extended care facilities are no longer places where the elderly while away the days, but are a bona fide area of specialty where the expertise of the nurse is desperately needed. In the spectrum of elderly care, GRNs can be extremely influential in the development and implementation of appropriate critical pathways. These may extend from an acute illness through home care or into the long-term care facility, providing a continuum of quality care for the aged.

HOME- AND COMMUNITY-BASED PROGRAMS

Group Homes

Groups homes are community-based programs designed to meet the long-term housing and care needs of those with physical and mental disabilities. Often, those adults living in group homes are those suffering from mental retardation from birth or as a result of disease, illness, or injury. Many of these adults have concomitant physical impairments that necessitate specially designed housing. Thus, most group homes utilize a ranch-style house, with the required accommodations made to allow easy access for those with disabilities.

The ideal group home has a low ratio of caregivers (who are usually not professionals) to clients. Homes are generally designed to accommodate from four to eight individuals. These types of care facilities may be found within the community, with many group home providers having purchased a home for this purpose.

Group homes provide assistance and constant supervision with ADLs for those who are unable to care for themselves. There is a sense of community, as the residents function in a home-like atmosphere. One of the dangers of such situations, however, is the potential for abuse of the residents, because many of the caregivers have little training, and policing of these homes is not as strict as for larger institutions.

Because of the advances in medical science, adults with cognitive impairments are living longer, and the need for adequate, competent long-term health care for these individuals is increasing. Group homes provide a non-threatening, less institutionalized solution to the needs of this population.

Senior Housing and Assisted Living

Many communities have built senior housing centers or apartment complexes that are specifically designed to meet the living needs of the elderly. These residences take a variety of forms, from ground-floor apartment clusters, such as senior communities for retirees, to high-rises in larger cities.

Senior housing projects also provide a diversity of services, from supervisory to assisted living. Many facilities are geared toward independent living but make services such as bus transportation, group trips, doctor's visits, meals, and church services more easily accessible to residents. For example, many such complexes have a chapel within the facility, as well as dining rooms that serve well-balanced meals or a clinic facility for doctors such as podiatrists to make "house calls."

Other facilities offer assisted living care. This level of care can be found within nursing homes or at sites supervised by a long-term care facility or hospital. Generally, assisted living services include private efficiency apartments, 24-hour-a-day supervision, some assistance with ADLs, medication monitoring, daily meal service, emergency call systems, social and recreational activities, and easy access to health care services.

One popular design for assisted living units is apartments emphasizing "clustered" living areas to provide a sense of community. Buildings may be constructed to emphasize a residential look and feel, having gathering places for members of the "neighborhood" where light meals may be served and socialization can take place. Many have a main dining room, and the living needs of couples can be accommodated. Social gathering and group activities are planned by the management.

There are several advantages to assisted living services provided in a home-like setting. One of the most significant is that these residences are not bound by the same government regulations as nursing homes and thus can be more flexible and creative in programming as well as building design. Also, residents have more independence and freedom of choice (DeYoung, Just, & Van Dyk, 1994; Patterson, 1995). Assisted living has been used successfully not only with the frail elderly but also for the mentally challenged, physically handicapped, and those with Alzheimer's disease (Widdes, 1995).

Nurses working with older adults living in these community-based settings face additional challenges. Assessment of needs is a primary concern. As trends in health care require nurses to take a more active role in maintaining health and wellness of elders, GRNs may find practice settings that require creativity and management skills to promote health and prevent disease among the community-dwelling elderly. This may be in the form of community care nursing through agencies, such as the YMCA, or through churches, as with parish nurse programs. Participation in health screenings and health fairs in these settings may also be part of the GRN role.

Adult Day Care

Another option available to the elderly is adult day care, also referred to as adult care or adult day. This form of comprehensive care is primarily for those who live at home with a family member but cannot be left alone during the day. These programs serve the needs of older adults who require supervision because of illness, disability, or the effects of aging. In addition to providing a wide range of services, this type of care can also give respite to the caregiver. For some individuals, the day care center offers intense care. For others, it represents an alternative to institutionalization and promotes their ability to continue living in the community (Masson, 1986). Participants can attend full- or part-time. Adult day care is a cost-effective program that allows the aged person requiring some assistance to interact with others under the supervision of trained professionals.

Admission requirements for adult day care facilities may vary slightly and are determined by the individual program. Most commonly, these facilities require that participants be (1) free from infectious or communicable disease, (2) able to participate in group activities, and (3) able to move independently or with the use of an assistive device. Guidelines for admission vary depending on the focus and location of the site. For example, a community- or church-based center may be more socially oriented, whereas a hospital-sponsored facility may provide more intense rehabilitative activities as a means of continuing care after discharge (Mehlferber, 1990).

As of 1985, the National Institute on Adult Day Care identified more than 1000 programs (Mehlferber, 1990). Some of these are free-standing, whereas others are hospital-based or sponsored by a health care facility at a community site. This model of care can be categorized into different types, including health-oriented and social services–oriented (Weissert et al., 1990). Weissert et al. also identified several variables that were associated with the increased probability of full-time day care use. Approximately 20% of day care users were 85 or older, with more women using the program than men. Another factor related to the increased use of adult day care was functional dependency, with about one quarter of the sample reporting the need for some assistance with ADLs, but nearly half being independent in ADLs. Mobility impairment is another factor related to day care attendance. Mental illness, stroke, and a history of nursing home use were additional significant factors. Being a private payer also contributed to the likelihood of full-time use. Although grants are becoming more available, the fear of many health care professionals is that adult day care programs, once established, will not be able to support themselves when funding runs out.

Intergenerational care is an emerging concept. These centers combine adult day care centers with child care centers. These programs provide separate facilities for the care of children and adults but strive to bridge the generation gap through group activities. This interaction helps both age groups grow intellectually and emotionally, while stimulating conversation and lively activity times.

Adult day care centers have a natural rehabilitation focus. Group care is provided in a supportive environment with the program designed to maximize independence while preventing deterioration (Hunter, 1992; Mehlferber, 1990). Such care is holistic and blends traditional health, social, and therapeutic services to promote optimum outcomes. Although these centers provide physical care, they also help reduce the participants' feelings of isolation and loneliness by fostering socialization in a safe, controlled setting. GRNs work with a team to incorporate rehabilitation principles into this environment.

A typical day care center for adults has several characteristics. Centers have practical, daytime hours during the work week. They are not designed to provide 24-hour care. Eligibility for adult day care is determined by criteria established within the individual program. Medicare and Medicaid, as well as other public and private sources, provide monies for day care. Many programs offer transportation. Nutritious meals are provided, made either at the center or brought in from the outside. State regulations determine staffing requirements, but employees of the center commonly include a director, a nurse, a social worker, an activities director, program assistants/aides, therapists, a secretary, drivers, and consultants (Mehlferber, 1990). Consultants to the program may be physicians, psychiatrists, dentists, nutritionists, business experts, lawyers, and the like.

According to Korhumel, most successful day care facilities share some specifics. The director, often a nurse, should be on site at all times. The professional staff follows an individualized plan of care for each client, complete with goals and documented outcomes that are reviewed regularly. A variety of services can be offered, such as physical and occupational therapy, behavior modification, music, and art therapy. Those centers that provide transportation and an attractive, clean environment are more likely to succeed (Korhumel, 1988).

Adult day care is a viable alternative for the elderly who wish to remain in the community but need additional assistance and socialization in a therapeutic setting. This area of health care represents a multidimensional field of practice for the gerontological rehabilitation nurse. The population of patients serviced within the framework of rehabilitation principles makes this an ideal specialization area.

Hospice

Although hospice care is not generally considered a rehabilitation option, the concept has strong self-care roots. There are occasions when an elderly individual moving through the health care system is diagnosed with a terminal illness. This may occur prior to or during the acute hospital stay. Sometimes patients who are terminally ill are rehabilitation candidates who enter the program with a desire to make their last days as meaningful as possible by regaining enough strength to care for themselves at home or allow a family member to help them. Of course, this is a situation about which much debate arises in the community. Health care professionals may ask why persons with a terminal illness would push themselves to participate in the rigors of therapy when the end of their life is so near. Nurses sometimes have difficulty understanding the reasoning behind encouraging such individuals to perform self-care for their latter days. But patients often choose to participate in rehabilitation despite a terminal diagnosis, and this decision can represent an act of self-care. Individuals may wish to attend therapy in order to improve their quality of life as well as the length of time they may spend at home before the end of their life. Similarly, the goal of hospice care is to "promote a high quality of life until the occurrence of biological death" (Koshuta, 1990, p. 311).

Of course hospice care is not exclusively for the aged patient, but it is an alternative health care option. According to Siebold (1992), "contemporary hospice programs are places or methods of care for dying patients, and the services they offer vary based on the predilection of the group establishing the program" (p. 1). Most of hospice care is provided in the home, but some health care facilities provide inpatient programs. That is, hospice is a program rather than a facility (Cohen, 1979). The purpose of hospice care is to allow a natural death to occur without efforts to prolong life, while providing comfort, care, and support to individuals in the last phase of life. Despite differences in the types of services provided by agencies or facilities involved with hospice care, each program desires to provide some form of support for patients and families affected by terminal illness (Siebold, 1992).

The approach to care is holistic, involving the active participation of many team members as well as the patient and family. Health professionals on the hospice team include physicians, nurses, nursing assistants, social workers, volunteers, counselors, therapists, and pastoral staff. As in rehabilitation, this interdisciplinary group of caregivers collaborate with the patient and family to meet their goals. Communication and consistency are key elements in promoting comfortable, holistic care in the secure home environment.

Gerontological rehabilitation nursing in the hospice setting may seem like a contradiction of terms. However, hospice nurses use rehabilitation concepts in daily practice. The therapeutic use of self, touch therapy, alternative methods of care, team dynamics, goal setting, promoting quality of life, and holistic care are common threads in both hospice and rehabilitation. The differences lie in perceived length of life and desired outcomes. The hospice nurse must be well educated in pain management techniques; have expert knowledge of the physical, emotional, and psychospiritual aspects of death and dying; and be adept at providing the needed support to the patient as well as family members. The GRN focuses on preparing individuals with a disability or chronic illness to face the rest of their lives, however long that may be. This involves returning control to the patient, whether it be control of physical function or decision-making. With home hospice care, the role of the nurse also shifts dramatically from that in the hospital, from providing basic care to being a consultant (Rossman, 1979). Hospice professionals understand that a person's decision to die with dignity is an exercise of control over his or her own destiny. As Schraff states, "the importance of dying at home seems to be coupled with the need for freedom and the need for preserving choice" (1984, p. x). Nurses who are experienced in rehabilitation but feel a special calling to work with the terminally ill may find this a rewarding field. The skills and knowledge gained in gerontological rehabilitation, such as effective listening, communication, goal setting, team work, acting as a patient advocate, working with the family and support systems, and providing comfort in difficult situations, can be applied in the hospice setting.

Home Health Care

Home health care refers to care of the person within the home. Whether services are provided by a home health agency or by family caregivers, care of the ill elderly in this setting presents unique challenges. Corbin and Strauss define the work of home care for the chronically ill as that which is "aimed at keeping the illness course stable and managing any associated disability" (1990, p. 60). Burdick suggested, "survival alone is not enough; the 'quality of survival' has become equally important" (1979, p. 206).

Home health care services are intended for patients considered "homebound." This word is used loosely in some settings, but it is strictly defined in the United States by the federal government for the purposes of Medicare reimbursement for services. Eliopoulos (1990) cited the major criteria for home health care under Medicare regulations: (1) the patient must be homebound, and (2) there must be a documented need for intermittent skilled care, ordered by a physician. Criteria may differ in other countries. The types of assistance available generally include skilled nursing care, physical therapy, speech therapy, occupational therapy, medical social services, homemaker or home health aide services, nutritional support, and medical equipment and supplies (Hogstel, 1985). Medicaid and some private insurance companies will reimburse for personal care in the home. Many patients needing home care have functional disabilities that prohibit transportation to a facility for treatment or necessitate assistance with ADLs. Others may require short-term teaching for a new disease or disability. Still others may need ongoing nursing care such as dressing changes for a wound or decubitus. Hospice care within the home is also an important component of home health care. The need for quality home health care for the aged is increasing, but millions of older Americans continue to go without care, forcing them to enter nursing homes (Hogstel, 1985) or be cared for by overwhelmed family members. Some estimate that families provide as much as 80% of the personal care required by the aged (Albert, 1990).

Although nursing is considered the backbone of the home health services, various other professionals and non-professionals make up the staff for an effective agency. Other types of personnel who may care for the older patient requiring home care include therapists (physical, occupational, speech), social workers, and home health aides. Home care through an agency is intended to be of limited duration, with a treatment plan determined by the physician and carried out by staff in the various disciplines as needed.

Home care nurses must have excellent assessment and documentation skills, as well as good judgment and effective communication. They provide a link between the patient, family, and the traditional health care system. Many nurses note a great deal of similarity between the role of the rehabilitation nurse and that of the home care nurse. Both specialties require a broad knowledge base, sound clinical skills, autonomous decision-making, case management, and practical interpersonal communication abilities (Neal, 1995).

The nurse specializing in gerontological rehabilitation may find home health care an exciting place to practice. The home care nurse must be able to work closely with family members experiencing a series of stressful life changes. The nurse's role is diverse and complex, involving teaching, counseling, caregiving, supervision, leadership, and case management, while fostering a creative, therapeutic environment. In fact, current trends suggest that rehabilitation nurses may in the near future assume an expanded role in home care, sharing many of the responsibilities previously fulfilled by therapists. This challenging field needs more nurses with expertise in the complexities of both gerontological and rehabilitative care to service the growing elderly population.

OUTPATIENT SERVICES

Outpatient services cover a wide variety of needs. These types of services generally refer to health care that can be obtained on an outpatient basis—that is, not requiring admission to a facility. Such offerings may include various types of therapy, such as physical, occupational, and speech therapy or cardiac rehabilitation. Outpatient therapy is a way of providing continuity of care after discharge from the hospital setting. Patients may return to the facility for continued care and progress toward optimal independence.

Laboratory tests, x-rays, and other diagnostic tests are increasingly done on an outpatient basis. Outpatient services are less costly than inpatient care and are generally used whenever possible. Many surgeries formerly requiring a hospital stay are now performed on an outpatient basis. This movement toward cost containment can benefit the elderly patient by decreasing length of immobility due to minor surgery, thus reducing possible complications.

Support groups can also be a form of outpatient service. Most hospitals have a wide variety of groups that provide socialization as well as education on specific topics or with certain patient populations. Typical organizations would be the Breather's Club or the Stroke Club, support groups for cancer survivors or families of Alzheimer's patients, groups focusing on living with Crohn's disease, and the like.

Many health care facilities have a wellness program for senior citizens, providing a vital link to the health care system. A nurse often coordinates this service through a large hospital or health care center. The GRN who also possesses an extensive knowledge of community resources can be invaluable to agencies offering preventive programming for the aged. Opportunities for public speaking, client education, and fostering community relations combined with administrative duties may make this an appealing position for a nurse desiring diversity within a "healthy aging" framework.

Wound care centers are gaining popularity as a mode of care for those experiencing "hard to heal" chronic wounds. Many clients utilizing these outpatient services are aged. Given the changes occurring with aging and the common chronic problems experienced by this population, wounds can be difficult to treat owing to impaired circulation and/or the presence of such conditions as peripheral vascular disease or diabetes. Wound centers fill a gap in health care by providing comprehensive medical, nursing, and rehabilitative therapy on an outpatient basis. Clinic settings such as this are another example of areas in which the GRN may practice. For those with additional expertise in skin care, or the enterostomal therapist desiring challenging work with the elderly, this presents a uniquely specialized field in which to work.

REFERENCES

Albert, S. M. (1990). The dependent elderly, home health care, and strategies of household adaptation. In J. F. Gubrium & A. Sankar (Eds.), *The home care experience: Ethnography and policy* (pp. 19–36). Newbury Park, CA: Sage Publications.

Aller, L. J., & Van Ess Coeling, H. (1995). Quality of life: Its meaning to the long-term care resident. *Journal of Gerontological Nursing, 21*(2), 20–25.

Bahr, R. T. (1993). Foreword. In M. Burke & S. Sherman (Eds.), *Gerontological nursing: Issues and opportunities for the twenty-first century* (pp. xi–xii). New York: National League for Nursing Press.

Brody, S. J., & Morrison, M. H. (1992). Aging and rehabilitation: Beyond the medical model. In

E. F. Ansello & N. N. Eustis (Eds.), *Aging and disabilities: Seeking common ground* (pp. 39–45). Amityville, NY: Baywood Publishing.

Burdick, D. (1979). On the nature of cancer: Continuing care of the cancer patient. In E. R. Prichard, J. Collard, J. Starr, J. A. Lockwood, A. H. Kutscher, & I. B. Seeland (Eds.), *Home care: Living with dying* (pp. 205–207). New York: Columbia University Press.

Burke, M., & Sherman, S. (Eds.). (1993). *Gerontological nursing: Issues and opportunities for the twenty-first century.* New York: National League for Nursing Press.

Cohen, K. P. (1979). *Hospice: Prescription for terminal care.* Germantown, MD: Aspen Systems Corporation.

Corbin, J. M., & Strauss, A. (1990). Making arrangements: The key to home care. In J. F. Gubrium & A. Sankar (Eds.), *The home care experience: Ethnography and policy* (pp. 59–73). Newbury Park, CA: Sage Publications.

Curry-Baggett, P. (1994). Long-term care: Resolution of a dilemma? *Nursing Management, 25*(9), 80R–80V.

Dewease, S. W. (1994). Paving the road to subacute care. *Nursing Homes, 44*(4), 35–38.

DeYoung, S., Just, G., & Van Dyk, R. (1994). Assisted living: Policy implications for nursing. *Nursing and Health Care, 15*(10), 510–513.

Eliopoulos, C. (1990). *Caring for the elderly in diverse care settings.* Philadelphia: J. B. Lippincott.

Garfinkle, S. W. (1994). Staffing the subacute care facility. *Nursing Homes, 44*(4), 20–23.

Gill, H. S., & Balsano, A. E. (1994). The move toward subacute care. *Nursing Homes, 43*(4), 6–11.

Glosner Walsh, G. (1995, March). How subacute care fills the gap. *Nursing95,* 51.

Heine, C. (1993). *Determining the future of gerontological nursing education: Partnerships between education and practice.* New York: National League for Nursing Press.

Hogstel, M. O. (1985). *Home nursing care for the elderly.* Bowie, MD: Brady Communications.

Hunter, S. (1992). Adult day care: Promoting quality of life for the elderly. *Journal of Gerontological Nursing, 18*(2), 17–20.

Korhumel, E. A. (1988, January/February). Creating an adult day care center. *Geriatric Nursing,* 35–37.

Koshuta, M. (1990). In C. Eliopoulos (Ed.), *Caring for the elderly in diverse care settings* (pp. 308–317). Philadelphia: J. B. Lippincott.

Masson, V. (1986, January/February). How nursing happens in adult day care. *Geriatric Nursing,* 18–21.

Mayer, G. G., Buckley, R. F., & White, T. L. (1990). Direct nursing care given to patients in a subacute rehabilitation center. *Rehabilitation Nursing, 15*(2), 86–88.

Mehlferber, K. (1990). In C. Eliopoulos (Ed.), *Caring for the elderly in diverse care settings* (pp. 284–289). Philadelphia: J. B. Lippincott.

Neal, L. J. (1995). The rehabilitation nursing team

in the home healthcare setting. *Rehabilitation Nursing, 20*(1), 32–36.

Patterson, D. (1994). Technology helping make subacute care a reality. *Nursing Homes, 44*(4), 40.

Patterson, D. (1995). Assisted living: A brave new world. *Nursing Homes, 44*(6), 40–41.

Peck, R. L. (1995). What's ahead for subacute? *Nursing Homes, 44*(4), 16–21.

Rossman, P. (1979). *Hospice.* New York: Fawcett Columbine.

Schraff, S. (1984). *Hospice: The nursing perspective.* New York: National League for Nursing.

Shaughnessy, P. W., & Kramer, A. M. (1990). The increased needs of patients in nursing homes and patients receiving home health care. *The New England Journal of Medicine, 322*(1), 21–25.

Siebold, C. (1992). *The hospice movement: Easing death's pains.* New York: Twayne Publishers.

Singleton, G. W. (1994). Transitioning to subacute: The keys to success. *Nursing Homes, 44*(4), 16–18.

Stahl, D. A. (1994). Subacute care: The future of health care. *Nursing Management, 25*(10), 34–40.

Waters, V. (1994). *Resources for teaching gerontology.* New York: National League for Nursing Press.

Weissert, W. G., Elston, J. M., Bolda, E. J., Zelman, W. N., Mutran, E., & Mangum, A. B. (1990). *Adult day care: Findings from a national survey.* Baltimore: The Johns Hopkins University Press.

Widdes, T. (1995). Assisted living for Alzheimer's patients: Is this the "missing link" in the continuum of care? *Nursing Homes, 44*(4), 32–33.

Chapter 3

Overview of Rehabilitation

■

DEFINITION

Rehabilitation is the process of adaptation or recovery through which an individual suffering from a disabling or functionally limiting condition, whether temporary or irreversible, participates to regain, or attempts to regain, maximum function, independence, and restoration. For some, this means a lifelong process. For others, rehabilitation is of short duration. For example, the process of recovery from a broken arm may require physical therapy for a time, with the end result being return to the individual's former state with full range of motion. If, however, an individual has been diagnosed with a stroke, the rehabilitation process may be continuous, even lifelong.

GOALS

"Rehabilitation goals are the desired outcomes for each rehabilitation client" (Habel, 1993, p. 3). Thus, the goals for each individual will be unique. Yet although this is true, there are definite underlying principles and objectives that guide the development of each plan of care. All members of the rehabilitation team, although concentrating on a particular area, share similar goals for the client. These include promoting self-care, maximizing independence, maintaining and restoring optimum function, preventing complications, and encouraging adaptation. Table 3–1 lists the common goals of the rehabilitation team. The client's achievement of these objectives is measured by considering outcomes based on the care planning of the interdisciplinary

team. More specific goals for each discipline are discussed later in this chapter.

PHILOSOPHY

Fawcett (1995) described a philosophy as a set of beliefs and values. Rehabilitation nursing books devote little discussion to the aspect of philosophy, concentrating more on goals, concepts, definition, and roles. The basic philosophy of rehabilitation, however, is that individuals have intrinsic worth and have the right to be experts in their own health care (Gender, 1998). Each person is a unique, complex, holistic being. Rehabilitation nurses, and the rest of the rehabilitation team, are responsible for providing the education and training that equip the person with the needed knowledge and skills to maximize self-care.

Table 3–1   GENERAL PATIENT GOALS OF THE INTERDISCIPLINARY REHABILITATION TEAM

Fostering self-care, self-sufficiency
Encouraging maximal independence level
Maintaining function
Preventing complications
Restoring optimum function
Promoting maximum potential of function
Emphasizing abilities
Adaptation/adjustment
Promoting acceptable quality of life
Maintaining dignity
Reeducation
Community reintegration, community reentry
Promoting optimum wellness

The specialty of gerontological rehabilitation nursing incorporates both the philosophy and concepts of rehabilitation and those of gerontological nursing. Gerontological nursing, like the broader field of gerontology, is an applied science in which nurses utilize knowledge of the aging process to provide individualized care to older people, assisting them to maintain independence. One might say that a foundational philosophical statement regarding gerontological rehabilitation is that older persons are unique, holistic beings whose adaptation after a functionally limiting disease or injury is affected by the aging process. Gerontological rehabilitation nursing strives to assist older persons toward achieving their goals and maximum level of independence through age-specific interventions, incorporating the roles of the gerontological rehabilitation nurse (GRN).

CONCEPTS

Although clinical reference books, texts, and health care research have provided a fine body of literature on the relatively recently accepted specialty of rehabilitation, those who are employed in this field understand that the concepts used, although they can be read, must be internalized in order for the professional to effectively work with the disabled client. There is a certain amount of abstraction inherent in the field of rehabilitation, in that physicians, nurses, and therapists become associated with their clients in the most intimate aspects of their lives. One cannot be effective in the rehabilitation specialty without empathizing with the client. This is not to say that the practice of rehabilitation does not have solid medical foundation, for this is certainly true. However, when one reads books such as Beisser's *Flying Without Wings* (1989), in which the author, a noted physician, reflects on his experiences as a patient with polio, or Baier's story of her bout with Guillain-Barré syndrome in *Bed Number Ten* (1985), one realizes that coping with a disabling condition is an intensely personal experience. Rehabilitation professionals understand that their role, no matter how great the contribution to the client's success, can only support and encourage the strength and resourcefulness within the client.

The health care literature is filled with many helpful rehabilitation quotes from a variety of sources. Most of these "sayings" can be placed into one of several categories. Examples of general principles used by rehabilitation professionals, with supporting concepts, follow.

Emphasize Adaptation, Not Just Recovery

All too often in health care terminology, one hears the word *recovery*. Of course, the notion that a patient can be completely restored to a former state is perhaps the goal of treatment, but such is often not the case with long-term illnesses or injuries. Indeed, when considering the concept of recovery, one must wonder whether a patient ever truly returns to the exact premorbid state, because a change has occurred necessitating care. Do humans ever remain the same in everyday life, or are we in a constant state of flux? Research has shown that the body has remarkable adaptive powers and is constantly adjusting to the changing environment. In this light, the term *recovery* takes on new meaning.

The process of rehabilitation helps individuals adjust or adapt to life-altering situations, without giving false hope of total recovery. In fact, some may argue that the term *recover* should be stricken from the long-term health care professionals' vocabulary. Rather, words such as *adaptation* suggest that clients may not return to the way they were but can learn to make adjustments in their lifestyle in order to cope with changes that have occurred as a result of an illness or injury.

Those who experience chronic illnesses or disability come to the hospital with quite different needs than those who arrive for acute care. Having a leg amputated is not akin to having an appendix removed. One condition may require a brief period of convalescence, and the other an extended period of rehabilitation. In the case of an amputation, the client does not "get fixed," go home, and then continue on with life as before. Adjustments must be made. From a long-term health deviation, there is often no complete "recovery" as most commonly think of it. But there is adaptation.

A person recently diagnosed with multiple sclerosis, or one who has suffered a spinal cord injury, is facing a life-altering situation. What has happened will change the way they live, think, and interact with others. For these individuals, the road of life will never be the same. They soon realize that they will not return to their former state. Their life has been forever altered, and they may experience feelings of hopelessness and powerlessness.

The rehabilitation team assists clients toward independence and the achievement of personal goals. If the individual's condition is acute, the services of the interdisciplinary team may be minimal. But if the state is chronic, a significant amount of therapy may be indicated. It is important to recognize that the client or patient is the most important member of the team. Keeping this in mind will promote collaborative care instead of taking control over decision-making away from the patient. This is one of the basic differences between an acute care philosophy and the rehabilitation mindset. In the acute phase of illness, health care professionals act on behalf of the patient, whereas in the rehabilitative setting, the team teaches and assists clients to care for themselves.

Rehabilitation often makes the difference between positive adjustment and negative coping. As patients participate in therapeutic activities, the likelihood of successful reintegration into the community increases (Dobkin, 1991; White, Richter, & Fry, 1992). Although this process may be long and arduous, patients and families who participate in it acknowledge feeling better about themselves and often express a greater ability to cope and improved acceptance of their new roles and self-image (Easton, Rawl, Zemen, Kwiatkowski, & Burczyk, 1995; Folden, 1993).

Emphasize Abilities, Accentuate the Positive

People who have experienced a major crisis in their life have reason enough to think negatively. If rehabilitation focused on what the individual had lost, then there would indeed be cause for despair. An amputated leg may not be restored, but an artificial one can return the function of ambulation. A hemiplegic arm may no longer be able to write, but it can help provide balance and stability. Likewise, individuals with severe physical impairments may choose to capitalize on their intellectual capabilities, exploring areas that were perhaps previously neglected. Many persons living with functional deficits no longer consider themselves disabled. There are things they cannot do, but other things they can do. Rehabilitation assists these individuals in making the most of abilities and strengths that remain and working with what they have. Thus, the process of adaptation and recovery engaged in by those with physical limitations must be optimistic and center on developing and maximizing the functions that remain.

Rehabilitation professionals offer hope and an optimistic outlook for the future to those whose lives have been devastated by a life-altering condition. Goal attainment is one way in which professionals can demonstrate a client's progress. Setting mutually agreed on, realistic, achievable goals, both short-term and long-term, allows the client to participate in the rehabilitation process. Having overcome obstacles to meet their objectives gives clients a sense of accomplishment. For some patients, being able to feed themselves again is a major step toward regaining independence. The rehabilitation team gives immediate feedback and constant encouragement throughout the client's tenure. Such positive reinforcement is necessary to combat feelings of despair and depression that may be part of working through the grieving process following a loss.

Treat the Whole Person

Each person is a unique individual, worthy of the same respect and courtesy as any other, regardless of age, race, gender, creed, or functional capacity. When a life-changing event such as a chronic illness or disability occurs, it is essential that health care professionals remember that the persons being treated bring with them all their past experiences, problems, values, and beliefs. The process of rehabilitation strives to utilize these prior experiences to the individuals benefit, not to remake the person. The concept of the person as a holistic being lends itself well to the rehabilitation process. Professionals treat the person, not the disease. Although this should be true in all of health care, it is one of the founding principles of rehabilitation. A disability affects not only the individual and the family, but everything about his or her body and life.

Rehabilitation professionals recognize that patients requiring a long period of treatment will experience multiple changes in their life. Financial considerations may be a great burden to some. Others will worry about role adjustments and the effect of their illness on the family. Still others struggle with anger and depression. Denial and non-acceptance of one's disability are barriers to successful adaptation.

Rehabilitation is one specialty in which knowledge of the principles of adult learning is essential. Assessing the patient's prior knowledge and experience provides insight into his or her life philosophy and goals. Utilizing this information, rehabilitation professionals can gain a better idea of the whole person and develop appropriate plans of care. Because team members engage in a large amount of educative activities, drawing on an individual's background as a basis for teaching and learning can be helpful.

A Disability Affects the Entire Family

Most health care professionals realize that grieving is a normal part of the rehabilitation process; however, it is important to emphasize that the client's family will also grieve. Research has demonstrated that the wives of stroke patients often remain in the depression phase of grieving longer than the patient (Rosenthal, Pituch, Greninger, & Metress, 1993). Those family members who become caregivers may also experience so much stress that they themselves also become patients. Coping with a chronic health problem requires many changes of the patient's entire support system. Thus, a long-term illness or disability affects the entire family.

The rehabilitation team members assist the patient and the family to attain a quality of life that is acceptable to them. Family members often have unrealistic expectations of the client, making comments such as "when he gets over this and things return to normal, then I'll be all right." It is wise to remember that the grieving process may take time and continue long after the patient is discharged. The health care professionals should never take hope away from patients or families; however, they can assist them in developing realistic, achievable goals as they work together to cope with sometimes devastating changes.

Support for the family should never be neglected. The interdisciplinary team works together to identify appropriate resources, whether financial, emotional, or spiritual, to assist the family. Times of respite for the caregivers may be indicated, and the nurse should be able to identify community resources for the family prior to discharge, anticipating future needs. Follow-up programs can also have a positive impact on coping skills (Easton et al., 1995).

Rehabilitation Begins "Day One"

Health care professionals today are becoming more aware of the need for preventive care. The push toward primary health care, health maintenance organizations, preventive medicine, and expanded roles for nurse prac-

titioners provides indications of this. In fact, gerontologists believe that prevention is the key to effective health care for the aged (Sommers, 1989). Most often, preventive medicine is associated with pre-illness conditions. Such concepts, however, also apply to the acute care phase of illness. For example, recognition of the negative consequences of prolonged immobilization have resulted in earlier ambulation of patients postoperatively and increased numbers of outpatient surgeries. Still, despite these changes in acute care, there is often little carryover of the same principles when dealing with the older adult who is experiencing a long-term condition.

Although it seems like common sense that prevention of secondary complications would be inherent in all health care, this is unfortunately not the reality. Although professional schools and colleges of nursing, medicine, therapy, and allied health have recently taken additional steps to promote preventive health education, this is not always practiced in many settings.

Take, for example, the situation of Mrs. Smith, who was admitted with the diagnosis of acute cerebral vascular accident to the intensive care unit (ICU) of a large, reputable hospital. As a result of the severity of her condition, Mrs. Smith twice experienced cardiac arrest and was successfully resuscitated. For 3 days, Mrs. Smith was essentially unresponsive and had to rely on others for all of her basic care needs. During this crucial time, however, Mrs. Smith developed darkened spots on her heels, indicating necrosis. Once medically stable, she was transferred to inpatient rehabilitation for concentrated therapy. After 1 week in rehabilitation, she stated, "In ICU, I died and they revived me twice, but I didn't feel alive after my stroke. The people in rehabilitation have brought me back to life in a different way. I feel alive inside again." Mrs. Smith's determination propelled her through the rehabilitation program, and she began gait training. However, the necrotic areas on her heels broke open once she became ambulatory. She told the rehabilitation nurses that she had not been turned for days while in the ICU. The stage IV wounds on both heels required whirlpool therapy twice daily to control the copious amounts of drainage. The pain, constant drainage, and bulky dressings greatly inhibited Mrs. Smith's ability to walk, setting her rehabilitation progress back. In addition, her wounds continued to require extensive treatment months after discharge, and Mrs. Smith and her family insisted that the hospital cover the cost, because her pressure ulcers had been acquired in the ICU. Aside from the obvious legal implications of this case scenario, Mrs. Smith experienced unnecessary pain, suffering, and impairment of her rehabilitation program as a result of events occurring in the acute care unit. Although such a statement may seem strong and even ungrateful, the fact remains that rehabilitation must begin as soon as the patient is hospitalized to prevent secondary complications that could have devastating consequences later.

Other examples that demonstrate how post-acute rehabilitation can be impeded if not practiced from "day one" include the development of contractures that can occur in the acute phase of illness and that may prevent ambulation or reduce function weeks later. The nurse in the acute care setting who does not educate an individual with a new below-knee amputation about the contraindication of using a pillow under the knee joint may well promote a contracture that prohibits the complete range of motion necessary for wearing a prosthesis to ambulate. When put in real terms, a nurse lacking sufficient knowledge in the area of rehabilitation can contribute to the likelihood of a patient's never being able to walk again. Likewise, a person with a complete spinal cord injury and paraplegia may be dependent on the acute care staff to maintain skin integrity. Should a sacral pressure ulcer form, that client, when entering long-term therapy, would be unable to develop needed wheelchair skills, perhaps being confined to a prone position until the wound is healed. In addition, stroke patients who have been in acute care even 1 week or less, if not being given proper range of motion exercises (whether active or passive), and those who are allowed to stay in the "stroke position," will have to undo the ill effects of immobilization while embarking on intensive therapy. All these conditions are likely to be preventable when the health care professional applies the concepts and principles of rehabilitation. It is particularly important that nurses practice preventive therapy with elderly adults, because even the normal effects of aging leave the older person more prone to secondary complications such as the hazards of immobility.

HISTORICAL INFLUENCES

The development of rehabilitation principles has occurred over a number of years, although rehabilitation was not recognized as a specialty until much later. As early as thousands of years ago, an Egyptian physician recorded his observations of a patient with a spinal cord injury, describing a dislocated vertebra in the neck, paralysis, and urinary incontinence (Martin, Holt, & Hicks, 1981). The earliest record of crutches on an Egyptian tomb was dated 2380 B.C. (Mumma, 1987). Even during 400 to 300 B.C., Hippocrates, known as the Father of Medicine, stated that "exercise strengthens and inactivity wastes," recording the use of artificial limbs in patients with amputations (Mumma, 1987).

Several nurses have had a significant role in the promotion of rehabilitation concepts. Florence Nightingale organized professional nursing in 1854 in England. Mumma states that Nightingale saved "more lives in the Crimean War than the entire British medical department, using hygiene and rehabilitation principles practiced by the ancient Romans" (1987, p. 5). Isabel Adams Hampton (1860–1910) was one of the leaders in the development of the nursing profession in North America. In a book on nursing principles and practice, Hampton pointed out to her pupils the importance of cleanliness and asepsis at all times to prevent secondary infections, saying, "no department of a nurse's work should appeal more forcibly to her than attention to the hygiene of the sick-room. She should thoroughly grasp the general principles which underlie the subject, and endeavor to apply them in the minutest detail" (Hampton, 1983, p. 93).

But although early records of the use of such principles exist, it was not until the World Wars ensued that significant gains were made in the field of rehabilitation. This first occurred through the armed forces, with rehabilitation services not generally being available to civilians. In fact, the increased number of disabled servicemen returning from battle provided the impetus for medical advancement and federal legislation. Prior to this time, the need for rehabilitation was not nearly as great.

World War I presented the United States with many casualties, but little hope of rehabilitation for injured soldiers. However, in 1917, the American Red Cross Institute for Crippled and Disabled Men was created in the United States to provide vocational training for wounded military personnel. Several federal as well as individual state laws were passed in an attempt to help the disabled, but nothing was done on a wide scale.

After World War I, the life expectancy of a spinal cord injured patient was less than 1 year. Mortality rates from these types of conditions were high, and rehabilitation was generally minimized. Howard Rusk, a pioneer in rehabilitation medicine stated that in those days, "they got terrible bed-sores, developed kidney and bladder problems, and simply lay in bed, waiting for death. It was almost the same with strokes" (Rusk, 1977, p. 43). Although the Veterans Administration was created after World War I to care for those with service-related disabilities, the initial care provided in the early 1940s was custodial, not rehabilitative. However, significant legislative decisions, such as the Vocational Rehabilitation Act of 1943, provided funding for training and research with the disabled. In addition, the United Nations Rehabilitation Administration drew the involvement of 44 countries in the planning of care for wounded and disabled veterans. As a result of the development of sulfa drugs and better medical treatment, more wounded had survived World War II, and the world now had to decide what to do with its disabled. According to Rusk (1977), although there had been many people concerned with the fate of the disabled, there was no organized movement to promote their rehabilitation. Fortunately, he persevered in his belief that there was quality of life beyond disability. Rusk's philosophy, which he developed and practiced during World War II, was to treat the whole man—that it was not enough just to heal the body. He pleaded his cause to any who would listen, pioneering a field that other doctors refused to accept as legitimate, until rehabilitative services were available to civilians as well as military patients. His experiences touched an entire nation, and his expertise influenced care of the disabled around the world.

The American Academy of Physical Medicine and Rehabilitation was established in 1938, and the American Board of Physical Medicine and Rehabilitation in 1947; however, it was not until well into the 1950s that rehabilitation began to be generally accepted as a viable medical specialty. During this time, books were published by physicians on the subject, and over the next two decades, several pieces of legislation were enacted, including many amendments to the Vocational Rehabilitation Act of 1943, the Architectural Barriers Act of 1968, and the Rehabilitation Act of 1973. The most significant piece of legislation passed in the 1990s was the Americans with Disabilities Act. This Act mandated employers to make reasonable accommodation for disabled workers, preventing discrimination on the basis of physical impairment. A summary of major historical and legislative highlights is presented in Table 3–2.

Although the roots of rehabilitation may have been slow to take hold, growth continues to be evident. By the early 1990s, rehabilitation was one of the top specialty choices of medical students. Certifications now exist for many types of specialists related to rehabilitation, including physiatrists, nurses, counselors, and insurance representatives. Rehabilitation nursing is a growing field.

As of 1995, there were more than 9500 members in the Association of Rehabilitation Nurses (established in 1974), many of whom are certified in this specialty.

THE INTERDISCIPLINARY REHABILITATION TEAM

"Teams are an essential aspect of health care today especially in rehabilitation or chronic illness where the course of care is frequently long, complex, and unpredictable" (Crepeau, 1994). The team approach to health care is not a new concept. However, there is no other area that exemplifies this idea more than rehabilitation. This concept is one of the great cornerstones of this specialty. While current trends lean toward generalization, cost efficiency, job merging, and role blurring, the interdisciplinary rehabilitation team continues to provide more combined knowledge and skill, clinical expertise, sensitivity, compassion, and understanding for individuals with disabilities than can be found in any other area of health care.

The term *interdisciplinary* is preferable to the formerly used word *multidisciplinary* in reference to the team, in that it denotes more of a cooperative, collaborative, and interactive partnership between team members rather than just multiple specialists acting as independent consultants. The individual team members each bring a unique perspective and expertise to the collective planning of the group. But the team shares similar goals for the patient (see Table 3–1).

There are many members who make up the usual caregiving group, or team, for long-term care patients. These include the physician, nurses, a variety of therapists, social worker, psychologist, and nutritionist. Additionally, there are auxiliary personnel, professionals and non-professionals, who contribute

Table 3–2 SELECTED MAJOR HISTORICAL AND LEGISLATIVE HIGHLIGHTS RELATED TO HEALTH CARE AND DISABILITY

1601	Poor Relief Act (England)—provided assistance for the poor and disabled.
1854	Florence Nightingale organized professional nursing (England)—used hygiene and rehabilitation principles.
1873	First school of nursing at Bellevue Hospital in New York.
1910	Nurse Susan Tracy published "Studies of Invalid Occupation"—beginning of occupational therapy.
1911	Workers' Compensation Laws enacted.
1914–1918	World War I American Red Cross Institute for Disabled Men provided vocational training for injured soldiers.
1918–1938	Post World War I—mortality rate of those wounded, particularly with spinal cord injuries, was high. Rehabilitation minimized. Veterans Administration created to care for those with service-related disabilities.
1919	First issue of Archives of Physical Medicine and Rehabilitation (APMR).
1920	First Civilian Rehabilitation Act passed by Congress (Smith-Fess Act)—provided vocational rehabilitation services. First civilian rehabilitation program formed.
1935	Social Security Act
1938	American Academy of Physical Medicine and Rehabilitation formed.
1939–1945	World War II
1941	Dr. Frank Krusen wrote first comprehensive book on physical medicine and rehabilitation.
1942	Sister Kenny Institute established. Sister Kenny's research led to development of profession of physical therapy and boosted support for physiatry as a specialty.
1943	Vocational Rehabilitation Act—provided funding for training and research with the disabled (amendments followed through 1960s). United Nations Rehabilitation Administration formed. Representatives from 44 countries met to plan care for disabled WWII veterans. Number of disabled veterans increased as a result of development of sulfa drugs and better medical treatment.
1945–present	Post World War II—greater number of disabled civilians because of increased industrialization and transportation accidents.
1947	Dr. Howard Rusk brings first medical rehabilitation services to a United States Hospital (Bellevue). American Board of Physical Medicine and Rehabilitation formed. Rehabilitation becomes a board-certified specialty.
1958	Dr. Rusk and collaborators first publish *Rehabilitation Medicine*.
1966	Medicaid enacted.
1968	Architectural Barriers Act—set accessibility standards for federal buildings.
1973	Federal Rehabilitation Act—increased awareness of the needs of those with disabilities; influenced accessibility and employability.
1990	Americans with Disabilities Act—mandated "reasonable accommodation" by employers for those with disabilities.

to the team approach on an individualized care plan basis. Examples of these would be the pastoral care provider, audiologist, prosthetist, orthotist, and other various specialists. However, many such team members are not included as a usual part of the team in a long-term care facility. As previously stated, each rehabilitation patient is different and may or may not require the services of additional team members according to his or her own unique situation. This is particularly true in the case of older adults, as many of them are retired and may not have the same concerns for returning to employment as younger patients. The roles of individual team members are discussed in the following sections.

Physiatrist

The physiatrist (not to be confused with the psychiatrist) is a doctor specializing in physical medicine and rehabilitation. This specialty was first recognized in 1947 with the formation of the American Board of Physical Medicine and Rehabilitation (Dittmar, 1989). The physiatrist possesses a medical degree and then completes an additional four years of training in the specialty including residency, and internship, with board certification following a year of practice or research in the specialty (Dittmar, 1989).

Physiatrists control the medical management of rehabilitation clients, evaluating their functional progress and making recommendations to the team. They prescribe appropriate medication, therapeutic aids, exercise regimens, and orthotic or prosthetic devices that may be needed by the patient. Physiatrists are ultimately responsible for the overall evaluation of the patient's functional progress as well as the comprehensive program for each patient. They confer with other physicians as needed and determine the length of stay for patients. Insurance coverage decisions are often based on the recommendations and documentation of this physician. Often the medical director of a rehabilitation unit is a physiatrist, providing education, structure, guidance, and leadership to the team.

Physical Therapist

The physical therapist (PT) is a professional with a minimum of 4 years of training and a bachelor of science degree in physical therapy. As of 1990, the entry level of education for a PT is a master's degree. Therapists licensed before this were grandfathered in and are not required to return for graduate training.

PTs assist the patient with several essential activities, particularly those involving the lower extremities. The PT assesses range of motion, mobility, strength, balance, and gait. Working on ambulation skills and fitting the client with necessary equipment for mobility are important jobs of the PT. This may include instructing the patient in the use of a wheelchair, walker, cane, or crutches. Some patients require the application of splints or casts to prevent or reduce contractures that inhibit mobility.

In addition to the common team goals, the PT aims treatment at restoring function, relieving pain, and preventing loss (Hasselkus, 1989). PTs are trained in pain management and may use a variety of methods, including massage, hot and cold packs, traction, splinting, whirlpool, and transcutaneous electrical nerve stimulation (TENS) units, to increase patient comfort. Therapists may also supervise daily whirlpool treatments for wounds and, in cooperation with the nurse, evaluate wound protocol and apply dressings.

PTs are an invaluable resource to the GRN. Their knowledge of muscle anatomy and physiology is far beyond what is taught in nursing school. Any area dealing with motion involves the PT. Each patient admitted for rehabilitation is evaluated by the licensed PT, who then develops a program specific to him or her. This plan includes exercises for balance and strengthening, particularly of the muscles that the individual will need to become mobile, whether through normal ambulation, with a prosthesis, or at wheelchair level. Utilizing the expertise of the PT in the area of gerontological care is particularly important because of the changes in bone mass and density that occur with aging. Most elderly also lose muscle power, strength, and some joint flexibility, so the recommendations of goals from the PT will be especially significant. In addition, elderly patients experiencing extreme changes in mobility status, such as occur with amputation, spinal cord injury, hip replacement, or trauma, require extensive work with the PT. The importance of a reciprocal working relationship between the PT and the nurse cannot be overemphasized.

Because a shortage of qualified PTs, many facilities employ physical therapy assistants (PTAs). The PTA works with the licensed PT to carry out the plan of care for the patient.

PTAs complete a 2-year program and are considered technical personnel. Although they may perform many of the duties of the PT, assistants cannot open a case, perform the initial evaluation of the patient, or formulate the comprehensive plan of care. Several PTAs may assist one PT. Many facilities use the PT as a supervisor or case manager in this area and have the PTAs work with the daily activities of the patient such as ambulating and exercise. This has proved to be a fiscally responsible arrangement in some departments. However, documentation and evaluation remain the ultimate responsibility of the PT, and other units pride themselves in using only "licensed professionals," although such a luxury may be a thing of the past.

Occupational Therapist

Occupational therapists (OTs) are degreed professionals, certified by the American Occupational Therapy Association (Dittmar, 1989). The goal of occupational therapy is to restore or maintain function, particularly in areas that promote community reentry and return to former roles. Much of the focus of occupational therapy activities is on work-related exercises. Mountford stated that "the twin tools of occupational therapy are purposeful activity and interpersonal relationships" (1971, p. 34).

Much of the work of the OT involves the client's upper extremities. In addition to assessing self-care capacity, such as feeding and dressing skills, the OT works with the client on vocational and home management tasks. Educating or reeducating the client about the activities of daily living is a large part of occupational therapy. This often takes place during morning care on the inpatient unit. Most facilities are equipped with a kitchen and/or transitional living apartment in which patients can practice homemaking skills such as cooking and doing laundry. Home evaluations are often done by the OT, prior to the patient's discharge, to ensure that proper equipment and supplies are ordered and that the home is accessible. The OT also helps plan leisure time and community outings that assist the client with reintegration into society after a disability.

Like PTs, OTs may have associates who help carry out the plan of care. Occupational therapy assistants may carry the title COTA, which stands for Certified Occupational Therapy Assistant. COTAs attend a 2-year training program. Their role is to aid the licensed OT

in completing the scheduled routine for each patient. Thus, in many facilities, the COTA sees the patients on a daily basis for each session, and the OT acts as a supervisor, formulating and directing the plan of care, attending team meetings, and performing evaluations. This means of care delivery is similar to nursing with the hierarchy of registered nurses, licensed practical nurses, nurse technicians, and certified nursing assistants.

Speech Therapist

The speech therapist is also called the speech-language pathologist. The minimal preparation required is a baccalaureate degree, and certification is mandatory. Most professionals are educated at the master's level. In fact, the speech therapist is often the most educated member of the rehabilitation team, aside from the physician.

The role of the speech therapist is diverse and complex. Speech pathologists assess swallowing, respiration, phonation, and language ability. They deal with communication disorders that may be secondary to disability, congenital or developmental problems, or postsurgical difficulties. Therapy is aimed at improving communication and may involve a variety of treatment modalities, including auditory, verbal, visual, and motor processing.

The speech-language pathologist not only helps patients having difficulty with verbal expression but also those experiencing cognitive problems as well. Treatment may include exercises involving the muscles of speech and swallowing, thermal stimulation, and memory cues. Because of the nature of this type of treatment, speech therapy sessions are conducted one-to-one in a controlled environment, limiting distractions and interruptions. However, family members, friends, and staff can assist the patient in goal achievement in this area by reinforcing what the patient has learned in private sessions.

Assisting patients to regain the use of oral-facial muscles needed for speaking and swallowing is a chief function of the therapist. They also evaluate barium swallows in conjunction with the radiologist to determine a safe and appropriate diet for patients with dysphagia. The rehabilitation nurse should take care to form a cooperative working relationship with the speech pathologist, because many of the exercises and precautions used daily by the inpatient therapist will need to be reinforced by the nurse on the off-shifts and weekends.

The speech therapist is an invaluable resource for GRNs concerned with the communication and swallowing abilities of their patients. Many elderly patients experience dysphagia, which can lead to aspiration and airway obstruction or pneumonia. It is the nurse's responsibility to request the consultation of a speech pathologist if there is any doubt as to the patient's swallowing ability or the appropriateness of the diet ordered. It is not unusual for elderly rehabilitation patients to have special swallowing instructions to prevent aspiration. This could include a sequence of steps such as tucking the chin, taking only one-half teaspoon amounts at a time, thickening liquids, or alternating solids and liquids. The entire nursing staff shares the responsibility of seeing that the patient strictly follows those instructions in the absence of the speech therapist. Likewise, the elderly patient with aphasia may be struggling with communication skills. The recommendations of the speech therapist, such as providing verbal cues, reality orientation, or assisting the patient with a journal as a memory tool, are important areas to reinforce. Continuity of the team plan of care is critical to the patient's overall success. Most speech therapists are willing teachers to those nurses interested in learning more about dysphagia and aphasia management.

Audiologist

The work of the audiologist complements the communication department and the roles of the speech-language pathologist. Audiologists perform hearing evaluations and provide alternative systems of communication, such as hearing aids, for patients. The audiologist may also teach sign language and lip reading and works with the speech therapist to develop aids of augmentative communication depending on the patient's needs. Many hospitals employ audiologists within the acute care setting to run hearing tests and screening. These services are especially convenient when a patient's speech or cognitive problems are complicated by hearing difficulties and are often used by elderly patients.

Dietitian/Nutritionist

Dietitians provide for the nutritional needs of patients. They possess a bachelor's degree in nutrition, and many are prepared at the master's level. Some of the duties of the dietitian include calculating calorie counts, monitoring the patient's overall nutritional health, and recommending various types of menu choices.

The dietitian is a good resource for the GRN, because the caloric needs of the aged are unique, especially when complicated by illness. Often, the older person's appetite is impaired during hospitalization, and finding appealing foods can be a challenge. Many dietitians have particular experience and training in the special needs of the older patient. Most professionals are eager to share information with the patient, family members, and staff, as well as answer individual questions.

Dietary counseling is a major role of the dietitian/nutritionist. Some elderly rehabilitation patients may be receiving tube feedings. Whether the cause is dysphagia, aspiration, or malnutrition, the dietitian is a ready source of information on the contents of various supplements. The nutritionist is prepared to educate others about necessary dietary modifications or restrictions, whether through inservice training sessions or on a one-to-one basis.

Social Worker

Social workers are master's prepared professionals, many of whom hold special certifications for clinical hospital work. They focus on assessment and evaluation of the patient's social situation. This involves taking a thorough psychosocial history, negotiating with insurance companies for medical coverage, arranging for placement in another facility, ordering equipment for home use, and arranging transportation from acute care. Social workers must be adept at diagnosing the overall social environment, as well as counseling patients and families through times of crisis, despite pre-existing family dynamics that may hinder smooth adjustment.

Social workers are a valuable link to community resources. They are knowledgeable about the quality of care provided in area extended care facilities and often must arrange for long-term care placement of the elderly patient requiring an additional convalescent period. The expertise of the social worker related to insurance policies, reimbursement protocol, and documentation can save the nurse much time and frustration. In addition to the services provided to the team, social workers often remain in contact with patients and families after discharge, providing follow-up and referrals to community resources as needed. This is a particularly valuable service for the elderly disabled client, who will require a longer period of adjustment and additional support.

Psychologist

Psychologists engage in counseling of patients and families in a wide variety of settings. The minimal academic preparation required for this profession is a master's degree, although most hold a PhD. Most rehabilitation facilities employ a psychologist more often than a psychiatrist. One reason for this is that psychologists, who are not medical doctors, focus on behavior modification and family adaptation, evaluating outcomes. Their treatment is more supportive and evaluative in nature. Many rehabilitation patients need the services of a psychologist to better cope with the adjustments required by a health crisis, but this normal experience of the grieving process usually does not warrant the attention of a psychiatrist. Psychiatrists possess a medical degree and are trained to diagnose and treat those with mental and emotional disturbances. The psychiatrist also can prescribe medications and perform more advanced medical treatment such as electroshock therapy.

Psychologists also may provide guidance to the interdisciplinary team about dealing with difficult patient problems. Assisting the staff in dealing with feelings that may arise during times of crisis can help them better cope with the daily stresses on the job. In addition, psychologists may help the team work more harmoniously by providing insight into the group dynamic process.

Recreational Therapist

Recreational therapy is an idea whose time has come. Some have compared it with the "play nurse" in pediatrics, only with a gerontological clientele. Although the role of the recreational therapist may have been minimized in past decades, the value of this professional within the long-term care setting is unquestionable. Dudish stated that "recreation can be referred to as the wise use of leisure" (Dudish, 1974, p. 87). Elderly patients in subacute or extended care facilities may have large amounts of "leisure" time. The aged resident of today is more educated and socially engaged than in the past. Recreation is a normal and necessary part of living for most Americans.

The goals of the recreational therapist working with the elderly include promoting a positive self-image, maintaining normal living activities, improving adjustment through a happy home-like environment, and adapting a specific plan of care to the unique needs of the patient (Allen, 1974). The recreational therapist must be able to plan and execute a wide variety of activities in order to appeal to the range of patients seen in these settings. Motivating and documenting patient participation are also important.

Recreational therapy may include activities such as crafts (e.g., painting, making decorations for a party), horticulture, pet therapy, or participation in musical events. Some patients prefer to do private hobbies such as crossword puzzles or crocheting. Others receive pleasure from more social functions such as movies, games like bingo or cards, or outings to a play or for shopping. Music, often called the universal language, can easily be incorporated into the recreational therapy program. Some facilities are fortunate enough to employ a music therapist, a professional with special education in music and health care. Unfortunately, budgetary restrictions may mean that not all facilities even have the luxury of a trained recreational therapist. Sometimes this role is filled by social workers, volunteers, or nurses. Fun and leisure activities are essential to maintaining health and happiness. For the aged and disabled, it promotes health and a positive self-esteem and contributes to maintaining their identity when other "normal" aspects of life may be closed to them (Dudish, 1974; Kraus, 1973).

Pastoral Care

The patient's spiritual leader can be an important resource for the nurse. This individual may be a priest, rabbi, minister, deacon, or layperson, but is someone whom the patient respects as a religious mentor or advisor. Many hospitals make it a routine part of admission to notify the patient's church or synagogue when the patient arrives. A number of facilities have chaplains, deacons, or sisters who are available 24 hours a day for those requesting spiritual guidance or prayer. In addition, some facilities offer chapel services or mass and televise them through a closed circuit system to rooms for residents who are unable to attend in person.

The nursing diagnosis of spiritual distress

is often recognized on the rehabilitation unit and in long-term care. Patients are frequently grappling with disturbing situations that make them question their previous beliefs. Nurses will find that pastoral care providers often can relate to the patient in a unique way and lend insight to the team. The area of spiritual care within the rehabilitation setting should not be neglected because it is a vital part of the holistic approach to health and wellness.

Prosthetist and Orthotist

Not every patient requires the services of the prosthetist or orthotist. The jobs of these two professionals often overlap, making good communication between the team members, patients, and families essential. The physician must prescribe the necessary equipment, after which these professionals begin work to measure, fit, and individualize devices for the client. The PT or OT will educate the client about the use of the equipment.

The skill of these individuals is essential for those needing a prosthesis (prosthetist) or an orthopedic brace (orthotist). They are valuable consultants to the interdisciplinary team, particularly when working with amputees or those needing corrective braces.

Nurse

The opportunities for nurses within the field of rehabilitation are many. Rehabilitation nursing is a dynamic, creative specialty that promotes the positive adaptation of individuals with disabilities through a holistic, nurturing environment by combining the clinical skills, advanced knowledge, and resourcefulness of the nurse with the perseverance, motivation, and strengths of the client to achieve maximal independence and acceptable quality of life. Nurses practicing in this setting use a broad knowledge base, combining expertise in work with those with disabilities and education in the nursing process to promote quality patient outcomes. The major goal of rehabilitation nursing, according to the Association of Rehabilitation Nurses, is "to assist persons with disability and chronic illness in attaining maximum functional ability, maintaining optimal health, and adapting to an altered lifestyle" (Habel, 1993, p. 13). Dittmar stated that "the goal of rehabilitation nursing is to facilitate the movement of individuals toward independence while helping them satisfy their needs" (1989, p. 6).

The major roles of the staff nurse include teacher, caregiver, advocate, counselor, consultant, and researcher. The emphasis on each of these titles varies depending on the nurse's educational background, job position, and the setting of practice. Nurses are a vital part of the interdisciplinary team, and they are the only team members who are with the patient 24 hours a day. The nurse brings expertise to the team in the areas of physical assessment, bowel and bladder management, skin care, nutrition, behavior, and family participation. No other team member will observe the family dynamics as much as the nurse. Rehabilitation nurses engage in a large amount of teaching and family education. They must be knowledgeable, patient, resourceful, creative, and non-judgmental. It is the nurse's responsibility to be aware of the patient's needs and goals and to act as a patient advocate to the rest of the staff if needed. Two mandatory qualities of the rehabilitation nurse are assessment and communication. The nurse must be able to recognize subtle changes in patients' conditions and properly and appropriately report them to the doctor.

Nurses working in rehabilitation may have received basic preparation at the associate degree (2-year), diploma (3-year), or baccalaureate (4-year) level. Some rehabilitation units require at least 1 year of medical-surgical nursing before hiring. Others prefer to educate graduate nurses directly out of school.

The Association of Rehabilitation Nurses (ARN), representing more than 8000 members, was founded in 1974, recognizing rehabilitation nursing as a specialty. Nurses can be certified in rehabilitation by passing a test administered by the American Psychological Association for the ARN. Any registered nurse with 2 years of experience in rehabilitation can sit for the examination, regardless of educational level. As of 2000, a bachelor's degree in nursing will be required to sit for the examination. The credential given on successful completion of the certification examination is CRRN (Certified Rehabilitation Registered Nurse).

The *nurse therapist* (NT) is a title used at several rehabilitation facilities. The definition and description of responsibilities may differ at each institution. For example, the world-renowned Rehabilitation Institute of Chicago (RIC) developed its nurse therapy role more than 20 years ago. At RIC, every registered nurse was a nurse therapist. Ideally, the NT performed the admissions assessment and formulated the nursing care plan, including long- and short-term goals. Monitoring and revising goals and nursing treatment, educating the patient and family, coordinating discharge planning and follow-up, and representing the patient's nursing needs to the interdisciplinary team all were components of the NT role.

Primary nurses were popular before budgetary cuts mandated a return to the team nursing approach, considered a more cost-effective method of care delivery. In the 1980s, with the opening of many rehabilitation units within acute care hospitals, primary nursing was the preferred model of care. Primary nurses were responsible for the 24-hour-a-day care of the patient on a unit with a low ratio of patients to nurses. They acted as case managers for the same team of patients on a daily basis. A major responsibility of these nurses was to represent nursing and the client's interests at the team meetings. The primary nurse functions similarly to the nurse therapist discussed previously.

The *clinical nurse specialist* (CNS) and *nurse practitioner* (NP) are advanced practice roles for rehabilitation professionals. The CNS is a master's prepared nurse with special expertise in a certain clinical area. The higher level of education and advanced skills of the CNSs allow them to deal with difficult patient situations that may arise. Some CNSs carry a caseload of the most challenging patients on the unit, acting as a case manager. Other facilities utilize the CNS for teaching and research, collaborating with other team members to problem solve and write policies and care plans. The CNS generally plays a major role in staff education, orientation, and development. Implementing programs on the unit and monitoring quality assurance are other possible duties of the CNS. The nursing supervisor or manager works closely with the CNS to provide comprehensive educational and administrative coverage for the unit.

NPs in rehabilitation have recently become more popular, particularly at larger rehabilitation facilities. NPs usually focus on physical assessment, diagnosis, and treatment of uncomplicated medical problems. The ways in which NPs are utilized on the team is based on collaborative practice agreements with physicians and/or administrators. Because the educational preparation of NPs does not generally have a tertiary care focus, their roles in rehabilitation settings may be quite diverse across geographical locations.

The core curriculum for advanced practice in rehabilitation nursing was published in 1997. In December 1997 and January 1998, the first advanced practice certification examination for rehabilitation nurses was offered. Both of these landmark events usher in a new era for advanced practice in the field of rehabilitation.

Nursing assistants and *nurse technicians* are important contributors to the interdisciplinary team. Most units, unable to economically support the primary nurse concept, utilize certified nursing assistants (CNAs) to perform much of the direct patient care under the supervision of the registered nurse. Nurse technicians are usually nursing students who have completed some, but not all, of their training and are given additional responsibilities beyond those of the assistant. CNAs may initially require additional guidance in rehabilitation techniques, because these concepts are only vaguely covered in nursing assistant courses, and the quality of their education depends largely on the instructor. Normal nurse's aide duties include helping patients with activities of daily living (ADLs) such as eating, bathing, dressing, toileting, and ambulation, as well as many other jobs to help the unit run efficiently. Most CNAs experienced in the care of patients with disabilities are adept at performing transfers, assisting the patient with ADLs, and reporting concerns or abnormalities to the nurse. In today's health care system, the CNA often spends as much or more time than the nurse as the direct caregiver of the elderly patient, depending on the module of care delivery of the facility. Working with a CNA provides the nurse with additional time to spend in patient and family teaching. Nurses should remember that the CNA is a valuable part of the team and can have a direct impact on patient care. The GRN should use every opportunity to help CNAs develop their skills and comfortably assume their role. Nurses can be excellent mentors for their assistants and nurse technicians. The quality of patient care, dependent on teamwork, can be promoted when *all* caregivers are instructed in rehabilitation principles and the unique needs of the elderly.

REFERENCES

Allen, E. C. (1974). The role of the recreation therapist in the long-term health care facility. In F. M. Robinson, Jr. (Ed.), *Therapeutic re-creation* (pp. 79–86). Springfield, IL: Charles C Thomas.

Baier, S., & Schomaker, M. Z. (1986). *Bed number ten*. Boca Raton, FL: CRC Press.

Beisser, A. R. (1989). *Flying without wings*. New York: Doubleday.

Crepeau, E. B. (1994). Three images of interdisciplinary team meetings. *The American Journal of Occupational Therapy, 48*(8), 717–721.

Dittmar, S. (1989). *Rehabilitation nursing: Process and application.* St. Louis, MO: C. V. Mosby.

Dobkin, B. H. (1991). The rehabilitation of elderly stroke patients. *Clinics in Geriatric Medicine, 7*(3), 507–523.

Dudish, L. T. (1974). Starting a recreation program with limited funding in nursing homes. In F. M. Robinson, Jr. (Ed.), *Therapeutic re-creation* (pp. 87–98). Springfield, IL: Charles C Thomas.

Easton, K., Rawl, S., Zemen, D., Kwiatkowski, S., & Burczyk, B. (1995). The effects of nursing follow-up on the coping strategies used by rehabilitation patients after discharge. *Rehabilitation Nursing Research, 4*(4), 119–127.

Fawcett, J. (1995). *Analysis and evaluation of conceptual models of nursing.* Philadelphia: F. A. Davis.

Folden, S. L. (1993). Effect of a supportive-educative nursing intervention on older adults' perceptions of self-care after a stroke. *Rehabilitation Nursing, 18*(3), 162–166.

Gender, A. (1998). Scope of rehabilitation and rehabilitation nursing. In P. A. Chin, D. Finocchiaro, & A. Rosebrough (Eds.), *Rehabilitation nursing practice* (pp. 3–20). New York: McGraw-Hill.

Habel, M. (1993). Rehabilitation: Philosophy, goals, and process. In A. E. McCourt (Ed.), *The specialty practice of rehabilitation nursing: A core curriculum* (pp. 2–5). Skokie, IL: Rehabilitation Nursing Foundation.

Hampton, I. A. (1993). *Nursing: Its principles and practice for hospital and private use.* Philadelphia: W. B. Saunders.

Hasselkus, B. R. (1989). Occupational and physical therapy in geriatric rehabilitation. *Physical & Occupational Therapy in Geriatrics, 7*(3), 3–21.

Kraus, R. (1973). *Therapeutic recreation service: Principles and practices.* Philadelphia: W. B. Saunders.

Martin, N., Holt, N., & Hicks, D. (Eds.). (1981). *Comprehensive rehabilitation nursing.* New York: McGraw-Hill.

Mountford, S. W. (1971). *Introduction to occupational therapy.* Edinburgh: E & S Livingstone.

Mumma, C. M. (1987). *Rehabilitation nursing: Concepts and practice* (2nd ed.). Evanston, IL: Rehabilitation Nursing Foundation.

Rosenthal, S., Pituch, M., Greninger, L., & Metress, E. (1993). Perceived needs of wives of stroke patients. *Rehabilitation Nursing, 18*(3), 148–153.

Rusk, H. A. (1977). *A world to care for.* New York: Random House.

Sommers, A. R. (1989). Foreword. In R. Lavizzo-Mourey, S. C. Day, D. Diserens, & J. A. Grisso (Eds.), *Practicing prevention for the elderly* (pp. xi–xiii). Philadelphia: Hanley & Belfus.

White, N. E., Richter, J. M., & Fry, C. (1992). Coping, social support, and adaptation to chronic illness. *Western Journal of Nursing Research, 14*(2), 211–224.

Chapter 4

Foundations of Gerontological Rehabilitation Nursing

HISTORICAL PERSPECTIVES

Nearly a century has passed since the *American Journal of Nursing* published the first article that declared that caring for the elderly required special skill and knowledge (Eliopoulos, 1997). Nurses were initially slow to develop gerontological nursing as a specialty—the first textbook on this subject was not published until 1950. In recent decades, however, gerontology has flourished. Today, a large body of literature from many disciplines focuses on the unique needs of the older population, with the field of nursing contributing resources, texts, and scientific research. More gerontological nursing books are currently published each year than ever before. Advanced practice programs have appeared throughout the country, and generous research funds are available for those engaging in research with the elderly.

Rehabilitation nursing, in comparison, is a newer specialty, first officially recognized in 1974 with the emergence of the Association of Rehabilitation Nurses. Since then, this organization has grown rapidly to include about 9000 members internationally. It is interesting to note that the subspecialty of gerontological rehabilitation nursing has emerged from this more recent group (Table 4–1) instead of the more established field of gerontological nursing, suggesting that gerontological rehabilitation nursing was born of necessity in answer to problems arising from nursing care of the elderly. The establishment of gerontological rehabilitation nursing is vital, because the future of health care for the elderly will rest largely on the shoulders of the nursing profession, and gerontological nurses will play a key role in the direction and quality of practice.

DEFINING GERONTOLOGICAL REHABILITATION NURSING

"Gerontological rehabilitation nursing is a specialty practice that focuses on the unique requirements of elderly rehabilitation clients" (Association of Rehabilitation Nurses, 1995). Because the needs of the aged adult differ from those of the rest of the population, the knowledge and skill needed to provide quality patient care warrant special attention. The gerontological rehabilitation nurse (GRN) is knowledgeable about both techniques of caring for the aged and rehabilitation concepts and principles. This unique type of nursing combines knowledge of both the aging process and rehabilitation practice to specialize in caring for the aging adult with a disability or long-term health problem.

GOALS OF GERONTOLOGICAL REHABILITATION NURSING

The main goal of gerontological rehabilitation nursing is to assist elderly patients in achieving their personal optimal level of health and well-being by providing holistic care in a therapeutic environment. This aim is similar to that of the general rehabilitation nurse, but with a special focus on the geriatric population, considering their special needs, roles, social relationships, and potential physical

Table 4–1   HIGHLIGHTS IN GERONTOLOGICAL AND REHABILITATION NURSING

1904	First article published on care of the aged in *American Journal of Nursing*.
1925	*American Journal of Nursing* suggests idea of a specialty in gerontological nursing.
1950	First textbook on geriatric nursing.
	Gerontological nursing emerges as a specialty.
1970	Standards for geriatric nursing practice first published.
1974	Association of Rehabilitation Nurses formed; rehabilitation nursing emerges as a specialty.
	American Nurses Association offers certification in gerontological nursing.
1981	*Rehabilitation Nursing: Concepts and Practice—A Core Curriculum* first published.
	American Nurses Association Division of Gerontological Nursing defines the scope of gerontological nursing practice.
1995	Association of Rehabilitation Nurses approves definition and scope of practice for gerontological rehabilitation nursing.
1997	Association of Rehabilitation Nurses publishes a core curriculum for advanced practice in rehabilitation nursing; first advanced practice nurse certification examination in rehabilitation offered.

limitations that may occur as a result of the aging process.

GRNs strive not only to provide rehabilitative care but also to teach prevention. Thus, GRNs may function within primary, secondary, and tertiary levels of care, with the universal goal of helping elderly patients to achieve optimum wellness and self-care.

ROLES OF THE GERONTOLOGICAL REHABILITATION NURSE

The roles of GRNs are many and diverse but typically include caregiver, teacher, leader, mediator, consultant, and researcher. Table 4–2 provides the complete role description for the GRN as set forth by the Association of Rehabilitation Nurses (ARN). The reader will note slight differences between this text and the ARN description regarding the labels attached to some of the roles. These terms are explained in the following sections. Nurses may engage in the practice of these roles in various proportions, depending on their level of education, experience, and practice setting. For example, staff GRNs in extended care may spend the majority of their time performing direct patient care, whereas those on inpatient rehabilitation units in the acute care hospital may devote more hours to patient and family teaching and consultation. Conversely, the GRN in the academic institution spends a vast majority of the time teaching students. The doctorally prepared GRN may divide time between teaching and research, with only a small portion given to the caregiving role.

Some GRNs practice almost exclusively within one role. Nurse managers, for example, may find their job description specifies leadership skills, with less emphasis on clinical practice, but this, of course, varies largely among institutions and clinical settings. Other nurses hold positions that are strictly research-oriented. But whatever the setting, most GRNs have participated in or will practice at some level within the roles described here.

Caregiver

The caregiver role is not unique to GRNs. All nurses participate in this physical care of patients, this nurturing aspect of the discipline of nursing. Caregiving is defined here as the provision of direct, hands-on physical care. GRNs bring to this role expertise in two subspecialties of nursing, gerontological and rehabilitation nursing, blending these to provide highly individualized nursing care to elderly patients with long-term health problems.

The caregiver role of gerontological rehabilitation nursing practice is often more time-consuming with the older adult than in other areas of nursing. Elderly patients with complex health care needs may require a longer period of time for direct caregiving than a young to middle-aged adult. Because sensory deficits are common, GRNs must be patient and willing to take the time to perform thorough assessments, including a detailed history and physical, cognitive appraisals, and/or mental status examinations. Units that cater to chronically ill elders should allow time for nurses and nursing assistants to give safe,

Table 4-2 SUMMARY OF GERONTOLOGICAL REHABILITATION NURSING

Definition of Gerontological Rehabilitation Nursing

Gerontological rehabilitation nursing is a specialty practice that focuses on the unique requirements of elderly rehabilitation clients. Elderly clients can be categorized into the following groups: the young-old (65 through 74 years of age), the old (75 through 84 years of age), and the old-old, or frail elderly (ages 85 and above) (Schrier, 1990*). The older a population is, the less homogeneous it is; therefore, more diverse care is required to meet the needs of the individuals within the population. Consequently, geriatric clients warrant special consideration.

Gerontological rehabilitation nurses consider the normal age-related changes and the functional limitations brought about by illness or injury in elderly people when they help an individual develop a plan of care. Specific disabling conditions and their concomitant medical issues dictate specific rehabilitation nursing interventions and techniques.

Goal

Gerontological rehabilitation nurses use a holistic approach in the assessment and provision of services to geriatric clients. Helping geriatric clients achieve their optimal level of physical, mental, and psychosocial well-being is the primary goal of the gerontological rehabilitation nurse.

Settings

Gerontological rehabilitation nursing services are provided in a wide variety of settings that include hospital-based rehabilitation units, freestanding rehabilitation hospitals, hospital-based skilled nursing facilities, acute care units, subacute units, long-term care facilities, residential care facilities, home health agencies, private and agency clinics, and governmental agencies. Nurses with advanced education and certification also can practice independently as gerontological nurse practitioners or clinical nurse specialists. Other nurses practice gerontological rehabilitation nursing by teaching or conducting research at the nursing school or at the university level.

Standards

Gerontological rehabilitation nurses adhere to the established rehabilitation nursing standards of care and scope of practice as published by the Association of Rehabilitation Nurses.

Roles of the Gerontological Rehabilitation Nurse

The gerontological rehabilitation nurse practices in a variety of roles, including, but not limited to, those outlined below.

Advocate: The gerontological rehabilitation nurse advocates for the rights of older persons and works to dispel the myths of aging.

Clinical Practitioner: The gerontological rehabilitation nurse practitioner demonstrates clinical expertise in the care provided to aging adults. This expertise includes assessing and identifying problems; planning, intervening in, and evaluating care; and participating in the interdisciplinary plan of care.

Educator: The gerontological rehabilitation nurse educator promotes activities that lead to healthy aging and prevent disability and also provides individualized education for clients and their families. The gerontological rehabilitation nurse is responsible for continually updating his or her knowledge base through in-service education, continuing education, or formal secondary education and training. Networking with other gerontological rehabilitation nurses to share ideas and experiences also expands the professional practice and knowledge base. The gerontological rehabilitation nurse also has a role in educating the public about issues related to aging by giving presentations and by publishing articles on related topics.

Manager: The gerontological nurse manager uses management skills when providing for patient care in a variety of hospital and community settings. The specialized skills and knowledge required for a management position include maintaining up-to-date information about federal and state regulatory statutes as well as information related to funding for elder care programs. The gerontological rehabilitation nurse manager must be proficient in the areas of quality assurance and quality improvement and must be familiar with the requirements of other accrediting bodies such as the Joint Commission on Accreditation of Healthcare Organizations and the Commission on Accreditation of Rehabilitation Facilities.

Consultant: The gerontological rehabilitation nurse consultant supports other healthcare practitioners who provide geriatric services. The consultant offers guidance in developing programs such as those on pressure ulcer prevention and care and on clinical issues such as Alzheimer's disease that typically pertain to an aging population.

Researcher: The gerontological rehabilitation nurse researcher communicates relevant research through presentations at continuing education programs and by writing articles for professional publications. The gerontological rehabilitation nurse researcher participates in rehabilitation research whenever possible and seeks opportunities to develop and conduct research projects.

---

*Schrier, R. W. (1990). *Geriatric medicine*. Philadelphia: W. B. Saunders.

efficient care without rushing the patient. Because gerontological rehabilitation nursing emphasizes the patient's performing self-care, time must be allowed for nurses to engage in patient/family teaching. Overworked and understaffed nursing teams can be pressured to take overwhelming assignments, resulting in less than adequate time to meet the patients' physical care demands, let alone allowing time for teaching. For those patients who rely on the nurse to compensate for their lack of self-care ability, such decreased time can lead to prolonged periods of immobility (and subsequent secondary problems such as skin breakdown, pressure sores, or decreased range of motion), impaired bowel and bladder function (such as incontinence related to lack of staff to promptly answer lights or follow through with toileting programs), or impaired safety (evidenced by higher fall rates or injury such as skin tears) related to a hurried feeling or inadequate staffing patterns.

Caregiving is an essential and indispensable component of the general nursing role. It is the essence of the specialty and one of the traits that distinguishes nursing from medicine or other disciplines. As important as this role is, however, GRNs emphasize the promotion of self-care. Helping the patient make the transition from the sick role to the disabled role should involve a gradual decrease in the amount of physical care provided by the nurse, while the patient assumes greater responsibility for self-care as he or she is able. The nurse then assumes a more supportive-educative role than in the acute care setting.

The nurse working with the aged in long-term care should be gentle, patient, thorough, and never rushed. As the primary caregiver, the GRN coordinates nursing care 24 hours a day, provides hands-on care, helps restore and maintain functioning together with other members of the rehabilitation team, creates a therapeutic environment for adaptation, and promotes self-care. This requires excellent assessment and communication skills. The nurse who does not possess both these qualities cannot successfully function in the caregiving role for older adults with chronic problems. Because the nurse is the only team member consistently present during off-shifts, the nurse's assessment skills must be finely tuned to the normalities and abnormalities of aging, as well as baseline data for each individual patient in his or her care. Yet, even with superb clinical expertise, the GRN will fall short of providing quality care if important observations are not effectively communicated to the physician and other team members. This is a crucial principle for all GRNs to grasp and essential to the smooth functioning of any rehabilitation program.

Mediator/Advocate

Advocacy connotes the effective protection of an individual's rights. According to Bandman and Bandman, "the nurse who understands the advocacy role promotes, protects, and thereby advocates patients' interests and rights in an effort to make them whole and well again" (1995, p. 24). All members of the rehabilitation team should be patient advocates. That is a reasonable expectation of every health care worker. The days are past when nurses should be thinking of themselves as the sole patient advocates, almost in an opposing role to the physician. Doctors are also patient advocates, and it is presumptuous to claim that the role of patient advocate belongs exclusively to nursing.

Thus, *mediator* may be a more appropriate description of this aspect of the GRN's role. Although every team member should defend the patient's best interest, not every health care worker has a primary role of mediating between the patient and other team members. This job, in which the nurse stands on behalf of the patient to others—whether physician, therapists, or family members—is certainly a large part of nursing care.

Because nurses are the only caregivers present 24 hours a day, this role goes beyond communicating with other disciplines. Nurses need to be the eyes and ears for the physician in reporting medical changes, but also the legs for the amputee, the voice for the aphasic patient, the steady hands for the patient with parkinsonian tremors, sight for the patient with glaucoma, hearing for the deaf older patient, and strength for the weak. Continuous nursing follow-through with techniques learned in various therapies, such as speech exercises and ambulation skills, is crucial to timely and efficient rehabilitation of the older adult. The notion of the nurse as a compensatory system, as described by Orem (1995), can easily be demonstrated within this role.

The elderly population particularly needs assertive, knowledgeable mediators. The nurse with expertise in rehabilitation techniques is already adept at communicating with team members and skilled at mutual goal setting. When these are combined with gerontological care principles, GRNs can effectively pass along important information to others, promoting high quality and continuity of care.

Leader

GRNs are leaders in gerontological care. By practicing gerontological nursing within a rehabilitative framework, the nurse establishes high standards and expectations for quality patient care. This aspect of the GRN role has two branches: (1) being a leader among health care professionals and the community, and (2) providing leadership for patients and family members struggling with adaptive changes in lifestyles and role adjustments.

GRNs distinguish themselves by using the concepts of rehabilitation in caring for older adults. They believe in the value and worth of all persons throughout the life span regardless of race, color, or creed, and that the elderly can and should continue to maintain independence and autonomy as long as possible. Care is focused on prevention of secondary complications (as well as primary prevention of problems that can occur with aging) and regaining optimum functional status.

There are several types of management roles used by GRNs. Some case management is inherent to every GRN position. All GRNs must learn to coordinate care. Indeed, the role of the primary nurse, or the nurse therapist, is quite similar in many facilities to that of a case manager.

Other nurses may function in a supervisory capacity, in which case, management skills such as balancing a budget, doing the payroll, dealing with staffing issues, making assignments, and staff development might take precedence over other roles.

Teacher

The GRN engages in a larger proportion of teaching time than do nurses in many other specialties. In this area, the nurse assumes a partnership role with the patient, assessing his or her level of knowledge, providing instruction, and evaluating learning. Knowledge of the principles of adult learning is essential. Older adults have different learning goals and styles than younger adults.

One of the most unique yet significant aspects of education for the GRN is reinforcing what patients have learned in therapies. This is essential to promote continuity of care and

an efficient rehabilitation program. GRNs should be in direct communication with all other team members and have knowledge of the patient's progress and goals in physical, occupational, and speech therapy and the like. Reinforcement may take the form of ambulating patients on the unit, supervising swallowing protocols at mealtime, practicing transfers, and other such tasks.

GRNs also teach skills falling within the medical/nursing domain, such as taking vital signs, medication management, tube feedings, and bowel and bladder programs. All the skills taught by nurses should be done with the knowledge that learning is highly individualized. Different persons learn better through different modalities. Some may prefer to have demonstrations and return demonstrations; others will wish to read instructions before attempting a new skill. The GRN is sensitive to the varied learning styles and needs of the older adult as well as the unique extraneous factors that may be involved in teaching an older patient, such as decreased vision, hearing impairments, or functional limitations.

Additional opportunities to engage in teaching present themselves in a wide variety of situations. GRNs may engage in educating other team members, particularly nursing assistants in the long-term care setting. Case Studies 4.1 and 4.2 provide examples of the GRN in the role of teacher.

CASE STUDY—4.1

A GRN from a temporary agency was assigned to work at a 100-bed nursing home on the day shift. She supervised five nursing assistants, who provided the direct patient care on her wing of 44 intermediate-level care residents. Most of the residents on this unit required minimal assistance with activities of daily living (ADLs), but several were bed-bound, necessitating maximal care by the nursing staff. The GRN was summoned to the nurse's station by a distraught certified nursing assistant (CNA), who explained that she had been taking a rectal temperature on a bed-bound resident and the plastic probe cover of the electric thermometer had come off and lodged high in the patient's rectum. The GRN performed a rectal check and was able to feel only the distal end of the plastic cover with the tip of her finger. Unable to remove the probe cover, the GRN administered a suppository and the patient expelled the plastic cover intact. The GRN used this opportunity to give a brief, impromptu inservice training session to all the CNAs working that shift on the proper way to take a rectal temperature using the electronic device. The GRN emphasized that only the tip of the probe needed to be inserted into the rectum to obtain an accurate reading, and inserting it farther was unnecessary and could harm the patient. According to the nursing assistants, they had been previously taught to insert the probe the entire length. The CNAs were given the opportunity to ask questions, which they did with enthusiasm, displaying a desire for further information on other topics. The relationship between the CNAs and the GRN was strengthened, and quality of patient care potentially improved.

CASE STUDY—4.2

A GRN working in a long-term care facility was checking vital signs taken by the CNA. Noting an isolated blood pressure of 240/120 recorded on an elderly woman with otherwise normal vital signs, the nurse suspected the measurement may have been in error. She approached the CNA about the reading and they went together to check the patient. The woman had an old mastectomy scar on the left side with lymphedema. After observing that the resident was in no apparent distress, the nurse asked the CNA which arm she took the blood pressure on. The CNA stated she had taken it on the left side. The nurse then explained why, for this person, the blood pressure should be taken on the opposite side, and she had the CNA recheck it on the unaffected right arm. The GRN also used this opportunity to observe the CNA's technique and give some helpful suggestions for obtaining more accurate blood pressure readings. The GRN rechecked the blood pressure with the CNA to ensure accuracy. The CNA thanked the GRN for taking the time to teach her something new, stating that she had never learned this before and "the other nurses were always too busy to help."

Consultant

A major goal of gerontological rehabilitation is for the patient to return home with optimum function and adjustment; therefore, GRNs engage in a large amount of discharge planning, often requiring consulting skills. GRNs may also be called on to share their expertise in a variety of settings (Case Study 4.3 provides an example). For the patient who is unable to return home, the nurse provides an important link to resources for families and promotes independence of the patient within a different setting. Although many jobs such as arranging for equipment needed at home, making initial doctor appointments for the patient after discharge, and arranging for transportation or placement in another facility have typically been the social worker's role, GRNs assume many of these tasks, depending on the setting in which they work. Good discharge planning is crucial to ensure a smooth transition to the home environment.

CASE STUDY—4.3

A GRN was asked to provide an inservice training session for nursing staff in a large nursing home, emphasizing safe transfer techniques. Acting as a consultant, the GRN developed an inservice session that discussed and demonstrated the use of three basic transfer techniques, as well as how to apply and use a gait belt. The staff was skeptical at first, expressing that they already knew how to move people. Through the GRN's use of humor, involving the group, and discussing ways to transfer the facility's most difficult residents, the staff became more receptive. The GRN was able to have all the participants give a return demonstration of the transfer techniques using a gait belt and teach them what to do if a gait belt was not available. The GRN also surveyed the staff to see whether they actually used gait belts to transfer. Most of the staff said they had never used a gait belt (resulting in their use of improper lifting techniques such as pulling under the resident's arms) but would use one if it were available. One of the charge nurses then volunteered to look for some gait belts and found that each unit had gait belts on the supply cart, but they had not been opened. This same staff nurse then passed gait belts out to the other nurses and urged everyone to start using them. The feedback from the session was that this inservice training had made an immediate positive impact on safety and quality of care for both the staff and the residents.

Many facilities now provide some mechanism of follow-up for these patients after discharge. Sometimes this consists of a telephone call, usually made within a few days, to see whether there are questions that have arisen. Some facilities use volunteers to make telephone calls and obtain satisfaction information without providing any real service to the patient or family. This is inadequate for the type of complex problems these individuals experience. Family members and patients often call the unit from which they were discharged to consult with their nurse (Easton, Rawl, Zemen, Kwiatkowski, & Burczyk, 1995; Rawl, Easton, Zemen, Kwiatkowski, & Burczyk, 1998). Typical questions include topics revolving around medications, equipment, procedures, and the like. So nurses, whether or not they may view themselves as counselors or consultants, may engage in advising or referral activities. Again, this requires that the nurse be informed about community and hospital services such as support groups, transportation availability, home health care services, and the like in order to maintain the patient's link to appropriate resources. Patients and family members may experience increased anxiety not only at discharge but especially several months later, when outpatient therapy and/or home care services may have ceased, and they are left "on their own" for the first time since the crisis occurred.

There are, of course, GRNs who work strictly as consultants. These professionals should have advanced education and additional expertise in the areas of gerontology, rehabilitation, and counseling. Advanced practice nurses (APNs) such as clinical nurse specialists and nurse practitioners are often used as consultants by the rehabilitation team to provide guidance for staff on program development or specific clinical problems. Those units fortunate enough to employ an APN on a regular basis may utilize this individual as a consultant, case manager, educator, researcher, practitioner, or, most commonly, a combination of all of these. Flexibility within the general description of the GRN role is necessary to meet the health care needs of the older adult in today's society (Staab & Hodges, 1996).

Researcher

Very few nurses in the specialty of gerontological rehabilitation have the opportunity to be full-time researchers. Recognition of the need for more nurse scientists in this area is emerging. The federal government, as well as national and local agencies on aging, provides research training grants for those specializing in gerontology. However, there continues to be a lack of qualified health care professionals who engage in research with the elderly population.

There are various levels of involvement in which GRNs may ideally participate in research. The full-time nurse researcher, sometimes called a *nurse scientist*, typically holds a doctoral degree (preferably in nursing) from an accredited university that emphasizes preparation of nurse researchers and advancement of nursing knowledge. The doctorally prepared nurse may act as a consultant to others in setting up research designs, analyzing and interpreting results, acting as primary investigator in studies, and collaborating with members of other disciplines conducting investigations. Knowledge of experimental design and analysis, exposure to various methods of both quantitative and qualitative research, theoretical foundations of nursing, and scholarly writing skills all should be part of the nurse scientist's background.

Nurses prepared at the master's level most typically participate in research at the level of clinical expert. This involves generating ideas for study that are prompted by real problems in the practice setting. The APN is a valuable part of the research team by virtue of his or her advanced clinical skills and knowledge and access to the needs of the patient population. Assessment, data collection, and suggestions of nursing implications will be valuable contributions to the study.

Bachelor's prepared nurses may also assist with data collection and generating ideas for research at their level of expertise and experience. Baccalaureate nurses may participate as members of a team led by an advanced practice nurse, nurse scientist, physician, or other health care professional.

All nurses and nursing staff can provide valuable support to the research team by offering suggestions and critiques and as consumers of nursing research. Often, the most significant questions for inquiry are raised by those who spend the most time at the patient's bedside. It is important to realize that all nurses who practice gerontological rehabilitation nursing need to be educated consumers of scientific research. Current practice and procedures should be supported and guided by sound scientific studies. Nurses should be aware of changes in practice prompted by new, reliable research findings and be prepared to modify care policies and procedures accordingly.

NURSING THEORIES APPLIED TO GERONTOLOGICAL REHABILITATION NURSING

The field of rehabilitation draws on theories from many different disciplines, including biology, psychology, sociology, anthropology, and others. Many of the frameworks and models used in rehabilitation nursing are derived from theories about health and wellness, adaptation, coping, change, family systems, and learning. For the purposes of this text, select nursing theories are discussed.

A nursing theory is one individual's ideas and concepts logically linked together to provide a framework, or blueprint, from which to view practice. All theories are subject to analysis, testing, and criticism and should generate ideas for research. The reader is encouraged to read the original work of the theorists presented here to obtain a clearer picture of each theory's use in their particular setting. Although nursing theory has often come under the scrutiny of other fields, theory development is an important aspect of any science. And while the debate about whether or not nursing is a science continues to rage, nurses have attempted, through the use of scientific inquiry and reasoning, to develop models that support and validate what nurses do as indeed being a science.

Fawcett (1995) identified four metaparadigm concepts of any nursing theory. These are person, health, environment, and nursing. Each theorist differs as to how the interaction between these concepts is viewed. Other theories and conceptual models can be derived from the theories presented here.

Several nursing theories pertain especially well to gerontological rehabilitation nursing. A brief overview of the work of the following nurse theorists will be included: Henderson, Hall, Roy, King, Rogers, and Orem.

Although the emergence of modern nursing theories did not begin until the 1950s, Florence Nightingale, the founder of the profession, wrote enlightening theses that defined the scope and practice of nursing. Her practice was based on hygiene and rehabilitation principles practiced by the ancient Romans (Mumma, 1987). In 1860, Nightingale's *Notes on Nursing* stated that what nursing needed to do was "to put the patient in the best condition for nature to act upon him" (1969, p. 133). This statement captures the essence of all nursing and marked the true beginning of nursing theory.

Virginia Henderson

Virginia Henderson was a pioneer in nursing theory. She delineated the basic principles of nursing care, which included helping patients with functions necessary to maintain life, prevent injury, support individuality and independence, and promote learning. Henderson stated that nursing's unique function is "to assist the individual, sick or well, in the performance of those activities contributing to health or its recovery (or to a peaceful death) that he would perform unaided if he had the necessary strength, will or knowledge. It is likewise her function to help the individual gain independence as rapidly as possible" (Henderson, 1960, p. 41).

Some key principles of gerontological rehabilitation nursing are supported within Henderson's conceptual model. It is humanistic and focuses on the nurse-client relationship. She emphasized the nurse's role in assisting the patient toward independence. Nurses do not impose their will on patients, but rather act almost as a catalyst in helping individuals to achieve their personal health goals.

A key principle of gerontological rehabilitation nursing can be seen in Henderson's definition of nursing. GRNs help patients to care for themselves as they would if they had the capacity to do so. This idea of nursing promotes the patient's autonomy and self-care, both basic goals in rehabilitation of the elderly adult.

Lydia Hall

Hall's theory of nursing was derived from her personal nursing experience. She was able to use her model at the Loeb Center of Montefiore Hospital in New York, where it is still in practice today, on a nurse-directed unit that emphasizes teaching and learning as well as mutuality (the nurse functioning with the patient). Hall's model promotes professionalism, autonomy, and creativity in nursing and provides a practical framework for practice in gerontological rehabilitation nursing.

Hall's model consists of three interlocking circles, each representing some aspect of health care: the *care, core,* and *cure.* Each circle may vary in size or emphasis, depending on the patient's point in the recovery process. The *care* circle represents the nurturing component of nursing. This involves the intimate bodily care, with a goal of patient comfort. According to Hall (1969), the nurse is the expert in care. The *core* circle has a rehabilitative focus, emphasizing the psychological, spiritual, and interpersonal aspects of the person. This circle stresses therapeutic use of self and that the motivation and energy needed for healing are within the patient. The third circle is called the *cure*. This represents the medical aspect of care. It is disease-oriented and involves more of an acute care nursing focus, that is, seeing the patient and family through medical care. The nurse participates in each of these levels of care to some degree, as the patient's condition warrants. Hall believed that although patients came to the hospital for care and cure, they often did not receive as much help with the core difficulties, but that nurses could help in this area through commitment to patient teaching (also considered a phase of medical care).

GRNs more often focus on the core component, because this has a rehabilitative emphasis. However, all three areas described by Hall are seen throughout rehabilitative care of the older adult with various emphases depending on the setting and patient progress. For example, the staff nurse working on a skilled unit in an extended care facility may practice within all three components nearly equally, whereas the nurse on an inpatient rehabilitation unit in the acute care hospital may find care being given largely within the core component. Hall's model is useful in providing flexibility within gerontological rehabilitation nursing practice and is straightforward enough to make it easily applicable to a variety of settings.

Sister Callista Roy

Roy's theory (Roy & Andrews, 1991) provides a holistic conceptual framework for nursing that focuses on the person's adaptation to stress in a constantly changing environment. The patient takes an active role in the adaptive process. The individual's response to stressful stimuli can be either positive (adaptive) or negative (ineffective). The goals of adaptation are survival, growth, reproduction, and mastery (Roy & Andrews, 1991). The goal of nursing is to promote adaptation.

The adaptive system, according to Roy, has two major control components: the cognator and the regulator. Cognator activities are manifested through four cognitive-emotive channels: perceptual/information processing, learning, judgment, and emotions (George,

1985). The regulator subsystem involves automatic physical, chemical, neural, and hormonal responses to internal and external stimuli.

The Roy adaptation model specifies adaptive responses in four interrelated behavioral modes: physiological (bodily responses such as activities of the cells and organs), self-concept (perception of self, such as body image and belief system), role function (place of function in society and relationships to others), and interdependence (feeling of security in relationship to significant others and support systems) (Fawcett, 1995).

Three levels of stimuli (focal, contextual, residual) give input to the person's adaptive system and prompt responses in the four behavioral modes. Focal stimuli are the immediate stressors that confront a person and require an adaptive response. Contextual stimuli, such as social isolation or immobility, contribute to the adaptation level of the individual. Management of contextual stimuli promotes adaptation. Residual factors are those unknown contributors such as historical factors that also influence the individual's response to stressors.

Roy's theory has been widely used and supported by a large body of research. Because adaptation is a primary concept of both the field of gerontological rehabilitation nursing and adaptations theory, it is not surprising that this would be a commonly used framework for nursing practice, although it has been more commonly used in the acute care setting. Roy's model has been used in several studies with elderly groups such as Alzheimer's patients (Thornbury & King, 1992), nursing home patients (Farkas, 1981), rehabilitation patients (Piazza & Foote, 1990), and women (Preston & Dellasega, 1990). The GRN referring to this model can find direction for provision of care through interventions that promote positive adaptive responses and enhance coping skills. Roy's theory certainly warrants more attention with this patient population in the future because of its well-developed perspective on the concept of adaptation.

Imogene King

King's theory of goal attainment focuses on the client as an open system interacting with the environment. King's conceptual framework for nursing is a dynamic interaction system consisting of three open systems: personal, interpersonal, and social (King, 1971).

The personal system consists of individuals. As individuals interact, they form groups, or interpersonal systems. Social systems are groups with special interests that make up communities or society (King, 1981).

The major concepts of King's theory are interrelated in all three systems. Key concepts include perception, self, growth and development, body image, space, and time (personal system); human interactions, communication, transactions, role, and stress (interpersonal system); and organizations, authority, power, status, and decision-making (social system) (King, 1981). According to King, the processes of human interactions involve perception, judgment, and action on the part of both the nurse and the patient. Actions then lead to reaction, interactions, and transactions, resulting in feedback and repetition of the process until mutual goals are attained (King, 1971). These goals, based on shared information between the nurse, client, and family, are developed mutually. King believed that when transactions occurred, goals were attained.

The goal of nursing is to help individuals maintain health so they can function in their roles. The nurse, through assessment, communication, interaction, and subsequent transactions with the patient, influences patient outcomes. Mutual goal setting is a key variable in this theory (King, 1992).

King's theory focuses on the individual's ability to function in social roles as an ultimate outcome. This may not be such an important goal for all elderly people. If social theories such as "disengagement" are true, then some elderly people may even desire to withdraw from previously held social roles. However, if the activity theory of aging holds true, then King's theory would well apply to gerontological rehabilitation nursing. Thus, this model should be used with caution when working with elderly adults in rehabilitation, realizing that aging is highly individualized and that returning to previous social roles may be neither possible nor desirable for some older individuals.

King's theory has not been widely researched for use with older adults or rehabilitation patients. However, because it is not situation-specific, the theory of goal attainment may be more generalizable (George, 1985). Because of its focus on mutual goals, this is a model that could be used in rehabilitation. Certainly the elderly rehabilitation patient is influenced greatly by social and interpersonal systems as well as the environment. Likewise, the rehabilitation process is centered on goal attainment, lending support to the use of King's theory.

Martha Rogers

Rogers' science of unitary human beings represents a major change in perspective from other more traditional nursing theories. This theory is highly abstract, and nurses often shy away from its use in practice. However, Rogers' ideas have merit in geriatric rehabilitation, when considering the significance and integrality of the environment to the person with a disability.

In Rogers' paradigm for nursing, she stated that the person and environment are inseparable (Rogers, 1992). The person is a unitary whole with pandimensional human and environmental energy fields forming a nonlinear domain. Rogers' many unique concepts and definitions emerged as a result of her belief that nursing science required a new way of thinking, a different worldview that went beyond typical systems theory (Rogers, 1992). She emphasized nursing as a learned profession that is both an art and a science. The purpose of nursing "is to promote health and well-being for all persons wherever they are" (Rogers, 1992, p. 28).

According to Rogers, the unifying fundamental unit of all things is the energy field, which has an infinite dynamic nature in continuous motion and is distinguished by a single wave called a pattern. The human field is irreducible, indivisible, nonlinear, and unitary, so that a person cannot be separated into parts and is not simply equal to the sum of those parts. Human beings manifest their energy fields through patterning. Changes in these field patterns are dynamic, unpredictable, and diverse and may manifest themselves through such rhythmical differences as unique sleep patterns and experiences of time passage. Individuals have their own ever-fluctuating patterns and manifestations that are different from others. The environmental field is integral with the human field and is also pandimensional and irreducible. Pandimensionality involves a shared consciousness and is considered a way of perceiving reality.

Rogers defines three principles of homeodynamics: resonancy, helicy, and integrality. Resonancy refers to the continuous change from lower to higher frequency wave patterns that occurs in all energy fields. The principle of helicy implies increasing diversity between human and environmental field patterns, which is continuous and unpredictable. Integrality involves a continuous mutual process between human and environmental fields.

Rogers' theory of nursing allows GRNs to view patients and the caring profession from a different perspective. Although most GRNs subscribe to the notion of holism—that is, treating each aspect of the whole person— Rogers' model goes beyond this. From her viewpoint, there is no separateness in the human experience. The practice and science of nursing should involve the realization that every aspect of the whole is bound up with the others and cannot be distinguished. Rogers' model can be used to help explain confounding outcomes in care of patients with disabilities or those factors that science cannot seem to justify in which individuals defy normal odds of recovery or adaptation. Differences in coping ability or perceived quality of life might be attributed to differences in field patterning.

A few published studies using Rogers' theory have involved the aging population, but demonstration of its usefulness with the general gerontological rehabilitation patient is yet to be seen. Gueldner (1986) studied the relationship between imposed motion and human field motion among elderly persons who lived in nursing homes. Malinski (1991) examined the use of humor in older couples. Rawnsley (1986) found that dying subjects, whether young or old, perceived time as passing more rapidly. Mason (1988) looked at circadian rhythms of body temperature relating to the well-being of older women. The mental health of older adults was considered by Reed (1989) in relation to Rogers' theory. One of the most widely investigated modalities is that of therapeutic touch. Human field motion and effects of light or sound on various outcomes have also been studied. Each of these areas can be a component of rehabilitative gerontic care and thus warrants further research with this specific population.

Dorothea Orem

Dorothea Orem's theories are probably the most widely used of the nursing theories in the area of rehabilitation. From her conceptual model, Orem delineates three theories: nursing, self-care deficit, and self-care. The theory of nursing systems encompasses the other two, and self-care deficit encompasses self-care theory. The major concepts within these three theories are self-care agency, self-care, and therapeutic self-care demand.

Orem includes many definitions in her propositions and assumptions that describe the relationship between and within her theories. Self-care is defined as "the voluntary regulation of one's own human functioning and development that is necessary for individuals to maintain life, health, and well-being" (Orem, 1995, p. 95). This suggests that self-care is the act of caring for oneself. Self-care agency is the ability or capacity of an individual to perform self-care. A self-care agent is a person who does the caring. Self-care deficit occurs when what one can do is less than what needs to be done, and self-care demand is the necessary, needed care (Orem, 1991).

Additionally, Orem identified what she believed were three types of self-care requisites, or "expressions of the purposes that individuals should have when they engage in self-care" (1995, p. 109). These are categorized as either universal, developmental, or health deviation. Universal self-care requisites include air, water, food, elimination, balance of activity and rest, balance of solitude and social interaction, safety, and normalcy.

Developmental self-care requisites relate to the diversity of human development and stages of the life cycle. These include provision of conditions that promote development, the engagement of self in the processes of development, and interferences with development. These may be part of primary or secondary health care.

Health deviations self-care is required when a person is ill, injured, or disabled. These needs refer to changes in human structure (such as edema or amputation), physical functioning (like decreased range of motion), and behavior (such as mood changes or loss of interest in life) (Orem, 1995). This level of care is most often considered tertiary and thus falls within the gerontological rehabilitation nursing scope of practice.

Orem believed in holistic persons interacting with their environment, which can positively or negatively affect the state of health and well-being. Nursing is seen in one of three systems (wholly compensatory, partly compensatory, or supportive-educative) that supplement or act in behalf of care an individual is unable to perform. A wholly compensatory nursing system is needed when the patient is unable to engage in necessary self-care actions. For example, a comatose patient will require the nurse to do total care to meet self-care requisites. Patients who can do some, but not all, of their own care require the nurse to partly compensate for them.

Lastly, in the supportive-educative system, the nurse helps the patient who is usually more physically able to care for himself or herself acquire the knowledge and skills necessary to maintain self-care.

GRNs most often work within the partly compensatory and supportive-educative systems. A combination of these nursing systems would represent typical gerontological rehabilitation care but will vary with the patient population. For example, nurses working in a nursing home setting on an assisted care unit may function as partly compensatory systems and, if the patient's self-care agency decreases, become more of a wholly compensatory system. The nurse on a freestanding rehabilitation hospital unit will aim at moving the patient toward increased self-care and a supportive-educative role for the nurse. Some nurses may believe that self-care agency decreases with age and thus overcompensate for the elderly patients' self-care deficits by doing more for them than they require. This can create an atmosphere that encourages learned helplessness (McDermott, 1993) or an unnecessary dependence on others. Further research is needed to determine the relationship between age and self-care capacity. But, as has been discussed in previous chapters, aging, although universal, is highly individualized, and care must be taken not to overgeneralize or oversimplify the complexities that come with increasing years.

All GRNs should emphasize the importance of self-care. This will become increasingly important as the number of elders in the population rises and the number of available caregivers becomes insufficient to meet the demands. Elders wishing to remain at home and live in the community will need to have a nursing mechanism that teaches self-care and prolonged independence, even in the face of chronic illness and disability. A nursing system for the elderly that allows for fluidity and flexibility to move in and out of supportive-educative and partially compensatory systems of care quickly and easily can promote the independence of older adults within the community setting.

However, the definition of self-care should not be limited to Orem's ideas. Some elderly rehabilitation patients may experience a period of adaptation during which they wish to be cared for. Orem's assumption that adults desire to engage in self-care may not be true in every situation. Elderly persons may feel the need to resign from self-care temporarily (often for their emotional well-being and the inability to adjust to role changes during the aftermath of a crisis), but this choice or decision may represent a form of self-care. In such a case, one would be reminded of Virginia Henderson's belief that nurses do for patients what they would do for themselves if they had the skill, *will*, or knowledge. So self-care may take different forms in unique situations.

SUMMARY

In conclusion, each of the theorists represented in this chapter emphasizes and expounds on different concepts applicable to gerontological rehabilitation nursing. No one theory encompasses the entire spectrum of care nor ideally addresses every situation or individual. But nursing theories, as well as

Table 4–3 RELATED PRINCIPLES OF GERONTOLOGICAL REHABILITATION NURSING AND THEORIES OF NURSING

Theorist	Theory	Related Gerontological Rehabilitation Nursing Principle
Hall	Philosophy of nursing	Nurses work with patients. Energy and motivation for healing are within the patient.
Henderson	Humanistic nursing	Nurses promote health, independence, and patient goals.
King	Goal attainment	Mutual goal setting is essential for quality patient outcomes.
Roy	Adaptation	Rehabilitation promotes effective responses and positive adaptation.
Rogers	Science of unitary human beings	Individuals are highly unique and integrally related to the environment.
Orem	Self-care deficit	Patient independence and self-care are primary goals of rehabilitation.

theories from related disciplines, can provide useful matrices from which to practice. Each different nursing model presents a unique viewpoint with respect to beliefs about the metaparadigm concepts of person, nursing, health, and environment. Table 4–3 displays a summary of the nursing theorists discussed in this chapter and concepts relating to gerontological rehabilitation nursing practice.

REFERENCES

Association of Rehabilitation Nurses. (1995). *The gerontological rehabilitation nurse: Role description* [Brochure]. Skokie, IL: Author.

Bandman, E. L., & Bandman, B. (1995). *Nursing ethics through the life span.* Norwalk, CT: Appleton & Lange.

Easton, K., Rawl, S., Zemen, D., Kwiatkowski, S., & Burczyk, B. (1995). The effects of nursing follow-up on the coping strategies used by rehabilitation patients after discharge. *Rehabilitation Nursing Research, 4*(4), 119–127.

Eliopoulos, C. (1997). *Gerontological nursing* (4th ed.). Philadelphia: J. B. Lippincott.

Farkas, L. (1981). Adaptation problems with nursing home application for elderly persons: An application of the Roy adaptation nursing model. *Journal of Advanced Nursing, 8,* 363–368.

Fawcett, J. (1995). *Analysis and evaluation of conceptual models of nursing* (3rd ed.). Philadelphia: F. A. Davis.

George, J. B. (Ed.). (1985). *Nursing theories: The base for professional nursing practice* (2nd ed.). Engelwood Cliffs, NJ: Prentice-Hall.

Gueldner, S. H. (1986). The relationship between imposed motion and human field motion in elderly individuals living in nursing homes. In V. M. Malinski (Ed.), *Explorations on Martha Rogers' science of unitary human beings* (pp. 161–171). Norwalk, CT: Appleton-Century-Crofts.

Hall, L. E. (1969). The Loeb Center for Nursing and Rehabilitation, Montefiore Hospital and Medical Center, Bronx, New York. *International Journal of Nursing Studies, 6*(2), 81–97.

Henderson, V. (1960). *Basic principles of nursing care.* London: ICN House.

King, I. M. (1971). *Toward a theory for nursing: General concepts of human behavior.* New York: John Wiley & Sons.

King, I. M. (1981). *A theory for nursing: Systems, concepts, process.* New York: John Wiley & Sons. (Reissued 1990, Albany, NY: Delmar)

King, I. M. (1992). King's theory of goal attainment. *Nursing Science Quarterly, 5*(1), 19–25.

Malinski, V. M. (1991). The experience of laughing at oneself in older couples. *Nursing Science Quarterly, 4,* 69–75.

Mason, D. J. (1988). Circadian rhythms of body temperature and activation and the well-being of older women. *Nursing Research, 37,* 276–281.

McDermott, M. A. N. (1993). Learned helplessness as an interacting variable with self-care agency: Testing a theoretical model. *Nursing Science Quarterly, 6*(1), 28–38.

Mumma, C. M. (1987). *Rehabilitation nursing: Concepts and practice* (2nd ed.). Evanston, IL: Rehabilitation Nursing Foundation.

Nightingale, F. (1969). *Notes on nursing.* New York: Dover. (Original work published 1860)

Orem, D. (1991). *Nursing: Concepts of practice.* St. Louis, MO: Mosby.

Orem, D. (1995). *Nursing: Concepts of practice.* St. Louis, MO: Mosby.

Piazza, D., & Foote, A. (1990). Roy's adaptation model: A guide for rehabilitation nursing practice. *Rehabilitation Nursing, 15,* 254–259.

Preston, D. B., & Dellasega, C. (1990). Elderly women and stress. Does marriage make a difference? *Journal of Gerontological Nursing, 16,* 26–32.

Rawl, S., Easton, K., Zemen, D., Kwiatkowski, S., & Burczyk, B. (1998). The effectiveness of a nurse-managed follow-up program for rehabilitation patients after discharge. *Rehabilitation Nursing, 23*(4), 204–209.

Rawnsley, M. M. (1986). The relationship between the perception of the speed of time and the process of dying. In V. M. Malinski (Ed.), *Explorations on Martha Rogers' science of unitary human beings* (pp. 79–93). Norwalk, CT: Appleton-Century-Crofts.

Reed, P. G. (1989). Mental health of older adults. *Western Journal of Nursing Research, 11,* 143–163.

Rogers, M. (1992). Nursing science and the space age. *Nursing Science Quarterly, 6*(2), 56–58.

Roy, C., & Andrews, H. A. (1991). *The Roy adaptation model: The definitive statement.* Norwalk, CT: Appleton & Lange.

Staab, A. S., & Hodges, L. C. (1996). *Essentials of gerontological nursing: Adaptation to the aging process.* Philadelphia: J. B. Lippincott.

Thornbury, J. M., & King, L. D. (1992). The Roy adaptation model and care of persons with Alzheimer's disease. *Nursing Science Quarterly, 5*(3), 129–133.

Part II

Promoting Wellness and Self-Care

■

Chapter 5

Improving Nutritional Status

■

COMPONENTS OF NUTRITIONAL ASSESSMENT

There are many factors to consider when assessing the nutritional status of any patient. Although there are many published studies on nutrition and the elderly, little research has been done on the nutritional status of elderly patients participating in rehabilitation. These individuals have unique needs and nutritional requirements, both from the standpoint of adaptation to a disease process as well as the extra nutrients needed for maintaining high levels of energy to support physical therapy and healing. Additionally, many rehabilitation patients experience dysphagia, "a disorder of the oropharyngeal or esophageal swallowing mechanism" (Lugger, 1994, p. 79). Considering age-associated changes in swallowing, elderly rehabilitation patients are particularly at risk for complications such as aspiration pneumonia or malnutrition.

For the older rehabilitation patient, some components are more significant than others. Assessment criteria may differ somewhat from those for middle-aged adults because of normal aging changes. Gerontological rehabilitation nurses (GRNs) working with elders in the community may be called on to rely on their own clinical expertise instead of laboratory results or diagnostic tests to initially detect a potential problem and report it to the physician so that further confirmation can be obtained.

A study by Sullivan and Walls (1994) sought to confirm results from Sullivan's previous studies, which showed a "strong independent correlation between the severity of protein energy undernutrition and the risk of subsequent morbidity in a population of elderly rehabilitation patients" (p. 471). The sample consisted of 350 randomly selected patients in a veterans hospital, with an average age of 76 years. The researchers, using logistic regression analysis, demonstrated that nine variables (out of 96 in the initial study) provided an overall predictive accuracy of 71%. In prioritized order those were the Katz Index of activities of daily living (ADLs) score, serum albumin, usual weight percentage, number of prescription medications, presence of renal disease, individual income, presence of decubitus, dysphagia, and mid-arm circumference. Additionally, the researchers suggested that protein energy nutritional deficits and functional disability had a cumulative effect on outcomes. Although the study had significant limitations in that the sample was 99% male and 75% white, the results provide interesting data.

Several of the variables used to predict morbidity are discussed in this chapter and throughout the text. Issues of particular importance to gerontological rehabilitation nursing assessment and interventions are discussed in this section.

Laboratory Values

Laboratory values that may be measured include complete blood count, hemoglobin, hematocrit, albumin, glucose, triglycerides, phosphorus, calcium, protein, cholesterol, and nitrogen balance. Urinalysis and stool tested for occult blood can provide additional information. Although it is possible to obtain such a profile in the acute care setting, this may be neither practical nor cost-effective for the long-term care patient.

Dietitians often rely on the albumin level as the most reliable single laboratory source to screen an individual's overall nutritional status. Albumin is a major serum protein formed mainly by the liver. It is responsible for maintaining plasma pressure and the normal balance of water within the body as well as aiding in the transport of drugs, dyes, and fatty acids (Nursing91 Books, 1991). Inadequate nutrition causes inhibition of the formation of plasma proteins, including albumin, which in turn can lead to edema and a weakened defense against infection. Serum albumin levels can provide a relatively inexpensive general picture of nutritional status for the older adult. Normal serum albumin levels are 3.2 to 4.5 g/dl. Sources vary as to suggestions for when nutritional interventions should be initiated based on serum albumin or what constitutes a deficiency. Recommendations range from less than 2.5 g/dl (Burns & Jairath, 1994) to 3.5 g/dl (Cope, 1994). Most physicians consider an albumin level of less than 3 g/dl in an older person to be deficient. This is referred to as hypoalbuminemic malnutrition (Lipschitz, 1995).

Several studies have confirmed the use of serum albumin to predict morbidity and mortality among older rehabilitation patients (Aptaker, Roth, Reichhardt, Duerden, & Levy, 1994; Sullivan, 1995; Sullivan & Walls, 1994; Sullivan, Walls, & Bopp, 1995). Aptaker et al. (1994) studied serum albumin level as a predictor of outcomes in geriatric rehabilitation patients with stroke. The results of their research demonstrated a relationship between medical complication rates and functional outcome in elderly stroke patients. Those with higher serum albumin levels (greater than or equal to 3.5 g/dl) experienced fewer medical complications than those with lower levels. Serum albumin is also considered a good predictor of hospital outcomes in the gerontological rehabilitation patient.

Weight

Another usual and relatively simple measurement of nutritional status is an individual's weight. It should be noted that weight should always be assessed in relation to height. Many frail elderly, particularly those who are hospitalized or suffering from chronic disease, experience an alteration in nutrition and subsequent weight loss. Even the older adult living in the community in relative independence is at risk for poor nutrition, in particular those who live alone and have lower income and educational levels.

Researchers have suggested that weight loss is a major predictor of morbidity and mortality for the elderly. So, although obesity is also a common problem among the elderly, physicians recommend a cautious and individualized approach to weight loss for elders. For those older than 70, it is indicated only for a medical condition that could be significantly improved by prudent dieting, such as obese individuals with hypertension, severe back pain, diabetes, or degenerative joint disease (Lipschitz, 1995). Keller stated that "a weight increase of at least 5% of body weight in previously undernourished patients is associated with a decreased incidence of death and may reduce morbidity events" (1995, p. 165). Accurate weights are thus essential in tracking the health status of older adults.

The exercise and activity associated with rehabilitation tend to promote appetite. An older person involved in intensive physical therapy will likely not need to be placed on a weight reduction diet unless obesity interferes with the person's ability to participate in such activities. The GRN should monitor the person's weight and work with the dietitian to make sure that excess weight loss does not occur and that adequate caloric intake is present to balance the increase in energy expenditure.

In the case of the gerontological rehabilitation patient, obtaining an accurate weight may be difficult. Many patients are unable to stand on a traditional scale without assistance because of hemiplegia, generalized weakness, or poor balance. This poses a particular problem for nurses working in the community.

For those individuals residing in a health care facility, there are a few options available. Earlier model chair scales still posed a problem because many older patients had trouble stepping up onto the chair and/or maintaining a sitting position. The emergence of the modern-day wheelchair scale (Fig. 5–1) has made accurate weighing possible for most patients. The wheelchair is weighed alone on the scale and its weight recorded on the bottom of the chair or in another secure, accessible place. The person can be rolled in the wheelchair directly onto the scale, which will provide a digital readout in kilograms or pounds. The patient can thus be weighed sitting in the wheelchair and the weight of the chair subtracted to provide a reliable measure of the individual's weight. This scale can of course provide weights for those who can

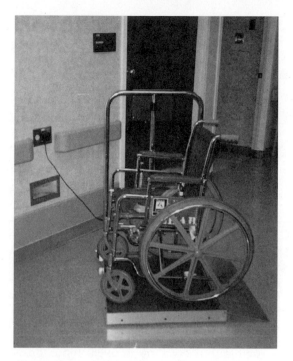

Figure 5–1   Modern wheelchair scale.

stand and has a ramp for those with difficulty negotiating steps.

An additional problem with weight as a comparative measure is that many older individuals who come to the rehabilitation setting do so because of functional limitations. It may have been quite some time since an accurate weight was obtained, because most acute care units do not have wheelchair scales and the patient was not likely up and about. The nurse should inquire from the transferring unit or facility whether and how the last weight was obtained. Some facilities have a type of Hoyer lift, which can be used to weigh the bed-bound patient.

Caution should be used when ascertaining baseline weight data from the patient or family. This information may not be accurate because of the length of time that may have passed between weighings or unreliable memories of the patient or caregiver. Thus, it is important to obtain an initial weight on admission to the rehabilitation unit or long-term care facility whenever possible to establish accurate baseline data.

History

A thorough nutritional history should include assessing past and current eating patterns, influence of cultural or religious practices or beliefs, and other psychosocial factors. Family members and caregivers can provide informa-

tion as to which foods the person seems to swallow more easily or whether some consistencies make the person cough.

The GRN should also determine what medications the person has been taking and whether alcohol is used regularly, as well as how much. Both medications and alcohol use can adversely affect appetite as well as ability to swallow or self-feed (Case Study 5.1). It is particularly important in achieving the goal of improving nutritional status in those without swallowing difficulties to ask the patient's food preferences and also to determine whether or not a special diet was followed prior to admission. The nurse should be constantly alert to those older adults who have been instructed by their physician to maintain a specific calorie diabetic diet but who do not consider themselves diabetic. These individuals may have been placed on a restricted diet to control blood sugar (yet take no medications for it) or to control weight. Many adults on special diets prior to admission may require reminders or additional teaching for dietary modifications while in rehabilitation. This is an opportunity for the nurse to reinforce appropriate eating habits and also to make referrals to the dietitian for those who desire or require additional education.

CASE STUDY 5.1

Mrs. Norris, a patient with myasthenia gravis, was noted to have a poor oral intake at breakfast each morning as a result of swallowing difficulties. The student nurse caring for Mrs. Norris also noted that she did not participate as well during her 8:30 A.M. physical therapy session as she did later in the day. On examination of her medication schedule, it was found that Mrs. Norris' Mestinon dose was being given at 8:00 A.M. but had a 30- to 60-minute onset of action period. The nursing instructor and the student acted as patient advocates by speaking with the physician to change the medication times, contacting the dietitian to have breakfast delivered a little later, and working with the physical and occupational therapists to reschedule therapy times for when Mrs. Norris would be feeling the maximum therapeutic effects of the Mestinon. Mrs. Norris' schedule was also modified to allow for alternate rest and therapy periods. Finally, the speech therapist was consulted for a swallowing evaluation.

CASE STUDY 5.2

Mrs. Smith was a 67 year old obese woman admitted to the inpatient rehabilitation unit of an acute care hospital after a right below-knee amputation secondary to severe peripheral vascular disease and diabetes. She also had a history of heart disease, hypertension, and anxiety.

When the nurse interviewed her about her knowledge regarding insulin injection related to her diabetes, Mrs. Smith stated that she had been a diabetic and had given her own insulin for over 10 years. After further discussion, the nurse seemed satisfied that Mrs. Smith had a solid basic knowledge about her disease process. However, later that day, Mrs. Smith remarked, "You know, the meals here are so good that I stay full all the time even though I'm on an 1800-calorie ADA diet. I must admit I haven't followed my diet at home like I should. I kind of forgot a lot of the things they taught us in the diabetic classes, but I would like to learn how to prepare my food better, like they do here. My daughter is coming to help me. Do you think someone could teach both of us?"

This presented a perfect opportunity for the GRN to further discuss Mrs. Smith's eating habits and nutritional requirements and to provide her with some written material to guide her at home. Additionally, the nurse arranged for the dietitian to spend some private teaching time with Mrs. Smith and her daughter before discharge. Mrs. Smith returned home shortly thereafter, not only rehabilitated after her amputation, but with new knowledge and increased motivation to maintain an appropriate diet, which could prevent further health problems.

Case Study 5.2 presents an example of the importance of being alert to the patient's knowledge level and future nutritional needs after discharge throughout the rehabilitative phase. Although patients are on a special diet while in the nurse's care, it should not be assumed that they have the needed knowledge, ability, or will to follow through with this after discharge. The GRN should continually be mindful of opportunities to incorporate primary prevention techniques and teaching with regard to nutrition in addition to tertiary prevention.

Physical Structures and Function

A usual physical assessment of the patient with regard to nutritional status would include inspection of the oral cavity, head, and neck, observing for facial symmetry, lip closure, gag reflex, and swallowing ability. The GRN should also assess voice quality, level of alertness, cranial nerve function (see later section), and the person's functional ability to feed himself or herself.

With regard to the oral cavity, it should be remembered that older persons often experience weight loss during a period of chronic illness or acute hospitalization. Weight loss is also reflected in a person's gums, so those who wear dentures may find them ill-fitting and uncomfortable. This poses a particular problem for the aged individual living in a long-term care facility or the community. The resident may inform nurses that his or her dentures no longer fit properly and that it causes pain to wear them. If an elderly patient is unable to chew a more usual food consistency, the staff or resident may select a pureed diet. This can result in further weight loss and nutritional deficiency because the resident finds it less appealing than his or her previous diet. Nurses should be aware that once an individual's weight has stabilized after a change in health status, a professional evaluation of the patient's dentures, if they appear to fit improperly or cause pain or soreness, would be indicated. Although a new pair of dentures may be costly, the long-term benefit to the patient's nutritional and overall health must be considered.

Older patients with neurological deficits resulting from such conditions as brain injury, stroke, Parkinson's disease (PD), myasthenia gravis (MG), multiple sclerosis (MS), or amyotrophic lateral sclerosis (ALS) may experience swallowing difficulties (Table 5–1). This may be due to a variety of factors. Several such conditions may involve poor head control and lip closure, making positioning of the food for swallowing difficult. Patients with hemiplegia or hemiparesis may be unable to maneuver the food bolus to the back of the pharynx and may pocket food, having decreased sensation and motor movement on one side. Differences may also be seen in the patterns and types of swallowing difficulties depending on location of the lesion in the brain (Robbins, Levine, Maser, Rosenbek, & Kempster, 1993).

Additionally, normal aging processes can contribute to swallowing problems in the

Table 5–1 NURSING DIAGNOSES AND COMMON ASSOCIATED DISEASES/DISORDERS OF REHABILITATION CLIENTS

Alteration in nutrition: less than body requirements
    Renal disease
    Stroke
    Diabetes
    Frailty (older than 85 years)
    Functional limitations
    Cognitive impairments

Alteration in nutrition: more than body requirements
    Obesity
    Heart disease
    Diabetes

Impaired swallowing
    Stroke
    Parkinson's disease
    Multiple sclerosis
    Amyotrophic lateral sclerosis
    Myasthenia gravis
    Guillain-Barré syndrome
    Post-polio syndrome
    Traumatic brain injury or brain tumor
    Patients who are fatigued

Knowledge deficit
    Any disease process, depending on patient and caregiver

Potential for fluid volume deficit
    Patients with impaired swallowing
    Frail elderly

neurologically impaired adult. A decrease in saliva makes forming the food bolus less efficient. Likewise, pharyngeal and esophageal peristalsis may be slower, causing even healthy elderly adults to sometimes complain that food feels as though it is "stuck" in their throat.

The absence of the gag reflex may indicate a potential swallowing problem. However, this is not a reliable assessment tool by itself. The gag reflex, although closely associated with swallowing, is separate and distinct from the swallowing reflex. The absence of one does not necessarily indicate the absence of the other, nor the presence of one, the presence of the other. For example, the 80 year old man with a diagnosis of right-sided stroke may lack a gag reflex on examination, but this does not necessarily mean that the barium swallow will show aspiration.

Swallowing Ability

Swallowing is a complex process. Although food preparation, selection, and anticipation certainly play an important role in eating and swallowing, this discussion focuses on deglutition, or the process of eating and swallowing. There are five phases involved in the swallow.

1. *Oral preparatory:* Food is voluntarily manipulated in the mouth. Lip closure and lateral tongue and jaw movement are needed to chew and form a food bolus.
2. *Oral (or lingual):* The bolus of food is voluntarily manipulated and directed posteriorly toward the oropharynx.
3. *Triggering pharyngeal:* The point at which the swallow reflex is triggered. This should occur in about 1 second.
4. *Pharyngeal:* Bolus is carried via the swallow through the pharynx. The reflex is initiated voluntarily, but the process is completed reflexively. The epiglottis protects food from entering the airway, and pharyngeal peristalsis moves the bolus into the esophagus.
5. *Esophageal:* Peristalsis carries the food to the stomach.

Aspiration can occur anytime before, during, or after the swallow. It is imperative that GRNs be able to recognize the signs and symptoms of aspiration (Table 5–2) in the older rehabilitation patient. Signs of aspiration in an elderly adult may be less obvious than in a younger person. The GRN should be particularly alert to a patient with a moist-sounding voice, one who clears the throat often after consuming food or drink, and those more frail elders who seem to require multiple swallowing to ingest even small amounts of liquids. The fatigue level of an older person can also contribute to difficulties, because the muscles used in speech and swallowing also become tired by the end of the day. The GRN should especially note those patients whose speech becomes more slurred as the day progresses.

Table 5–2 SIGNS AND SYMPTOMS OF SWALLOWING DYSFUNCTION

Coughing
Eyes watering
Asthma attacks
Choking
Gurgling or moist-sounding voice after eating or drinking
Breathing difficulties
Multiple swallowing
Clearing throat

Some elderly persons exhibit few to no signs of choking although material is entering the airway. This is often referred to as "silent" aspiration and poses a unique challenge for health care professionals. Noting the quality of the voice and whether or not any expressive aphasia or dysphasia is present may alert the nurse to potential swallowing problems, because the muscles used for speech and swallowing are closely associated. Early identification and treatment of dysphagia can prevent serious complications such as aspiration pneumonia or even death from choking.

Diagnostic Tests

The best and most efficient way to determine swallowing ability and difficulties in the older rehabilitation client is through a barium or modified barium swallow. Barium swallows are done by a radiologist, sometimes with the speech therapist in attendance. The patient is given various consistencies of food mixed with barium, such as applesauce, thin or thick liquids, or a cookie (thus the common term *cookie swallow*). A modified barium swallow would require the use of a smaller amount of liquid, paste, or other material for those in whom aspiration is suspected. The act of swallowing is observed via fluoroscopy and recorded on videotape so that it can be replayed and watched in slow motion later. This diagnostic test measures the efficiency of the swallow, allowing the physician and therapist to see areas of aspiration. From the results of this test, the speech therapist can determine an appropriate diet and fluid consistency modification for the patient as well as set up a swallowing protocol to prevent aspiration. Barium swallows may be repeated after a period of speech therapy when the therapist feels that enough progress has been made in strengthening or retraining the swallowing muscles to indicate a possible advance in the diet.

Level of Alertness

Arousal and attention are important factors to consider when assisting the patient with swallowing problems. Trying to feed a patient who is only partially awake, or insufficiently alert to eat, is unsafe. This is particularly important for the older patient who may have experienced a head injury resulting in variable neurological arousal states. Distractions may cause emotional upset, and the patient may need to be assisted to focus on the task at hand without interruptions. Increased time may be necessary to assist the patient with feeding.

Safety and supervision are other factors to consider. Some patients are unaware of their swallowing problem, or choose to ignore it. This may result in unsafe eating habits such as gulping thin liquids when thickener is needed or eating rice or peas on a mechanical soft diet. Many facilities group residents with special swallowing protocols at a certain table in the dining room so they may be more closely supervised by a staff member who can provide verbal cues or assistance during meals. Proper assessment of the patient with unsafe behavioral practices or neurological impairments can help prevent aspiration.

Functional Ability

Many patients with neurological impairments also need functional assistance with eating. The nurse should ascertain the patient's ability to view the food, open containers, unwrap foods, pour milk, grasp utensils, and the like. Changes often occurring with aging, such as arthritis, can compound the person's existing medical problems, making these tasks more difficult. The presence of an intravenous line in a hemiplegic patient's unaffected arm may inhibit the ability to self-feed. Tremors in the resident with Parkinson's syndrome may make drinking hot liquids unassisted a hazard. Although every effort should be made to encourage patients to feed themselves, the nurse must assess a variety of factors to promote success as well as safety.

Nurses should also realize that various assistive devices may be available or developed, based on the person's unique needs, to promote self-feeding. Many acute rehabilitation facilities have equipment for the tetraplegic person to perform self-feeding using ball bearings and gravity to help raise and lower food to the patient's mouth. Occupational therapists and clinical engineers are continually devising unique systems to assist patients in maintaining the capability of feeding themselves. Through the use of adaptive spoons, plates, magnetic holders, dishes, and the like, even patients with severe chronic injuries can perform this activity. Patients report this to be preferable than being fed by a caregiver, despite the extra time needed for meals (Yuen, 1993).

Cranial Nerves

There are six cranial nerves involved in eating and swallowing: trigeminal (V), facial (VII), glossopharyngeal (IX), vagus (X), spinal accessory (XI), and hypoglossal (XII). Assessment of these during the admission physical examination can alert the GRN to potential swallowing problems.

The trigeminal cranial nerve is tested by instructing patients to clench their teeth and observing for temporal, facial, and jaw symmetry and strength. These functions would be related to the motor ability to chew and manipulate food in the mouth. The facial nerve (VII) can be tested by asking persons to smile and show their teeth, raise the eyebrows, or wrinkle the forehead, while the nurse observes for symmetry.

The glossopharyngeal and vagus nerve functions are tested together. The patient is asked to open the mouth and say "ah." The uvula is observed for any deviation from midline. The quality of the voice is noted, as well as the patient's ability to swallow. The gag reflex is also tested. Cranial nerve IX controls secretion of saliva, the movement of swallowing, taste on the posterior third of the tongue, and reflexes such as breathing and blood pressure. The vagus nerve controls both motor and sensory functions for the heart, digestive organs, and larynx.

The spinal accessory cranial nerve involves the movement of the head, shoulders, and voice-producing parts of the larynx. It is tested by asking persons to shrug their shoulders and to turn their head against the nurse's hand, thus assessing sternocleidomastoid muscle strength. Patients with impairment of the pharyngeal and laryngeal structures may experience a delayed swallowing and/or aspiration from inadequate protection of the airway (Price & DiIorio, 1990). Patients with these difficulties may include those with ALS, MS, PD, and various types of head injury (stroke, aneurysm, trauma).

Lastly, the hypoglossal cranial nerve, which controls tongue movements, is also important in food manipulation. Assessment includes noting the quality of the patient's speech and tongue control. Parkinson's patients may experience rigidity in the tongue muscle as with other muscles, which can make the formation and manipulation of the food bolus difficult. With hemiplegic patients, the tongue may deviate toward the paralyzed side. The tongue is considered one of the strongest muscles in the human body. Yet with disease processes, it may be affected like other muscles. Patients with a weakened tongue muscle may include those with ALS, MG, stroke, or head injury (DiIorio & Price, 1990; Price & DiIorio, 1990).

Other Assessment Criteria

Other components of a thorough nutritional assessment may include measuring triceps skinfold and performing a calorie count. The triceps skinfold is a less reliable test in older people because of the redistribution of adipose tissue that occurs as a normal part of aging. Calorie counts may be inaccurate if they are based on reporting by the patient or caregiver, whose methods of measurement and recording information may vary. Calorie counts done within the hospital setting provide more dependable information, because the amounts and types of food taken by the patient are carefully recorded by health professionals and then the calories are computed by the dietitian.

The impact of culture, ethnicity, and religious beliefs must also be assessed. Many societies associate health and wellness with the ability and desire to eat. The role that food plays is of particular importance when assessing patients who require tube feedings. The values and beliefs of the family and community likewise play a part in the patient's feeling of acceptance or rejection when parenteral feeding methods are involved.

In the case of stroke patients with dysphagia, the location and nature of the lesion may be significant in assessment of swallowing ability. A study by Robbins et al. (1993) suggested that patients with left hemisphere stroke tended to have fewer problems with swallowing than those with right-sided stroke. Although they may experience apraxia with swallowing or difficulty with manipulating food in the oral phase, these patients may require no direct swallowing treatment. They appear to eat well spontaneously yet can have an abnormal videofluoroscopy result, showing an increased length of time for the bolus to travel through the pharynx, which is believed by researchers to occur because of the apraxia (Robbins et al., 1993). Patients with right hemispheric stroke tend to experience longer pharyngeal stages and longer swallowing times (Robbins et al., 1993). This puts them at increased risk for aspiration and subsequent pneumonia. These patients may not demonstrate a strong cough or usual audible signs of aspiration.

It should be noted here that these findings may not be consistent with some clinical beliefs. That is, the person with right hemispheric stroke and left-sided weakness is often thought of as having fewer problems with swallowing than the right hemiplegic patient, who often has aphasia and obvious difficulty with weakened speech muscles. This is an area in which further research is needed. Additionally, those with right unilateral stroke and anterior unilateral stroke may have more significant swallowing problems than those with left or posterior strokes. However, Robbins' study emphasizes the importance of paying particular attention to the potential of problems with apraxia, delayed swallowing, pharyngeal emptying, and decreased peristalsis of the bolus in persons with stroke.

Many tools for nutritional screening are available to nurses. One such aid is the Nutritional Health Checklist, a self-administered test that can also be used for educational purposes or screening. This tool lists the warning signs of poor nutritional health using the acronym DETERMINE: disease, eating poorly, tooth loss/mouth pain, economic hardship, reduced social contact, multiple medicines, involuntary weight loss/gain, needs assistance in self-care, elder years (older than age 80) (Cope, 1994). Using this as a reference, it is not difficult to see that the majority of elderly rehabilitation patients are at moderate to high nutritional risk. Primary prevention must be practiced to ensure optimal outcomes.

Nursing diagnoses are made as a natural part of assessment. The GRN should look at all subjective and objective data to formulate diagnoses. These will then guide planning and interventions.

GOALS

One overriding principle and goal in promoting nutrition for elderly persons with chronic health alterations is to make the eating and swallowing process as close to "normal" as possible while providing adequate nutrition and preventing aspiration. Nursing interventions will thus be aimed at assisting the patient to regain normal eating and swallowing abilities, and until this is possible, to provide adequate nutrition without compromising the airway. This may cause a number of important modifications to be added to one's daily routine.

In the case of tube feedings, appropriate positioning of the patient, as well as the administration of water in addition to the nutritional supplement ordered, would be indicated. "The goal of enteral hyperalimentation is to maintain ideal weight while minimizing muscle mass loss and assuring adequate hydration" (Lipschitz, 1995). Further interventions related to tube feedings are discussed later in this chapter.

A great deal of patient and family teaching may be required to meet the nutritional goals. Thus, another goal related to nutritional status is increased knowledge of the caregiver in this area. In addition to education about diet, nutritional needs, signs of aspiration, use of adaptive equipment, and swallowing techniques prescribed by the speech therapist, the nurse should be prepared to teach clients about tube feedings and medication administration through the tube if needed. The prospect of having to perform tube feedings may cause the caregiver anxiety, and multiple structured learning sessions may be necessary for the family whose loved one is returning home with a tube in place.

Another goal related to nutritional status is to develop functional skills to enhance the older adult's abilities to meet nutritional needs through self-care activities. This is done in a variety of ways, including promoting physical exercises and activities and by working with the occupational and speech therapists to see that appropriate adaptive equipment is used as needed. Upper extremity exercises are particularly important for self-feeding and should be included as part of ADLs in rehabilitation.

NURSING INTERVENTIONS FOR IMPROVING NUTRITION AND MANAGING DYSPHAGIA

As previously stated, nursing interventions center around providing the patient with adequate nutrition and hydration as well as promoting as close to normal process of eating and swallowing as is safely possible. It is expected that with speech therapy the patient will progress and may experience different levels of swallowing ability during adaptation after a health-altering crisis. Special dysphagic diets, such as those in Table 5–3, may be indicated to prevent aspiration. Patient and family teaching about dietary restrictions, as well as healthy eating patterns, is part of a comprehensive teaching program (Table 5–4).

The role of the interdisciplinary team in the care of the patient with dysphagia is crucial (Emick-Herring & Wood, 1990). All staff members in the rehabilitation setting, as well as the family, should be aware of the specific swallowing protocol set up by the speech

Table 5–3   EXAMPLES OF SPECIAL DIETS FOR PATIENTS WITH DYSPHAGIA

Food	Preparation/Consistency Requirements and Examples
Pureed Diet	
Breads	No breads or crackers.
Cereals	Cooked, refined cereals such as strained oatmeal, Cream of Rice, and Cream of Wheat. No cereals with nuts, fruit, or raisins. No ready-to-eat cereals.
Vegetables	All must be pureed. No vegetables with skin, strings, or seeds (such as string beans and cucumbers).
Fruits	All pureed or applesauce. No fruits with seeds or skins (such as fresh apples or oranges).
Meats	Pureed meats and poultry or macaroni and cheese. No whole or ground meats of any kind.
Eggs	Only eggnog if allowed by speech therapist. No other preparations of eggs (such as scrambled, fried, or boiled).
Soups	Creamed, strained, or thickened soups if approved by speech therapist. No soup with chunks or pieces of vegetables, meats, or potatoes.
Potatoes	Whipped only. No pasta, rice, or other types of potatoes or potato preparations.
Dairy	Ice cream, sherbet, plain yogurt, cream cheese spread, and smooth cheese sauces. No ice cream with fruit pieces, nuts, or other chunks. No yogurt with fruit. No cottage cheese.
Desserts	Pudding, custard, whipped cream, and other pureed desserts without pieces. Honey and sugar. No gelatin, tapioca, rice puddings, bread puddings, or coconut. No hard candy, cakes, pies, gumdrops, or any other candy pieces.
Beverages	As instructed by speech therapist.

Rule of thumb for pureed diet: All foods must be smooth and free of lumps or pieces. No foods allowed that contain chunks, pieces, seeds, skins, or strings. Consistency of liquids determined on an individual basis by speech therapist. Liquids are more often aspirated than semi-solids.

Food	Preparation/Consistency Requirements and Examples
Mechanical Soft Diet	
Breads	No breads or crackers.
Cereals	Cooked refined cereals such as strained oatmeal, Cream of Rice, and Cream of Wheat. No cereals with nuts, fruit, or raisins. No ready-to-eat cereals.
Vegetables	Vegetables should be canned or well cooked and chopped (beets, carrots, squash, and spinach). No tough vegetables with skin or seeds. No raw, dried, or fibrous vegetables (such as peas, beans, broccoli, or asparagus).
Fruits	Canned or well-cooked fruit (such as pears, peaches, apricots, cranberry sauce, and pureed fruits). Ripe, mashed bananas, nectar. No fruits with seeds or skins (such as fresh apples or oranges).
Meats	Thoroughly ground, soft meats and poultry or macaroni and cheese.
Eggs	Only eggnog, or egg salad, if allowed by speech therapist. No other preparations of eggs (such as scrambled, fried, or boiled).
Soups	Creamed, strained, or thickened soups if approved by speech therapist. No soup with chunks or pieces of vegetables, meats, or potatoes.
Potatoes	Mashed, boiled, or creamed. Soft noodles such as spaghetti. No rice or potato skins.
Dairy	Ice cream, thick milk shakes, sherbet, smooth yogurt, cream cheese spread, smooth cheese sauces, and cottage cheese. No ice cream with fruit pieces, nuts, or other chunks.
Desserts	Pudding, custard, whipped cream, and other desserts without pieces. No hard candy, cakes, pies, gumdrops, or any other candy pieces.
Beverages	As instructed by speech therapist.

Rule of thumb for dysphagic mechanical soft diet: This diet is a slight upgrade from the pureed diet. More food choices are allowed, but all foods must be free of pieces that could be aspirated. No foods allowed that contain seeds or skins. Consistency of liquids determined on an individual basis by speech therapist.

Table 5–4 CLIENT/CAREGIVER TEACHING: SUBSTITUTING FOODS LOWER IN FAT AND CHOLESTEROL

Avoid	Substitute
Organ meats	Lean meats, skinless chicken, and turkey; tuna fish packed in water; fresh and frozen fish (not breaded)
Frankfurters and sausage	Non-fat hot dogs, turkey hot dogs
Luncheon meats	Tuna fish, egg substitutes, peanut butter (in moderation)
Canned foods/fruits	Plain fresh fruits and vegetables; fruit juices
Cheese	Low-fat or non-fat cheese
Ice cream	Frozen yogurt or low-fat ice cream
Bacon grease, butter, lard	Reduced-fat margarine or butter; use cooking sprays instead of oils
Rich desserts	Angel food cake, frozen yogurt, fresh fruits
Potato chips, other snack foods	Pretzels (also low in sodium), boxed cereal, graham crackers
Whole/buttermilk	1% or skim milk

pathologist for each individual patient. Nursing staff members who supervise clients during meals should strictly follow instructions for assisting the patient with safe swallowing. There are several general techniques for safe swallowing, but the best method for each patient is determined by the speech therapist after assessing the person and viewing the barium swallow. For those persons who may be living in a long-term care facility or the community setting, general rules may be followed. However, for any person experiencing a new disease process that impairs swallowing, there is no substitute for the services of the speech therapist and the diagnostic test of the barium swallow.

General Guidelines

When the entire team is dedicated to facilitating the patient's ability to eat and swallow, certain rules will always be followed. Whether or not all staff members adhere to these principles can mean the difference between a patient's potential to be independent with eating and having to have a tube inserted to prevent aspiration. General rules to guide all nursing interventions related to improving nutritional status include the following:

1. Always check the patient's plate or tray to make certain the patient has been given the appropriate diet. Some patients will eat what is put in front of them, whether it is part of their diet or not.
2. Give repeated cues to patients who are self-feeding to go slowly. Mealtimes should never be rushed. Adequate time and care may be needed for them to swallow appropriately.
3. Make certain that any adaptive equipment that assists the patient with self-feeding is clean and available for each meal.
4. Consult with the occupational therapist if it appears that modifications in adaptive feeding utensils may be needed.
5. Listen to patients when they request certain foods or complain about meals. Allow family members to bring in food from home when possible to stimulate a sluggish appetite by providing familiar foods. If certain items are questionable on their particular diet, consult with the dietitian and see what modifications could be made to make meals more palatable.
6. Make community dining a pleasant experience. Many long-term care facilities, resident homes, community apartments, and rehabilitation units provide group dining. This fosters a sense of socialization and normalcy that most are accustomed to as a part of usual dining. Nurses can make this experience more enjoyable by ensuring a clean, well-kept, home-like environment. Playing appropriate background music or inviting a local pianist to provide dinner music on occasion can promote a sense of warmth and relaxation, essential elements for promoting positive eating experiences in what can seem like a negative environment for those with swallowing problems.
7. Patients should take meals sitting up straight in a chair. When this is not possible, the head of the bed should be raised to the maximum tolerable (and safe) level (preferably 90 degrees), taking care to avoid shearing force that can cause skin

breakdown. When the neck is hyperextended, even with the patient at a 45-degree angle, the risk of aspiration is increased, particularly in the pharyngeal and esophageal phases (Damon, 1988).

8. Set up meals immediately for those who can feed themselves but have trouble opening cartons or packets because of physical limitations such as hemiplegia, weakness, or arthritis. This encourages them to do what they can while still acknowledging and accepting their present limitations.

Additional considerations for those with dysphagia include the following:

9. Thicken liquids as indicated before placing the tray in front of the patient. Necessary mixing equipment and thickeners should be readily available. Giving a patient thin liquids when they aspirate such is dangerous, but many individuals forget this and will drink as they were formerly accustomed to.

10. Seat all those with special swallowing instructions at the same table and assign one staff member to supervise them. Cards can be placed at the tables (in a plastic cover to preserve them) to remind staff members of each individual's specific swallowing protocol. This is more efficient than having individuals scattered throughout a dining room or unit with inadequate supervision. In acute rehabilitation, the speech therapist often supervises the noon meal for those who are working on improving swallowing, but nursing personnel are more often required to help with this at breakfast and dinner as well as snacktime.

Additional nursing interventions to manage patients with dysphagia and promote self-feeding should be noted. Nurses must be alert to the patient's signs of fatigue, which can affect both the ability to manipulate food and the efficiency of the swallowing process. Older patients participating in several hours of therapy per day will likely be tired by the end of the day, and many experience decreased endurance and deconditioning secondary to their rehabilitation diagnosis.

Thermal stimulation is a method commonly used by speech therapists that involves the use of cold to stimulate a swallow response. A dental-type mirror is placed in ice until chilled, then the sides of the throat (the anterior faucial arches) are touched lightly with the cold mirror five times each. This may stimulate a swallow but does not always. The procedure is repeated about five times, several times per day. This, in effect, exercises the muscles involved in swallowing and speech. The GRN may be required to perform thermal stimulation on patients during off-shifts or supervise a family member or other caregiver learning this activity. The speech therapist will give detailed verbal and written instructions to both the nurse and the caregiver to maintain consistency and proper technique. Other sensory stimulation techniques as researched by nurses, such as icing or brushing the lips, jaw, or cheeks, have been unsuccessful in decreasing dysphagia (Williams, McDonald, Daggett, Schut, & Buckwalter, 1983).

For patients with a delayed swallow or delayed pharyngeal or esophageal peristalsis, a thermal gustatory technique using lemon ice may be used. This involves administering a half teaspoon of lemon ice between bites of regular food to stimulate a swallow and promote pharyngeal and esophageal peristalsis. This relatively simple procedure can be taught to family caregivers who assist with feeding. In some facilities, lemon ice technique is used during the modified barium swallow procedure to determine whether this assists the person with delayed swallowing or peristalsis.

Manipulation and control of the environment is a relatively simple but effective nursing measure to promote self-feeding. Van Ort and Phillips (1995) found that nursing interventions could improve the functional feeding status of older, cognitively impaired adults in an institutionalized setting without increasing the length of time for meals. Results, although based on a small sample of seven, indicated that reducing interruptions, minimizing distractions, having residents eat at a dining table, using placemats and namecards, using finger foods, positioning food directly in front of patients, and maintaining consistent mealtime activities all promoted self-feeding behaviors. These results support traditional gerontological rehabilitative nursing techniques used with dysphagic patients. More specific nursing interventions may be indicated in various situations. Several suggestions and examples appear below.

Specific Gerontological Rehabilitation Nursing Interventions

Some patients, as a result of extreme weakness, contractures, medical apparatus, trauma, or other physical problems, are unable to feed themselves. Such is the case with many frail elderly in long-term care settings. It is the goal of the GRN then to provide what Orem refers to as a wholly compensatory service (1995), that is, performing a function that the patient would do for himself or herself if able. As such, the nurse should strive to simulate the normal eating process as closely as possible, promoting patient involvement as much as is feasible, even if this involves such simple things as the patient's choosing which food to eat next. During all such interventions, the GRN should try to return to patients as much control as possible without overwhelming them. For example, patients with severe Parkinson's syndrome or MS may experience tremors that prevent them from being able to handle utensils or even get food into their mouth. Although they may not be able to perform this task, they might be able to wipe their own face with a napkin or perform some other task associated with eating. Even such small activities involve them in the meal process.

Feeding Patients Who Cannot Feed Themselves

1. Position the patient appropriately; sitting up in the chair is preferable. Use pillows to support those who may lean to the side because of hemiplegia from stroke or general poor balance.
2. Assess the patient's fatigue level. Changing mealtimes may make a difference in the patient's level of alertness as well as his or her ability to assist in the meal. Fatigue may particularly affect self-feeding capabilities of persons with MS, PD, and stroke.
3. Offer choices, however small, if the patient is able to make them. Even though patients may lack the ability to feed themselves, they can be given some control over what they eat.
4. Recognize that many patients may have the desire to feed themselves but are physically unable to do so. Involve the patient in the meal process in whatever ways possible, such as holding a glass or spoon or putting the utensil to the mouth after a small amount of food has been put on it.
5. Monitor closely for signs of dysphagia or aspiration. Teach other caregivers, staff, and family members these signs and symptoms. Pay particular attention to those diagnosed with PD or stroke.
6. Have suction equipment nearby for patients who are at high risk for aspiration.
7. Know (and have posted in the dining room) instructions for helping a person who is choking.
8. For patients who experience cognitive difficulties or dementia in addition to physical impairment, frequent cues may promote functional feeding behaviors (Van Ort & Phillips, 1995).
9. Give positive reinforcement for any patient attempts toward self-feeding. Patients unable to feed themselves can still be given positive feedback for food consumption.

Other nursing interventions can assist the debilitated elderly person in meeting the goals of improving nutrition, even when progress in self-feeding is unlikely. The GRN can continually assess an individual's physical status and report any significant changes in swallowing patterns to the physician, requesting a speech therapy evaluation. This could be referred to as either primary or tertiary prevention, depending on whether or not the person had a pre-existing medical condition affecting swallowing ability. About half of all elderly stroke patients experience dysphagia, so are considered at particularly high risk for aspiration (Lugger, 1994). The nurse can also teach patients and families to recognize signs of aspiration and encourage visitors to the patient to respect the dietary guidelines set up for the patient.

Additionally, techniques such as the supraglottic swallow (Table 5–5) or a simple head tilt can facilitate swallowing for the older person. The supraglottic swallow is used for patients who have undergone surgery that may have affected the neck structures and also for patients who have weakness of certain throat

---

Table 5–5 CLIENT TEACHING: SUPRAGLOTTIC SWALLOWING TECHNIQUE FOR THOSE WITH WEAKENED THROAT MUSCLES

1. Take a deep breath and hold it.
2. Take a bite of food.
3. Tip chin toward chest, holding bolus in mouth.
4. Swallow (may need to swallow more than once) until oral cavity is empty.
5. Raise chin and clear your throat by coughing as you exhale.
6. Swallow again and clear your throat or cough.
7. Breathe.
8. Repeat steps 1 through 6 with every bite.

Table 5–6   CLIENT/CAREGIVER TEACHING: SAFE SWALLOWING

1. Follow the swallowing guidelines prescribed by your speech therapist. (In the event that no specific guidelines are available, implement general guidelines as discussed in this chapter or other procedures such as supraglottic technique.)

2. Avoid water, milk products, and other thin liquids. Thin liquids are easily aspirated. Milk products can thicken secretions. Thicken liquids to a nectar-like consistency (or consistency specified by the speech therapist).

3. Be patient with yourself. Allow time to eat. Remember that the retraining of swallowing muscles is a gradual process.

4. Heavy, moist foods that are easily made into a ball (like applesauce) will be easiest to swallow.

5. Weigh yourself regularly. Report weight loss to your physician or speech therapist.

6. Sit up when eating meals or drinking fluids. Continue to sit up at least 45 minutes to an hour after meals.

7. Eating smaller meals 5–6 times per day may be helpful in decreasing fatigue levels, yet promoting good nutrition.

8. Avoid use of straws unless directed otherwise by the speech therapist. If you have difficulty swallowing liquids, taking small amounts by teaspoon or half-teaspoon is recommended. Remember, however, that you still need to drink enough fluid to promote hydration and prevent bladder infections and constipation. This may mean you should plan to take liquids frequently during the day.

9. Take smaller amounts of food at a time.

10. Alternate solids and liquids.

11. Use adaptive equipment as instructed by the occupational therapist.

12. Family members can assist the patient with head control or lip closure if this is a problem.

13. Place food on the unaffected side of the mouth where the patient can sense it and manipulate it more effectively.

14. Have a family member inspect your mouth, or look in a mirror to be sure food or medication was swallowed, not pocketed. Have the client perform a tongue sweep to ensure that food was swallowed.

15. Stroking the sides of the trachea and neck can help stimulate a swallow response.

16. Family members and staff may need to give verbal cues, or reminders, to patients about swallowing, slowing down, and the like.

muscles. For bed-bound neurologically impaired patients, placing them in a high Fowler's position with the head slightly forward and tilted downward toward the chest can reduce risk of aspiration by protecting the airway. The nurse can provide positioning support with his or her hands for those with poor head and neck control.

Older bed-bound, debilitated patients were often formerly fed in a recumbent position using a bulb syringe. This unsafe practice used to be common in nursing homes and was referred to as "force-feeding" those who could not or would not eat on their own. The intention was to avoid intubation. However, such methods contributed to choking and aspiration and are unacceptable nursing practice.

Instructing the Hemiplegic, Dysphagic Patient

The GRN may be responsible for teaching the patient and family to follow swallowing precautions at home after discharge. At the least, the nurse reinforces the instructions given by the speech therapist during meals on the off-shifts. An example of typical education that the nurse may provide to stroke patients and families regarding swallowing appears in Table 5–6.

The patient with more serious swallowing problems may go home with a feeding tube but continue speech therapy and home exercises with the goal of having the tube removed when adequate nutrition can be taken safely orally. Thus, patients may be discharged with a feeding tube and on a special diet with swallowing protocol. In cases such as these, it may be necessary for the GRN to teach both tube feeding skills and care as well as reinforcing proper nutrition and swallowing. Whereas in the acute care setting, the presence of a feeding tube usually indicated an NPO (nothing by mouth) status, this is not often the case in long-term care. Patients may experience advances in diet and eat food while still having a tube in place (usually a gastrostomy tube) for nutritional supplements or additional hydration when needed. The tube is removed as soon as possible once the patient is no longer aspirating and has an adequate nutritional intake. These things need to be explained to patients and family members who will, of course, have concerns. Modifications may need to be made in the usual procedures for tube feedings and medication administration when a patient returns home with a feeding tube (see later discussion).

Be particularly alert to the effects that hemianopia or other visual disturbances may have on the person's ability to complete a meal. The person with hemianopia may see only half of the plate or have difficulty getting food from the plate to the mouth. Turning the plate to visualize the entire 360 degrees of it, teaching scanning, and using adaptive devices may assist these individuals in self-feeding.

Setting Up and Directing a Meal for the Patient with Brain Injury

Several additional nursing interventions may be needed to assist persons with traumatic brain injury to feed themselves. Although the actual physical ability to eat and swallow may be present in many of these patients, cognitive issues may inhibit the performance of safe self-feeding.

Experts state that pre-feeding activities can be initiated with patients when they reach a level III on the Rancho Los Amigos [Medical Center] Levels of Cognitive Function Scale. Patients rated as a level IV (confused and agitated) are usually able and ready to begin eating, but complete oral intake should not be expected before level VI (Avery-Smith & Dellarosa, 1994). Further explanation of the Rancho Scale is given in Chapter 11.

Persons recovering from brain injury tend to be impulsive, socially uninhibited, forgetful, and in need of repeated cues. They can be easily distracted and/or agitated depending on the phase of recovery. The environment should be well controlled, calm, and unhurried. This is best done initially in a private room in a one-on-one setting, rather than the noisy, distracting community dining room. Once the patient has acquired suitable and safe eating habits, community dining is appropriate. The following interventions should be used in conjunction with those previously discussed.

1. Minimize or eliminate distractions. Turn off the television or radio. Ask visitors to return after the meal (unless family teaching is being done).
2. Make sure the individual is alert enough to eat. Be sure the person is sitting upright in a chair. Talk to the person and make certain he or she is awake and ready to participate. Assessing level of arousal is particularly important. Preparations for the meal such as turning off the television, positioning the patient, and speaking to him or her during this time can help.
3. Get the patient's attention. Say the patient's name and speak slowly and distinctly. Make eye contact.
4. Prepare the tray, removing all wrappings, cutting foods, and thickening liquids as needed.
5. Place only one food at a time in front of the patient. It may be necessary to place the food or utensil in the patient's hand.
6. Offer liquids between solids, but be careful of spills, and especially avoid hot liquids.
7. Give continual cues using short, simple, one-step directions to guide the patient through the meal. For example: "John, take a bite of bread" (pause while John does this, or repeat until he does). "Now, pick up the cup."
8. Avoid multi-step instructions such as "Take a bite, then swallow, and have a drink of milk." Such instructions may only confuse the patient further.
9. Remember that overstimulation is a common cause of agitation for the brain-injured person. Use a calm, quiet, and nonthreatening manner.
10. Plan to allow increased time for meals until the patient has an established routine and is able to feed himself or herself with less stringent supervision.
11. Be aware that you may frequently need to repeat instructions.

Many persons with brain injury are physically capable of feeding themselves. However, cognitive processes such as distraction, agitation, and frustration may make it appear as though they need to be fed. With careful planning, the nurse can direct or cue patients to do this for themselves and thus promote self-care and independence.

Tube Feedings

There are several ways in which enteral nutrition is provided to patients. The most commonly used tubes for feeding in older patients include nasogastric (NG), nasointestinal (NI), percutaneous endoscopic gastrostomy (PEG), percutaneous endoscopic jejunostomy (PEJ), gastrostomy (G-tube), and jejunostomy (J-tube). Little research has been done on elderly persons' tolerance to these types of nutritional support measures (Galindo-Ciocon, 1993). However, their use is common among gerontological rehabilitation clients, so the GRN should be familiar with related clinical implications.

PEG tubes have been in use for some time. They are becoming increasingly popular for use with the geriatric rehabilitation patient. PEG tubes are the preferred route of insertion for most rehabilitation patients who will have a tube for more than a few weeks. There are fewer complications and less risk of aspiration than with NG tubes. Insertion can be done under local anesthetic and has a lower infection rate than with G-tubes. Readers are encouraged to refer to a medical-surgical textbook if further review of traditional enteral feeding methods is needed.

Nasogastric Tubes

Nasogastric and nasointestinal tubes were intended for short-term use. Complications as a result of these tubes abound, particularly with use in the elderly. These tubes are inserted, usually by the nurse, through the nose and into either the stomach (NG) or the intestines (NI). The major adverse reactions cited in the literature include aspiration pneumonia, undernutrition or delay in receiving nutrition, clogging of the tube, agitation and self-extubation, irritation of the nasal and esophageal passages, and diarrhea (Burns & Jairath, 1994; Galindo-Ciocon, 1993; Sliwa & Marciniak, 1989; Stechmiller, Treloar, Derrico, Yarandi, & Guin, 1994).

Rehabilitation patients may have an NG tube if it is expected that they will be able to resume taking nutrition orally during the rehabilitation stay. The physician selects the insertion route based on factors such as the patient's risk of aspiration, underlying gastrointestinal pathology, level of consciousness, cognitive state, recommendations of the nurse and speech therapist, and estimated length of time it will remain in place (Bockus, 1993). In situations in which either an NG or a PEG

tube could be appropriate, the GRN can provide important input into this decision process by relating family preferences and knowledge level, knowing the patient's desires and level of cooperation, and considering the patient's coping ability as well as self-esteem issues.

With length of stays being significantly shortened at the present time, most patients who require long-term therapy as a result of dysphagia will have a G-tube or PEG tube inserted relatively soon, usually before discharge from rehabilitation. This allows time for the nurses to teach family members tube feeding skills if the patient is discharged home or gives the patient time to adjust to enteral nutritional measures before moving to a long-term care or subacute facility. It is preferable that a patient who is discharged home with a feeding tube have a G-tube or PEG tube in place. NG tubes are more easily displaced than gastrostomy tubes, require greater skill on the part of the caregiver to ascertain proper position, and carry a greater risk of aspiration.

Several suggestions may help the GRN with NG tube insertion on the older adult (Table 5–7). In addition to gaining skill with insertion, checking for tube placement is an important task and should be done each time before the tube is used. Aspiration of stomach contents is a good method, but this is not always possible with the small-bore flexible tube often used. Confirmation by auscultation is probably the most practical, if not the most widely used method, for bedside clinical practice. This is done by placing the stethoscope over the area on the left side of the abdomen just below the ribs. When a bolus of air is injected through the tube, a gurgling sound (like bowel sounds) should be heard. However, if the patient has hyperactive bowel sounds, these sounds can be confused. Recent research has also suggested that auscultation is an unreliable method for differentiating gastric from respiratory placement of feeding tubes, citing a 34.4% average of correct tube placement classifications in a sample of 85 acutely ill adults, age 21 years and older (Metheny, McSweeney, Wehrle, & Wiersema, 1990). Nurses reported hearing air insufflation sounds even when the tube was positioned in the lungs. Such commonly accepted techniques may be less reliable with small-bore feeding tubes (Martyn-Nemeth & Fitzgerald, 1992). Some say litmus paper tests are preferable, but this also is inefficient if no stomach contents can be aspirated through

Table 5–7   TIPS ON NASOGASTRIC TUBE INSERTION IN THE OLDER ADULT WITH SWALLOWING PROBLEMS

- Explain the procedure to the patient and ascertain the patient's ability to understand and cooperate. Explain that the patient can help make this process much easier by following your instructions.
- Use a flexible tube with a weighted tip if possible. This will help with ease of insertion.
- Use the smallest bore possible, considering the type and viscosity of intended feeding, length of duration of tube placement, and types of medications that may need to be given via the tube.
- Check both nares before beginning. Older adults often have septal deviation, making one naris much easier to pass a tube through than the other.
- Use plenty of water-soluble lubricant. Older adults tend to have more dry mucous membranes, making insertion more uncomfortable.
- Have the patient swallow several times prior to tube insertion so that you can see what the throat looks like during the swallow. This is particularly difficult when the individual has a poor swallow reflex. It may be hard to visualize the rise and fall of the larynx in these patients.
- Pause once the tube has been inserted through the naris toward the pharynx but before the gag reflex is triggered. Cue the patient to "swallow the tube." If allowed, have the patient take a sip of water, or place an ice chip in the mouth. Observing the rise and fall of the larynx (or "Adam's apple"), insert the tube as the patient swallows. Avoid attempting insertion during respiration, because this will more likely result in misplacement.
- The tube should thread the rest of the way easily if the patient has swallowed it.
- Any signs of the patient's choking, gagging, or coughing or the eyes watering usually mean the tube is entering incorrectly or is misplaced. However, not all older patients will exhibit such signs (similar to silent aspiration).
- Once the tube is secured and placement has been confirmed, mark the tubing with an indelible marker at the spot it exits the nose. This can be used later for comparison to see whether the tube has moved.
- Check tube placement several ways to ensure correct positioning, realizing that radiographic evaluation is the only totally reliable method for confirmation of correct tube location (Sliwa & Marciniak, 1989). Auscultation of insufflated air, pH of aspirated contents, measurement of the tube, and visual inspection of aspirated contents are the most popularly used methods at present.
- Anchor the tube securely. Older patients often cough or sneeze out their feeding tubes, resulting in displacement. Patients who are cognitively impaired may pull out their tubes, posing a particular danger if this occurs during a feeding. Mitts for the hands to prevent this are available if necessary. Commercially available products such as devices that adhere to the nose and provide a clamp for the tube will work for some patients, but not all. Taping the tube with a chevron-type anchor that hangs down from the nose is the usual method. Some sources recommend anchoring the NG tube only to the cheek to prevent irritation of the nasal mucosa (Eliopoulos, 1997). However, this does not prevent displacement if the patient sneezes, coughs, or rubs the nose.

---

the small tube at the time needed. When this method can be used, the gastric pH of the stomach will be significantly lower (3.02) than intestinal readings (6.57) (Metheny et al., 1993). Another, less reliable, method is to place the end of the tube in a cup of water. The water should not bubble with the patient's respirations, because this could indicate placement in the lungs. The problem with this method is that many feeding tubes are not transparent, so if the patient were to inspire, water could be sucked into the lungs through the tube without the nurse's seeing it, posing aspiration hazard. Thus, this method should not be used alone or with colored feeding tubes. The most reliable method to ensure correct tube placement is radiographic confirmation, but this is inconvenient, costly, and inaccessible in many long-

term care facilities. Hospital-based rehabilitation units with appropriate resources may find this a preferable method of assessment. Obviously, more research needs to be done to provide safe, cost-efficient, and practical ways to ensure correct tube placement, particularly for those patients being cared for in long-term care facilities or community settings.

Also of particular importance for the patient with an NG or NI tube are nursing interventions related to patient comfort. Dry mouth and nose, sore throat, and hoarseness are common complaints (Eisenberg, 1994a). Frequent oral hygiene is essential. Some patients find that having a damp rag to wipe lips, tongue, and gums allows them to maintain comfort on their own. Others are permitted to chew gum or suck hard candy to maintain moisture in the oral mucosa. Bacteriostatic mouthwashes or sprays can also be helpful.

Psychosocial issues associated with having an NG tube should be addressed with the patient. Many patients find it extremely embarrassing to have a tube hanging out their nose, and this may inhibit their desire to participate in group activities or therapy. Additionally, being deprived of oral intake, and the cultural implications this can carry for many ethnic groups, can be overwhelming to patients and families. Frank discussions between nurses, patients, and family members can help alleviate anxiety, reassure, and give hope.

Percutaneous Endoscopic Gastrostomy Tubes

PEG tubes are a type of gastrostomy tube that are not inserted and maintained in the usual manner. The typical gastrostomy tube is inserted directly into the stomach in the operating room under sterile conditions and general anesthesia. This is a more costly procedure and carries greater risk for the elderly person. The tube is secured with sutures, which pose an additional infection hazard.

There are several advantages to the PEG tube over the usual gastrostomy tube. The PEG tube can be inserted in an endoscopic suite and requires only local anesthetic and usually intravenous conscious sedation. The endoscopist usually is a physician specializing in internal medicine and gastrointestinal disorders. Via endoscopy, the physician is able to visualize the ideal place for the tube to be positioned. The entire procedure is relatively quick (less than 30 minutes). Feedings and medications can usually be given within 24 hours after placement (Eisenberg, 1994b). Checking placement is also simpler. A mark can be made on the tube's insertion site that can be observed before each use to ensure that the tube is in the same position. Additionally, gastric contents can be aspirated and observed and residual amounts monitored much more easily than with NG tubes.

Disadvantages to use of the PEG include the fact that candidates for this procedure must be free of esophageal obstructions, and previous gastrointestinal disorders such as ulcers would not make this a method of choice. Obesity may preclude its use if percutaneous puncture is not possible (Eisenberg, 1994b).

Insertion and Care: Understanding the procedure for PEG tube insertion can assist the GRN in educating family members and other caregivers about possible complications and care of the tube. The patient is placed in a supine position on the table. A minimum staff of the physician and a nurse is present. Once the patient is sedated and the throat sprayed with an anesthetic, the physician inserts a flexible fiberoptic scope into the patient's mouth, down the esophagus, and into the stomach. Using this equipment, the physician can inspect the entire inner stomach wall and observe for any signs of ulceration or disease. The ideal spot for tube placement can be directly determined through this method. Once this spot is determined, the light from the fiberoptic is shined from the inside of the stomach out toward the skin, where it is marked on the outside. The scope is then removed, but a guidance tube (or guide wire) is left in place. The PEG tube is then inserted through the mouth and threaded down the esophagus via the guidance tube to the stomach, where a stab wound has been made in the marked spot on the skin. The tube is then pulled out through the small stab wound, with the larger bulb-type end remaining inside the stomach taut against the stomach wall. A T-bar or triangular type of plastic bumper on the outside against the patient's abdominal skin (Fig. 5–2) helps secure the tube against the stomach wall. The guide wire is also removed.

The PEG tube is anchored to the abdominal wall according to hospital policy. A dressing may or may not be required or desired. It is common for the patient to initially have some crusty, brownish drainage around the insertion site. If a dressing is ordered, it should be only one layer in thickness under the external bumper. This bumper should not be pulled on or raised, because it holds the PEG tube in place. There are no sutures present. As fibrous or scar tissue forms around the bulb-like end of the tube in the stomach, it helps secure the tube, but this does not take place for more than 1 to 2 weeks, so extra care must be taken during this time for securing the outside part of the tube, which may be rather long and can easily be pulled on during therapy sessions. Newly inserted tubes are often taped to the abdomen. Thus, skin checks are particularly important, not just at the insertion site but also at the tape.

The main complication of PEG tubes is infection at the insertion site. Signs of infection include purulent or other unusual discharge at the stoma site (small amounts of crusty, brownish drainage are common), redness, warmth, fever, chills, swelling, and sore-

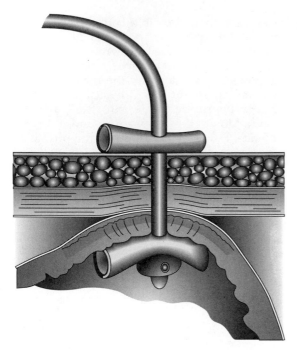

Figure 5–2 PEG tube. (From Starkey, J. F., Jefferson, P. A., & Kirby, D. F. (1988). Taking care of percutaneous endoscopic gastrostomy. *American Journal of Nursing, 88*(1), 42–45. Robert Shepherd, artist.)

ness at the site. Although infection can occur at any time, it is more likely to happen within the first 2 weeks of insertion. This can often be prevented by prudent nursing care, including careful cleaning of the site according to the physician's directions or hospital policy. A common cleansing solution is half-strength peroxide and half-strength water. Although it is often acceptable practice to use tap water for cleansing (and family members will use tap water if doing this at home), the nurse should use sterile water and sterile Q-tips to cleanse the wound in the hospital setting, where the risk of infection may be highest. However, once the stoma has healed or the patient is being discharged from an acute rehabilitation setting, this becomes impractical, expensive, and unnecessary.

If the stoma has healed and there are no signs of infection, family members can clean the stoma daily at home with mild soap and warm water using a cotton swab or gauze, or even a soft, clean washcloth. They should be instructed in proper procedures for this, such as cleaning in a circular motion from the stoma outward, then using a different area of gauze or new cotton swab for each subsequent return to the insertion site. Dressings

are not needed over the tube, and many patients prefer not to have the ends of their tubes taped at all because of subsequent skin irritation. If the PEG tube is pulled out, place a sterile dressing over the stoma, and notify the physician.

Feeding and Medications: There are two basic methods of feeding through the PEG tube: continuous and intermittent (also called bolus feedings). Although some patients are able to tolerate bolus feedings right away, this is not preferable. It is common for the elderly rehabilitation patient to initially be placed on a continuous feeding schedule. This allows the nutritional goals to be met more quickly and is often better tolerated by the patient (Bockus, 1993).

Bowel sounds must be present before tube feeding is initiated. Patients are often started on water at about 50 cc/hr to assess tolerance, after which continuous feedings may be slowly initiated (beginning at about 50 cc/hr). The amount of feeding is advanced about 25 cc/hr each day until the patient's caloric requirements are being met. Intermittent, or bolus, feedings may be attempted if the patient is tolerating continuous feedings of 100 to 125 cc/hr (Starkey, Jefferson, & Kirby, 1988). The GRN should always watch for abdominal distention and any other signs of intolerance. Checking for gastric residual material is another nursing measure. Residual amounts more than twice the hourly infusion volume indicate poor absorption. Residual amounts are always replaced after checking unless otherwise directed by the physician (Starkey et al., 1988).

The continuous feeding method uses gravity or a pump to provide constant infusion of the nutritional supplement over a longer period of time. This could be 24 hours a day or a portion of the day, say 12 to 16 hours. For rehabilitation patients, the latter schedule is often used—from the time therapy is ended, through the night, until morning, when therapy begins again. This eliminates the cumbersome pump and equipment that is used for continuous feeding, so that the patient may more fully participate in therapy without fear of dislodging the tube or interrupting feeding. In addition, those patients who are beginning to receive oral intake but do not consume enough calories for proper nutrition may benefit from cyclic feedings (Bockus, 1993). Continuous feedings may provide more nutrition quickly; however, they are less like normal eating, so can have adverse effects on the body system and are not as likely to promote goals of independent feeding. Diarrhea is a common problem with tube feedings, but moreso with those receiving bolus doses (Ciocon, Galindo-Ciocon, Thiessen, & Galindo, 1992). Bacterial contamination from manipulation of formulas and administration bags can also contribute to diarrhea (Burns & Jairath, 1994). This type of adverse reaction would be less likely with bolus feedings.

Bolus feedings are preferred for older rehabilitation clients for many reasons. First, these intermittent feedings eliminate the need for bags, pumps, and extra equipment. Bags used in continuous feedings are changed every 24 hours in the hospital, but this is not cost-effective for the home environment. Furthermore, the chance of bacteria forming in hanging solutions or being present in bags inadequately cleaned and reused is a likely risk. The equipment for continuous feeding may dissuade those otherwise able from reintegrating into the community or socializing with others. Second, bolus feedings are administered in a more convenient manner and simulate more of a normal eating pattern than continuous feedings. Patients who are able to tolerate bolus feedings find it preferable because there is less equipment to carry around, making it less noticeable that they are receiving enteral supplements through a tube. The PEG tube is tucked into their clothes so that it is not obvious, enhancing self-esteem more than a continuous feeding apparatus. Another quite significant advantage of bolus feedings over continuous feedings is that patients need to be continuously monitored while tube feeding is taking place. The danger of aspiration is still present for those with gastrostomy tubes. It is highly unlikely that a caregiver will be present constantly during a continuous feeding, but this is mandatory by the very nature of a bolus feeding via syringe, unless the patient is doing it himself or herself, in which case it is assumed the patient will recognize signs and symptoms of aspiration. Sometimes bolus feedings are given via a bag and tubing, but the syringe method is more cost-effective for those living in the community.

Not all patients are able to tolerate bolus tube feedings. Success in this area can be promoted by giving feedings slowly and using smaller, more frequent feedings to begin with until the patient's tolerance is established. Nutritional requirements must be closely monitored also.

Nurses are the primary teachers of patients, family members, and other caregivers who need to learn how to do a tube feeding. The client or caregiver who will be performing this task needs clear, consistent instructions. It is most helpful to use a booklet or brochure that can be given to the person and followed by all. Some such materials are available through manufacturers such as Bard or in educational books that can be purchased, but facilities may wish to produce their own. Table 5–8 gives suggestions for teaching clients or caregivers to perform PEG tube bolus feeding via the syringe method.

There are also two different approaches to the way in which medications are given through enteral feeding tubes. Within rehabilitation and long-term care settings, there is great variation as to how nurses administer medications through a tube, as well as how they teach clients and family members to do this. First, it should be emphasized that traditional, preferred methods are clear in nursing texts. That is, medications are measured into separate cups and given individually one at a time through the tube, flushing with water in between. This is the safest and most recommended method and probably the most common hospital policy. Medications are not mixed with each other prior to administration because of potential interaction effects. Unfortunately, this procedure is not practical, or functionally possible, for many elderly patients and their caregivers, so modifications may need to be made.

In some long-term care facilities it is commonplace to mix all the medications and give them together. The reasons for this are several. Older adults may receive many medications throughout the day. The process of giving them all separately with water in between is time-consuming, particularly if a nurse is caring for several patients with tubes who all receive many medications several times per day. Another reason is that in teaching patients or family members to perform this task when a patient is discharged home, it is much simpler for them to combine medications in one cup with water and give them together than to try to manipulate many cups, flushing with water between each. Using the traditional method prohibits some elderly caregivers from being able to perform this task, because they cannot manipulate the multitude of cups, resulting in spillage and frustration. If the choice is between giving medications together at home or giving them separately but the patient going to a nursing home, the

Table 5–8 CLIENT/CAREGIVER TEACHING: PEG TUBE BOLUS FEEDING AT HOME VIA THE SYRINGE METHOD

1. Gather all the equipment you need for this procedure: a 60-cc syringe, a towel, tube feeding solution, at least one cup with measurements on it, and fresh warm tap water. A stethoscope and/or ruler are optional depending on which method for checking tube placement is used. Keep supplies in the same place, such as on a TV tray, in a box, or in a large plastic container. Supplies should be kept clean and covered, although this is not a sterile procedure.
2. Position the client upright if possible, or at least at a 30- to 45-degree angle.
3. Prepare the feeding by opening the cans or mixing the powder, whichever method you are using. Refrigerate any unused portion. Discard if not used within 24 hours.
4. Have your designated amounts of warm water premeasured in a cup nearby, as well as any medications that will be given at this time (see Table 5–9).
5. Place a towel underneath the area in which you are working, to protect clothing.
6. Check tube placement. The doctor or nurse will tell you which method is preferred for you (auscultation, checking tube length, aspiration of gastric contents).
7. Check residual stomach contents if your physician has asked you to. This is done by attaching the syringe to the tube and drawing the plunger back to observe the stomach contents. Reinject the contents and flush the tube with approximately 30 cc of water and cap the tube. Do not give the feeding if there is more in the syringe than the physician has specified. Wait about 30–60 minutes and check the residual amount again. If it is still high, report the problem to your physician or home health care nurse.
8. Once the previous steps are completed, you are ready to begin the feeding. Remove the plunger from the syringe.
9. Pinch the tubing prior to uncapping the tube. You can do this by folding the tube over one of your fingers with the hand that will be holding the syringe. The nurse can demonstrate this for you. This is an important point to remember. If you forget to do this, leaving the tube uncapped without pinching or clamping the tube, the stomach contents can leak or spray out onto you if the client sneezes, coughs, or turns.
10. Once the tube is pinched, uncap it and insert the tip of the syringe into the end of the tube (plunger is not present).
11. Hold the syringe upright in one hand and pour the feeding solution into the syringe with the other hand until it is about ¾ full. Continue to pinch the tube until this is done.
12. Unpinch the tube and control the flow rate by raising or lowering the syringe. The feeding should be given slowly. This system works by gravity, so the higher you raise the syringe, the faster the fluid will go in.
13. Keep the syringe about ¾ full during the entire process. If you let the syringe empty before pouring more liquid in, air will enter the stomach and can cause discomfort. It will take practice to be able to do this smoothly, but the nurse will guide you through it until you feel comfortable on your own.
14. Once the entire amount for that particular feeding has been given, flush with at least 30–50 cc of warm, but not hot, water. The amount of water that is used to flush can vary. Remember that the client may only be getting fluids through the tube, so the nurse or doctor can give you a specific amount of water that is to be given after each feeding. This will help keep the client hydrated.
15. Once the feeding is given and the tube flushed with water, pinch the tube, remove the syringe, and replace the cap.
16. Rinse and clean supplies so they are ready for the next feeding.
17. If the tube feeding seems to be sluggish, as if the tube were becoming plugged, use about 30 cc of cola or other carbonated beverage (diet cola for diabetics) to flush the tube. The carbonation will often clear residual material from the inside of the tube. Then flush again with warm water. Always remember to flush with warm water after anything has been put down the tube. This will help prevent clogging.
18. The client should not lay down for 30–60 minutes after the feeding.

decision is generally made to change the technique for one more practical so the patient can return home. Another argument for administering medications all at once through the tube is that when patients take pills orally, they often swallow them together, either whole or crushed in applesauce. Certainly, crushing pills and putting them in applesauce together is also mixing, yet this is commonly done. If the choice is made to give medications together through the tube, then it is wise to consult with both the physician and the pharmacist regarding drug interactions using this procedure and what alternatives can be

Table 5–9   CLIENT/CAREGIVER TEACHING:
ALTERNATIVE PEG TUBE MEDICATION ADMINISTRATION

1. Follow all the steps in Table 5–8 for preparation, client positioning, and checking tube placement.
2. Have two cups of warm water ready: one for mixing medications (about 30–50 cc, depending on number and consistency of medications) and one for flushing the tube (30–50 cc).
3. Prepare medications. Measure prescribed dosage of liquid medication separately, emptying them into the cup with warm water as each is measured. Crush pills that are in tablet form to fine powder. Place them in the cup of warm water with the other medications. Stir to mix thoroughly.
4. Draw the medications up in the syringe.
5. Because tube placement has already been checked, crimp the end of the tube and open the cap.
6. Place the tip of the syringe in the end of the PEG tube.
7. Unpinch the tube and slowly inject the medications.
8. Pinch the tube again, remove the syringe, and replace the clamp.
9. Draw up the 30–50 cc of warm water in the second cup you set up at the beginning and flush the tube, pinching the end until the syringe is attached as directed before. (If a tube feeding is to be given, it can be done at this time, after the medications.) Replace the cap.
10. Rinse the syringe and cups for reuse.
11. The client should not lay down for at least 30 minutes after medications are given.

used. Table 5–9 further describes how to teach clients or family members to administer medications via a PEG tube. Most often, a person other than the client will give the tube feeding. However, if the patient is able, both cognitively and functionally, to perform this self-care activity, this should be encouraged. The GRN should be knowledgeable about which medications cannot be crushed or given via the tube. Alternative forms of medications should be discussed with the doctor and pharmacist as soon as possible if the patient is going home with a tube in place, as well as the implications of mixing medications together for administration at home. There are pages of lists at any hospital of those medications that should not be crushed; Table 5–10 provides an easy reference for GRNs to use.

EVALUATION

The effectiveness of nursing interventions is evaluated in terms of the overall goals. The GRN would expect to see the patient maintaining an appropriate weight, as indicated by regular recording of such on the patient's chart. The assessment criteria discussed in the beginning of this chapter should be monitored regularly throughout the care of the patient. Other signs of improved nutrition one would expect to see include better skin turgor, increased hydration, moist mucous membranes, higher serum albumin level, and improvement in skin integrity.

Improved functional outcomes would include activities that demonstrate an increase in self-care. This could mean an upgrade in diet as a result of improved swallowing muscle function or increased participation (according to ability) in the eating process. Continued presence of active bowel sounds and radiofluoroscopic studies that show a decrease in aspiration and improvement in swallowing ability are also measurable outcomes that demonstrate maintenance or improvement of nutritional status.

Desired educational outcomes would include demonstration by the client and caregiver of sufficient knowledge about dietary requirements and restrictions to maintain these standards in the home environment. Essential outcomes include the caregiver's ability to recognize signs of aspiration and steps to prevent and treat it. For those who require tube feedings, sufficient skill in enteral feed-

Table 5–10   SIMPLIFIED GUIDE TO MEDICATIONS THAT SHOULD NOT BE CRUSHED

Do not crush:

- Medications that have the following abbreviations or terms in their name, which would indicate slow or sustained release: SR (sustained release), SA (sustained action), XL (extended release), -bid, -dur, -ten, -slow (examples: Cardizem SR, Procardia XL, Ten-K, Slow-K, Nitro-Bid, Nitro-Dur).
- Capsules that contain liquid (examples: Colace, Procardia).
- Capsules that are sealed (example: Dilantin).
- Tablets with enteric coating (example: Ecotrin).

ing techniques (and medication administration) to safely perform these tasks unsupervised is the desired objective.

REFERENCES

Aptaker, R. L., Roth, E. J., Reichhardt, G., Duerden, M. E., & Levy, C. E. (1994). Serum albumin level as a predictor of geriatric stroke rehabilitation outcome. *Archives of Physical Medicine and Rehabilitation, 75,* 80–84.

Avery-Smith, W., & Dellarosa, D. M. (1994). Approaches to treating dysphagia in patients with brain injury. *American Journal of Occupational Therapy, 48*(3), 235–239.

Bockus, S. (1993). When your patient needs tube feedings: Making the right decisions. *Nursing93, 23*(7), 34–42.

Burns, P. E., & Jairath, N. (1994). Diarrhea and the patient receiving enteral feedings: A multifactorial problem. *Journal of Wound, Ostomy, and Continence Nursing, 21*(6), 257–263.

Ciocon, J., Galindo-Ciocon, D., Thiessen, C., & Galindo, D. (1992). Comparison of intermittent vs. continuous tube feeding among the elderly. *Journal of Parenteral Enteral Nutrition, 16*(6), 525–528.

Cope, K. A. (1994). Nutritional status: A basic "vital sign." *Home Healthcare Nurse, 12*(2), 29–34.

Damon, J. (1988). Nutritional considerations. In M. A. Matteson & E. S. McConnell (Eds.), *Gerontological nursing: Concepts and practice.* Philadelphia: W. B. Saunders.

DiIorio, C., & Price, M. E. (1990). Swallowing: An assessment guide. *American Journal of Nursing, 90*(7), 38–41.

Eisenberg, P. G. (1994a). Nasoenteral tubes. *RN, 57*(10), 62–69.

Eisenberg, P. G. (1994b). Gastrostomy and jejunostomy tubes. *RN, 57*(11), 54–59.

Eliopoulos, C. (1997). *Gerontological nursing* (4th ed.). Philadelphia: J. B. Lippincott.

Emick-Herring, B., & Wood, P. (1990). A team approach to neurologically based swallowing disorders. *Rehabilitation Nursing, 15*(3), 126–132.

Galindo-Ciocon, D. J. (1993). Tube feeding: Complications among the elderly. *Journal of Gerontological Nursing, 19*(6), 17–22.

Keller, H. H. (1995). Weight gain impacts morbidity and mortality in institutionalized older persons. *Journal of the American Geriatrics Society, 43,* 165–169.

Lipschitz, D. A. (1995). Approaches to the nutritional support of the older patient. *Clinics in Geriatric Medicine, 11*(4), 715–724.

Lugger, K. E. (1994). Dysphagia in the elderly stroke patient. *Journal of Neuroscience Nursing, 26*(2), 78–84.

Martyn-Nemeth, P., & Fitzgerald, K. (1992). Clinical considerations: Tube feeding in the elderly. *Journal of Gerontological Nursing, 18*(2), 30–36.

Metheny, N., McSweeney, M., Wehrle, M. A., & Wiersema, L. (1990). Effectiveness of the auscultatory method in predicting feeding tube location. *Nursing Research, 39*(5), 262–267.

Metheny, N., Reed, L., Wiersma, L., McSweeney, M., Wehrle, M. A., & Clark, J. (1993). Effectiveness of pH measurements in predicting feeding tube placement: An update. *Nursing Research, 42*(6), 325–331.

Nursing91 Books. (1991). *Diagnostics.* Springhouse, PA: Springhouse Publishing.

Orem, D. E. (1995). *Nursing: Concepts of practice.* St. Louis, MO: C. V. Mosby.

Price, M. E., & DiIorio, C. (1990). Swallowing: A practice guide. *American Journal of Nursing, 90*(7), 42–46.

Robbins, J., Levine, R. L., Maser, A., Rosenbek, J. C., & Kempster, G. B. (1993). Swallowing after unilateral stroke of the cerebral cortex. *Archives of Physical Medicine and Rehabilitation, 74,* 1295–1300.

Sliwa, J. A., & Marciniak, C. (1989). A complication of nasogastric tube removal. *Archives of Physical Medicine and Rehabilitation, 70,* 702–704.

Starkey, J. F., Jefferson, P. A., & Kirby, D. F. (1988). Taking care of percutaneous endoscopic gastrostomy. *American Journal of Nursing, 88*(1), 42–45.

Stechmiller, J., Treloar, D. M., Derrico, D., Yarandi, H., & Guin, P. (1994). Interruption of enteral feedings in head injured patients. *Journal of Neuroscience Nursing, 26*(4), 224–229.

Sullivan, D. H. (1995). The role of nutrition in increased morbidity and mortality. *Clinics in Geriatric Medicine, 11*(4), 661–674.

Sullivan, D. H., & Walls, R. C. (1994). Impact of nutritional status on morbidity in a population of geriatric rehabilitation patients. *Journal of the American Geriatrics Society, 42,* 471–477.

Sullivan, D. H., Walls, R. C., & Bopp, M. M. (1995). Protein-energy undernutrition and the risk of mortality within one year of hospital discharge: A follow-up study. *Journal of the American Geriatrics Society, 43,* 507–512.

Van Ort, S., & Phillips, L. R. (1995). Nursing interventions to promote functional feeding. *Journal of Gerontological Nursing, 21*(10), 6–14.

Williams, H., McDonald, E., Daggett, M., Schut, B., & Buckwalter, K. C. (1983). Treating dysphagia. *Journal of Gerontological Nursing, 9*(12), 638–647.

Yuen, H. K. (1993). Self-feeding system for an adult with head injury and severe ataxia. *American Journal of Occupational Therapy, 47*(5), 444–451.

Chapter 6

Maintaining and Promoting Skin Integrity

■

The skin is the largest organ in the body. It serves several key roles in the regulation of important physiological functions. The skin helps control body temperature, so any neurological damage within the control centers of the brain or the periphery can result in temperature regulation problems such as are seen in those with spinal cord injuries, multiple sclerosis, or Guillain-Barré syndrome. The skin also contains nerve receptors that signal pain, hot, cold, and pressure. However, in the person with neurological damage, these sensations may not be intact, or even present. For example, the patient with spinal cord injury does not tolerate prolonged exposure to the sun and can easily experience severe sunburns and fever in a short period of time, regardless of age. This is even more of a problem in the older adult, whose skin perspires less and is more frail. The nurse must take extra measures to compensate for those patients who no longer have the protective mechanisms they relied on before their injury or illness, particularly when complicated by age.

One of the major functions of the skin is to protect the underlying tissues, but significant changes occur with aging. The skin is the body's first line of defense against infection and is particularly important in the older individual. The epidermal layer prevents dehydration of the underlying tissues and keeps fluids and nutrients in the skin. However, the epidermis of an older person is thinner and has a decrease in local inflammatory response when damaged, with less ability to repair itself (Levine, Simpson, & McDonald, 1989).

When only the epidermis or upper part of the dermis is damaged, these layers usually heal by regeneration with no scar tissue formation. With total destruction of epidermis or dermis, subcutaneous tissue, muscle, or bone, healing involves scar formation, as discussed later in this chapter. This occurs more slowly and less efficiently in the older adult. Even after healing, the skin of an older person continues to be relatively weak and more prone to subsequent breakdown.

Older persons are also less sensitive to light touch or pressure, so may not realize when skin breakdown begins, particularly if other circulatory problems or peripheral neuropathies are present. The elderly have less reserve in all body systems to fight off infection. When the skin is broken, harmful bacteria may enter and cause infection and chronic wounds that are slower to heal in the older adult. Such wounds can easily lead to sepsis and even death.

Skin changes alone that occur with aging may not adversely affect the health of an aged person. However, the presence of neurological deficits, immobility, and adaptive equipment increase the potential for skin breakdown. Having a system or protocol to assess risk for pressure ulcer development is especially important for the gerontological rehabilitation patient.

Several skin problems are common in gerontological clients with chronic conditions seen in extended care settings. The nature of long-term care of the elderly with disabilities makes the maintenance of skin integrity a particular challenge. In addition to the normal skin changes associated with aging, rehabilitation patients may be dealing with paralysis, amputation, hemiparesis, edema, pre-existing conditions such as peripheral vascular disease or diabetes, as well as the presence of multiple splints, tubes, or other equipment. It is essential that the gerontological rehabilitation nurse (GRN) continually practice preventive techniques to prevent skin breakdown and be knowledgeable in the treatment of pressure sores, which are a common complication among these patients.

ASSESSMENT

There are many factors to consider when performing a skin assessment. Looking at the most commonly acknowledged risk factors for skin breakdown provides the best clues for obtaining an accurate picture of both the patient's risk and the present skin condition. Several good risk assessment scales are used in facilities today. Risk factor scores have been shown to be useful in identifying patients at high risk for pressure sore development (Levine et al., 1989; Pajik, Craven, Cameron-Barry, Shipps, & Bennum, 1986).

Visual inspection of the skin and proper documentation of observations are essential. Many facilities require or advise that color photographs be taken of any wounds or pressure areas present at the admission assessment. All areas of breakdown or redness should be measured, staged, and photographed. This record should remain with the patient's chart until discharge. Not only does concise documentation provide a baseline from which to judge the effectiveness of treatment, but it can also protect the staff from legal action that may arise months or years later from lawsuits pertaining to hospital costs from decubitus ulcer treatment. Case Study 6.1 provides just such an example.

CASE STUDY 6.1
Wound Assessment and Documentation

Mrs. Case was a 67 year old woman admitted to the inpatient rehabilitation unit after a right-sided stroke. She had spent 7 days in a different hospital, 3 of those in the intensive care unit, prior to transfer. On admission to rehabilitation, Mrs. Case was alert and oriented, had a good appetite, but required moderate assistance to transfer because of left

hemiparesis. The GRN performed a thorough skin assessment including assignment of a Braden risk score of 18, scoring mostly 3's in each of the six categories. However, the GRN noted a large, black area on each of the patient's heels. The skin was intact, but black eschar was present. The nurse took photographs and measurements, precisely documenting the condition of the heels and the surrounding skin. Even though the risk scale assessment indicated a low risk, the GRN knew Mrs. Case could be prone to further breakdown.

From the GRN's assessment data, several nursing diagnoses were delineated. Goals for Mrs. Case included maintaining adequate nutrition, increasing ambulation, preventing further skin breakdown, healing of the heel wounds, and education of the patient and family in each of these areas.

The GRN promptly began interventions to address the problems and meet the identified goals. Interventions included a turning schedule when in bed, teaching Mrs. Case to perform wheelchair leans and push-ups throughout the day, education of the husband and daughter about reducing risk factors for skin breakdown, ensuring that adequate nutritional status was maintained by working with the dietitian, and instituting pressure relief devices. The enterostomal therapist was also consulted regarding treatment of the heel ulcers, and immediate measures were taken to reduce further risk.

Although the GRN implemented the nursing care as planned, some complicating factors arose in Mrs. Case's situation. About 1 week after Mrs. Case began to ambulate in therapy, her heel ulcers opened and became stage III–IV draining wounds, causing severe pain that prevented her from completely participating in physical therapy. She was discharged shortly thereafter, receiving outpatient therapy and whirlpool treatments to her heels once a day. Several weeks after her discharge from rehabilitation, the nursing supervisor of the rehabilitation unit was called by the patient representative of the hospital. Mrs. Case and her husband claimed that since her heel sores had been acquired in the hospital, the hospital should pay for her treatments, which were frequent and costly. The physical therapist predicted that the wounds would take up to 6 months to heal. The patient representative was to find out which unit was responsible and to take appropriate action with those involved.

The nursing supervisor was able to assist

the patient representative in locating the area of the patient's rehabilitation chart, in medical records, which contained pictures and a detailed description of the patient's admission with the black heel sores already present. The GRN's accurate and detailed documentation cleared the rehabilitation unit of any wrongdoing, malpractice, or neglect. The ulcers were found to have developed in the intensive care unit, where the patient stated she was "not turned for three days." That hospital had to cover the cost of treatment and was found liable for the patient's injuries.

The nurses on the rehabilitation unit received a commendation from the hospital administration and the family for their thorough documentation and care of the patient while in rehabilitation.

Identifying Risk Factors

One of the most common tools is the Braden Risk Assessment Scale (Bergstrom, Braden, & Laguzza, 1987), which is used to determine which patients are at risk for the development of pressure ulcers. Patients are rated 1 to 4 on each of six risk factors (except for friction and shear, rated as 1 to 3): sensory perception, moisture, activity, mobility, nutrition, and friction and shear. The total of the numbers for each category is then applied to an overall scale (with a range from 4 to 23), which identifies patients at increased risk of skin breakdown (score of 16 or below). The Braden scale is considered highly reliable and valid (Levine et al., 1989).

Another scale commonly used for measuring the risk of pressure sore formation is the Norton scale (LaMantia, 1996). The patient is rated 1 to 4 in each of five categories: general physical condition, mental state, activity, mobility, and incontinence. For those with a total score of less than 15, pressure sore prevention methods should be instituted. Patients scoring less than 12 points on this scale are thought to be particularly at risk.

Although risk scales are convenient and provide consistency in treatment as well as documentation, they should be used with caution for older rehabilitation patients. The sensitivity of risk assessment tools even in general rehabilitation is uncertain (LaMantia, 1996). The Braden scale has been found to be reliable when used by a registered nurse, primary nurse, or graduate students. However, the reliability is less when used by licensed practical nurses and nursing assistants (Bergstrom & Braden, 1987). With a smaller number of advanced professionals working in long-term care facilities, risk factor tools must be used with caution, because they are only as useful and reliable as the person performing the assessment.

Neither the Braden nor the Norton scale lists age as a risk factor. Yet, the normal changes that occur with aging make the elderly more prone to skin breakdown, even when the other factors listed provide minimal risk. The Norton scale does not cite malnutrition as a risk component, unless the person performing the assessment includes this judgment under general physical condition, a broad, vague term. Yet the literature suggests that poor nutrition is one of the most significant factors in pressure ulcer development in older rehabilitation patients, and serum albumin level may be a predictor of geriatric rehabilitation outcomes after stroke (Aptaker, Roth, Reichhardt, Duerden, & Levy, 1994).

The use of adaptive equipment is a frequent source of pressure sore development in persons with disabilities, but it is not mentioned under mobility or activity in either scale. This could result in a compromised individual receiving a rating that shows low risk even though sound clinical judgment would suggest otherwise. For example, a 75 year old stroke patient with mild hemiparesis could be alert, continent, ambulate with minimal assistance, and have slightly limited mobility and thus be assigned a low risk score on both the Braden and Norton scales. However, in addition to her age, this same person could have diabetic neuropathy and a hemisling for transfers, all factors that would alert a clinician to a higher risk for skin breakdown than indicated by either scale.

Other risk factors have been identified by several researchers. Pajik et al. (1986) found a clear linear relationship between skin integrity and age and that women developed pressure sores more often than men. Their data suggested significant relationships between age, gender, and the incidence of skin breakdown, all patient characteristics not cited in the Braden or Norton scales. Other studies cite men being more prone to skin breakdown or no significant gender differences (Gosnell, 1973; Williams, 1972). A pressure ulcer prevalence study by Gawron (1994) suggested that although the staff readily identified high-risk patients, those with moderate risk scores (11–16) on the Braden scale were more likely to "fall through the cracks" (pp. 237–238). When assessing the scores of many older rehabilitation patients, it is likely that their scores will fall into a moderate risk category. So although risk assessment scales are useful in predicting pressure sore development, they do not account for all possible variables, many of which play a part in rehabilitation.

Other variables have been found to have an effect on skin integrity. Serum albumin level of less than 3.0 has been associated with increased incidence of pressure ulcers, as has been poor hydration and a body weight 80% to 85% less than ideal (Buelow & Jamieson, 1990; Lipschitz, 1995; Miller, 1995; Pinchcofsky-Devin & Kaminski, 1986). The presence of friction, being dependent in self-care, being confined to bed or a chair, elevated temperature, and certain medications have also been cited as discriminators for pressure ulcer risk (Gosnell, 1973; Sparks, 1993; Williams, 1972).

A better approach to maintaining skin integrity in older long-term care patients is to treat them all as if they are at risk or create a high-risk profile. Although the institution of preventive devices such as Spenco boots or pressure relief mattresses may be costly, the expense of pressure sore treatment is much greater. The GRN must develop clinical expertise to judge those patients who are more likely to develop skin breakdown and use this advanced clinical skill in combination with existing risk assessment tools. More research is needed to identify and isolate other factors unique to the disabled elderly, yet common among this population. Based on the literature available, a summary of risk factors that should be considered when assessing the skin of the older rehabilitation patient appears in Table 6–1.

Physical Inspection and Documentation

The initial physical inspection of a patient's skin must be meticulous and thorough. Most facilities use a standard form for baseline assessment, such as that in Figure 6–1. Although the GRN may perform the initial admission assessment, an interdisciplinary approach to skin care is preferable in the rehabilitative setting. Any health care professional finding signs of skin breakdown should record these observations on such a form. The nursing staff typically uses this tool to document assessments of wound improvement on a regular basis, at least twice weekly. However, skin checks should be done on each shift, as skin breakdown can begin in a short

Table 6–1 POTENTIAL RISK FACTORS FOR PRESSURE SORES IN THE GERONTOLOGICAL REHABILITATION PATIENT

Decreased level of consciousness
Albumin less than 3.0 g/dl
Body weight less than 80%–85% of ideal
Impaired cognitive state
Altered sensory perception
Incontinence of bowel or bladder
Decreased activity level
Impaired physical mobility
Altered nutritional status (thin or obese)
Frail general physical condition, atrophy, or
  anemia
Presence of pressure, friction, or shearing force
Use of adaptive equipment
Cardiovascular disease
Increased age (older than 65)
Pain or sedative medications
Presence of skin breakdown
Inability to change positions per self
Elevated temperature
Chairbound
Cancer
Diabetes
Transmetatarsal amputation
Dependence in self-care

time (even minutes) in the compromised individual. Any new areas of breakdown should be recorded on the flow sheet for continued monitoring.

Several items should be noted on the documentation form. These include the date and time, location of the area, wound assessment (size, color, odor, drainage, amount), surrounding skin temperature and color, treatment, amount of pain reported by the person, and whether or not certain treatments have improved the wound condition. Most flow sheets include a picture of the front and back of the body so that areas of breakdown can be marked, in addition to pictures being taken. Nutritional consults should be obtained for any breakdown beyond stage I (redness with intact skin). The enterostomal therapist should be consulted for treatment recommendations if the GRN is uncertain what the preferred treatment would be. In the long-term care setting or the community, where a nurse specializing in skin care is not available, GRNs must develop clinical expertise in the treatment and management of wounds.

There are many types of skin problems that the GRN might observe in the elderly rehabilitation patient. These include rashes,

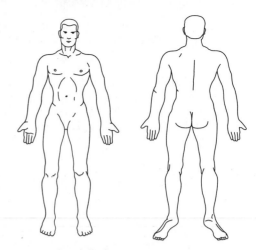

MULTIDISCIPLINARY WOUND
ASSESSMENT FORM

Assessment: Record all pressure/vascular ulcers on admission, 2 times per week and discharge.
Wound assessment: Record size in cm. Record anything unusual or undermining by using a clock as orientation
           e.g., pts. Head=12:00. (LxWxDxU).
           Stage I: Reddened area. **Stage II**: Dermis exposed; blister. **Stage III**: Subcutaneous exposed.
           Stage IV: Muscle/bone exposed. Wnd. color: r=Red, y=Yellow, b=Black, g=Green.
Drainage: Type: ser=Serosanguineous, s=Serous, p=Purulent, g=Green. Odor: O=None, M=Mild, F=Foul.
        Amount: sm=Small, mod=Moderate, lge=Large.

Date/Time							
Location							
Wound assessment LxWxDxU Stage/Color							
Drainage Type/Odor/Amount							
Surrounding skin condition Color/Temp./Width							
Cleansing/dressing method							
Assessment Improvement							
No improvement							
Deteriorating							
Nutritional consult							
Special equipment							

Figure 6–1 Multidisciplinary wound assessment form. (Courtesy of Geri Smith, St. Margaret Mercy Healthcare Centers, Hammond, IN.)

bruises, skin tears, chronic leg ulcers, pressure ulcers, and the pressure or friction effects of adaptive equipment.

Rashes are a common skin disorder in the elderly, and the itching that they cause can easily lead to skin breakdown from the patient's scratching. The most common site for this skin irritation is the groin area. Women also experience rashes under the breasts. Obese individuals or those with poor hygiene often develop a rash in various skinfolds. Rashes should be noted and described on the skin flow sheet. Although minor skin irritations alone may seem relatively insignificant, involved areas that are broken from the patient's scratching can be difficult to treat. Patients in therapy perspire as activity is increased, thereby irritating pre-existing skin conditions. Incontinence of bowel or bladder aggravates rashes and makes healing difficult if areas are not kept clean and dry.

Bruising of the skin is seen in many older people, even those who are healthy. Areas of bruising should be noted on the admission assessment sheet, because new bruises often appear during the course of rehabilitation. Places of bruising where the patient has bumped the wheelchair, walker, or bed when transferring and ambulating should be noted. These are not uncommon, yet with many rehabilitation patients receiving anticoagulant therapy this can be significant and must be monitored.

Skin tears are often caused by improper transfer techniques such as grabbing the patient's arm instead of using a gait belt. Many such tears occur on the patient's arms and hands, where the skin is very thin and fragile. Skin tears are difficult to treat because of their irregular nature and are often serious, painful wounds. When the GRN assesses an individual whose skin is particularly fragile (sometimes called "paper-thin"), additional measures should be taken to prevent skin tearing. The use of tape or bandages, even Band-Aids, on the skin should be restricted or prohibited. Removal of bandages must be done carefully so as not to pull the skin in any way. Likewise, staff should not hold onto or twist the patient's hands or forearm, because this can cause skin separation and tearing.

Ulcers, or sores, of various types are common problems. Acute wounds present less of a challenge than chronic wounds. Chronic leg ulcers may be present as a result of venous insufficiency or arterial occlusion, taking months or even years to heal. The majority of these chronic ulcers are managed by home health nurses in the community (Flett, Harcourt, & Alpass, 1994).

Pressure ulcers are especially common among the institutionalized elderly. The most common sites for pressure ulcer development are the coccyx, or sacrum, and heels. Older patients with disabilities have several other areas in which breakdown is seen, including head, ears, scapula, vertebrae, elbows, iliac crest, trochanters, ischia, lateral and medial condyles, lateral malleolus, lateral edge of foot, and several areas of the feet (Gawron, 1994; Iverson-Carpenter, 1988; Levine et al., 1989; Pajik et al., 1986). A primary diagnosis of cardiovascular disease has been linked with a significant risk for pressure necrosis (Gawron, 1994).

Persons with diabetes should be asked about circulation and sensation in their lower extremities. The feet of persons with diabetes should be of particular concern. Footwear should be carefully inspected, and the use of adaptive devices thoroughly evaluated. In elders with transmetatarsal amputation (TMA), many of whom experience diabetes, a high risk of skin breakdown or higher amputation has been noted, especially in the first 3 months after surgery (Mueller, Allen, & Sinacore, 1995). Education of amputee patients in skin care and prevention techniques is a necessity.

The heels of all older patients should be inspected and palpated, especially those with immobilizers, casts, paresis, or paralysis, because this site of breakdown is often neglected or overlooked. Shoes and socks must be removed and the leg lifted to examine the heel properly. The report of the patient with regard to pain, redness, or soreness should not be relied on. All footwear should also be inspected for proper fit and smoothness next to the patient's skin.

The use of adaptive equipment presents another potential problem in addition to the common skin disorders seen in the elderly. Patients may use orthoses, prostheses, splints, slings, casts, hemi-walkers, and wheelchairs, all of which can cause skin irritation and breakdown if improperly fitted. The orthotist and prosthetist, in addition to the physical and occupational therapists, are resources for the GRN in ascertaining proper fit of adaptive devices. Anytime a piece of equipment is used that comes in contact with the patient's skin, all team members should watch for areas of redness, friction, or pressure (Baxter & Mertz, 1990). Many older rehabilitation clients experience decreased sensation in the extremities; therefore, it is particularly important that the GRN monitor the skin condition each shift and throughout the day, because participation in activities can cause breakdown from friction during activity.

Ankle-foot orthoses (AFOs) are often used for those who have experienced lower extremity weakness, such as occurs with stroke or multiple sclerosis, and require additional lower extremity support in the affected leg. Typical AFOs are made of a firm yet flexible, plastic-type material, fitting under the patient's foot inside the shoe and coming up behind the lower leg, attaching below the knee with Velcro or other closure. Because of the location of the AFO, skin irritation and breakdown can occur in the feet, heels, and legs. All these areas should be inspected before donning the brace and when removing it. Likewise, splints are worn by many patients to prevent contractures, especially on the hands. Areas of redness should be reported to the therapist or orthotist immediately, because it does not take long for small areas of breakdown to become large problems in the compromised patient. These same guidelines hold true for assessment of prosthetic devices.

Slings are often worn by the patient with hemiplegia. Although there are many variations of slings, all are designed to support the affected limb and generally do so by straps that fit over the neck or shoulders. Thus, not only should the skin of the affected arm be assessed for redness from the sling but also the places around the neck, shoulders, or back that provide the support. For those with casts, the GRN should follow the usual, accepted protocol for assessing circulation and sensation in the affected extremity to ensure the cast is not too tight.

Wheelchairs ideally should be fitted to the individual's size and weight. If a patient does not have enough room at the sides of the wheelchair, friction areas may be seen on the hips and buttocks, as well as the lateral knees where rubbing has occurred from parts of the chair. This is especially important for patients who have had hip surgery. An ill-fitting chair may cause the surgical wound to be rubbed and irritated if the width is too small for the patient.

Wound Staging

The GRN may see many types of wounds in the rehabilitation unit, long-term care facility, or community. The cause of injury should be the first assessment factor considered. Causes can be mechanical (pressure ulcers), thermal (heat or cold), chemical, radiation, or vascular insufficiency. Wounds are commonly described as contusions, abrasions, lacerations, punctures, burns, bites, tears, or pressure ulcers.

The most common cause of skin injuries among elderly rehabilitation patients is from pressure ulcers. This is the type of wound for which nurses often have primary management, because treatment involves long-term planning, interventions, and evaluation. Thus, this discussion focuses on assessment and nursing management of pressure ulcers.

A traditional approach, although not the only method, to documentation of pressure ulcers is to categorize wounds into four stages. These are based on recommendations from the National Pressure Ulcer Advisory Panel (NPUAP) (1989).

Stage I: These pressure areas appear as nonblanchable redness of intact skin. This is a pinkness or redness that does not go away, yet the skin is not broken. Stage I ulcers are sometimes difficult to assess in patients with darkly pigmented skin, because areas of redness do not have the same appearance as in lighter skin. Preventive measures should be instituted immediately, but preferably before this occurs. If preventive measures have been used and a stage I ulcer still occurs, interventions should be reevaluated for effectiveness.

Stage II: A stage II ulcer involves partial-thickness loss of the epidermis and/or the dermis. This is a superficial wound, which appears as a blister, abrasion, or shallow crater. The skin is no longer considered intact, and exudate may be present.

Stage III: When no skin is present over the wound and subcutaneous tissue is seen, the wound is stage III. The tissue damage may extend down to the fascia, but not into the muscle. This appears to be a deeper crater and may or may not have exudate.

Stage IV: These wounds are the most extensive. There is full-thickness skin loss, as well as tissue necrosis and/or damage to muscle, bone, and other supporting structures (such as tendons or joint capsules). These wounds also may have exudate or appear dry.

Black Wounds: Another type of pressure ulcer that occurs, particularly on the feet and heels, is a black wound. Black wounds are generally considered to be stage IV wounds because they contain necrotic tissue that looks like a thick, dried, black eschar (Krasner, 1995). Sometimes a black wound appears as a dark blister, with the skin intact. This is seen on the heels of aged patients with some frequency, but makes staging difficult. Obviously, a black area most likely indicates a severe wound, yet with intact skin the nurse cannot observe the amount of damage present to categorize the area into one of the four stages. For purposes of documentation, the ulcer should be charted in detail, but staging is not recommended (Bergstrom et al., 1994). This wound may be categorized automatically as stage IV, intact, if this provides the best assessment according to the facility's protocol.

Wound Healing

There are three overlapping phases of wound healing: inflammatory, proliferative, and maturation. These occur on a continuum but follow a predictable course in a healthy, well-nourished individual. The GRN should be able to recognize abnormalities in this normal process of healing to improve assessment and evaluation of elderly rehabilitation patients with difficult-to-manage wounds.

Phase I: The inflammatory phase occurs immediately after an injury. There is first a short period of vasoconstriction in which platelets aggregate around the injured vessels to clot and prevent hemorrhage. Then the capillaries are dilated as leukocytes gather around the site within 20 minutes to eradicate bacteria and begin tissue repair. Phagocytosis also occurs at this stage. Clinical observations indicating this process are edema, redness, warmth, and pain. This internal cleansing and healing, first involving neutrophils, then macrophages, continues for about 3 days, at which time new tissue has begun to form (Rudolph & Shannon, 1990).

The inflammatory phase is slower in burns and some chronic wounds. This may be caused by a deficiency of proteins that stimulate epithelialization. A decrease in collagen with age may prolong this phase in the older adult as well.

Phase II: During the proliferative phase, granulation tissue forms and epithelialization occurs. Granulation tissue can be recognized by its bright red, beefy, raised, thick appearance. This is due to capillary dilation and the formation of collagen. A thin, silvery border of new epithelium forms around the periphery of the wound and eventually migrates across the wound bed over the granulation tissue. The granulation tissue has contracture properties that are used to close the wound. This decrease in wound size can be measured and documented. For those with large, extensive wounds, contracture of the granulation tissue can cause distortions in the skin and limit range of motion.

Fibroblasts are the key cells in this phase of wound healing. They produce strands of the protein collagen and weave it together to form a matrix of connective tissue that holds the wound together and increases tensile strength. The skin of an older person after wound healing has lower tensile strength than in younger individuals. This means that the wound has less ability to withstand pressure or disruption without breakdown (Levine et al., 1989; Rudolph & Shannon, 1990).

Phase III: The last phase of wound healing begins about 3 weeks after the injury and can continue up to several years. During this maturation phase, the wound becomes stronger through the arrangement of the scar tissue formed by the collagen network. The collagen bundles with other proteins and lends strength to the healing tissues. The nurse will observe a shrinking and thinning scar. The color of the scar will fade and become less red as capillaries regress. A mature scar is thick and palpable and either hyper- or hypopigmented. Even after the maturation phase is complete, the wound of an older, debilitated person will not be as strong as that of a healthy, younger individual, and the skin can still be prone to breakdown long after the wound appears to be healed.

Wound Closure

Three types of wound closure are distinguished that may be seen in the rehabilitation setting. *Primary closure,* or *first intention closure,* is when the skin is incised, with clean edges, and closed with sutures or staples, such as occurs with surgery. Tissue repair and regeneration are modest with this type of closure. Little granulation tissue is formed because of the less traumatic nature of the wound and closure. *Secondary closure* refers to open wounds that take longer to heal than those with primary closure. Also called *second intention closure,* these wounds are usually left open and treated without surgical intervention. This results in greater amounts of scar tissue than either other type of closure and longer healing times. *Delayed primary closure,* or *third intention closure,* is when a wound is left open for several days, then sutured as in first intention closure. This is done in cases where drainage of the wound to treat or prevent infection (such as the case of a ruptured appendix or peritoneal abscess) is important.

All three methods of wound management are seen in rehabilitation. Most older rehabilitation clients are managed with secondary closure for pressure ulcers. However, GRNs will see postsurgical patients who have had hip replacements or amputations and primary closure. On occasion, patients may have wounds that are open, as in the case of peritoneal abscess from an infected percutaneous endoscopic gastrostomy (PEG) tube site that was opened and drained. The physician may elect to delay closure, instead irrigating and packing the wound with a sterile dressing until the infection has begun to subside. These patients are generally transferred to a medical-surgical unit but sometimes continue in acute rehabilitation, depending on the extent and nature of the wound.

Factors Affecting Wound Healing

A variety of factors affect wound healing, but some are more prevalent or significant than others for older adults with disabilities. General factors include age; nutritional status; infection; vascular insufficiency; metabolic factors; immunosuppression; glucocorticoid therapy; use of steroids, anticoagulants, or immunosuppressives; smoking; obesity; neurological and psychological factors; and clotting disorders. Pre-existing conditions inhibiting wound healing that occur with some frequency in the older rehabilitative population include diabetes, renal insufficiency, malnutrition, arterial insufficiency, anemia, impaired physical mobility, decreased sensory perception, medication regimen, cancer, and obesity. Cancer, when associated with protein deficiencies, has also been linked to a greater risk of pressure sore development (Waltman, Bergstrom, Armstrong, Norvell, & Braden, 1991).

GOALS

There are several goals for skin maintenance of the older rehabilitation client. The most important is to maintain skin integrity through primary preventive measures. Clini-

cal practice guidelines list four major goals for prevention of pressure ulcers in adults. These include (1) identifying at-risk individuals and the specific factors that place them at risk; (2) maintaining and improving tissue tolerance to pressure in preventing injury; (3) protecting the skin against adverse effects of external forces such as pressure, friction, and shear; and (4) reducing the incidence of pressure ulcers through education (Bergstrom et al., 1994). If wounds are present, then prevention of infection is also a priority. Healing of wounds is another goal, but may be long-term depending on the nature of the injury.

More specific educational goals are that the patient and/or caregiver implements pressure-reducing techniques, practices safety measures, recognizes signs of skin breakdown, and provides good skin hygiene. Additionally, the patient or caregiver may need to learn treatment methods such as the use of Granulex spray, wound care, and the proper application of adaptive devices.

INTERVENTIONS

Prevention of unrelieved pressure and skin breakdown is the most important nursing intervention in promoting skin integrity. General nursing interventions for the older adult include implementing devices that reduce pressure, promoting activity, encouraging a high-protein, vitamin-rich diet, teaching good skin care and hygiene, treating incontinence, managing existing wounds, providing emotional and educational support, and promoting a positive self-image. Nurses have identified the need for more education in the prevention and treatment of pressure ulcers as being extremely important (Brower & Crist, 1985).

Prevention

Geriatric patients are immediately at an increased risk for pressure ulcers and potential for impaired skin integrity because of the more fragile nature of aged skin. Considering that most older rehabilitation clients experience some degree of altered activity levels or immobility, this is a group whose risk is automatically higher than the general population. Although it may be unnecessary and certainly not cost-effective to institute extensive prevention methods on the entire gerontological rehabilitation population, it is wise to acknowledge that this is a high-risk group. Some patients may require more preventive measures than others, but all are at risk. Assessment tools that help identify risk factors assist the GRN in focusing resources on those patients who need them most. However, this does not mean that those who rate lower on a risk scale are not at risk. They may only be at a lesser risk, and then only if the tool and the person using it are reliable.

General Nursing Measures

Preventive nursing measures are aimed at reduction of controllable risk factors for skin breakdown. General preventive measures can be found in any nursing text and include pressure relief, proper positioning, good hygiene, adequate nutrition, decreasing friction and shearing force, monitoring fluid and electrolyte balance, daily skin inspections, ambulating as able, and client/family education. Specialty beds, such as those that use air, water, gel, sand, or a combination of these, can be extremely helpful in preventing skin breakdown for the high-risk person. However, they are costly, and the benefits should be weighed against the person and family's financial resources.

Patients seen by the GRN in a variety of settings require special interventions to promote skin integrity and prevent breakdown. These patients may include those with diagnoses of stroke, Guillain-Barré syndrome, Parkinson's disease, amputation, hip fracture, multiple sclerosis, spinal cord injury, and nearly all other common disorders associated with gerontological rehabilitation. As patients become increasingly knowledgeable about skin care, and their status has improved and stabilized, self-care in this area increases, allowing the GRN to focus attention on those less capable of self-management. More specific nursing interventions for elderly patients with rehabilitative needs are addressed here.

Focus of Gerontological Rehabilitation Nursing Interventions

Most nursing interventions within gerontological rehabilitation nursing are multidimensional and interrelated. That is, nursing care that helps promote skin integrity includes such things as bowel and bladder training to prevent moisture, encouraging adequate nutrition, and promoting activity such as assisting the patient to ambulate as pressure relief and for promotion of circulation. All of these interventions work on many body systems simultaneously. Thus, the development of comprehensive nursing care plans that address the many integrated problems seen in this field is a necessity. Just as impaired skin integrity can inhibit progress in mobility (see Case Study 6.1), so can impaired mobility create problems with skin integrity. Although these interventions are common sense, their implementation in the clinical setting is crucial.

Promoting Activity and Mobility

Persons with impaired physical mobility experience a decrease in activity after the onset of a "disabling" condition. The elderly, particularly those older than 85 years, usually experience some limitations in movement from that of their younger years. Additionally, many of these individuals have decreased circulation and sensation, whether from paralysis or paresis or a chronic condition such as vascular disease or diabetes. The combination of these factors puts the patient at considerable risk for impaired skin integrity. One of the key nursing interventions, which is carried out within a team framework, is to increase the person's endurance and activity. Gerontological patients in the acute rehabilitation setting may be participating in 3 or more hours of therapy per day; however, those in the long-term care setting and the community will probably have far less activity, making the GRN's role even more important.

Patient positioning for bed-bound patients is important in preventing skin breakdown. General rules of thumb tell the nurse that patients' bony prominences should be padded and pressure-reducing surfaces such as mattress overlays, gel pads, air mattresses, water, and kinetic beds should be used appropriately. Heel and elbow protection should be used on nearly all older patients with any kind of mobility impairment, realizing that most heel devices provide inadequate security against breakdown and that additional measures will be necessary for the older adult. Donuts are not recommended for any body parts, because they cause increased pressure in areas not supported by the device. Likewise, eggcrate mattresses do not provide sufficient cushioning against breakdown for frail skin. The efficacy of air, gel, or alternating air mattresses is uncertain, because without additional measures, skin breakdown is still likely to occur (Conine, Choi, & Lim,

1989; Mikulic, 1980). However, pressure-reducing devices are believed to significantly reduce the incidence of pressure ulcers, particularly when other measures are also used.

Shearing force and skin tears can be avoided by careful positioning and patient education (Maklebust, 1987). Proper body alignment can be maintained without placing bony prominences over other body surfaces. An example is the 30-degree lateral side-lying position with upper leg flexed to avoid pressure points, especially direct pressure over the trochanter (Kemp & Krouskop, 1994; La-Mantia, 1995). Pillows should always be available for support and comfort in repositioning. Turns should be done at least every 2 hours, but this is not a magic number, and turning schedules should be individualized according to patient risk factors. All these interventions should be followed, but there is no substitute for actual physical activity in preventing skin breakdown. The mobile patient has much less risk for breakdown than the immobile one.

The GRN should aim interventions at those that cause the patient to be more active and mobile. Further discussion of interventions to promote mobility appear in Chapter 7. Repositioning the patient in bed is essential, but it does not provide the same pressure relief that sitting up in a chair, standing in a standing box, or ambulating does. The nurse should use different chairs for the patient to sit in, because each will cause slightly different pressure points. It is important to remember, however, that no position or chair is so good that a person can be left for hours without repositioning. All sitting furniture should be appropriately padded, and the patient must be taught to perform pressure reliefs such as wheelchair lifts and leans. Assisting the patient with ambulation to the dining room on off-shifts is a simple way to promote mobility. This is often done by nursing assistants. However, some facilities recruit volunteers to participate in a walking program with older residents. Recreational therapists can work with occupational therapists to design entertaining, yet appropriate, activities for older adults that strengthen the upper extremities for those in wheelchairs. A strong upper body can help assist in pressure reliefs for the lower body. Any attempts at improving activity should be encouraged, because the benefits to health and well-being are many, and this is a key to promoting healthy skin as well.

Educating Patients, Families, and Caregivers

Education of patients in their role in skin care is essential. Older adults need to be informed about the effects of the aging process on their skin. Increased dryness, fragility, and decreased elasticity are common. All older individuals should also be instructed in repositioning methods. Good guidelines for this are the techniques taught to patients of all ages with spinal cord injury. Pressure reliefs or position changes for those in a wheelchair should be done every 15 minutes.

Observation of paraplegics who have mastered pressure relief will show that they appear to be constantly shifting and moving within the chair. It should be noted, however, that patients with spinal cord injuries gradually can increase their "sitting time." One study demonstrated that younger quadriplegics were able to tolerate multi-hour periods without pressure relief (with capillary pressures of 32 mmHg) without skin breakdown (Patterson, Cranmer, Fisher, & Engel, 1993; Patterson & Fisher, 1986).

Wheelchair leans are simpler than wheelchair lifts for most older people. Leans involve shifting the weight to one side so that at least 1 inch is between the body and the support surface. Wheelchair lifts are more difficult for the elderly patient, because they require the ability to lift the torso with both hands placed on the wheelchair rests. Many older people do not have this upper body strength, only have the use of one side, or have arthritic changes that could make this method painful. Bending over at the waist is another pressure relief technique sometimes used. This takes pressure off the ischia, but it is a less desirable method for older patients. Such bending would be contraindicated for the postoperative hip fracture patient and those with dizziness or poor balance. This forward lean also causes many older patients to perform a Valsalva maneuver and could result in increased intra-abdominal and intra-cranial pressure, undesirable results for those with stroke, cardiac problems, and incontinence. Table 6–2 gives suggestions for teaching older clients to perform wheelchair lifts and leans.

Patients and caregivers also need to be taught to inspect the skin at least twice daily. This is best remembered on awakening and going to bed. Patients with adaptive devices should be instructed to check their skin where the equipment makes contact, both on donning and removing the device. A mirror may

Table 6–2 CLIENT TEACHING: PERFORMING WHEELCHAIR LEANS AND PUSH-UPS

Wheelchair Leans

Make sure your chair is well fitting and the leg rests keep your legs in proper position for stability.

Lock wheelchair brakes.

Shift weight to one side, lifting hips and buttocks at least 1 inch off the chair, yet not leaning so far as to tip over. You are leaning far enough to the side if you can slide your hand under your buttock and upper thigh.

Maintain this leaning position for at least 15 seconds.

Shift weight to the opposite side and repeat the procedure.

Do this every 15 minutes throughout the time you are in the chair.

Wheelchair Push-ups or Lifts

Make sure your chair is well fitting and the leg rests keep your legs in proper position for stability.

Lock wheechair brakes.

Make sure armrests are securely locked to the wheelchair.

Place both forearms on the wheelchair armrests, grasping them with both hands.

Push up with both hands/arms at the same time to raise hips and buttocks off the chair surface.

Hold this position for as long as is safely comfortable.

This technique puts pressure onto the shoulders, arms, hands, and elbows, so it may not be practical for those with upper extremity impairment or arthritis.

Repeat this pressure relief every 15 minutes throughout the time in the chair, or alternate with wheelchair leans, repositioning, or other methods.

---

be used for those doing self-inspection. However, it is wise to have another person help monitor the skin periodically in places that are difficult to visualize. Additionally, patients need to be reminded that when impaired circulation or sensation is present, pressure ulcers can develop and no pain may be felt. Inspection must take the place of pressure and pain receptors that can no longer warn the patient of an impending problem.

Managing Moisture

Another factor to consider in prevention of skin breakdown is managing moisture that can occur as a result of perspiration or incontinence. Perspiration can cause rashes, particularly in skinfold areas of the older person. Although elders do perspire less, the absence of air conditioning in many homes in the community as well as long-term care facilities makes skin problems from overly warm conditions a challenge to treat. Inadequate drying in places such as the groin, under the breasts, or between the toes can maintain a moist environment that promotes fungal growth.

The groin area is the most common place for a rash to develop in both males and females. Women often develop excoriation under the breasts, particularly those who are obese and have poor hygiene. The nurse should examine these areas when performing an initial assessment and take proper steps to prevent even minor skin irritation. The best treatment for a rash remains keeping the skin clean and dry and open to air when possible. Creams and powders can be effective in treating rashes, but cleansing of the skin must be done between applications. This is sometimes difficult and can result in further irritation. If not properly instructed, patients and family members can complicate skin problems by rubbing the fragile areas too hard during bathing or using a rough washcloth in cleansing, causing breaks and bleeding in the already compromised area. If this occurs, the area should then be treated as a wound and no longer simply as a rash.

Bowel and bladder incontinence are significant contributors to skin breakdown in older rehabilitation patients. The ultimate goal here is for continence to be achieved so that this is no longer a problem. Bowel and bladder training should be instituted as soon as rehabilitation begins, although this is highly dependent on the patient's physical condition at that time. As a general rule, Foley catheters are discontinued as soon as possible during rehabilitation (see Chapter 8). However, in serious situations, if the patient has a wound or chronic skin condition and is incontinent, the decision may be made by the rehabilitation team (particularly the nurse and the physician) to leave the catheter in place until skin integrity can be improved. If a patient with skin breakdown develops urinary incontinence, it is sometimes preferable to insert an indwelling Foley catheter into the bladder until the wound has time to heal than to try to manage both confounding problems at once. All factors should be considered carefully before making such a decision, realizing that insertion of a Foley catheter is one of the least desirable methods for bladder maintenance in rehabilitation patients. The use of an external catheter is a less invasive option for males, but little success has been shown with female external devices.

For patients with fecal incontinence, bowel retraining is essential. Although there are some devices for managing bowel incontinence and diarrhea available on the market, their application and maintenance make them difficult to use. The best way to remedy bowel incontinence is through establishment of a bowel program. Once other causes of incontinence have been ruled out, such as bacteria (e.g., *Clostridium difficile*) or other pathologic causes, the nurse begins a management program by balancing controllable factors such as diet, fluids, activity, timing, positioning, and medications. These are discussed further in Chapter 8.

Promoting Nutrition

Nutrition is another key in preventing skin breakdown in the older adult, as well as in promoting wound healing. Adequate nutrition and vitamins improve the health of the skin and its ability to withstand adverse forces such as pressure. Malnutrition has been associated with greater incidence of pressure sores in elderly orthopedic patients (Closs, 1993). Elders should receive 35 kcal/kg body weight as a goal, with at least 20% of those calories as protein. An increase in protein (to 25% of caloric intake) has been shown to significantly improve pressure ulcer healing in those receiving enteral hyperalimentation (Lipschitz, 1995). Albumin levels of less than 3.5 g/dl, total lymphocyte counts of less than 1800 mm³, and weight less than 80% of ideal are considered nutritional risk factors (Bergstrom et al., 1994). Significant relationships have been found between low serum protein levels and the development of pressure sores (Winslow, 1992) as well as increased morbidity and mortality in elderly rehabilitation patients (Sullivan & Walls, 1994; Sullivan, Walls, & Bopp, 1995). Adequate dietary protein is essential in healing pressure ulcers (Waltman et al., 1991). Vitamins A, E, and C as well as iron and zinc are especially important in wound healing (Gogia, 1992; Silane & Oot-Giromini, 1990). An example of a flow chart for nutritional assessment and support appears in Figure 6–2.

Adequate hydration is another need (Warren et al., 1994). Most institutionalized elders do not consume enough fluids per day to maintain good hydration without reminders or assistance from staff. Those chronically ill elderly living in the community, particularly those with functional disabilities that affect activities of daily living (ADLs), may find it difficult to meet the needed requirements. Although the recommended 2 to 3 L of fluid per day can seem overwhelming, older rehabilitation patients can be taught to consume smaller amounts of liquids throughout the day to meet these goals. This is discussed in subsequent chapters.

Managing Additional Sources of Friction, Pressure, Shearing Force, or Trauma

As previously mentioned, sources of friction and pressure for those with disabilities may also come in the form of adaptive equipment. Splints may be applied to prevent contractures or provide stability. Slings are used to support hemiplegic upper extremities. Ankle-foot orthoses are often provided to stroke or brain-injured patients to assist with stability in ambulation. Temporary casts may be applied in cases where spasticity threatens to permanently decrease range of motion. Immobilizers or casts may be issued for patients with fractures. Wheelchairs are used by many patients with impaired physical mobility. All of these helpful pieces of adaptive equipment aid healing or make life easier for individuals with functional impairments yet pose a significant threat to skin integrity for patients who have decreased circulation and sensation and more fragile skin.

Even the rehabilitation process itself with all the turning, transferring, positioning, and ambulating done by patients as they learn to care for themselves again can cause bumps, bruises, and tears. Nurses need to identify these potential hazards related to skin breakdown and take necessary steps to prevent injury. The skin should be checked frequently throughout the day whenever any type of adaptive equipment is being used.

Causes of skin and tissue damage from equipment used in rehabilitation can be categorized as friction, pressure, shearing force, or trauma. Friction occurs when the skin moves against another surface, producing abrasions and tears, such as the rubbing of a hand splint against the wrist. Pressure injuries occur when tissues are subjected to a prolonged period of unrelieved pressure. These are the most common sources of wounds in the debilitated elderly. Shearing force refers to injury to tissues when the skin remains

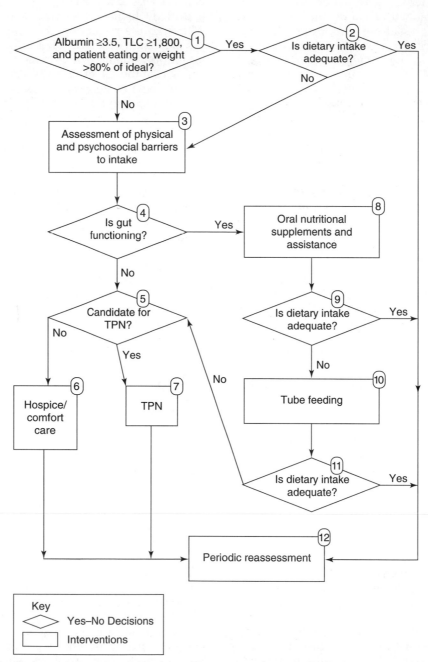

Figure 6–2 Flow chart for nutritional assessment and support. (From Bergstrom, N., Bennett, M. A., & Carlson, C. E., et al. (1994, December). *Pressure ulcer treatment. Clinical practice guideline.* Quick Reference Guide for Clinicians, No. 15 (AHCPR Pub. No. 95-0653). Rockville, MD: U.S. Department of Health and Human Services, Public Health Service, Agency for Health Care Policy and Research.)

stationary while other tissues slide. Examples include when a patient slides down in bed as the head of the bed is raised, or when a sliding board is used for transfers.

The term *trauma* can be used to refer generally to any other injury that occurs to skin that does not fall into the other categories. Examples include bruising, lacerations, or abrasions from hitting, bumping into, or falling onto furniture such as a table, bed, or chair, as occurs when patients who are unsteady are transferring or ambulating. Although these injuries could probably be technically classified as pressure, friction, or shearing force, the word trauma is used to better describe the cause of injury.

One significant source of trauma in the rehabilitation of older adults is the wheelchair. Patients with hemiplegia or with one-sided neglect can unknowingly catch their fingers in the spokes or pinch body parts when repositioning. The GRN must take special care during transfers to keep body parts properly aligned and free from harm. Table 6–3 lists commonly used items that could cause injury to the patient's skin.

An additional source of potential skin im-

Table 6–3 POTENTIAL SOURCES OF SKIN IMPAIRMENT FROM DEVICES USED IN REHABILITATION

Equipment	Type of Force
Sliding boards	Friction
Wheelchair	Pressure, shearing, trauma
Splints	Pressure, friction
Ankle-foot orthoses	Pressure, friction
Immobilizers	Pressure, friction
Continuous passive motion machines	Pressure, friction
Furniture	Trauma
Bed	Shearing force, pressure
Casts	Pressure, friction
Nasogastric tubes	Friction
Slings	Pressure, friction
Prostheses	Pressure, friction, trauma
Reachers, grabbers	Trauma
Long-handled shoe horn	Shearing force
Universal cuffs/ adaptive eating utensils	Pressure, friction
Tub chair	Shearing force
Lift chair	Pressure, friction
Lifting by staff	Shearing force, friction

pairment is the activities that are necessary when staff is assisting the older patient to transfer from one place to another. Skin tears, abrasions, and bruises are likely possibilities even when precautions are taken, just by virtue of the active nature of the rehabilitation regimen. A patient's risk can be reduced by following a few simple guidelines. A gait belt over clothing should be used for all transfers to avoid pulling on the patient's skin, a significant risk factor for skin tears. The gait belt allows the nurse to guide and stabilize the patient who requires assistance to stand or transfer, but it decreases the risk of trauma to the frail skin that may occur with arm-to-arm or other "pulling" types of transfers. Using safe transfer techniques and good body alignment is essential. Proper transfer techniques are discussed in later chapters. Additionally, patients with tendencies to bruise easily, or with particularly delicate skin, can dress in clothing that provides additional protection during therapies, such as long-sleeved shirts, sweat pants, or even Isotoner gloves. Lift sheets should always be used to move patients in bed, and mechanical lifts can help minimize friction and shearing force for those who require total assistance to transfer.

Some research has been done on pressure relief devices and the development of pressure ulcers on older patients with limited mobility. Although it has been demonstrated that pressure-reducing surfaces help reduce the risk of pressure sores, results have been inconclusive with regard to which types of pressure-relieving/reducing support surfaces are most effective (Kemp et al., 1993; Lazzara & Buschmann, 1991; Pase, 1994).

Treatment of Pressure Ulcers

The GRN, in many settings, is largely responsible for management of pressure ulcers if a clinical nurse specialist (CNS) consultant is not available. However, nursing assistants and licensed practical nurses may carry out the care at the bedside in long-term care facilities. Physicians often look to nurses for recommendations on protocol to treat wounds. Home health care nurses have more autonomy, and thus greater responsibility, for managing wounds, as well as documentation and educating clients and caregivers.

One way for GRNs to become acquainted with proper wound management is to develop guidelines for practice based on staging, color, and amount of drainage. Following proper skin care protocols reduces the prevalence of pressure ulcers in older patients (Hunter et al., 1995; Kemp & Krouskop, 1994; Levine & Totolos, 1995). Table 6–4 gives an example of a protocol used on a rehabilitation unit, using currently recommended guidelines from the Agency for Health Care Policy and Research (AHCPR).

Basic Guidelines for Treatment of Pressure Ulcers

There are some general wound care principles that will help guide care of pressure ulcers. The goal of treatment is to promote wound healing by establishing a suitable environment for the body to heal itself (Dimant & Francis, 1988; Gosnell, 1987). Preventive measures should be practiced with all elderly rehabilitation patients. Purulent wounds should be cultured. Necrotic wounds should be debrided. Red areas should not be massaged, and heat lamps are no longer used, because both these formerly acceptable interventions

cause further damage to surrounding tissue. Normal saline is the best wound irrigant, and all wounds should be regularly cleansed. Povidone-iodine solutions (such as Betadine) or hydrogen peroxide should not be used on any open wound because they damage granulation tissue and are considered cytotoxic. Other commercially available wound cleansers should be used with caution, because they may impair wound healing if used in certain concentrations (Bergman-Evans, Cuddigan, & Bergstrom, 1994). Topical therapy is also controversial, and the role of antibiotics in open wound treatment has not been established (Baxter & Rodeheaver, 1990; Fowler, 1982; Stone, 1991). In the case of smaller, shallow wounds in a relatively healthy patient, topical therapy can be effective (Doughty, 1992). Chemical debriding ointments (e.g., Santyl, Elase) are placed in the wound on necrotic tissue, not on the surrounding skin. Such enzymatics will deteriorate healthy tissue as

Table 6–4 SKIN CARE PROTOCOL BASED ON STAGE AND AMOUNTS OF WOUND DRAINAGE

	Stage I	Stage II	Stage III–IV		
			Red wound	Yellow wound	Black wound
Cleansing	Normal saline	Normal saline	Normal saline	Normal saline	Normal saline
Pressure relief	Air mattress Heel protectors	Air mattress Heel protectors	Special mattress (e.g., ROHO) or bed (e.g., KinAir) Heel protectors Rotation clock	Special mattress (e.g., ROHO) or bed (e.g., KinAir) Heel protectors Rotation clock	Special mattress or bed Heel protectors Rotation clock
Dressings	Occlusive or film Thin hydrocolloid	Occlusive or film Thin hydrocolloid with/ without border	Hydrogels Hydrocolloids Silvadene cream (for small amounts of drainage)	Hydrogels (for small amounts of drainage) Absorptive (for moderate amounts of drainage) Wound filler or absorptive dressing (for heavy drainage) Gauze	Occlusive or film (for small wounds or intact skin) Hydrocolloids Hydrogels Gauze
Debridement	None	4 × 4 NS wet-to-damp	4 × 4 NS wet-to-damp	4 × 4 NS wet-to-dry Chemical debridement (e.g., Santyl)	4 × 4 NS wet-to-dry Chemical debridement (e.g., Elase ointment)

NS, normal saline.
Adapted from Geri Smith, St. Margaret Hospital and Healthcare Centers, Hammond, IN.

well. Discussion of how to choose the type of dressing for specific wounds is contained in following sections.

A healthy wound bed looks red and fleshy. This signifies the appearance of granulation tissue (phase II, proliferative). The wound needs to be protected from further insult. A wet-to-dry dressing would not be used on a wound with this type of tissue, because the gauze can tear the new granulation tissue out of the wound bed. An exception should be noted in the case of the wound that appears healthy but does not heal over a long period of time. This non-healing wound should be cultured and closely examined for the presence of unusual fibrotic tissue (Krasner, 1995). If a subtle infection or abnormal tissue is present, consult a physician specializing in wound care. Chronic wounds need to be treated as a disability (Neal, 1995). Such wounds affect a person's health, sense of well-being, susceptibility to infection, risk of further complications, and ability to rehabilitate and perform self-care.

Familiarity with the mechanisms of various types of dressings aids in understanding which types to use. Two basic types are gauze and occlusive. Gauze-type dressings include commonly used products such as Telfa, Kling, and Adaptic. Impregnated gauze dressings include Vaseline, Aquaphor, and Xeroform. These dressings are useful for absorbing wound exudate and debriding surface necrotic tissue (Mertz, 1990). However, they are not as effective in wound healing as occlusive dressings. A more thorough discussion related to choosing dressings follows.

There are specific advantages to occlusive, or moisture-retentive, dressings. Occlusive dressings speed wound healing by facilitating a moist, protected environment for new tissue to grow. They also reduce pain, tenderness, and scarring. The most commonly used occlusive dressings can be categorized as films (e.g., Bioclusive, Op-Site, Tegaderm), hydrogels (e.g., elastogel, Spenco, Vigilon), hydrocolloids (e.g., DuoDerm, IntraSite, Tegasorb), copolymers (e.g., Lyofoam, Epilock, Kontour), and wound fillers in the form of beads, gels, granules, or pastes (e.g., Debrisan, DuoDerm granules, IntraSite gel, Comfeel paste).

Film dressings are transparent and usually waterproof. They provide an additional "skin" to cover the wound, are conforming and flexible, and facilitate autolytic debridement. Hydrogel dressings are also transparent or translucent and are composed mainly of water. They cool the wound, may reduce inflammation and pain, and are easier to remove unless allowed to dry. Hydrocolloids provide protection to the wound, shielding it from external bacteria, are waterproof and comfortable, and promote autolytic debridement by maintaining a moist environment. Hydrocolloids have been shown to enhance wound healing (Yarkony et al., 1984). Copolymers, or composite polymeric dressings, have different layers that serve different functions—with one layer being absorbent and another occlusive—to maintain a suitable wound environment. Wound fillers are used for absorption of exudate for heavily draining wounds.

Because there is such a vast array of products available for wound care, it is wise for the GRN to develop and follow a particular protocol, such as the hospital or facility policy. An example is shown in Table 6–4. This ensures continuity and allows better evaluation of the effectiveness of certain products. Most facilities order those dressings to be available for use but will evaluate new products on a regular basis.

Historically, different types of wound treatments have been used effectively in a variety of settings, but GRNs should search the research literature for current studies on less traditional treatments. Some less traditional topical treatments have included Maalox, sugar, insulin, cornstarch, egg white, honey paste, and various combinations of items commonly found in one's kitchen. Maggots were commonly used for wound debridement, particularly on servicemen during times of war. When current traditional methods fail, the GRN should be mindful that there are many options for care that have been used with success in the past. The nursing interventions discussed here are based on current recommendations of wound care experts.

Specific Nursing Interventions

Stage I Ulcers: A transparent dressing for reddened areas provides an additional layer of protection for the skin. These dressings are permeable to moisture but keep bacteria out. They provide the added benefit of allowing the nurse to visualize and monitor the area. However, these dressings are often flimsy and are difficult to keep in place, especially in areas such as the coccyx or on patients who are actively participating in therapy. Patients with incontinence require more frequent dressing changes. Stage I ulcers have intact skin and can be cleansed per hospital routine. Sprays such as Granulex are used routinely in some facilities to prevent breakdown. It is particularly important to follow preventive measures before further injury occurs. Strict adherence to skin care protocol, especially pressure relief techniques, is often all that is needed in a well-nourished, rehabilitating elder to eliminate stage I pressure areas.

Stage II Ulcers: Cleansing is done with normal saline. Stage II ulcers are treated with a variety of dressings. Film dressings may be the choice if there is little or no drainage, particularly for dry blisters. A thin hydrocolloid dressing with a tape border is another option, depending on the size and appearance of the wound. Taping or "picture framing" dressings must be done with care, because the tape can cause additional trauma to already compromised elderly skin. If any debriding is needed, a gauze dressing with wet-to-damp normal saline can be used.

Stage III or IV Ulcers: The color (red, yellow, black) system is useful here in choosing treatment methods. Red wounds need a clean, protected, moist environment to promote wound healing. Red wounds can be treated with a variety of dressings. For those with small amounts of drainage, a hydrocolloid dressing such as IntraSite or DuoDerm has been shown to be effective (Krasner, 1995; Levine & Totolos, 1995). These dressings form a soft gel over the wound, which generally can be removed without injury. However, there is a danger that newly formed skin can also be removed, so care should be taken. It must be noted that hydrocolloid adhesive dressings are designed to stay in place for up to 7 days. If dressing changes must be done daily because of incontinence or increased amounts of drainage, a different dressing should be selected. Taping around all four sides of the hydrocolloid dressing to form a seal may help it remain in place during therapeutic activities. Silvadene cream, commonly used for burns, is also quite effective for some patients. Wet-to-damp dressings may also be used. Wet-to-dry dressings are contraindicated because the dry gauze can tear the new granulation tissue when the dressing is removed.

Yellow wounds indicate either infection or fibrous slough (Krasner, 1995). Any such material must be removed from the wound bed to encourage growth of healthy tissue. Yellow wounds often are malodorous and have larger amounts of drainage. If infection is suspected (Table 6–5), a culture should be done (Table 6–6). Frequent dressing changes and cleansing via irrigation with saline may be necessary. Irrigation is best done with a device that provides pressures between 4 and 15 pounds per square inch (psi) (Bergstrom et al., 1994). Bulb syringes are not adequate, because they provide too little pressure for proper cleansing, whereas devices such as the Water Pik deliver excessive pressure, which can damage the wound bed. A saline squeeze bottle with irrigation cap (4.5 psi) or a 35-ml syringe with a 19-gauge needle (8.0 psi) is preferable (Bergstrom et al., 1994). Choices of dressings for yellow wounds depend on the amount of drainage present. Absorptive dressings such as wound fillers with a sea-

Table 6–5 SIGNS OF WOUND INFECTION

Increased erythema
Edema
Purulence
Warmth at the site
Elevated temperature (this can be slight in the older adult, even as low as 99°F)
Elevated white blood cell count
Pain
Bacterial concentration of greater than 100,000 organisms per gram of tissue

Table 6–6 SUGGESTIONS FOR OBTAINING A WOUND CULTURE

Obtain a swab culture only if unable to aspirate wound tissue fluid or have tissue biopsied.

Cleanse the wound first with saline. Any purulent exudate may contain bacteria that is not the primary cause of infection.

Using a sterile calcium aginate swab (not cotton), swab around the wound and edges 10 times, or 30 seconds, in a diagonal pattern. Try to cover the entire wound surface of clean, granulating tissue, rotating the swab as you go. This will ensure a better and more accurate culture of the wound bed.

Avoid swabbing the wound margins.

Do not swab over any hard, black eschar.

Immediately put the culture swab in a gel-based container and label properly.

Based on guidelines by Baxter & Rodeheaver, 1990; Burdette-Taylor & Taylor, 1993.

weed base are often used. Occlusive dressings are not used over areas of infection or extensive necrosis (Levine & Totolos, 1995). Wet-to-dry gauze dressings aid in debridement and may be less costly than other products. If bleeding occurs when removing the dry gauze dressing, treatment must be reevaluated, because this indicates that circulation has improved in the wound bed and granulation tissue has formed. Some long-term care physicians use this sign as an indicator for when the GRN should call them for further wound treatment orders. The GRN knowledgeable in the field of wound care can provide information to the physician and the health care team about the appearance of the wound without waiting for signs of bleeding as occurs when the new granulation tissue is stripped from the wound bed on removal of wet-to-dry dressings.

Black wounds generally require removal of necrotic tissue to promote healing. Necrosis can be debrided using several techniques: surgical, enzymatic, mechanical, or autolytic. Choice of debridement method depends on the nature and extent of the wound. An enzymatic debriding ointment such as Elase may be ordered. A large absorptive dressing, such as Kaltostat, can be used for an ulcer with heavy drainage. Black wounds that are intact (as in heel blisters) are not generally punctured or debrided, but protected. If such wounds become open, more aggressive treatment and debridement is indicated. Standard treatment protocol for treatment of closed black wounds varies throughout the country and according to available resources.

Wound Clinics/Wound Care Centers

Wound clinics, or wound care centers, are now popular in the United States as a place for interdisciplinary treatment of difficult-to-heal chronic wounds. These clinics treat mainly outpatients with stubborn, complicated wounds and are overseen by a physician with expertise in this area. The newest and most recent research techniques, sometimes experimental, are used for those whose wounds have not healed with any conventional methods. It is not unusual for patients attending a wound clinic to report wounds that have taken longer than a year to heal.

EVALUATION

Evaluation of skin integrity is an ongoing process. Thorough assessment and identification of risk factors are the first steps in preventing skin breakdown. Risk assessment tools such as those by Braden and Norton are useful in documenting the likelihood of pressure ulcers. However, the use of these scales in the gerontological rehabilitation population is questionable. Examination of the tools in use and their appropriateness for the types of patients being cared for should be discussed among the nursing staff. Tools are helpful for documentation purposes, but more research is needed to identify key problems for the older and disabled patient whose unique deficits are not included in traditional forms.

The outcomes related to maintaining and improving skin integrity that the GRN would expect to see include the patient being free from skin breakdown as well as signs and symptoms of this occurring (such as redness, edema, and pruritus). This is evaluated by daily assessment. Symptoms such as itching can be controlled with creams or medication. If breakdown is found to occur, reevaluation of preventive measures in use is indicated, as well as treatment of existing problems. The reduction of identified controllable risk factors is another desired outcome. The nurse can develop appropriate interventions and also observe improvements for all factors that compromise skin integrity and impede wound healing, such as poor nutrition, poor hygiene, smoking, obesity, the presence of adaptive devices, and lack of activity.

With regard to wound healing, the GRN would expect a decrease in wound size and the amount of drainage. Evidence of the stages of wound healing can be observed. Precise documentation of these observations is extremely important, not only from an evaluative standpoint, but also because of reimbursement issues. Home visits made by nurses for wound care are reimbursable under Medicare and Medicaid, yet evidence of progress in wound healing must be shown. This is documented through decreased amounts of wound drainage and progressively smaller size of the wound.

The nurse will not be able to prevent every pressure ulcer. A few debilitated and malnourished patients will experience skin breakdown regardless of strict nursing interventions. However, most pressure ulcers can be prevented, and this is largely a nursing measure. Appropriate preventive measures and continuous, thorough evaluations are necessary to ensure desired outcomes.

REFERENCES

Aptaker, R. L., Roth, E. J., Reichhardt, G., Duerden, M. E., & Levy, C. E. (1994). Serum albumin level as a predictor of geriatric stroke rehabilitation outcome. *Archives of Physical Medicine and Rehabilitation, 75*, 80–84.

Baxter, C. R., & Mertz P. M. (1990). Local factors that affect wound healing. In W. H. Eaglstein (Ed.), *New directions in wound healing: Wound care manual* (pp. 25–37). Princeton, NJ: Squibb & Sons.

Baxter, C. R., & Rodeheaver, G. T. (1990). Wound assessment and categorization. In W. H. Eaglstein (Ed.), *New directions in wound healing: Wound care manual* (pp. 55–69). Princeton, NJ: Squibb & Sons.

Bergman-Evans, B., Cuddigan, J., & Bergstrom, N. (1994). Clinical practice guidelines: Prediction and prevention of pressure ulcers. *Journal of Gerontological Nursing, 20*(9), 19–26.

Bergstrom, N., Bennett, M. A., Carlson, C. E., et al. (1994). *Pressure ulcer treatment. Clinical practice guideline.* Quick reference guide for clinicians, No. 15 (AHCPR Pub. No. 95-0653). Rockville, MD: U.S. Department of Health and Human Services, Public Health Service, Agency for Health Care Policy and Research.

Bergstrom, N., Braden, B.J., & Laguzza, A. (1987). The Braden Scale for predicting pressure sore risk. *Nursing Research, 36*, 205–210.

Brower, H. T., & Crist, M. A. (1985). Research priorities in gerontological nursing for long-term care. *Image, 17*(1), 22–27.

Buelow, J. M., & Jamieson, D. (1990). Potential for altered nutritional states in the stroke patient. *Rehabilitation Nursing, 15*(5), 260–263.

Burdette-Taylor, S., & Taylor, T. G. (1993). Wound cultures: What, when and how. *Ostomy/Wound Management, 39*(8), 26–32.

Closs, S. J. (1993). Malnutrition: The key to pressure sores? *Nursing Standard, 8*(4), 32–36.

Conine, T. A., Choi, A. K., & Lim, R. (1989). The user friendliness of protective support surfaces in prevention of pressure sores. *Rehabilitation Nursing, 14*(5), 261–263.

Dimant, J., & Francis, M. E. (1988). Pressure sore prevention and management. *Journal of Gerontological Nursing, 14*(8), 18–25.

Doughty, D. (1992). Topical therapy: From concepts to results. *Ostomy/Wound Management, 38*(8), 16–24.

Flett, R., Harcourt, B., & Alpass, F. (1994). Psychosocial aspects of chronic lower leg ulceration in the elderly. *Western Journal of Nursing Research, 16*(2), 183–192.

Fowler, E. (1982). Pressure sores: A deadly nuisance. *Journal of Gerontological Nursing, 8*(12), 680–685.

Gawron, C. L. (1994). Risk factors for and prevalence of pressure ulcers among hospitalized patients. *Journal of Wound, Ostomy, & Continence Nursing, 21*(6), 232–240.

Gogia, P. P. (1992). The biology of wound healing. *Ostomy/Wound Management, 38*(9), 12–22.

Gosnell, D. J. (1973). An assessment tool to identify pressure sores. *Nursing Research, 22*(1), 55–59.

Gosnell, D. J. (1987). Assessment and evaluation of pressure sores. *Nursing Clinics of North America, 22*(2), 399–415.

Hunter, S. M., Langemo, D. K., Olson, B., Hanson, D., Cathcart-Silberberg, T., Burd, C., & Sauvage, T. R. (1995). The effectiveness of skin care protocols for pressure ulcers. *Rehabilitation Nursing, 29*(5), 250–255.

Iverson-Carpenter, M. S. (1988). Impaired skin integrity. *Journal of Gerontological Nursing, 14*(3), 25–29.

Kemp, M. G., Kopanke, D., Tordecilla, L., Fogg, L., Shott, S., Matthiesen, V., & Johnson, B. (1993). The role of support surfaces and patient attributes in preventing pressure ulcers in elderly patients. *Research in Nursing and Health, 16*(2), 89–96.

Kemp, M. G., & Krouskop, T. A. (1994). Pressure ulcers: Reducing incidence and severity by managing pressure. *Journal of Gerontological Nursing, 29*(9), 27–34.

Krasner, D. (1995). Wound care: How to use the red-yellow-black system. *American Journal of Nursing, 95*(5), 44–47.

LaMantia, J. G. (1996). Skin integrity. In S. P. Hoeman (Ed.), *Rehabilitation nursing: Process and application*. St. Louis, MO: C. V. Mosby.

Lazzara, D. J., & Buschmann, M. T. (1991). Prevention of pressure ulcers in elderly nursing home residents: Are special support surfaces the answer? *Decubitus, 4*(4), 42–44, 46.

Levine, J. M., Simpson, M., & McDonald, R. J. (1989). Pressure sores: A plan for primary care prevention. *Geriatrics, 44*(4), 75–90.

Levine, J. M., & Totolos, E. (1995). Pressure ulcers: A strategic plan to prevent and heal them. *Geriatrics, 50*(1), 32–37.

Lipschitz, D. A. (1995). Approaches to the nutritional support of the older patient. In D. A. Lipschitz (Ed.), *Clinics in Geriatric Medicine, 11*(4), 715–724.

Maklebust, J. (1987). Pressure ulcers: Etiology and prevention. *Nursing Clinics of North America, 22*(2), 359–377.

Mertz, P. M. (1990). Intervention: Dressing effects on wound healing. In W. H. Eaglstein (Ed.), *New directions in wound healing: Wound care manual* (pp. 83–96). Princeton, NJ: Squibb & Sons.

Mikulic, M. A. (1980). Treatment of pressure ulcers. *American Journal of Nursing, 80*(6), 1125–1128.

Miller, L. (1995). Maintaining skin integrity: Setting the standard in a rehabilitation facility. *Rehabilitation Nursing, 20*(5), 273–277.

Mueller, M. J., Allen, B. R., & Sinacore, D. R. (1995). Incidence of skin breakdown and higher amputation after transmetatarsal amputation: Implications for rehabilitation. *Archives of Physical Medicine and Rehabilitation, 76*, 50–54.

National Pressure Ulcer Advisory Panel (NPUAP). (1989). Pressure ulcers prevalence, cost and risk assessment: Consensus development conference statement. *Decubitus, 2*(2), 24–28.

Neal, L. J. (1995). The rehabilitation nurse in the home care setting: Treating chronic wounds as a disability. *Rehabilitation Nursing, 29*(5), 261–264.

Pajik, M., Craven, G. A., Cameron-Barry, J., Shipps, T., & Bennum, N. W. (1986). Investigating the problem of pressure sores. *Journal of Gerontological Nursing, 12*(7), 11–16.

Pase, M. N. (1994). Pressure relief devices, risk factors, and development of pressure ulcers in elderly patients with limited mobility. *Advances in Wound Care: The Journal for Prevention and Healing, 7*(2), 38–42.

Patterson, R. P., Cranmer, H. H., Fisher, S. V., & Engel, R. R. (1993). The impaired response of spinal cord injured individuals to repeated surface pressure loads. *Archives of Physical Medicine and Rehabilitation, 74*(9), 947–953.

Patterson, R. P., & Fisher, S. V. (1986). Sitting pressure-time patterns in patients with quadriplegia. *Archives of Physical Medicine and Rehabilitation, 67*(11), 812–814.

Pinchcofsky-Devin, G. D., & Kaminski, M. V., Jr. (1986). Correlation of pressure sores and nutritional status. *Journal of the American Geriatric Society, 34*(6), 435–440.

Rudolph, R., & Shannon, M. L. (1990). The normal healing process. In W. H. Eaglstein (Ed.), *New directions in wound healing: Wound care manual* (pp. 7–24). Princeton, NJ: Squibb & Sons.

Silane, M., & Oot-Giromini, B. (1990). Systemic and other factors that affect wound healing. In W. H. Eaglstein (Ed.), *New directions in wound healing: Wound care manual* (pp. 39–53). Princeton, NJ: Squibb & Sons.

Sparks, S. M. (1993). Clincial validation of pressure ulcer risk factors. *Ostomy/Wound Management, 39*(4), 40–41, 43–46.

Stone, J. T. (1991). Pressure sores. In W. C. Chenitz, J. T. Stone, & S. A. Salisbury (Eds.), *Clinical gerontological nursing: A guide to advanced practice* (pp. 247–265). Philadelphia: W. B. Saunders.

Sullivan, D. H., & Walls, R. C. (1994). Impact of nutritional status on morbidity in a population of geriatric rehabilitation patients. *Journal of the American Geriatrics Society, 42*(5), 471–477.

Sullivan, D. H., Walls, R. C., & Bopp, M. M. (1995). Protein-energy undernutrition and the risk of mortality within one year of hospital discharge: A follow-up study. *Journal of the American Geriatrics Society, 43*(5), 507–512.

Waltman, N. L., Bergstrom, N., Armstrong, N., Norvell, K., & Braden, B. (1991). Nutritional status, pressure sores, and mortality in elderly patients with cancer. *Oncology Nursing Forum, 18*(5), 867–873.

Warren, J. L., Bacon, W. E., Harris, R., McBean, A. M., Foley, D. J., & Phillips, C. (1994). The burden and outcomes associated with dehydration among U.S. elderly, 1991. *American Journal of Public Health, 84*(8), 1265–1269.

Williams, A. (1972). A study of factors contributing to skin breakdown. *Nursing Research, 21*(3), 238–243.

Winslow, M. N. B. (1992). Commentary on intrinsic factors associated with pressure sores in elderly people. *ONS Nursing Scan in Oncology, 1*(4), 3.

Yarkony, G. M., Kramer, E., King, R., Lukane, C., & Carle, T. V. (1984). Pressure sore management: Efficacy of a moisture reactive occlusive dressing. *Archives of Physical Medicine and Rehabilitation, 65*(10), 597–600.

Chapter 7

Promoting Mobility and Functional Independence

Activity may be the single most important factor for older adults in maintaining or recovering health and wellness. The person who has experienced functional deficits as the result of chronic illness or a physical insult may have lost the ability to ambulate independently. Yet this basic skill of being able to walk is often the chief goal of patients in rehabilitation. Ambulation has been associated with survival, and "recovery of ambulation is an excellent index of rehabilitation outcome" (Kauffman, Albright, & Wagner, 1987). A positive relationship has been found between health and movement, particularly walking cadence (Engle, 1986).

Although an age of older than 75 years has often been considered a negative factor in rehabilitation, many studies have suggested that older patients can improve functional outcomes with rehabilitation (Engle, 1986; Williams, Oberst, & Bjorklund, 1994). Persons 90 years and older with hip fracture have also shown improvement with the guidance of a physical therapist (Kauffman et al., 1987). However, prognosis for rehabilitation depends greatly on the prefracture functional status of these patients (Cheng et al., 1989; Thorngren, 1994). Stroke patients who practiced weight bearing exercises showed improved walking outcomes (Nugent, Schurr, & Adams, 1994). Likewise, early and intense gait therapy is critical to facilitate early ambulation in the elderly after a stroke (Richards et al., 1993). Increased ambulatory skills have also been associated with a decrease in the number of falls experienced (Galindo-Ciocon, Ciocon, & Galindo, 1995b; Koroknay, Werner,

Cohen-Mansfield, & Braun, 1995). Table 7–1 lists several nursing diagnoses common to elderly rehabilitation patients with regard to functional capacity.

ASSESSMENT

There are many factors related to assessment of function and mobility. These include the ability to perform a variety of tasks related to activities of daily living (ADLs). These tasks include grooming, dressing, toileting, walking, eating, and getting in and out of the bed or chair. Other activities are also important to the health and well-being of adults (Atwood, Holm, & James, 1994). The ability to perform instrumental activities of daily living (IADLs) is also important to include in any assess-

Table 7–1 COMMON NURSING DIAGNOSES RELATED TO FUNCTIONAL DISABILITIES

Impaired physical mobility
Activity intolerance
Decreased endurance
High risk for injury
Impaired balance
Dysfunctional gait pattern
Deconditioning
Self-care deficit syndrome
Disuse syndrome
Impaired home maintenance management
Diversional activity deficit
Fear
Alteration in urinary elimination: incontinence

ment. Such activities include shopping, handling money, preparing food, using the telephone, doing housework, and the like. For the older person with a functional limitation, some of these chores can seem impossible, because so many day-to-day routines require the ability to ambulate.

There are several components to consider when assessing the functional capacity of the aged. The gerontological rehabilitation nurse (GRN) should consider what the person was able to do a month ago, a week ago, and currently. Framing questions in this manner allows for comparisons across time. Additionally, the person's potential functional status, both short-term (for example, in 2 weeks) and long-term (in 6 months), should also be projected. Assessment scales have been developed to ascertain a person's functional status and to measure improvement during and after treatment. For seniors in general, rehabilitative treatment should ideally begin when the person first has difficulty completing IADLs and before diminished capacity for performing ADLs occurs.

In addition to using reliable tools, GRNs should observe patients for the effects of immobility. With general deconditioning, immobility negatively affects nearly every body system. Falls are another significant problem that can be related to decreased endurance, poor balance, and a variety of other factors. GRNs should be able to judge the patient's functional status by observing the patient's ability to transfer, perform ADLs and IADLs, and ambulate. The presence of poor trunk control, lack of balance, or general weakness should be evident during these activities.

Functional Scales

The purposes of functional assessment are to "determine physical functional status, document the need for interventions and services, devise a treatment plan, and assess and monitor progress" (Kelly-Hayes, 1996, p. 146). There are many types of scales, measuring different abilities, from physical functioning to socioeconomic factors to cognition. The scales used most often in gerontological rehabilitation to measure ADLs are the Barthel Index and the Functional Independence Measure (FIM) (from the Uniform Data System) (Appendix 7-A). Both instruments are considered reliable and valid. Table 7–2 gives a comparison and summary of both scales.

The FIM scale measures disability in several categories. It includes both cognitive and motor functions. Many rehabilitation facilities take an interdisciplinary approach to completing the FIM scale. Coding is done according to the set FIM levels of 1 to 7. The number rates the individual from total assistance (1) to complete independence (7). Each discipline is responsible for documenting a different section. For example, the GRN would complete scores for bladder and bowel management, whereas the speech therapist would document scores under communication and social cognition. In this way, an interdisciplinary team approach to care is maintained.

The FIM scale is also useful for measuring progress in the rehabilitative program. As overall scores are obtained on a regular basis, progress should be seen by higher FIM scores. Goals can be established, and predictions made, using quantitative measures. This is also helpful for insurance coverage purposes, to show progress in the rehabilitation program.

The evaluation of the FIM scale has been based mainly on its use with patients who have suffered a stroke or spinal cord injury. However, the use of the FIM to evaluate rehabilitation progress and predict outcomes with other disabilities is being explored. For example, in a study by Muecke, Shekar, Dwyer, Israel, and Flynn (1992) of nontraumatic, lower-limb amputees, the predictability of FIM scores was variable. Although modifications to the scale might better tailor it to this specific condition, it provided valuable data. In the case of lower-limb amputation, it was found that the lower scoring patients benefited most from hospitalization and had short stays, yet individual outcomes were highly variable. Additionally, not all tools work equally well in all settings. For example, the FIM tool may not work well for geriatric outpatients, although it is still used for these patients. Researchers continue to explore and develop new instruments to measure functional ability and to revise ones currently in use.

The Barthel Index measures mobility, self-care, and bowel and bladder control. Scores are assigned according to whether the patient needs assistance or is independent. Scores may range from 0 (complete dependence in all areas) to 100 (complete independence). This tool is useful in obtaining data and monitoring progress in ability to perform personal care ADLs as well as mobility.

More than 50 scales that measure functional status are available. Inpatient rehabili-

Table 7-2 MEASURES OF DISABILITY IN BASIC ACTIVITIES OF DAILY LIVING (ADLs)

Instrument	Description	Uses	Time Required to Administer	Strengths	Weaknesses
Barthel Index	Ordinal scale with total scores from 0 (totally dependent) to 20 (totally independent) (or 0 to 100 by multiplying each item score by 5). Ten items include bowel, bladder, feeding, grooming, dressing, transfers, toilet use, mobility, stairs, bathing.	Screening Assessment Monitoring Maintenance	5–10 min	Excellent reliability and validity. Widely used with stroke patients.	Ceiling effect in detecting change at higher level of functioning. Only fair sensitivity to change.
Functional Independence Measure (FIM)	18 items scored on a 7-point ordinal scale (7 = complete independence, 1 = total assistance). Total score ranges from 18–126. Subscores for motor function and cognition. Domains for self-care, sphincter control, mobility, locomotion, communication, and social cognition.	Screening Assessment Monitoring Maintenance	<40 min	Measure social cognition and functional communication as well as mobility and ADLs. Use of 7-point scale increases sensitivity as compared with other disability scales. Widely used in the United States and other countries.	Ceiling and floor effects at upper and lower ends of function. Clinician needs to be certified in use of tool.

Adapted from Gresham, G. E., Duncan, P. W., Stason, W. B., et al. (1995, May). *Post-stroke rehabilitation* (Clinical Practice Guideline, No. 16) (AHCPR Publication No. 95-0662). Rockville, MD: U. S. Department of Health and Human Services, Public Health Service, Agency for Health Care Policy and Research.

tation units and long-term care facilities regularly use functional assessment instruments. For home care GRNs, tools are useful, but they may be cumbersome and impractical given the community situation, unless being used for the purpose of research. Thus, physical indicators related to mobility and function may be more heavily relied on when planning care.

Physical Indicators

Endurance

Decreased endurance, which occurs commonly in elderly rehabilitation patients, can be the result of both the effects of age and the exhaustion or fatigue that a physical insult brings to the body. Activity intolerance is a common problem, especially with geriatric stroke patients (Mol & Baker, 1991). Fatigue is also a problem for persons with post-polio syndrome, multiple sclerosis, myasthenia gravis, and rheumatoid arthritis as well as those with chronic pain (Habel, 1996; Hymovich & Hagopian, 1992). Age-related issues such as polypharmacy, multiple interacting pathologies, depression, or the presence of cancer as well as expectations of endurance in old age are other factors to consider. Additionally, persons may become deconditioned from the effects of bedrest, so rehabilitation must be initiated early.

Little research has been done on the relationship of patients' feelings of fatigue to rehabilitation outcomes. More studies have focused on fatigue of persons other than the patient, such as the results of caregiver stress. However, the role of patients' fatigue in adaptation to chronic illness has recently received increased attention.

Daily exercise can improve endurance, particularly when muscle strength is increased, because these two factors are related (Jirovec, 1991; Milde, 1988). In one study, endurance training in a small sample of elderly nursing home patients showed a positive effect, but moreso in the upper extremities than the lower extremities. Pre-existing functional limitations may have resulted in a lack of training effect in this group (Naso, Carner, Blankfort-Doyle, & Coughey, 1990). This would not be surprising, because muscle strength and mass commonly decrease with age, even in the absence of disability, but especially with inactivity. In another study by Fisher, Pendergast, Gresham, and Calkins (1991a), a majority (75%) of a small sample of impaired nursing home residents completing a muscle strengthening program (n = 14) experienced a 35% improvement in endurance. This study used isometric and isotonic exercises, whereas the study by Naso et al. involved the use of equipment such as the stationary bicycle and treadmill. Both studies are limited in generalizability because of the small sample sizes and careful selection of patients. Still, these programs provide good examples of types of methods that need to be explored in relation to older patients and means of increasing endurance.

Muscle Strength

With a decrease in muscle strength comes less endurance and increased muscle fatigue. The rate of muscle strength loss is related mainly to activity, so the more movement present, the less a person should experience muscle weakness (Kasper, Maxwell, & White, 1996; Milde, 1988). Muscle rehabilitation, through a carefully constructed and implemented program, can help nursing home residents improve functional levels and increase independence (Fisher et al., 1991a). Older adults reported positive outcomes with strength training, such as improved body image, greater flexibility, increased strength, and increased self-confidence (Tinetti, 1986; Topp, Mikesky, & Bawel, 1994). Building endurance, muscle strengthening, and promoting ambulatory activities are, therefore, essential team activities.

Gait Speed/Walking Cadence

Gait speed is considered a useful indicator of ADL function in elderly patients (Engle, 1986; Gehlsen & Whaley, 1990a; Potter, Evans, & Duncan, 1995). The number of steps walked per minute, also known as walking cadence, has been shown to be stable for an individual over time. Using the Sickness Impact Profile (SIP), Engle (1986) found a positive relationship between health and walking cadence.

Although speed, or velocity, is not thought to improve in older adults in an activity program, such a factor is more useful as an indicator than a goal. The aged may have no desire or motivation to walk quickly; just to walk smoothly and "get there" may be enough. However, ambulatory ability is related to a decreased incidence in falls and remains of extreme importance in preventing untoward effects of immobility. A more intense, task-specific approach to physical therapy seems to correlate with optimal gait recovery in acute stroke patients (Richards et al., 1993).

Range of Motion

With increased age often comes a decrease in joint mobility and flexibility. Certain degrees of motion are necessary to perform specific skills. Treatment goals will be aimed at the patient's achieving at least the minimal recovery of function needed to perform ADLs. For example, the patient with a total knee replacement will be unable to ambulate without 0 to 90 degrees of extension/flexion at the knee. This is because it is difficult to walk without being able to straighten the knee (although some do) and difficult to get up from a chair without being able to put the legs underneath enough to stand from a sitting position.

Amputees face unique problems with regard to range of motion and ambulatory ability. Persons with transtibial prostheses are considered to have a greater risk of developing osteoarthritis in the non-affected leg (Lemaire & Fisher, 1994). This is mainly caused by the larger than normal load on the affected joint over a long period of time. Likewise, those patients living with lower extremity disabilities (spinal cord injury, amputation) since their younger years are almost certain to experience more arthritis in the upper extremity joints, particularly the shoulders, because the upper body was not designed to support the additional weight, for years, required to transfer independently.

The GRN must assist the patient and therapist by reinforcing the exercises done in therapy that prevent complications and improve function. Contractures can easily occur with the onset of a chronic problem. Such secondary losses must be prevented. Active and/or passive range of motion exercises must be done diligently, especially in the bed-bound patient who is unable to ambulate or perform self-care.

Patients with hemiplegia or hemiparesis may find their range of motion greatly affected. Subluxation can occur from atrophy of the shoulder muscles after stroke. This is not only painful but generally considered permanent, although it is often preventable. The GRN must be alert to the additional weight placed on the shoulder from the pulling of an unsupported arm. Shoulder slings or lapboards should be used at all times when the patient is out of bed. Reports from stroke patients indicate that range of motion exer-

cises were also helpful in reducing pain associated with the stroke or long periods of lying in bed.

Balance and Coordination

Good trunk control is needed for safe transfers and ambulation. Many elders experience dizziness and ataxia, even in the absence of disease or disabilities. Yet in the case of the person with acute stroke, an unsteady gait is common. Impaired balance has also been associated with fall risk, predicting the occurrence of multiple falls, and correlating with functional and motor performance in stroke patients (Berg, Wood-Dauphinee, Williams, & Maki, 1992).

Balance is critical for safe mobility (Patla, Frank, & Winter, 1992). Older persons are known to improve and maintain balance with physical therapy. Most successful methods seem to include individualized physical therapist–assisted gait training (Galindo-Ciocon et al., 1995b; Harada, Chiu, Fowler, Lee, & Reuben, 1995).

Socioemotional and Perceptual Factors

Mobility is a complex process. A decrease in mobility is not inevitable with age, but many older adults believe that going to a nursing home means becoming wheelchair bound (Tinetti, 1986). Fewer than half of nursing home residents can walk (Jirovec & Maxwell, 1993). Fear of falling may cause some elderly persons to restrict activity, even subconsciously.

Psychosocial factors such as depression, delirium, dementia, or other cognitive factors can inhibit mobility and activity. A decreased desire to socialize is often attributed to withdrawal as a result of depression. Social isolation or lack of access to appropriate resources and assistance may also contribute to decreased physical mobility, especially in minority populations.

Other factors that may influence mobility include the presence of complicating physical problems such as visual loss, whether from cataracts, glaucoma, or another disease process. Decreased proprioception may contribute to fear of falling when ambulating. Polypharmacy, or use of multiple medications, can impair mobility indirectly secondary to side effects, particularly those that contribute to fall risk.

Fall Risk Assessment

Patient falls remain responsible for the largest category of hospital inpatient incident reports published since the 1940s (Grant & Hamilton, 1987). Falls are the second leading cause of accidental death in the elderly (Brady et al., 1993). Falls can have other damaging effects on the persons involved, including injury, decreased confidence, insecurity, increased dependence, extended length of stays due to complications, greater expense to the hospital and patient, increased provider liability, and potential lawsuits.

Because falls tend to occur more frequently in the older population, fall risk assessment and prevention are relevant nursing issues. The nursing literature regarding fall risk factors is abundant. Many studies have been done on older long-term care and rehabilitation patients. The elderly between 70 and 80 years of age have been reported to fall more often than the general population (Pablo, 1977). In 1964, one tenth of accidental deaths in those age 75 to 84 years were related to falls that occurred in homes for the aged, nursing homes, long-term care facilities, and hospitals (Rodstein, 1964). Other researchers have estimated that falls account for half of the accidental deaths in the elderly (Kalchthaler, Bascon, & Quintos, 1978). In 1991, falls were ranked as the second leading cause of accidental death in the United States, accounting for 9300 deaths of persons age 65 and older within that year (Kippenbrock & Soja, 1993). Mortality from falls rises with increased age (Ross, 1991). Several sources report from 43% to 68% of nursing home patients falling more than once (Hogue, Studenski, & Duncan, 1990; Ross, 1991; Tinetti, 1987).

Because of these staggering statistics, many research studies have been conducted, especially since the 1970s, to identify factors associated with falls (DeVincenzo & Watkins, 1987; Grant & Hamilton, 1987; Janken, Reynolds, & Sweich, 1986; Mion et al., 1989; Pablo, 1977; Roberts & Wykle, 1993; Tutuarima, de Haan, & Limburg, 1993). (Many of these studies, although conducted decades ago, provided the essential data on which present fall risk interventions are based, so are included here.) The available nursing research on falls in long-term care and rehabilitation identifies several key risk factors, which can be used to develop fall risk tools that guide GRN interventions.

Mion et al. (1989) reported that general medical rehabilitation units have a higher incidence of falls when compared with acute medical units (38% versus 2%). Mion's study found that 32% of rehabilitation patients fell at least once, and 68% of falls were from wheelchairs. Factors associated with falling included longer average length of hospital stay, psychiatric illness, inability to understand or follow directions, impaired memory or judgment, week of hospitalization, and limited use of the call light.

Ashley, Gryfe, and Amies (1977) identified many circumstances associated with elderly falls. This longitudinal study described the following factors contributing to falls in the aged: impaired balance and sway, visual deficits, complications of illness, hypotension, age, non-psychotropic medications, decreased functional ability, severe ill health, number and type of medical diagnoses, and altered bowel and bladder function. Morton (1989) stated that patients were at risk for falls if they had a known fall before or after admission, altered mental state, recent seizures, decreased mobility or abnormal gait, sensory deficits, history of escape from restraints, hesitation to call for help, or a history of dizziness. Balance, leg strength, and flexibility may also be factors contributing to falls in the elderly (Gehlsen & Whaley, 1990b). Peripheral neuropathy has also been associated with falling (Richardson, Ching, & Hurvitz, 1992).

In 1987, DeVincenzo and Watkins stated that age and diagnosis were the two most critical variables in determining fall risk in rehabilitation. Stroke patients were identified as having the highest incidence of falls. Other environmental variables associated with falls were the week of hospitalization (patients fell more often at the beginning and end of their hospital stay), day of the week, activity levels, site, and equipment. The most common locations were the bedroom and bathroom. Garcia et al. (1988) also found that most patients fell on the way to the bathroom.

Although there is a large body of research available on fall risk criteria, not all studies have similar results. Tutuarima et al. (1993) found that stroke patients in acute care settings fell most often on the day shift when most nursing staff were present. More cases of falls (35%) occurred within the first week of admission. DeVincenzo and Watkins (1987) found that patients in the rehabilitation settings fell most during the first week and after the fourth week of hospitalization. This may be due to an increased level of false confidence after a period of therapy. Rogers (1994) specified the days 5 to 7 of the rehabilitation stay as the most likely time for falls. Falls also occurred more often at shift change, especially around 8:00 A.M. on the day shift.

Many studies report that women were more likely to fall than men (Berry, Fisher, & Lang, 1981; Louis, 1983; Morgan, Mathison, Rice, & Clemmer, 1985; Morse, Prowse, Morrow, & Federspeil, 1976; Schested & Severin-Nielsen, 1977). Several other studies dispute this, stating that men fall more often than women (Gryfe, Amies, & Ashley, 1977; Morris, Isaacs, & Brislen, 1981; Walshe & Rosen, 1979).

Several researchers found psychosocial factors related to falls. Some persons who fell were hesitant to ask for assistance (Pablo, 1977). Some long-term care residents express a strong need for independence (preservation of autonomy, self-esteem, and control) (Kippenbrock & Soja, 1993; Wright, Aizenstein, Vogler, Rower, & Miller, 1990). Such clients would deny that they had fallen, stating they only "slipped" or "tripped." Many were reluctant to "bother" the staff for assistance or expressed a fear of being restrained.

Fall prevention strategies have been shown to decrease the incidence of falls (Brians, Alexander, Grota, Chen, & Dumas, 1991; Fife, Solomon, & Stanton, 1984; Morton, 1989). Specific unique risk factors should be identified for the unit or population for which a risk assessment tool is being developed. The GRN should be aware of the most commonly reported risk factors among rehabilitation patients as well as factors associated with certain patient groups. For example, stroke patients with right cerebrovascular accident who fell had a higher rating of impulsivity, suggesting this as a significant risk factor (Rapport et al., 1993). Additionally, factors identified with rehabilitation patients sustaining a fracture as a result of falls include advanced age, female gender, ability to ambulate, disorientation, use of vitamins, and use of anti-ulcer medications (Mayo, Korner-Bitensky, & Levy, 1993). Environmental factors, such as pieces of furniture, have been associated with a majority of falls by residents in adult day care facilities (Fleming & Pendergast, 1993). More nursing research studies related to fall prevention done with specific patient populations are needed.

GOALS

The goals of mobility and activity for older adults with chronic health alterations may not be as ambitious as those for younger persons. Goals should be attainable and mutually established. The physical capability of the individual to perform certain activities will depend on both age and whether functional deficits are permanent or rehabilitative. The 80 year old with a new above-knee amputation and a history of hip fracture in the unaffected leg may have decidedly different ambulatory goals than the 65 year old with mild hemiparesis after a stroke.

Although there are a wide variety of factors that affect the functional outcomes of elderly rehabilitation patients, several overriding goals remain constant. Rehabilitation goals include improving range of motion, improving endurance and tolerance for activity, promoting better functional outcomes, improving ambulation, and maintaining safety. With physical and occupational therapy, as well as the interventions of the GRN and other team members, older patients can and do experience better functional outcomes and improve in the area of self-care. The demands that a chronic illness or disability place on the body are exhausting. It is the challenge of rehabilitation professionals to assist individuals in returning to their maximum potential functional level and the greatest independence possible. Such outcomes are achieved not only through a few weeks in rehabilitation but through concentrated efforts to teach clients, family members, and caregivers to continue their own progress at home and in the community.

Tolerance to activity is built gradually. As the individual's endurance increases, so does the ability to participate more fully in therapeutic activities that enhance self-care skills and mobility. Ambulation is the main objective of mobility training. But this is not possible in all cases, so alternative goals will be made to help the individual attain some level of independent mobility, whether through a wheelchair or other mechanism.

Safety, particularly in the form of fall prevention, is a continuous goal. Aged rehabilitation patients are at particular risk for falls because of the many factors inherent in conditions that necessitate this type of treatment. In order to keep patients free from falling injuries, as well as other trauma that can occur during exercise and the rehabilitation regimen, constant vigilance must be maintained. This is often done in the form of fall risk assessment tools as discussed previously.

INTERVENTIONS

In addition to the usual and accepted nursing interventions for preventing immobility, there are several techniques that, when used by the

GRN, promote mobility in older adults. The GRN's care should go beyond the maintenance level, emphasizing regaining mobility, building strength, and increasing endurance. Skills that assist in the accomplishment of these positive outcomes are initially taught by physical and occupational therapists during rehabilitation. Patients practice these skills during therapy sessions, and these techniques should be reinforced by nurses and nursing assistants throughout the rest of the day. Communication between team members is crucial to promote quality outcomes related to mobility and function.

One area in which GRNs must be skilled is that of patient transfers. Nurses with an acute care background may have a different perspective on assisting patients with ambulation than GRNs who work with patients who have severe physical mobility limitations. Much of the patient's progress in several different areas of rehabilitation relates to the staff's ability and willingness to assist the patient in transfers and regaining independent mobility. Improvements in bowel and bladder training are facilitated through many trips to the bathroom, all of which may require ambulation assistance from nursing staff. Skin integrity is promoted by activity and reducing immobility. The GRN can use thoughtful and careful transfer techniques that will also help the patient take an increasingly larger role in self-care as strength returns.

There are many ways to perform patient transfers. The technique chosen depends on the patient's level of function, physical deficits, and weight as well as the ability of the person assisting with the transfer. Transfer techniques can be modified to fit individuals' unique needs and the abilities of the caregiver. The nurse should be in constant communication with the physical therapist so that consistent transfers are used. Both team members can share information on what works and what does not for a variety of different situations (Malzer, 1988). An important task of the GRN is to teach the caregiver to assist the patient with safe transfers. Although this may initially be done by the physical therapist, the GRN is the professional present on the off-shifts, when most family members visit. The GRN may also need to teach other nursing staff members, such as new nursing assistants, to perform transfers. It should be noted, however, that many rehabilitation nursing assistants do the bulk of the patient transfers, particularly related to toileting

needs, and may be more proficient at this skill than the nurses, so a mutual sharing of information may be indicated. Mechanical lifts are often used to move patients who are totally unable to bear weight or when a person's weight prohibits safe transfers according to the resources and personnel available to assist. Several types of transfers commonly used, as well as mechanical supports, are discussed here.

Several guidelines provide a foundation for the discussion of transfer techniques. Proper body mechanics are always used for both patients and staff. The use of a gait belt is preferable. The GRN can structure the approaches used so that each transfer provides exercise for the patient, promotes self-care, and enforces correct techniques at all times. Incorrect transfers, on the other hand, reinforce poor, unsafe patterns and lead to undesirable outcomes.

Utilizing Principles of Body Mechanics to Promote Self-care in Transfers

Although nearly all nurses are familiar with proper body mechanics, and may even be required to attend annual inservice sessions focused on preventing staff injuries, assisting the physically challenged individual with mobility skills requires careful attention to detail and special skills. The principles of body mechanics should be applied by *both* the nurse and the patient during transferring. Older rehabilitation patients have unique needs. Some may have the use of only one side of their body, causing poor trunk control and balance problems. Others have spasticity, paralysis, weakness, functional debility, deconditioning, fractures, or other deficits that affect mobility. All these factors, in addition to normal aging changes, make promoting mobility a challenge for the entire team.

When preparing to move a patient, it should be clear that certain principles are always followed by both the patient and the caregiver (or person assisting with the transfer). Lifting is done with the stronger muscles of the legs, not the weaker back muscles. Feet should be at least 12 inches apart, providing a wide base of support. Having feet too close together promotes sway, too far apart makes taking steps difficult. Pulling should be avoided. That is, the patient should not reach up and grab the caregiver's shoulders to pull himself or herself up. Nor should the caregiver pull the patient, but rather guide the transfer using the patient's own momentum.

The caregiver should never pull on the patient's arm or shoulders. Older patients have fragile skin, and pulling could result in skin tears. Additionally, arthritic changes may cause pain with pulling. Using the transfer belt allows the staff to have a secure hold without causing the patient pain.

The patient and the caregiver must remain close together throughout the transfer, particularly if the patient requires more than minimal assistance. The gait belt is used to guide the transfer. The caregiver's hips and knees should be bent, and movements should be in the direction in which the transfer is going.

The GRN's interventions are centered on performing safe, effective, mobility-promoting transfers. A primary goal is to assist patients in accomplishing a transfer or movement that is most like the way they did it unaided prior to requiring assistance. This is done by cueing the person to perform as much of the motion as is possible at that time.

A helpful guideline to staff is the use of descriptors in the nursing care plan to communicate how a person transfers. The terms *independent, supervised, contact guard,* or *min, mod,* and *max* are often used. *Independent* means no help is required. *Supervised* indicates a caregiver should be in attendance. *Contact guard* suggests that the caregiver be touching the patient or standing right next to him or her for safety, but the effort is entirely the patient's. If the Kardex indicates that the patient transfers with *min x 1* assist, this means that the person needs the minimal assistance or effort of one helper. The designations *mod* and *max* assist mean that moderate or maximal assistance of the caregiver, respectively, is required. A *"max assist of 3"* indicates a difficult transfer during which three caregivers expend their maximal energy and the patient does little. For the purposes of this discussion, the term *desired surface* refers to the place where the transfer is heading or where the patient is to go.

Most transfers go to the patient's strong side. That is, the patient's unaffected or stronger side is positioned next to the desired surface. For example, when transferring a patient with left hemiplegia from the bed to the wheelchair, the chair is placed on the patient's stronger right side. This facilitates the transfer, because it is difficult for most patients to move toward the weaker side. However, in the community, patients will have to transfer to both sides, so training in both directions is desirable. The exception to the rule of transferring to the stronger side is the patient who severely pushes to the involved side when transferring. These patients sometimes transfer better toward the weaker side. Additionally, patients with spasticity problems that may be aggravated with such movements sometimes find it easier to transfer toward the affected side.

Other general rules of thumb include locking the wheelchair brakes. No transfer should be attempted until both surfaces involved are secure to the ground. The wheelchair should be properly positioned, at about a 30-degree angle from the desired surface. This provides the least distance for a more efficient transfer. The leg rests should be removed from the wheelchair or commode. The patient and caregiver should have on firm-soled shoes, with non-skid bottoms. Tennis shoes are generally ideal. The gait belt should be applied snugly around the patient's middle.

Using a Gait Belt

The gait belt, also called a transfer belt, is a very helpful device used to assist the patient and caregiver with transfers and ambulation. Such belts are made of a thick, durable material that fastens with a metal or plastic clasp and allows the nursing staff to obtain a secure hold of the patient. Failure to use transfer or gait belts appropriately can result in patient falls, injury, and lawsuits (Case Study 7.1).

CASE STUDY 7.1

Mrs. Smith was a 76 year old woman who was admitted to inpatient rehabilitation with a diagnosis of functional debility as a result of a prolonged hospital stay for pneumonia and other resulting medical complications. The activity-related team goals included improved exercise tolerance and endurance as well as strengthening for the purpose of regaining independent ambulatory skills. Early in her rehabilitation stay, Mrs. Smith had graduated to the use of a walker and was ambulating with contact guard to minimal assistance using a gait belt. She was steady on her feet but had a history of dizziness.

One evening Mrs. Smith used her call light and expressed an urgent desire to use the bathroom. The nursing assistant, wishing to assist the patient quickly to the toilet, did not apply the gait belt, as the team had deemed appropriate, judging that Mrs. Smith had been steady on her feet for several days. After ambulating several steps, Mrs. Smith suddenly fell forward, apparently fainting. The nursing assistant had been holding onto her gown, which tore, and Mrs. Smith fell, sustaining a minor concussion, bruises on her face, and several lacerations requiring sutures. Because the nursing assistant had not applied the gait belt, the patient suffered unnecessary injuries and emotional distress, and the hospital and the nursing assistant were liable for the accident.

The gait belt is positioned around the patient's waist, closest to his or her center of gravity. This is around the belt line, not under the shoulders. For women, be certain the belt is placed under the breasts, close to the waist (Fig. 7–1). The belt is not intended to be used as a device for pulling on the patient, but rather for guiding the transfer. In the case of older individuals who have difficulty with a forward weight shift, as is needed to rise from the chair, the nurse will provide only the extra energy needed to make that movement. Belts, such as the Posey belt, are designed to help provide safety and protection during transfers and ambulation. If more than one person is required to help steady the patient, caregivers can be positioned one on either side, and both hold the transfer belt. However, this requires careful planning on the part of all involved to develop a smooth transfer.

Using Four Basic Types of Transfers

Although there are many variations of ways to transfer a patient, four basic methods are discussed here: the stand-pivot, modified stand-pivot, sliding board, and mechanical lifts. Again, the choice of transfer method depends on several variables, with the best method often being decided on by the physical therapists, then communicated to the nurses. However, in the interim of deciding which method to use, or in the case of nurses working in the community setting or extended care, these guidelines should prove helpful. It should be noted that these transfers are quite similar and use consistent and correct approaches to transferring.

Stand-Pivot

This type of transfer is often used for higher level patients who can perform some of the activity themselves (Fig. 7–2). Once the chair is positioned and locked, with leg rests removed, and the gait belt is put on, the patient is assisted, or instructed, to move forward in the chair until the feet are flat on the floor. Transfers should never be initiated without both of the patient's feet on the floor. The patient's legs should be positioned so that the toes are approximately under the knees. The knees should be flexed to 90 degrees if possible, but the feet should not be underneath either surface. Once the patient is in this position, the forward weight shift can occur. The caregiver should stand facing the patient, providing cues during the transfer. The caregiver should have a wide base of support with knees bent and back straight. The gait belt should be grasped firmly on either side to help steady the patient. The patient is instructed to place his or her hands on the armrests of the chair or on the surface from which he or she is rising. This mimics "nor-

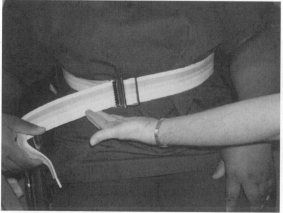

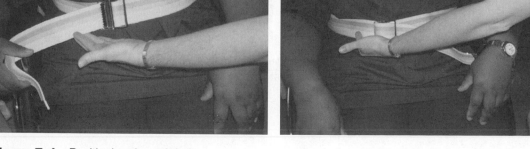

Figure 7–1 Positioning the gait belt.

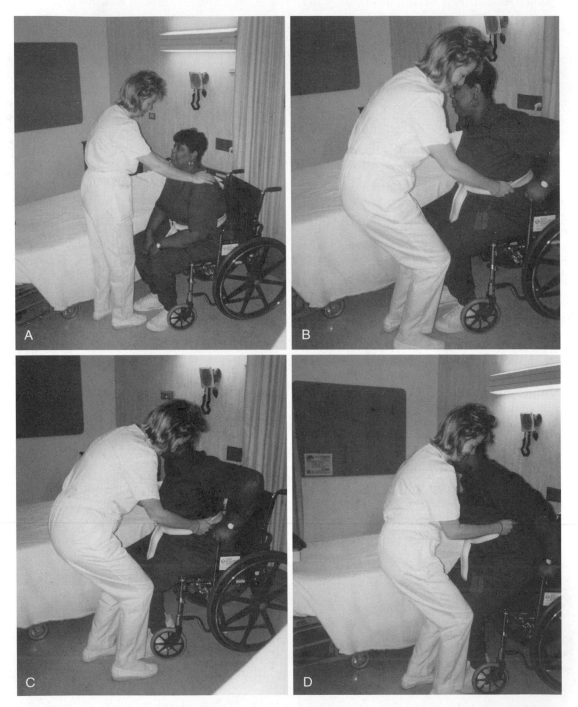

Figure 7–2 Performing a stand-pivot transfer. *A,* Patient slides forward in chair, feet flat on the floor. *B,* Nurse bends at knees and hips; patient pushes off from the chair. *C,* Patient leans forward and pushes up from the chair, as nurse blocks weaker leg. *D,* Nurse helps steady patient until she comes to a full stand.

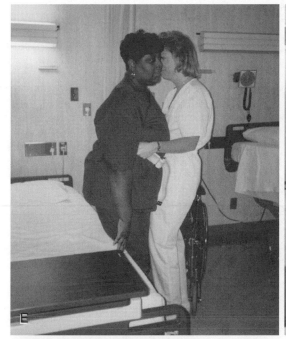

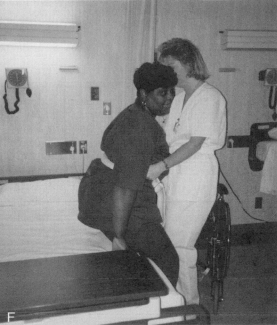

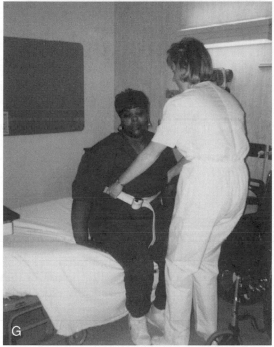

Figure 7–2 *Continued E,* After pivoting to desired surface, patient feels bed at back of legs. *F,* Patient reaches for the bed and sits down with guidance of nurse. *G,* Transfer safely completed.

mal" movement. The patient should not hold onto the caregiver above the waist before rising. This promotes a pulling motion and imbalance and can result in injury to the caregiver. In addition, it does not promote self-care in any way.

After counting "1-2-3," the patient is assisted to a standing position. Older individuals find it helpful to rock back and forth prior

to standing on "3," in order to gain some momentum. The GRN may have observed this technique being used unknowingly by healthy elders. A forward weight shift is essential. If the patient does not get his or her weight forward over the legs, the transfer will fail, resulting in the patient falling backward.

Once in a standing position, the patient should be encouraged to stand straight and tall. Elders tend to stay bent somewhat at the waist at this point, whether from fear or poor habits. At this point, a lower level patient can pivot and reach for the desired surface. A higher level patient should be encouraged to take steps to the desired surface. The nurse stabilizes the patient as needed through using the gait belt, which is situated at the patient's center of gravity for maximum usefulness. If a gait belt is not available or cannot be used for some reason, the nurse's hands may be placed around the patient's middle, or beneath the scapulae, and used like a gait belt. This is not as safe as using a gait belt. Patients may steady themselves by placing a hand on the nurse's shoulder or waist, if needed, but only after they are standing.

The patient should be instructed not to sit down until the chair or other desired surface is felt at the back of the legs. He or she may then reach back to touch the chair, and only then lower himself or herself slowly down. This technique requires some use of the upper and lower extremities. A hemiplegic arm should be placed in a sling during transfer or tucked between the patient and the caregiver. An affected arm should never be left dangling during transfers.

Modified Stand-Pivot

In this transfer, used for lower level patients such as those who have a tendency to push backward (sometimes called "pushers"), the patient does not come to a full stand but does attempt to use the lower extremities. The patient is positioned as before, but a gait belt may or may not be used, because of the different placement of the nurse's hands. The armrest closest to the desired surface can be removed. The patient should be assisted far forward in the chair, with the nurse directly in front of the patient, preventing sliding or falling before the transfer. The leading leg is blocked firmly with the nurse's knee (one or both). If the patient is known to "buckle," or have the knee or knees drop suddenly during the transfer, the nurse should take care to block appropriately. The patient's head must lean forward and over the nurse's shoulder, or to the side, but always away from the desired surface and in front of the knees. The nurse's hands can be positioned in a few different ways for this transfer. Different hand positions should be tried to find what works best for each patient and the nurse. Common hand positions include under the patient's buttocks at the area of the ischia, from the

front, or the same area from over the patient's back. If the patient is at home and wearing pants, some caregivers grasp the pants to transfer. If the gait belt is used, it is gripped from underneath, with the caregiver supporting the patient's knees with his or her own knees and using the belt to help lift the buttocks up and onto the desired surface.

This transfer obviously requires more practice and skill than a regular stand-pivot transfer. Having to block the patient's legs can confound the nurse's balance and proper body alignment, so care must be taken to set things up properly before the transfer is attempted.

On the count of "1-2-3," the patient moves forward, lifting the buttocks off the chair. As the patient pivots, the nurse then guides the buttocks to the desired surface. The nurse uses the patient's forward momentum to rock backward and pivot the patient to the desired surface. The nurse's main concern should be where the buttocks are headed.

With this method, the patient does not try to take steps. Care should be taken that the patient does not grab onto the nurse during the transfer. Patients can be instructed to hold the affected upper extremity or hold at the nurse's waist, but nowhere else. If an additional helper is available, he or she may be positioned between the two surfaces from behind (such as between the wheelchair and the bed) and help guide the hips.

Sliding Board Transfers

Sliding board transfers are used for patients who cannot stand or bear weight on both lower extremities. This is a commonly used transfer for patients with paraplegia and for some individuals with amputation. One advantage of this transfer is that it can be performed independently and thus promotes self-care. The main disadvantages are the shearing force it places on the skin and the potential for falls.

Correct positioning of the sliding board is a key factor in safe transfers of this type. The board must be securely sitting on both the surface from which the patient is transferring and the desired surface. The patient is positioned, or positions himself or herself, in the wheelchair as for the stand-pivot transfer. The sliding board acts as a bridge between surfaces. Approximately one third of the board should be placed under the patient's buttock, with the ischial tuberosity on the board. The opposite one quarter to one third of the board must be on the desired surface. The patient's trunk must remain forward during the transfer or the patient can slide off. Flexing at the waist and bracing the knees help prevent this when practicing this transfer. The patient's legs should be even with the floor if possible. The shoulders should be over the hips, and the patient should assist with his or her arms (and legs, if possible).

This transfer can be practiced slowly with the assistance of the staff. Older patients may experience more difficulty with this type of transfer because it requires a good deal of upper body strength to perform it independently. In addition to a decrease in muscle strength that may occur with age, arthritic changes in the shoulder and elbow joints can make this transfer painful. Also, a sliding board transfer would be contraindicated in any patient with a sacral, coccygeal, or ischial pressure ulcer or for those at higher risk of skin breakdown, because of high shearing forces resulting from sliding on the board. Sliding board transfers should not be done on bare skin. Shearing forces can be minimized by making sure the patient has on a soft, cotton-like or slick material that will slide easily. Some patients find that sprinkling baby powder on the board helps reduce friction. When patients are transferring to the tub or shower, pants can be removed after the transfer. Occasionally, patients place a towel on the board to transfer after clothes have been removed, but this may result in a higher risk for falls.

Persons who have mastered the sliding board transfer, and who have long-term deficits, may no longer require the use of the board. These individuals often perform lateral transfers with ease, such as from the car to the wheelchair, in one or two swift movements. This is more practical for long-term maintenance but runs a greater risk of falls.

Mechanical Lifts

There are many kinds of mechanical lifts on the market today. Two of the most commonly used are the Hoyer lift and the Sara lift. These types of lifts are generally used for large or obese patients who require maximal assistance in transferring or for the dependent patient. They should be used only when other types of transfers are physically impossible or unsafe, because dependency should not be promoted. If lifts are used, patients should be instructed that this is only temporary until their strength and endurance have been built

and other techniques can be learned. The Sara lift is a more recent invention and differs slightly from other lifters in that patients can be transferred to the toilet or commode easily, because the lift support goes under the shoulder blades instead of the entire trunk and torso. Both types of lifts are discussed here briefly.

All GRNs should be familiar with safe use of the Hoyer lift. The base of the Hoyer lift should be wide for stability. This device comes with a sling, which should be positioned from behind the patient's knees to the shoulder blades. It cradles the patient during the transfer. The hooks are placed facing outward from the patient. The longer chains are for the leg fasteners and the shorter ones for the shoulders. The patient, once positioned on the sling, is raised slowly by pumping a lever, and the device is checked for areas that may pinch the patient, knots in the chain, and the like. Patients should not hold onto the chains, because their fingers can become pinched. Once the patient is raised, the lift is slowly wheeled to the desired surface; swinging is avoided, because this can tip the device over. A valve is slowly released to lower the patient, and then the chains are removed. Several disadvantages to the traditional Hoyer lift are apparent. It requires turning and positioning of the patient properly upon the sling, which may require several caregivers' assistance. Although some slings have a hole cut out for use with toileting, this is difficult and generally messy and does not provide the same support to the buttocks as an intact sling. Additionally, either the patient must sit on the sling while up in the chair or it must be removed and replaced, which is difficult for a patient who is using it because he or she cannot stand. Hoyer lifts are useful but can present a danger if used improperly. Tipping of the device and patients' catching their fingers on the chains are potential sources of injury.

A more recent lift being used in gerontological rehabilitation is the Sara lift (Fig. 7–3). This is best used for patients who are able to bear a small amount of weight or at least able to stabilize themselves with their legs. The Sara lift has an adjustable base, much like the Hoyer lift, but can extend around a wheelchair, close to wheel into a smaller entryway, and widen to go around the toilet or commode. The Sara lift does not use a sling, but rather a wide, sheepskin-type band that is positioned beneath the patient's shoulder blades. The lift is positioned facing the pa-

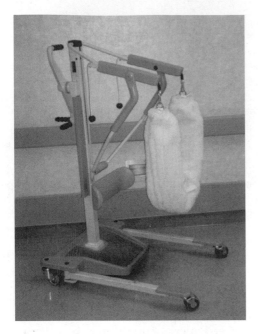

Figure 7–3 Sara mechanical lift.

tient, with the patient's feet placed directly on the non-skid, inclined base surface of the lift. The strap is positioned around the patient's back and under the scapulae. The patient is instructed to hold onto the lift bars as it is raised. As the staff member pumps up the lift, the patient is pulled out of the chair to a partial-standing position. The lift is rolled over the desired surface and lowered via a valve, much like the Hoyer lift.

There are several advantages of the Sara lift. Its usefulness in toileting is unquestionable. With no sling apparatus, even dependent patients can be taken to the bathroom to void on the toilet. This advantage alone is of great worth in terms of patient privacy, self-esteem, and bowel and bladder management. Another advantage to this type of lift is that it promotes a more natural posturing than the dependent posture of the Hoyer lift. Patients assume a standing or near-standing position. Pressure is placed only over the back area, not under the knees, as with those lifts using a sling. The legs do not hang from the sling as with the Hoyer lift. This approach is in keeping with the principles of gerontological rehabilitation nursing care, that is, promoting activities that are as close to normal bodily functions as possible. One disadvantage to the Sara lift is that patients with knees that buckle could potentially slide out of the strap if they cannot support themselves or hold on to the bars with the upper extremities. The

nurse should evaluate each patient carefully before deciding which type of lift would be most appropriate.

Promoting Ambulation

Promoting ambulation, or walking, is one of the most significant contributions nursing staff in long-term care can make toward a patient's independence. As discussed previously, ambulation has many benefits to the entire body. As mobility increases, the incidence of falls decreases, even in a frail elderly population (Galindo-Ciocon et al., 1995b; Koroknay et al., 1995). Fractures (especially of the hip) as a result of falling are associated with high morbidity and mortality (Davis, 1995). Even with cognitively impaired elderly nursing home residents, Jirovec's study (1991) showed that exercise and increased mobility significantly reduced the incidence of urinary incontinence. It stands to reason, then, that measures to increase ambulatory skills would be appropriate for all elderly, regardless of setting, but particularly when the focus is rehabilitative.

Several nursing interventions related to promoting ambulation can be initiated in most settings. Those in nursing homes can also improve their ambulatory status, even when the services of a physical therapist are unavailable. Koroknay et al. stated, "nursing home staff often do not pursue walking as a therapeutic goal once a loss has been experienced in this area" (1995, p. 21). Staff may not even be aware of a patient's ability to ambulate (Spier & Meis, 1994). Milde further stated that in the prevention of physical immobility, the "attitudes of the nurse are important because unless the nurse values preventative interventions, none will be initiated" (1988, p. 21). GRNs who work in long-term care settings can educate other staff members in therapeutic transfer techniques and ambulation skills so that the focus of care can be rehabilitative, not custodial.

Some suggestions for improving ambulation status in the elderly appear in Table 7–3. Goals for ambulation should be set individually and mutually. Using rehabilitation principles, the nurse and client should discuss and establish goals that are the client's, not just the nurse's, and are designed with that particular person's present abilities in mind. To promote goal attainment, activities can be centered around unit activities or ADLs. Examples of goals might include: "Mrs. Smith will ambulate 20 feet to the dining room for

Table 7–3 SUGGESTIONS FOR PROMOTING MUSCLE STRENGTH AND AMBULATION

- Begin slowly. It will take time for the deconditioned patient to regain muscle strength.
- Range of motion exercises should be done several times daily, whether active or passive.
- Select the appropriate exercise (isometric, isotonic, or a combination) for patients who lack the guidance of a physical therapist but are bed-bound.
- Be sure that all transfers are performed with attention to maximizing the patient's self-care potential.
- Avoid techniques that promote patient dependence, such as pulling on the caregiver during transfers.
- Make ambulation a primary goal when the patient's physical status allows it. Encourage exercises that foster walking as a long-term goal.
- Assist patients to ambulate whenever possible instead of using the wheelchair for convenience.
- Institute a walking program in your facility. If staffing is insufficient, consider training volunteers to assist with walking protocol.
- Promote even minimal weight bearing using assistance or a standing box.
- Communicate regularly with the interdisciplinary team. Follow and reinforce activities, exercises, and transfer techniques designed by the therapists for each individual. Help the patient practice these techniques throughout the day and on off-shifts. Encourage family members and other caregivers to attend therapy and practice what they have learned with the nurse's supervision on off-shifts.

lunch and dinner," or "Mr. Jones will ambulate with his quad cane and supervision to the bathroom twice per shift." If a clinical nurse specialist is available, he or she may assist the staff in identifying those patients who have the ability to walk, and focus interventions accordingly.

Strengthening exercises can be done in groups or individually. The GRN can work with the recreational therapist or activity director to plan social activities that promote muscle strengthening and ambulatory skills (Hamilton & Lyon, 1995). Even when many of the patients are in wheelchairs, activities such as mock Olympics, wheelchair volleyball or basketball, dances, and other forms of entertainment can be modified to accommodate various types of abilities and physical challenges. Most rehabilitation units have groups that meet with the occupational therapist on a regular basis for home management skills or upper extremity exercises. The social stimulation and support provided by the group setting is also therapeutic.

Ambulation should take place whenever safely possible. Instead of transporting patients via the wheelchair to the bathroom or community dining room, staff should be encouraged to assist them with ambulation. This takes planning ahead so that time is allowed for walking. Many facilities have walking programs in which volunteers come in just to help patients ambulate around the unit. Nursing home residents may feel a sense of loss of control and that they have less choice than they desire. An increase in functional abilities has been associated with an increase in actual as well as desired choice in older nursing home residents (Jirovec &

Maxwell, 1993). Persons who can ambulate independently obviously have more of a choice in their activities, because this ability of personal locomotion decreases dependency on the caregivers.

When walking is not immediately possible, other measures must be instituted to preserve ambulation potential. Isometric muscle exercises are tightening contractions that help maintain muscle strength. These can be done even when a patient cannot ambulate, because they do not involve movement, but a tightening and relaxing of the muscle. Patients should breathe through their mouth when performing these exercises, to prevent accidental use of the Valsalva maneuver, which increases intrathoracic pressure. Isometric exercises are especially useful when it is necessary to avoid additional stress on the cardiovascular system (Milde, 1988).

Isotonic exercises can also be helpful, but they should be used cautiously for those with cardiac diagnoses. Isotonic exercises involve pushing or pulling against a stationary object, such as pushing off from the bed, or lifting up using a trapeze in bed. When GRNs promote proper transfer and positioning techniques, the patient is automatically engaged in isotonic exercising.

Range of motion (ROM) exercises are necessary to maintain joint mobility and prevent contractures in the compromised patient. Active ROM is, of course, preferable and most beneficial to all body systems, but passive ROM (that done by another person) is focused on maintenance instead of improvement. ROM can improve flexibility and strength in addition to preventing complications. Such exercises involve taking each joint through its entire range of motion. This should be done consistently in any setting where mobility is impaired and can be incorporated into the resident's daily routine. This, however, does require a concerted effort and dedication on the part of the entire staff to have therapeutic potential.

Other exercises that can be beneficial in promoting ambulation are those that encourage the patient to practice balance and coordination. Balance and trunk control are necessary for safe transferring and subsequent walking. For patients who have poor balance, medication effects should be evaluated. Commonly used medications such as antihypertensives and diuretics can alter fluid balance, contributing to dizziness, weakness, or orthostatic hypotension. Assisting themselves to an upright position in bed and dangling the legs over the side of the bed with supervision or assistance are good practice situations for balance and trunk control. They also allow the nurse to evaluate some of the patient's potential problems that could affect the ability to transfer and ambulate safely.

No exercises can take the place of ambulation for an older individual with impaired physical mobility. Safe ambulation should always be the overriding goal when physically possible. Weight bearing helps prevent osteoporosis, deep vein thrombosis, and a myriad of other complications. Thus, even when walking is not currently possible, every effort should be made to assist the patient to stand several times per day. Ambulation has been associated with survival, and lack of it with the hazards of immobility and disability (Kauffman et al., 1987). GRNs can work with physical and occupational therapists to provide a 24-hour-a-day therapeutic environment for rehabilitation patients. Even in the absence of other professionals, GRNs can use self-care promoting strategies to improve a patient's ambulatory status.

Oxygen Therapy

It must be noted in any discussion on mobility that an older person's ability to participate in such activities can be greatly affected by complicating respiratory disorders. Many older adults have chronic respiratory problems, which, when combined with the normal effects of aging, leave lesser amounts of oxygen available with each breath and higher CO_2 levels. Those with cardiac problems may have additional limitations to activity. Thus, the importance of finding optimal medication

times (when medication effects are at the peak onset) and the time of day when endurance is greatest is crucial in planning nursing care. Correctly timing when inhalation therapy or respiratory treatments are done in relation to a person's optimum ability to participate in exercise is essential. Likewise, the benefits of oxygen therapy during exercise should be considered. Remembering these simple tips will help promote an individual exercise prescription that is best for each person.

Promoting Function in Specific Populations

Some specific information and interventions found in the literature may assist the GRN in setting appropriate goals. Although individuals are unique and each recovers or adapts somewhat differently, some generalizations about commonly seen medical and nursing problems related to rehabilitation may be helpful.

Hip Fracture

Most older patients with hip fracture do not recover full function, but they do experience improvement with rehabilitation (Williams et al., 1994).

The usual treatment for hip fracture is surgery, but medical researchers suggest that because of poor outcomes with the frail elderly, this should be reevaluated (Folman, Gepstein, Assaraf, & Leberty, 1994). The most common fracture after a fall is that of the proximal femur, and falls occur more often from an upright position (Kauffman et al., 1987; Mayo et al., 1993). Approximately 40% of patients with hip fractures die within 6 months (Tideiksaar, 1988). A high risk for confusion after hip fracture can also impede a patient's progress in rehabilitation (O'Brien, Grisso, Maislin, Chiu, & Evans, 1993). Cheng et al. (1989) found that important factors affecting ambulation included age and preoperative ambulatory level.

Social support has been shown to play a role in recovery after hip fracture. Cummings et al. (1988) found that those patients who reported more social support experienced a more complete recovery of function measured at 6 months after injury. Other predictors of recovery were arm strength, mental status, and serum albumin level.

Although several of these factors cannot be controlled by the GRN, others can be. Assisting patients in increasing balance, leg strength, and flexibility should decrease the risk for falls (Gehlsen & Whaley, 1990b). The social support system of patients should be evaluated and family participation encouraged. Nurses must help the patient and caregivers realize that a sedentary lifestyle in the elderly contributes to falls because of the increased skeletal fragility and greater tendency to fall with advancing age (Thorngren, 1994). Rehabilitation and muscle strengthening need to begin in the acute care setting. Patients and caregivers should also be instructed in the importance of a proper diet with adequate protein, vitamins, and minerals. In addition to promoting healing, good nutrition can prevent many untoward effects of aging.

Stroke

Certain expectations can help guide GRN care of the stroke patient. These should be used only as guidelines, not as hard and fast rules, because improvement in function has been seen in stroke patients for many months, to even years, after onset. However, new research from the large Copenhagen Stroke Study has led researchers to conclude that "recovery of walking function occurs in 95% of the patients within the first 11 weeks after stroke" (Jorgensen, Nakayama, Raaschou, & Olsen, 1995, p. 27). In patients with no paresis or mild to moderate leg paresis, optimum progress is often made in 3 weeks, with no recovery after 9 weeks in most patients. For those with severe leg paresis, a prognosis can be made in 6 weeks regarding walking function, with little recovery after 11 weeks after stroke onset. These physicians also found that with mild upper extremity paresis, a relatively accurate prognosis could be made in 3 weeks, and that further return of function should not be expected after 6 weeks (Nakayama, Jorgensen, Raaschou, & Olsen, 1994). For those with severe upper extremity paresis, a prognosis would be made in 6 weeks, with no further expectation of function after 11 weeks (Jorgensen et al., 1995). These statistics have enormous implications for rehabilitation professionals who wish to maximize the patient's potential in these areas. With average lengths of stay for stroke patients in rehabilitation becoming shorter, the window of opportunity for concentrated rehabilitation is small, yet crucial. One must wonder, then, whether those patients discharged before the time when maximal function is reached receive the same intensity of treatment as they did as inpatients in the United States health care system.

There is also some support to indicate that non-traditional approaches, such as the Bobath techniques, may be more effective in treatment of stroke patients (Lewis, 1986). But perhaps this effect was found more because nurses were consciously focusing on providing round-the-clock therapeutic treatment than because of the treatment itself. Much more research is needed to determine the ideal approaches to nursing care of stroke patients.

Arthritis and Osteoporosis

Patients with osteoarthritis of the knees experienced significant improvement in muscle function and better functional performance with an exercise program (Burckhardt, Moncur, & Minor, 1994). Increased muscle function was associated with decreased dependency; decreased difficulty with tasks; improved strength, endurance, and speed; as well as less pain. Aerobics did not improve muscle function (Fisher, Pendergast, Gresham, & Calkins, 1991a). Patients who participated in an intensive, interdisciplinary, 6-day inpatient arthritis program experienced significantly less pain, less disability, and a decreased need for assistance (Orr & Bratton, 1992).

The management of pain in patients with arthritis is a significant factor in rehabilitation progress. Arthritic pain is a common complaint among the elderly, because arthritis ranks as the number one chronic illness experienced in the aged. Pain can affect one's ability to perform self-care. Elderly women with back pain from osteoporotic vertebral fractures have been shown to have functional limitations in ADLs such as bathing, toileting, dressing, and transfers as a result of high amounts of pain (Galindo-Ciocon, Ciocon, & Galindo, 1995a). The GRN can promote comfort by assisting with pain relief techniques or providing appropriate medications before therapy. Patients should be instructed that increasing muscle strength through exercise and increased mobility can actually help reduce pain. Low-impact exercise is best, and swimming provides a good aerobic workout. Physical and occupational therapy, which include practice in ADLs, help with adaptation. GRNs can help the patient learn to cope with stress and pain and develop positive, realistic attitudes toward problem solving and goal setting. The social worker can help address social support, family and role adjustment, sexuality, and self-esteem issues as well (Orr & Bratton, 1992).

Amputation

Most amputees improve in function with rehabilitation, and the majority are discharged home (Heafey, Golden-Baker, & Mahoney, 1994). Patients with leg amputation are generally discharged at a more independent level in ADLs than those with stroke (Gregor, McCarthy, Chwirchak, Meluch, & Mion, 1986). However, they may need family assistance with ADLs and tend to experience problems with tasks such as yard care, showering, gardening, and athletic activities (Medhat, Huber, & Medhat, 1990). Nurses should encourage exercises that promote balance and coordinated movement for those who are learning to use a prosthesis. The patient's sense of balance will be decidedly different postoperatively, and time will be needed to learn to balance with and without the prosthesis. The importance of upper extremity strength cannot be overlooked for a patient with lower extremity amputation. The GRN should expect to see arthritic changes in the upper extremities occur with age over time, not only because of effects of aging but also because of additional wear and tear placed on the joints.

CASE STUDY 7.2

Mr. Stanford has been living with multiple chronic illnesses and disabilities for more than 50 years. He sustained a service-related injury at the age of 19, resulting in an above-knee amputation and impaired use of the opposite leg. Mr. Stanford spent much of his life adapting his environment to make life easier and more fulfilling for him and his family (a wife and two children). Through normal aging processes combined with the onset of diabetes, hypertension, renal disease, and aging with a disability, Mr. Stanford taught himself techniques that worked best for him at home. His house, built by special architects and provided by the Veterans Administration, is ground level, making it possible for him to go inside or out independently. All the doorways and hallways were built larger to accommodate a wheelchair comfortably. All the walkways are 40 inches wide. There are no stairs, no steps, and no throw rugs. A

hospital bed in his room, which he shares with his wife, promotes self-positioning. The bathroom is equipped with hand rails, a shower chair and hand-held shower head, and a sink whose cabinet opens to allow the wheelchair to roll underneath, yet closes for attractiveness when not in use. His lift chair (adapted for those with physical limitations) in the family room has electric controls that can be used to make the chair lift him to a standing position. With his increasing age, some tasks have become more difficult. He is no longer able to ambulate with his prosthesis because of severely impaired circulation in the non-amputated leg, which causes venous stasis and fainting. Mr. Stanford states that he can do almost anything that anyone else can do if he can sit, but it just takes longer and requires additional planning. He maintains a garden, fixes things around the house, spends time with his family, attends church, and drives an electric wheelchair that looks more like a bicycle (to get around the backyard). He has outlived seven prostheses and many more wheelchairs. He recently sold his boat, also complete with adaptations, because of recent health complications. Mr. Stanford is an excellent example of how persons can modify their environment to lead a satisfying life with multiple physical challenges.

Recognizing Adaptive Equipment for Self-care and Improving Function

Many types of adaptive equipment are available to enhance self-care (Case Study 7.2). "Grabbers" and "reachers" can be used to help extend a patient's reach and grasp things that he or she may be unable to. Extensions of various kinds such as handles for bath sponges or long-handled shoe horns can ease ADLs (Fig. 7–4). A hand-held shower head is essential for those with hemiparesis. Tub and shower chairs promote self-bathing activities (Fig. 7–5). Suction cups can be secured on the sink or in the tub to hold items such as nailbrushes, soap containers, and the like. Raised toilet seats can be used for those with hip fractures or arthritis, when sitting and rising is a problem.

A wide variety of utensils with built-up grips to facilitate eating can be obtained from the occupational therapy department. Plate guards, special drinking cups, mirrors, and

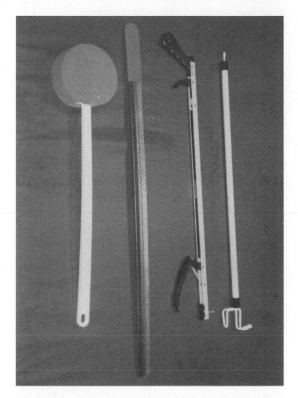

Figure 7–4 Adaptive devices used to promote self-care: reacher, long-handled shoe horn, bath sponge.

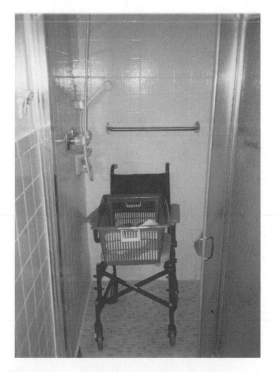

Figure 7–5 Modified shower in the home with hand rail, hand-held shower head, separate temperature controls, and rolling shower chair.

the like all serve to facilitate self-care (Fig. 7–6). However, none of these devices are useful if the patient is not informed that they are available. The GRN must be constantly alert to patients in long-term care facilities and the community who could benefit from self-help equipment. Something as simple as a medicine box (Fig. 7–7) that organizes pills can make the difference between taking medication correctly and independently and requiring a caregiver's assistance.

A trip to the facility's occupational therapy department could be enlightening. One may observe many unique adaptive devices available for patients, such as those pictured in Figures 7–8 and 7–9. Collaborative efforts between disciplines can yield tailor-made equipment for those with special needs. Medication administration is an important area for which adaptive equipment is available. Figure 7–10 shows a type of stabilizer for drawing up insulin that is also equipped with a magnifier. Stroke patients may use similar devices that have suction cups that can attach to the refrigerator or cabinet door, allowing the drawing up of medication into a syringe with the use of only one hand.

Other special adaptations to furniture and the like can also foster independence in the home and community. Lift chairs that both recline and straighten to help a person up to a standing position (Fig. 7–11) can be used in the home. However, lift chairs are controversial in that their use may promote muscle atrophy. Motorized chairs that look like three-wheel bicycles (Fig. 7–12) are good for traveling distances difficult with a standard manually propelled wheelchair, yet do not look like

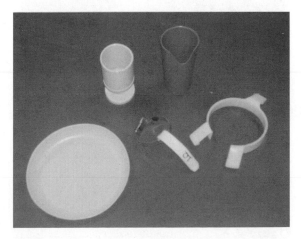

Figure 7–6 Adaptive plate guards, cup holders, and cups.

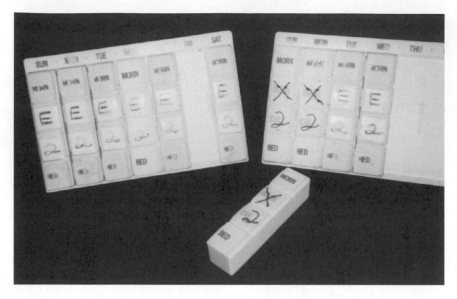

Figure 7–7 Medication boxes promoting self-management.

a regular wheelchair. These battery-powered mobility devices and others, such as the golf cart (Fig. 7–13), can help older persons with disabilities or functional limitations to get around in their backyard or to enjoy activities that would be prohibited by standard wheelchairs or that require walking long distances. Additionally, adaptive and exercise equipment used in rehabilitation can be taken home for continued use. For example, sponges (Fig. 7–14) with different stiffnesses provide increasingly greater resistance for the patient practicing hand grips. The various colors represent different resistance levels. Likewise, the red rubber-like band in Figure 7–14 provides resistance exercises. Anti-spasticity splints also shown in Figure 7–14 may need to be worn at home to prevent contractures until more active ROM is attained.

Once again, the need for patient and family

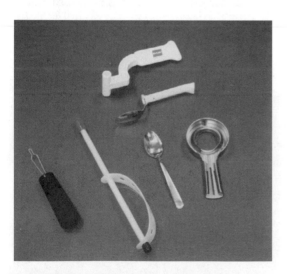

Figure 7–8 Other adaptive utensils for self-care: button-fastener, pointer with grip, swivel spoons, universal bottle opener and handle.

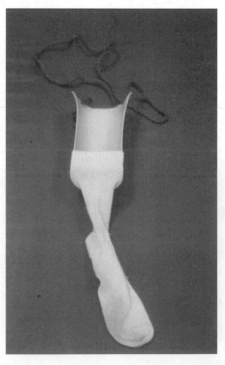

Figure 7–9 Assistive device for donning a sock.

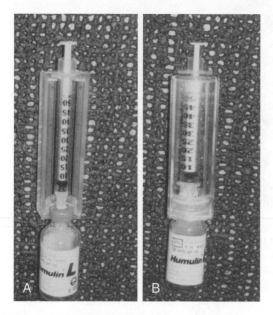
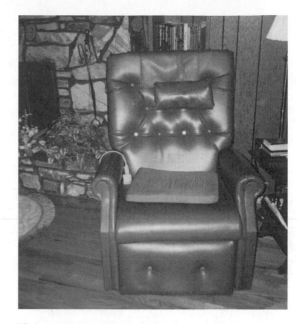

Figure 7-10 *A*, Plastic guide for drawing up insulin. *B*, Opposite side is a magnifier.

Figure 7-11 Lift chair for home use.

education is apparent. The GRN must know what resources are available within both the facility and the community. Social workers and case managers are excellent consultants for these types of questions. The nurse can also learn from patients and their caregivers what modifications they have invented at home to adapt to their new situation. A simple example is the case of a caregiver whose loved one was incontinent at night, requiring frequent changing of the sheets and mattress

soiling. While working on the incontinence problem with the home health nurse, the caregiver found that cutting an old shower curtain in half and using it as a "rubber draw sheet" on the bed saved her time and money and was much easier to clean. Other examples are the modifications made in the home of an older person who depends largely on a wheelchair for mobility. Note the hand rails on either side of the toilet and the "roll under" feature of the sink (Fig. 7-15).

Figure 7-12 Motorized vehicle for those with ambulation difficulties.

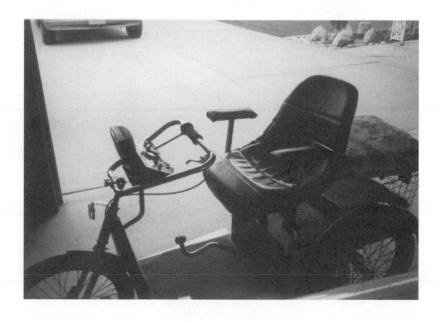
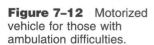

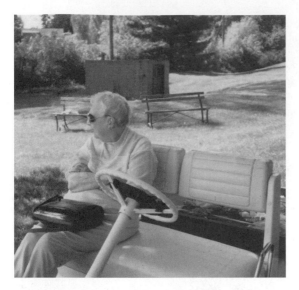

Figure 7–13 An elderly woman is able to visit with her family at the lakeside by riding in an electric golf cart.

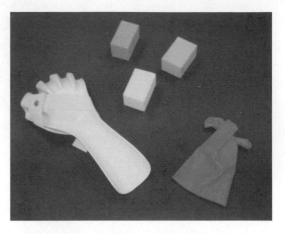

Figure 7–14 Sponges for hand exercises, elastic rubber band for resistance exercises, and an anti-spasticity splint.

Preventing Falls

The creation of an assessment tool to evaluate fall risk is a major step in fall prevention. Through examination of the literature, the GRN is able to devise a relatively well-established list of fall risk criteria. Fall statistics should be reviewed. Once the need is identi-

fied, prevention of falls (or safety promotion) follows directly from the assessment of the nursing problem. It is no secret that falls in rehabilitation are a costly problem, affecting patients' health and outcomes and staff/facility liability and finances. Many hospitals have fall committees that regularly evaluate the incidence of falls, precautions taken, and the effectiveness of prevention measures. Constant monitoring of these statistics is necessary to control these hazards. An example of a

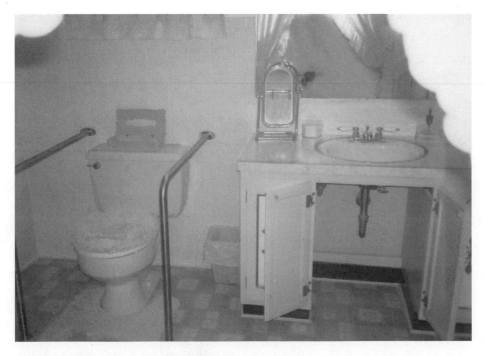

Figure 7–15 Adaptations in the bathroom at home.

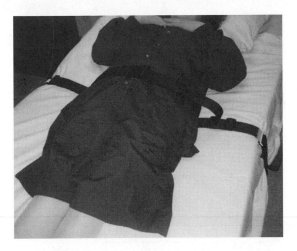

Figure 7–16   A new type of safety device that is less restrictive than vest restraints.

report form that could be used for committee evaluation appears in Table 7–4. GRNs should be active members of groups that strive to reduce fall incidence within their facilities (Commodore, 1995). Such committees help ensure good patient care through quality assurance or continuous quality improvement.

Development of a useful tool to reduce falls should begin with assessment on the unit on which it will be used. Effective fall prevention programs should include components such as less restraint use, increased patient autonomy and better self-esteem, in addition to safety education (Brady et al., 1993). Not all units experience the exact same fall patterns. Much of this depends on staffing policies, restraint use, assistance with toileting for patients, medical diagnoses, type of unit, and other factors. Of course, if safety devices are used, they should be the least restrictive possible. New devices are available that, because they fasten with Velcro, are not actually called restraints, because the patient is free to turn side to side and can easily remove them (Fig. 7–16). However, these types of belts, which may be used in place of vest restraints, provide the patient with an additional reminder not to get out of bed without assistance.

Once individual unit patterns have been identified, these may be combined in a tool that incorporates known risk factors with the unique ones for that particular setting. A search of the literature as discussed previously revealed many risk factors for falls. These have been incorporated into the example of a rehabilitation client's fall risk assessment sheet as seen in Table 7–5. A check is placed in each box where a risk factor is present. These checks are totaled, and the individual is assigned a score. This is then used as a guide for use of safety devices. Other methods weigh each risk factor and then obtain a total score. When used with a safety promotion tool such as in Table 7–6, continuity of care and good interdisciplinary communication are encouraged. In today's health care environment, where many facilities use agency staff who are not familiar with specific units or patients, a tool that provides information about transferring and ambulation skills, as well as safety needs, decreases the likelihood of injury to clients or staff.

It is my opinion that the tool itself is not as important as the awareness it creates within the staff as they use it on a regular basis. This notion is supported by studies that showed that a simple warning or arm bracelet is inadequate to prevent falls and that no one strategy works for all patients (Mayo, Gloutney, & Levy, 1994). Tailor-made strategies and fall risk assessment tools should promote better outcomes than using a standardized form.

The fall risk tool, of which there are many available in the literature, should be completed on specific days of the week for continuity. The nursing staff may decide which safety devices are appropriate for which scores. However, it must be emphasized that use of safety devices in the form of restraints should be minimized and must be appropriately documented according to the facility's policies. Restraints should be used only when a patient is a danger to others or himself or herself.

One additional factor should be mentioned. The fear of falling may cause a decrease in mobility (Steinmetz & Hobson, 1994). Caregivers also report a great fear that their loved one might fall. This fear of falling "was primarily related to the emotional rather than the physical status of the patient" (Liddle & Gilleard, 1995, p. 110). Education of patients and family members on how they can reduce the risk for falls in the hospital, in the long-term care facility, and in the community is essential (Tideiksaar, 1989; Tideiksaar & Kay, 1986). Knowledge of what can be done to prevent falls, instead of decreasing mobility, can help patients and families cope with the fear of falling. Suggestions for teaching about a safe environment that promotes improved functional outcomes appear in Table 7–7.

Table 7-4 EXAMPLE OF A FALL COMMITTEE EVALUATION FORM

Pt. Name	Age	Dx	Time of Fall	Cause of Fall	Location of Fall	Fall History	Activity Order	Mental Status	Meds	Sensory Deficits	Safety Measures	Results of Fall

Table 7-5   REHABILITATION FALL RISK ASSESSMENT TOOL

	Admission	Date	Date	Date
Age older than 60 years				
Diagnosis of CVA or TBI				
Altered physical capabilities (limited mobility, abnormal gait, impaired balance, sway, weakness, motor deficits, hemiparesis, hemiplegia, decreased endurance)				
Altered mental state (confused, restless, sedated, disoriented, sleepless, TIAs, depressed, history of seizures, history of loss of consciousness, complaint of dizziness, demented, psychiatric diagnosis)				
Altered bowel/bladder elimination (incontinence, urgency, frequency, nocturia)				
Cognitive/sensory impairments (impaired memory or judgment, decreased ability to understand and/or follow directions, impaired vision or hearing, aphasia, neglect)				
Altered proprioception				
Day of hospitalization (first week or after fourth week)				
Medications that affect fluid balance or sensorium (diuretics, narcotics, sedatives, hypnotics, tranquilizers, antidepressants, antihypertensives, laxatives, history of drug/alcohol abuse)				
Psychological factors (denies falls, denies condition, hesitant to call for assistance, impulsive, demonstrates high value of independence, fear of restraints, history of escape from restraints or crawling out of bed)				
Total Score				
List safety devices to be used: Score of 1–5: generally may need lap belt, side rails up Score of 6–10: generally may require additional safety devices as deemed necessary				

CVA, cerebrovascular accident; TBI, traumatic brain injury; TIA, transient ischemic attack.

Table 7–6 SAFETY PROMOTION CHECKLIST

Directions: Circle all that apply. Post on door, or in Kardex.

Fall risk rating:	1 2 3 4 5 6 7 8 9 10
Transfer status:	Independent
	Supervision
	Contact guard
	No weight bearing
	Partial weight bearing _____
	Min assist × 1
	Mod assist × 1 Mod assist × 2
	Max assist × 1 Max assist × 2
	Max assist of more than 2 persons
	Mechanical lift
	Other _____
Ambulation status:	Independent: in room, in hallway
	Supervision
	Contact guard
	Hand-in-hand
	Min assist × 1
	Mod assist × 1
	Partial weight bearing _____
	Wheelchair bound
	Ambulates only in therapy
	Ambulates to dining room
	Ambulates to bathroom
	Other _____
Devices for transfer/ ambulation:	None
	Gait belt
	Quad cane
	Ankle-foot orthosis/splint
	Sling
	Walker
	Straight cane
	Prosthesis
	Other _____
Safety devices/restraints:	Side rails up × 4
	Side rails up × 2
	Call light in reach
	Lap belt in chair
	Gait belt for transfers
	Gait belt for ambulation
	Lapboard on wheelchair
	Nurse alert at all times in room
	Nurse alert at bedtime
	Vest restraint in wheelchair
	Vest restraint at all times
	Crotch safety device
	Padded side rails
	Seizure precautions
	Check q _____ hr
	Other _____

Table 7–7   CLIENT/CAREGIVER TEACHING: PROMOTING A SAFE HOME ENVIRONMENT FOR A PERSON WITH A FUNCTIONAL DISABILITY

- Install hand rails in the bathroom and along stairs.
- Lower medicine cabinets to wheelchair level.
- Arrange the kitchen and bedroom so that the person can reach commonly used household items.
- Remove all throw rugs.
- Use two knobs in the shower for singular hot and cold.
- If moving or building another home, consult an architect who specializes in "handicapped homes." Have hallways built at least 48 inches wide and doorways 36 inches wide if accommodating a wheelchair. Homes can be built, even with a basement, at ground level so there are no steps to the outside.
- Install a lower tub.
- Obtain adaptive equipment to make life easier and promote independence, such as shower chairs, rolling commodes, tub chairs, reachers, walkers, and the like.
- Place tables and other furniture purposely in the room to keep walkways clear and free from clutter.
- Be careful of small animals and children, which can accidentally cause a person to lose balance.
- Mark steps clearly. Bright colored tape can be placed on the edge of steps as a warning.
- Use low-pile carpeting instead of shag.
- Make certain non-skid shoes are worn, but be careful with rubber soles that can stick to the floor and also cause slipping.
- Be sure trousers and pants are hemmed well above the shoes.
- Leave lights in hallways on at night. Remember an older person may require more light to see, so tiny night lights may be insufficient.
- Place the person's room close to the bathroom if possible, or use a commode if necessary at night.
- Monitor effects of medication that could cause dizziness or poor balance. Notify your primary health care provider of any changes in alertness or balance.
- Encourage the person to change positions slowly and sit at the edge of the bed or chair for a minute before rising.
- Place needed items near the bedside at night. A portable or rolling bedside table, as used in the hospital, works well for some.
- Remember that falls are often associated with needing to go to the bathroom. Make sure these needs are taken care of before bed.
- Have a system for the person to use to call for help at home if needed, such as a bell or whistle, if the caregiver happens to be in a different room. For those living alone, various types of devices, such as the Lifeline, are available.
- Have emergency numbers close to the phone.
- Always lock wheelchair, bed, commode, or shower chair brakes before transferring.

Use of Restraints

The use of restraints remains a controversial topic in long-term care and rehabilitation. Restraints may be chemical, as in medications that restrict activity, or physical, as in the application and use of safety devices to prevent falls. Safety devices come in many forms, but they should be used only in cases in which the patient is a danger to himself or herself or others. Even so, all other methods to keep the person safe should be tried first, because there are many viable alternatives to restraints.

In considering the use of safety devices that restrict mobility, a careful balance must be struck between the need to keep persons safe in order to keep them mobile and the need for them to be active without harm.

Both sides of this dilemma have the goal of keeping the person safe and mobile. However, restraints do not contribute to mobility, unless they do so indirectly and temporarily by preventing a fall that could cause an injury, such as a hip fracture. Sometimes restraint use is warranted to prevent a further cycle of immobility that could be caused by such fractures. On the other hand, use of restraints for the purpose of safety surely contributes to the hazards of immobility, particularly if great care is not taken to promote mobility in every other way. GRNs must be knowledgeable about the current guidelines for restraint use in the facility in which they work, including the proper documentation needed. A more thorough discussion surrounding the ethics of restraint use appears in Chapter 15.

EVALUATION

Evaluation of improved outcomes related to mobility and functional capacity can be seen by the increase in FIM or other such scores. Quantitative criteria are assigned on patient evaluation, and goals are set for discharge. On discharge, or reevaluation, scores should reflect rehabilitative progress. These numbers are also used by insurance carriers to ascertain an individual's present status, weekly or monthly progress, and predicted discharge abilities. Another method of evaluation is increased endurance time such as tolerance to activity or ability to remain sitting up in the chair for longer intervals. The nurse can assess the patient's ability to ambulate progressively farther distances as another sign of achievement of desired outcomes. Additionally, when evaluating results of an exercise program, the GRN can assess the tone, strength, and size of muscles, as well as the participant's range of motion (Milde, 1988). All rehabilitation team members share the responsibility for improved functional outcomes.

The use of fall risk tools to concentrate efforts on prevention of injury is another method of documentation of outcomes. Although the risk assessment criteria may not change significantly throughout the rehabilitation stay, factors such as poor balance and sway, incontinence, and the like should show improvement. Assignment of a rating on the fall risk scale and the monitoring of such scores are other ways to demonstrate better outcomes.

Perhaps the best way to evaluate whether a person has met his or her goals is to set mutually agreed on goals at the outset and periodically monitor progress toward those objectives. For example, the patient's main desire might be to "walk out of the hospital." Knowing this is the patient's motivation, the rehabilitation team can set their individual specialty objectives accordingly. The GRN can work with the physical therapist to help the patient achieve this practical goal by setting smaller, short-term goals along the rehabilitation path. This could include supervising the patient in ROM activities, practicing transfers, and eventually ambulating with assistance to the dining room or around the unit.

REFERENCES

Ashley, M. J., Gryfe, C. I., & Amies, A. (1977). A longitudinal study of falls in an elderly population. II: Some circumstances of falling. *Age and Ageing, 6,* 211–220.

Atwood, S. M., Holm, M. B., & James, A. (1994). Activities of daily living capabilities and values of long-term-care facility residents. *American Journal of Occupational Therapy, 48*(8), 710–716.

Berg, K. O., Wood-Dauphinee, S. L., Williams, J. I., & Maki, B. (1992). Measuring balance in the elderly: Validation of an instrument. *Canadian Journal of Public Health, 83,* S7–S11.

Berry, G., Fisher, R., & Lang, S. (1981). Detrimental incidents including falls in an elderly institutional population. *Journal of the American Geriatric Society, 29*(7), 322–324.

Brady, R., Chester, F. R., Pierce, L. L., Salter, J. P., Schreck, S., & Radziewicz, R. (1993). Geriatric falls: Prevention strategies for the staff. *Journal of Gerontological Nursing, 19*(9), 26–32.

Brians, L. K., Alexander, K., Grota, P., Chen, R. W. H., & Dumas, V. (1991). The development of the RISK tool for fall prevention. *Rehabilitation Nursing, 16*(2), 67–69.

Burckhardt, C. S., Moncur, C., & Minor, M. A. (1994). Exercise tests as outcome measures. *Arthritis Care and Research, 7*(4), 169–174.

Cheng, C. L., Lau, S., Hui, P. W., Chow, S. P., Pun, J. N., & Leong, J. C. Y. (1989). Prognostic factors and progress for ambulation in elderly patients after hip fracture. *American Journal of Physical Medicine and Rehabilitation, 68*(5), 230–233.

Commodore, D. I. B. (1995). Falls in the elderly population: A look at incidence, risks, health-care costs, and preventive strategies. *Rehabilitation Nursing, 20*(2), 84–89.

Cummings, S. R., Phillips, S. L., Wheat, M. E., Black, D., Goosby, E., Wlodarczyk, D., Trafton, P., Jergesen, H., Winograd, C. H., & Hulley, S. B. (1988). Recovery of function after hip fracture: The role of social supports. *Journal of the American Geriatrics Society, 36,* 801–806.

Davis, A. E. (1995). Hip fractures in the elderly: Surveillance methods and injury control. *Journal of Trauma Nursing, 2*(1), 15–21.

DeVincenzo, D. K., & Watkins, S. (1987). Accidental falls in a rehabilitation setting. *Rehabilitation Nursing, 12*(5), 248–252.

Engle, V. F. (1986). The relationship of movement and time to older adults' functional health. *Research in Nursing and Health, 9*(2), 123–129.

Fife, D. D., Solomon, P., & Stanton, M. (1984). A risk/falls program: Code orange for success. *Nursing Management, 15*(11), 50–54.

Fisher, N. M., Pendergast, D. R., Gresham, G. E., & Calkins, E. (1991a). Muscle rehabilitation in impaired elderly nursing home residents. *Archives of Physical Medicine and Rehabilitation, 72,* 181–185.

Fisher, N. M., Pendergast, D. R., Gresham, G. E., & Calkins, E. (1991b). Muscle rehabilitation: Its effect on muscular and functional performance of patients with knee osteoarthritis. *Archives of Physical Medicine and Rehabilitation, 72,* 367–374.

Fleming, E. R., & Pendergast, D. R. (1993). Physical condition, activity pattern, and environment as factors in falls by adult day care facility residents. *Archives of Physical Medicine and Rehabilitation, 74,* 627–630.

Folman, Y., Gepstein, R., Assaraf, A., & Leberty, S. (1994). Functional recovery after operative treatment of femoral neck fractures in an institutionalized elderly population. *Archives of Physical Medicine and Rehabilitation, 75,* 454–456.

Galindo-Ciocon, D., Ciocon, J. O., & Galindo, D. (1995a). Functional impairment among elderly women with osteoporotic vertebral fractures. *Rehabilitation Nursing, 20*(2), 79–83.

Galindo-Ciocon, D. J., Ciocon, J. O., & Galindo, D. J. (1995b). Gait training and falls in the elderly. *Journal of Gerontological Nursing, 21*(6), 10–17.

Garcia, R. M., Cruz, M., Reed, M., Taylor, P. V., Sloan, G., & Beran, N. (1988). Relationship between falls and patient attempts to satisfy elimination needs. *Nursing Management, 19*(7), 80v–80x.

Gehlsen, G. M., & Whaley, M. H. (1990a). Falls in elderly: Part I, gait. *Archives of Physical Medicine and Rehabilitation, 71,* 735–738.

Gehlsen, G. M., & Whaley, M. H. (1990b). Falls in elderly: Part II, balance, strength, and flexibility. *Archives of Physical Medicine and Rehabilitation, 71,* 739–741.

Grant, J. S., & Hamilton, S. (1987). Falls in a rehabilitation setting: Incidence and characteristics. *Rehabilitation Nursing, 12*(2), 74–76.

Gregor, S., McCarthy, K., Chwirchak, D., Meluch, M., & Mion, L. (1986). Characteristics and functional outcomes of elderly rehabilitation patients. *Rehabilitation Nursing, 11*(30), 10–14.

Gryfe, C. I., Amies, A., & Ashley, M. J. (1977). A longitudinal study of falls in an elderly population. I: Incidence and morbidity. *Age and Ageing, 6,* 210–220.

Habel, M. (1996). Sleep, rest, and fatigue. In S. Hoeman (Ed.), *Rehabilitation nursing: Process and application* (pp. 508–525). St. Louis, MO: C. V. Mosby.

Hamilton, L., & Lyon, P. S. (1995). A nursing-driven program to preserve and restore functional ability in hospitalized elderly patients. *Journal of Nursing Administration, 25*(4), 30–37.

Harada, N., Chiu, V., Fowler, E., Lee, M., & Reuben, D. B. (1995). *Physical Therapy, 75*(9), 830–838.

Heafey, M. L., Golden-Baker, S. B., & Mahoney, D. W. (1994). Using nursing diagnoses and interventions in an inpatient amputee program. *Rehabilitation Nursing, 19*(3), 163–168.

Hogue, C. C., Studenski, S., & Duncan, P. (1990). Assessing mobility: The first step in preventing falls. In S. G. Funk, M. T. Tournquist, M. T. Champagne, L. A. Copp, R. A. Weise (Eds.), *Key aspects of recovery: Improving nutrition, rest, and mobility.* New York: Springer.

Hymovich, D. P., & Hagopian, G. A. (1992). *Chronic illness in children and adults: A psychosocial approach.* Philadelphia: W. B. Saunders.

Janken, J. K., Reynolds, B. A., & Sweich, K. (1986).

Patient falls in the acute care setting: Identifying risk factors. *Nursing Research, 35*(4), 215–219.

Jirovec, M. M. (1991). The impact of daily exercise on the mobility, balance and urine control of cognitively impaired nursing home residents. *International Journal of Nursing Studies, 28*(2), 145–151.

Jirovec, M. M., & Maxwell, B. A. (1993). Nursing home residents: Functional ability and perceptions of choice. *Journal of Gerontological Nursing, 19*(9), 10–14.

Jorgensen, H. S., Nakayama, H., Raaschou, H. O., & Olsen, T. S. (1995). Recovery of walking function in stroke patients: The Copenhagen Stroke Study. *Archives of Physical Medicine and Rehabilitation, 76,* 27–32.

Kalchthaler, T., Bascon, R. A., & Quintos, V. (1978). Falls in the institutionalized elderly. *Journal of the American Geriatrics Society, 26,* 424–428.

Kasper, C. E., Maxwell, L. C., & White, T. P. (1996). Alterations in skeletal muscle related to short-term impaired physical mobility. *Research in Nursing and Health, 19,* 133–142.

Kauffman, T. L., Albright, L., & Wagner, C. (1987). Rehabilitation outcomes after hip fracture in persons 90 years old and older. *Archives of Physical Medicine and Rehabilitation, 68*(6), 369–371.

Kelly-Hayes, M. (1996). Functional evaluation. In S. Hoeman (Ed.), *Rehabilitation nursing: Process and application* (pp. 144–155). St. Louis, MO: C. V. Mosby.

Kippenbrock, T., & Soja, M. E. (1993). Preventing falls in the elderly: Interviewing patients who have fallen. *Geriatric Nursing, 14*(4), 205–209.

Koroknay, V. J., Werner, P., Cohen-Mansfield, J., & Braun, J. V. (1995). Maintaining ambulation in the frail nursing home resident: A nursing administered walking program. *Journal of Gerontological Nursing, 21*(11), 18–24.

Lemaire, E. D., & Fisher, F. R. (1994). Osteoarthritis and elderly amputee gait. *Archives of Physical Medicine and Rehabilitation, 75,* 1094–1099.

Lewis, N. A. (1986). Functional gains in CVA patients: A nursing approach. *Rehabilitation Nursing, 11*(2), 25–27.

Liddle, J., & Gilleard, C. (1995). The emotional consequences of falls for older people and their families. *Clinical Rehabilitation, 9*(2), 110–114.

Louis, M. (1983). Falls and their causes. *Journal of Gerontological Nursing, 9,* 142–149.

Malzer, R. L. (1988). Patient performance level during inpatient physical rehabilitation: Therapist, nurse, and patient perspectives. *Archives of Physical Medicine and Rehabilitation, 69,* 363–365.

Mayo, N. E., Gloutney, L., & Levy, A. R. (1994). A randomized trial of identification bracelets to prevent falls among patients in a rehabilitation hospital. *Archives of Physical Medicine and Rehabilitation, 75*(12), 1302–1308.

Mayo, N. E., Korner-Bitensky, N., & Levy, A. R. (1993). Risk factors for fractures due to falls. *Archives of Physical Medicine and Rehabilitation, 74,* 917–921.

Medhat, A., Huber, P. M., & Medhat, M. A. (1990).

Factors that influence the level of activities in persons with lower extremity amputation. *Rehabilitation Nursing, 15*(1), 13–18.

Milde, F. K. (1988). Impaired physical mobility. *Journal of Gerontological Nursing, 14*(30), 20–24.

Mion, L. C., Gregor, S., Beuttner, M., Chwirchak, D., Lee, O., & Paras, W. (1989). Falls in the rehabilitation setting: Incidence and characteristics. *Rehabilitation Nursing, 14*(1), 17–21.

Mol, V. J., & Baker, C. A. (1991). Activity intolerance in the geriatric stroke patient. *Rehabilitation Nursing, 16*(6), 337–342.

Morgan, V. R., Mathison, J. H., Rice, J. C., & Clemmer, D. I. (1985). Hospital falls: A persistent problem. *American Journal of Public Health, 75,* 775–777.

Morris, E. V., Isaacs, B., & Brislen, W. (1981). Falls in the elderly hospital. *Nursing Times, 77,* 1522–1524.

Morse, J. M., Prowse, M. D., Morrow, N., & Federspeil, G. (1976). A retrospective analysis of patient falls. *Canadian Journal of Public Health, 76*(2), 116–118.

Morton, D. (1989). Five years of fewer falls. *American Journal of Nursing, 2,* 204–205.

Muecke, L., Shekar, S., Dwyer, D., Israel, E., & Flynn, J. P. G. (1992). Functional screening of lower-limb amputees: A role in predicting rehabilitation outcome? *Archives of Physical Medicine and Rehabilitation, 73,* 851–858.

Nakayama, H., Jorgensen, H. S., Raaschou, H. O., & Olsen, T. S. (1994). Recovery of upper extremity function in stroke patients: The Copenhagen Stroke Study. *Archives of Physical Medicine and Rehabilitation, 75,* 394–398.

Naso, F., Carner, E., Blankfort-Doyle, W., & Coughey, K. (1990). Endurance training in the elderly nursing home patient. *Archives of Physical Medicine and Rehabilitation, 71,* 241–242.

Nugent, J. A., Schurr, K. A., & Adams, R. D. (1994). A dose-response relationship between amount of weight-bearing exercise and walking outcome following cerebrovascular accident. *Archives of Physical Medicine and Rehabilitation, 75,* 399–402.

O'Brien, L. A., Grisso, J. A., Maislin, G., Chiu, G. Y., & Evans, L. (1993). Hospitalized elders: Risk of confusion with hip fracture. *Journal of Gerontological Nursing, 19*(2), 25–31.

Orr, P. M., & Bratton, G. N. (1992). The effect of an inpatient arthritis rehabilitation program on self-assessed functional ability. *Rehabilitation Nursing, 17*(6), 306–309.

Pablo, R. (1977). Patient accidents in a long-term facility. *Canadian Journal of Public Health, 3,* 237–247.

Patla, A. E., Frank, J. S., & Winter, D. A. (1992). Balance control in the elderly: Implications for clinical assessment and rehabilitation. *Canadian Journal of Public Health, 83,* S29–S33.

Potter, J. M., Evans, A. L., & Duncan, G. (1995). Gait speed and activities of daily living function in geriatric patients. *Archives of Physical Medicine and Rehabilitation, 76*(11), 997–999.

Rapport, L. J., Webster, J. S., Flemming, K., Lindberg, J. W., Godlewski, M. C., Brees, J., & Abadee, P. S. (1993). Predictors of falls among right-hemisphere stroke patients in the rehabilitation setting. *Archives of Physical Medicine and Rehabilitation, 74,* 621–626.

Richards, C. L., Malouin, F., Wood-Sauphinee, C., Williams, J. I., Bouchard, J. P., & Brunet, D. (1993). Task-specific physical therapy for optimization of gait recovery in acute stroke patients. *Archives of Physical Medicine and Rehabilitation, 74,* 612–620.

Richardson, J. I., Ching, C., & Hurvitz, E. A. (1992). The relationship between electromyographically documented peripheral neuropathy and falls. *Journal of the American Geriatrics Society, 40*(10), 1008–1012.

Roberts, B. L., & Wykle, M. L. (1993). Pilot study results: Falls among institutionalized elderly. *Journal of Gerontological Nursing, 19*(5), 13–20.

Rodstein, M. (1964). Accidents among the aged: Incidence, causes, prevention. *Journal of Chronic Diseases, 17,* 515–526.

Rogers, S. (1994). Reducing falls in a rehabilitation setting: A safer environment through team effort. *Rehabilitation Nursing, 19*(5), 274–276.

Ross, J. E. R. (1991). Iatrogenesis in the elderly: Contributors to falls. *Journal of Gerontological Nursing, 17*(9), 19–23.

Schested, P., & Severin-Nielsen, T. (1977). Falls by hospitalized elderly patients: Causes and prevention. *Geriatrics, 32,* 101–108.

Spier, B. E., & Meis, M. (1994). Maintenance ambulation: Its significance and the role of nursing. *Geriatric Nursing, 15*(5), 277–281.

Steinmetz, H. M., & Hobson, S. J. G. (1994). Prevention of falls among the community-dwelling elderly: An overview. *Physical and Occupational Therapy in Geriatrics, 12*(4), 13–29.

Thorngren, K. (1994). Fractures in older persons. *Disability and Rehabilitation, 16*(3), 119–126.

Tideiksaar, R. (1988). Falls in the elderly: An approach to management. *Physician Assistant, 12*(10), 114, 117–118.

Tideiksaar, R. (1989). Home safe home. Practical tips for fall-proofing. *Geriatric Nursing, 11,* 280–284.

Tideiksaar, R., & Kay, A. D. (1986). What causes falls? A logical diagnostic procedure. *Geriatrics, 41*(12), 32–49.

Tinetti, M. E. (1986). Performance-oriented assessment of mobility problems in elderly patients. *Journal of the American Geriatrics Society, 34*(2), 119–126.

Tinetti, M. E. (1987). Factors associated with serious injury during falls by ambulatory nursing home residents. *Journal of the American Geriatrics Society, 35,* 644–648.

Topp, R., Mikesky, A., & Bawel, K. (1994). Developing a strength training program for older adults: Planning, programming, and potential outcomes. *Rehabilitation Nursing, 19*(5), 266–273.

Tutuarima, J. A., de Haan, R. J., & Limburg, M.

(1993). Number of nursing staff and falls: A case-control study on falls by stroke patients in acute-care settings. *Journal of Advanced Nursing, 18,* 1101–1105.

Walshe, A., & Rosen, H. (1979). A study of patient falls from bed. *Journal of Nursing Administration, 9*(5), 31–35.

Williams, M. A., Oberst, M. T., & Bjorklund, B. C. (1994). Early outcomes after hip fracture among women discharged home and to nursing homes. *Research in Nursing and Health, 17,* 175–183.

Wright, B. A., Aizenstein, S., Vogler, G., Rower, M., & Miller, C. (1990). Frequent fallers: Leading groups to identify psychological factors. *Journal of Gerontological Nursing, 16*(4), 15–19.

Appendix 7A

UDSMR^{SM} FIM^{SM} Instrument

UDSMR^{SM} FIM^{SM} Instrument

	ADMISSION*	DISCHARGE*	GOAL
SELF-CARE			
A. Eating			
B. Grooming			
C. Bathing			
D. Dressing-Upper			
E. Dressing-Lower			
F. Toileting			
SPHINCTER CONTROL			
G. Bladder			
H. Bowel			
TRANSFERS			
I. Bed, Chair, Whlchair			
J. Toilet			
K. Tub, Shower			
LOCOMOTION	W-Walk C-Wheelchair B-Both ⊥		
L. Walk/Wheelchair			
M. Stairs	A-Auditory V-Visual B-Both ⊥		
COMMUNICATION			
N. Comprehension			
O. Expression	⊤ V-Vocal N-Nonvocal B-Both		
SOCIAL COGNITION			
P. Social Interaction			
Q. Problem Solving			
R. Memory			

*Leave no blanks. Enter 1 if not testable due to risk.

FIM LEVELS

No Helper
   7 Complete Independence (Timely, Safely)
   6 Modified Independence (Device)

Helper - Modified Dependence
   5 Supervision (Subject = 100%)
   4 Minimal Assistance (Subject = 75% or more)
   3 Moderate Assistance (Subject = 50% or more)

Helper - Complete Dependence
   2 Maximal Assistance (Subject = 25% or more)
   1 Total Assistance or not testable (Subject less than 25%)

Chapter 8

Establishing Bowel and Bladder Patterns

■

Bowel and bladder problems are not typically the topic of public discussion. In fact, in many societies subjects like incontinence are avoided, indicating there is a negative stigma associated with it. In the past, some facilities used systems of reward and punishment to try to manage incontinence, but significant progress has been made in our understanding of the physiological mechanisms behind these problems (Wells, 1988). Despite these advances, myths about bowel and bladder habits persist. The notion of needing to have a daily bowel movement in order to be healthy is one example. The function of a person's elimination system is often used as a judge of overall health, and sometimes this is appropriate. However, through cultural norms, the value is conveyed that control of feces and urine is important, and the loss of control is humiliating. Pressure to maintain control in this area may make it particularly devastating for an older adult to experience problems. Many elders hide the problem of incontinence (Simons, 1985). Some have expressed that incontinence was as much a problem as the disability that contributed to it. Incontinence is a significant predictor for institutionalization of the elderly. It is estimated that half of all institutionalized aged are incontinent (Simons, 1985; Tunink, 1988). Approximately 31% of stroke patients experience bowel incontinence, although this usually resolves within 2 weeks after the stroke (Lorish, Sandin, Roth, & Noll, 1994). Generally speaking, the reestablishment of bowel function or continence is quicker and more easily attained than that of the bladder. The literature sup-

ports this notion; there are many more studies and clinical articles available on managing urinary incontinence than on bowel function.

BOWEL MANAGEMENT

Mechanism of Defecation

The process of defecation is complex and involves both voluntary and involuntary mechanisms. Certain physiological events, such as getting up in the morning or eating or drinking, initiate involuntary reflexes. For example, the gastrocolic and gastroileal reflexes, strongest within the first 15 minutes after breakfast, are triggered by ingestion of food or fluids. These reflexes, mediated by several different nerves such as the pelvic splanchnic or intrinsic nerves, start a general peristalsis that propels the fecal mass into the rectum. Stretch receptors in the rectum signal the brain, via the spinal cord, that it is time to have a bowel movement. In healthy persons, inhibitory reflexes allow them, in combination with memory and habit, to wait until an appropriate time and place to defecate is found. Much of the ability to retain feces until a toilet or other suitable place can be used occurs voluntarily with the contraction of the external sphincter and levator ani muscles. The act of defecating itself involves the coordinated effort of no less than nine specific nerves, the diaphragm, the abdominal muscles, and multiple other muscles. It is no wonder that an elderly individual with a disability should have problems maintaining control in this area.

In the case of an older person, gastric motility has already slowed. There is a decreased production of digestive enzymes such as hydrochloric acid, pepsin, and those from the pancreas. A lack of roughage in combination with these factors may make constipation a recurring problem. If a disease or illness that affects the brain or spinal cord is added to this clinical picture, the inhibitory reflexes that prevented incontinence may no longer be receiving messages as a result of interruptions in the pathways that communicate from the body via the spinal cord to the control centers of the brain. The person with stroke may experience the effects of an uninhibited neurogenic bowel. The client with damage to the S2–S4 area of the spinal cord may have a flaccid, atonic bowel that is quite difficult to manage. Anytime there is an interruption in the mechanism by which the body via stretch receptors and the like transmits messages to the brain, there may be problems with bowel management. However, certain factors make the prognosis good for regaining bowel control for most elderly rehabilitation patients.

The importance of reestablishing a bowel program cannot be overlooked. Not only is it of physical benefit, but the lack of continence has serious social implications as well. Gerontological rehabilitation nurses (GRNs) will attest to the fact that the patient with constipation often has a difficult time focusing on anything else except the need to have a bowel movement. Constipation can also lead to loss of appetite, dehydration, abdominal discomfort, and depression. This interferes with the ability to participate in therapy and can cause undue anxiety to the patient and caregivers. Many medications can also contribute to constipation (Table 8–1).

Understanding the Effects of a Neurogenic Bowel

Neurogenic bowel generally means a person has difficulty voluntarily controlling bowel movements. There are several types of neurogenic bowels. The three most commonly seen in gerontological rehabilitation are discussed here: uninhibited, reflexic, and areflexic (or autonomous). Table 8–2 presents a summary of these three bowel types.

Uninhibited: Uninhibited neurogenic bowel is the name given to the bowel activity seen with lesions above C1 or those that occur within the brain. This is probably the most common type of bowel dysfunction seen in

Table 8–1   MEDICATIONS COMMONLY USED IN GERONTOLOGICAL REHABILITATION THAT CAN CONTRIBUTE TO CONSTIPATION

Medication/Purpose	Example
Analgesics	Tylenol with Codeine, Demerol
Anticholinergics	Cogentin
Anticonvulsives	Dilantin
Antidepressants	Ludiomil, Elavil
Antiparkinsonians	Levodopa
Antihypertensives	Diuril, Aldactone
Diuretics	Lasix
Opiates	Morphine, codeine
Iron supplements	Feosol
Muscle relaxants	Lioresal

older persons. Bowel sensation and reflex activity are intact, but the brain does not have the same control over inhibitory processes that prevented incontinence before. This is called an upper motor neuron disorder. Characteristics of this type of bowel function may include involuntary stools, a lack of awareness of need, urgency, smearing, constipation (more than 3 days with no bowel movement), impaction, hypoactive bowel sounds, and decreased sphincter control. This is the type of function most stroke patients have. Other persons who may present with this type of function include those with head injury, brain tumor, Parkinson's disease, and multiple sclerosis (MS). Treatment for patients with uninhibited neurogenic bowel includes establishing a consistent schedule for toileting, managing controllable factors, and using suppositories and/or stool softeners as needed. Most of these patients experience good success with regaining bowel control.

Reflexic: As the name suggests, in this type of bowel function the defecation reflex located in the S2–S4 spinal cord segments is retained. Persons with this problem have injury in the upper spinal cord (thus, an upper motor neuron disorder). This may be due to spinal cord tumors, infarct, lesions (as in MS), or other trauma. Characteristics of reflexic bowel function include loss of urge to defecate, incontinence, automatic emptying, and impaired external sphincter control. Most quadriplegics fall into this category and may require a caregiver to assist with the bowel program. Nursing management includes capitalizing on the intact reflex for defecation.

Table 8–2 SUMMARY OF THREE TYPES OF NEUROGENIC BOWEL

Type	Associated Diagnoses	Traits	Treatment
Uninhibited	Stroke TBI Brain tumor MS Parkinson's disease Alzheimer's disease	Urgency Incontinence Smearing Constipation Intact reflexes Hypoactive bowel sounds Decreased awareness of need Lesions above C1	Managing controllable factors Toileting schedule Suppositories p.r.n.
Reflexic	SCI SC tumors SC infarct Quadriplegia MS Trauma High thoracic paraplegics	Incontinence Loss of urge S2–S4 intact Empties automatically Impaired external sphincter control Lack of voluntary control Damage above T12–L1	Bowel program Digital stimulation Dulcolax suppository
Areflexic	Spina bifida Cauda equina injury Diabetes Intervertebral disk problem Trauma to S2–S4 Paraplegia	Incontinence Sensory loss of need to defecate Flaccid external sphincter Leakage of stool Damage below T12–L1	High-fiber diet Valsalva maneuver Manual removal Suppository

MS, multiple sclerosis; p.r.n., as needed; SC, spinal cord; SCI, spinal cord injury; TBI, traumatic brain injury.

Digital stimulation, use of gravity, and control of other factors as previously discussed are indicated. Suppositories are frequently used.

Areflexic (Autonomous): The autonomous bowel is caused by injury to the lumbosacral cord and spinal root. This lower motor neuron disorder results from damage to the S2–S4 segments. This could be caused by a cauda equina injury, spina bifida, diabetes, or intervertebral disk disease. Traits seen include recurring and frequent incontinence, a flaccid external sphincter that results in leakage of stool, and the sensory loss of the need to defecate (Gender, 1996). The spinal reflex arc has been damaged, making this the most difficult bowel problem to manage. Many paraplegics experience this bowel type. Treatment includes strict adherence to a bowel program, plenty of fiber and fluids in the diet to maintain a firm stool and prevent diarrhea, use of suppositories and manual removal of stool, and the Valsalva maneuver to promote defecation. Of course, use of the Valsalva maneuver should be judicious, taking into consideration other factors that result, such as increased intra-abdominal and intracranial pressure.

Assessment

The main tasks in assessment of bowel and bladder function are taking a thorough history, observing the patient, performing a physical assessment, and keeping good records. Recording patterns before initiating treatment will assist the GRN in identifying the nature of the problem. The best place to begin retraining is in the acute rehabilitation setting. Until this time, the patient receiving acute hospital care may not have been stabilized, and this process requires the patient's cooperation and participation. Those in long-term care facilities may require long-term management, and some have a poor prognosis for regaining control.

Within the area of bowel management, factors that should be assessed are categorized as controllable or uncontrollable. Controllable factors are those that the GRN can influence through planned nursing interventions to promote patient self-care. Uncontrollable factors are those that the patient presents with that cannot be influenced by treatment. The GRN should perform a complete assessment of both sets of factors to obtain a clear picture of the patient's present bowel status.

The premorbid habits of the individual are particularly important and are used to plan care in the rehabilitation setting. These include the time of day when the individual normally defecated prior to the health crisis and how often this occurred. Normal bowel function can be bowel movements anywhere from twice per day to once every 3 to 4 days. The assessment of abnormality is based on the person's premorbid patterns. Additionally, the GRN should ask information about the patient's use of laxatives, suppositories, or enemas. Laxative abuse is not uncommon among those in the community with chronic constipation.

Uncontrollable factors include previous bowel diseases or surgery, such as a history of diverticulosis or colon cancer or the presence of a colostomy. The disease with which the patient is admitted is also beyond the nurse's control; for instance, the person has already been diagnosed with a stroke, MS, diabetes, head injury, or spinal cord injury (SCI). Additionally, a family history of any problems related to bowel management is considered an uncontrollable factor.

Interventions regarding a patient's bowel status center around managing controllable factors. These factors include diet, fluids, timing, activity, positioning, environment, and medications. Nursing interventions in these areas will promote reestablishment of effective bowel patterns through a carefully planned program.

Physical assessment of the patient related to bowel status involves observation and documentation of general appearance and nutritional and hydration status. Auscultation of bowel sounds should be done on admission and during every shift. Palpation of the abdomen may also be indicated. The color, odor, amount, and quality of stools should be documented.

If the patient cannot remember when the last bowel movement occurred, or expresses concern over possible constipation, the nurse should perform a rectal check. Any stool present within the rectum is removed at this time if possible, or if not, then other steps are taken to clean out the bowel. These are discussed in the section on interventions. A rectal check is also useful in determining whether the patient with spinal cord involvement has an autonomous or reflexic bowel. If the reflexes for defecation are intact, the sphincter will tighten around the finger. If the rectal sphincter does not tighten, the bowel is likely flaccid or autonomous. A flaccid sphincter has significant implications for the type of bowel program that will be necessary for that patient.

Goals

The goals of any bowel program are simple. First, a bowel program must be predictable. To avoid incontinent episodes, the person must be able to accurately predict when the bowel movement will occur, even in the absence of sensation or motor function. For the stroke patient, this may mean having a set time each day for a bowel movement, as well as increasing fluids and fiber. The patient with SCI may use a different approach, such as daily evacuation after a suppository in the morning before beginning activities of daily living (ADLs).

A second goal of any bowel program is that it be convenient. Several effective pieces of equipment or suppositories have been designed to assist with evacuation of stool; however, many are cumbersome and inconvenient. This decreases the likelihood that they will be used appropriately. Expense is another consideration. The least expensive method is generally best. If at all possible, all other factors should be considered before starting the patient on medication. Enemas are a last resort and should never be used regularly. Many patients can achieve bowel continence relatively quickly by using more natural methods such as those discussed in this chapter.

As with any program, it is essential that it be realistic and mutually agreed on. That is, the program must fit the patient's or caregiver's abilities, desires, personal goals, and socioeconomic resources. To plan a nursing-based protocol with which patients must comply is to set oneself up for failure. Care must be individualized if it is to be effective. Still, certain guidelines will assist the GRN with planning an appropriate bowel program.

Interventions

Most of the nursing interventions discussed here are based on accepted protocols that have been shown to work with elderly patients. The main factors that the GRN can influence with regard to establishing a bowel program include diet, fluids, timing, activity, positioning, and medications. Several approaches to bowel management can be taken, but most focus on manipulation of these controllable variables.

Several statistics related to elderly rehabilitation patients also help plan more specific care. The GRN should expect to find compromised bowel elimination in patients with MS, stroke, brain injury or tumor, intervertebral disk disease, diabetes, post-polio syndrome, SCI, and any other disorders that affect the brain or spinal cord (such as Alzheimer's disease). For those with stroke, constipation and impaction are the most common bowel problems (versus diarrhea and incontinence) (Gresham, Duncan, Stason, et al., 1995). Fecal incontinence does occur often, but usually resolves within 2 weeks in most stroke patients (Brocklehurst, Andrews, Richards, & Laycock, 1985). Patients with right hemiplegia may take more time to establish bowel continence, but most stroke patients can achieve effective bowel training without incontinence within 1 month after the stroke (Munchiando & Kendall, 1993; Venn, Taft, Carpentier, & Applebaugh, 1992). Persons with SCI experience different types of problems depending on the completeness and level of injury. More specific interventions with SCI patients are discussed in Chapter 11. Individuals with progressive health alterations affecting the inhibitory reflexes that help control incontinence may experience acute or gradual chronic loss of bowel function.

Basic Principles

When beginning any bowel program, start with a clean bowel. Patients may be admitted to rehabilitation or long-term care settings with constipation or impaction. This immediate problem should be remedied before any bowel program is initiated. This may mean that the GRN needs to manually remove the impaction and/or give enemas to cleanse the bowel.

Most units have a protocol for bowel management, but if one is not available, these guidelines can be followed. However, it is recommended that a procedure be developed and documented as standing orders in collaboration with the advanced practice nurse, staff nurses, and physicians. Use the least-invasive method for control. Factors such as diet, fluids, activity, and timing should be modified first. Medications, suppositories, and enemas are a last resort. Following the

unit policy, change only one or two factors at a time until a satisfactory, effective regimen has been established. If designing a bowel program in the community or home care setting, more time can be allowed to determine the effectiveness of altering one factor at a time. For example, if the GRN recommends that the patient increase fluids by 500 ml per day and drink one glass of prune juice each morning, reevaluation can be done a week later. However, in the acute care setting, where the patient's length of stay is too short to change only one factor at a time with proper evaluation in between, the GRN must seek to set up an appropriate program from the start and promote continuity of care by communicating the need for follow-up to the home health care nurse or other caregivers.

Diet

One of the key factors related to establishment of bowel control is the amount of fiber in the diet. Some believe that lack of dietary fiber is the underlying cause of all constipation. A study by Venn et al. (1992), however, found that food and fluid intake were better predictors of constipation than age or fiber. A diet high in fiber promotes absorption of water into the intestines to make the stool softer and more easily passed. One might observe the effect of "natural fiber" laxatives such as Metamucil. When mixed with water, this fibrous powder-like material turns into a gel in the glass if not consumed immediately. This is similar to the effect that occurs in the intestines. The fiber draws water into the fecal mass, increasing weight and forming a gelatin-like bolus that distends the colon. Colonic distention stimulates further intestinal activity and peristalsis, thereby decreasing constipation.

Fiber is contained in such food as nuts, shredded wheat, popcorn, bran, various cereals, prunes, apples, root vegetables (such as potatoes and carrots), green leafy vegetables, cabbage, oranges, and whole wheat bread. Despite the availability of these food items, many elders do not take in enough to prevent constipation. Although sources vary as to the recommended amount of fiber needed per day, an optimal amount would be 20 to 30 g (Stone, 1991). Elders may find that adding a bowl of cereal high in fiber to the daily diet may be all that is needed to prevent constipation.

Several different remedies have attempted to combine foods to make a "magic" recipe

that will eliminate constipation. One popular mixture combines 1 cup of applesauce, 1 cup of unprocessed bran, and ½ cup of 100% prune juice to form a food that is taken at bedtime (2 tablespoons) with a glass of fluid (Behm, 1985). This and other proportions of the same or similar food items have been used with success. Gibson, Opalka, Moore, Brady, and Mion (1995) recommended 1 cup of Kellogg's All Bran, 1 cup of applesauce, and 1 cup of prune juice (1 ounce per day) to be given with meals. Brown and Everett (1990) found that 30 ml (2.2 g of fiber) of a mixture of 2 cups Kellogg's All Bran, 2 cups applesauce, and 1 cup prune juice added to the diet decreased use of laxatives and resulted in cost savings to the patient. Prune juice has been used alone with some success, but daily use of this received criticism because it was thought to decrease rectal tone. Miller's Bran added to cereal is another common remedy. Drinking a cup of hot liquid half an hour before supper, then toileting after the meal, is another method that may be tried, because the warm liquid is thought to stimulate peristalsis. GRNs should also consider the issue of palatability. If the recipe used does not look, smell, or taste appealing, it may not be the best choice. Extra fiber can be added to other foods such as blueberry muffins or various types of cookies to help prevent constipation.

Increasing fiber in the diet results in use of fewer suppositories and less constipation. Expert opinion does emphasize the need for adequate fluids, however, whenever fiber recipes such as this are in use; otherwise, side effects can occur. Overuse can cause diarrhea, cramping, and loss of essential electrolytes. Generally, the GRN must be creative and resourceful to determine which approach works best for each patient.

Fluids

Adequate fluid intake is essential to any bowel program. Water is the best liquid for this, but many elders prefer to take other fluids such as tea or coffee. Older adults may experience a diminished thirst, making it unlikely that they will feel a need to increase fluid intake unless instructed to do so. The GRN may need to be creative to encourage elders to consume the needed amount of liquid to prevent constipation. An intake of 1500 to 2000 ml/day is recommended and should provide needed fluids without fluid overload in most cases. By dividing this fluid intake

into small amounts throughout the day, time is still allowed for limiting fluids at night if nocturia is a problem.

When teaching patients about proper fluid intake, nurses should make sure that patients understand the role of fluids in preventing constipation and urinary tract infection. Patients using suppositories or taking bulk laxatives must understand that an adequate amount of fluids is needed for those medications to work (Davis, Nagelhout, Hoban, & Barnard, 1986). Interestingly, patients who have an intake of 1500 to 2000 ml/day are less likely to require medications for bowel management. Nurses can use a graduated cylinder (which holds 1 L) and a plastic drinking cup with measurements on it to demonstrate to patients how much they need to drink each day and how this amount can be broken down. Older patients are often overwhelmed when viewing how much water they need to be drinking. However, if the average elderly person drinks a 300-ml cup of coffee or tea in the morning, the same amount with each of three meals, and three other times during the day, he or she will have consumed 2100 ml. If unable to drink large amounts at a time, 100 ml/hr from the time of waking until dinner plus the normal drinks taken with meals should come close to the recommended amount. Nurses can make a conscious effort to promote fluid consumption by providing choices of beverages and reminding the patient to take them during the day. Extra water can be taken with medications. If medications are taken three to four times per day and a habit is made to drink at least 8 ounces with the medications, then the person has consumed nearly half the fluids he or she needs for the day, and the rest may be taken with meals.

For patients with dysphagia, getting the recommended fluid intake per day is a particular challenge. Those with feeding tubes can add the needed amount of water through the tube, but those with swallowing problems and problems with oral intake may find this particularly difficult and time-consuming. In addition to attempting to increase liquid intake, the GRN can assist the patient with dysphagia by offering fluids with thickener, as well as other forms of liquid such as gelatin, soup, broth, or fluids with a thicker consistency. These patients are often in more need of adequate hydration and thus require special planning on the part of the nurse to ensure essential fluid intake. Smaller amounts should be offered more frequently to those

with swallowing problems. Help can also be obtained from the family and caregivers in meeting fluid goals.

Timing and Habits

Taking advantage of the person's premorbid bowel habits can save time and increase the efficiency of the bowel program as well as the patient's satisfaction with it. The body is already accustomed to certain patterns and will recall these in most instances, particularly in the case of stroke. Although there are relatively few studies of bowel function after stroke, some researchers found that use of premorbid habits in the establishment of a bowel program resulted in 85% of patients achieving effective bowel training within 1 month (Venn et al., 1992). The GRN must obtain an accurate picture of previous bowel habits from either the patient or family members. This may be a subject the patient is reluctant to discuss, particularly if cultural influences discourage it. The GRN should, in this event, explain the importance of having this information to help develop a program that will promote control of the bowels in the most efficient manner. A consistent habit and time is recommended for establishing a bowel program with all three major types of neurogenic bowels.

If no information is available, or the patient is having difficulty establishing a program based on premorbid habits, then the GRN should try to take advantage of natural reflexes. Knowing that the gastrocolic reflex is strongest shortly after the breakfast meal, the GRN could choose this time to begin toileting and plan other interventions around this, such as offering warm liquids with breakfast and encouraging fiber at this first meal. A regular schedule for toileting should be a primary goal.

Positioning

Positioning is particularly important for individuals with rehabilitative problems. In addition to the normal effects of aging, patients in rehabilitation experience a variety of mobility difficulties of different levels. The temptation to use the easiest form of toileting procedure for the caregiver should be resisted. The use of bedpans for the immobile patient who is hard to transfer is contraindicated in all but the most exceptional circumstances. Bedpans were not designed to promote self-care in bowel training. They are not a substitute for the use of a bedside commode or toilet. Even

with proper positioning in bed (e.g., head of the bed raised), the feelings associated with eliminating in bed in this manner are against most cultural norms. Additionally, bedpans are uncomfortable and place undue pressure on the buttocks and sacrum. Persons with impaired circulation or sensation or with coccygeal skin breakdown should not use a bedpan. Older persons may require anywhere from 15 to 60 minutes to experience the effects of a suppository. This is too long a time to remain in such a position. Patients should be transferred to the toilet or a bedside commode when toileting, if at all possible. This body position is most like "normal" and has the additional benefit of letting gravity assist with defecation and stool expulsion.

Privacy should be provided for all patients, and giving assistance to the bathroom shows respect for their basic needs. Many older persons feel emotionally uncomfortable at the lack of privacy provided in some bathroom facilities. Having to be assisted with this basic human function, whether through the use of suppositories or in being helped to the toilet, may cause feelings of helplessness and distress. Generally, the more privacy that can be provided, the better the person's comfort level and bowel program outcomes.

Patients with SCI and paraplegia or quadriplegia frequently complete their bowel programs in bed. Those using digital stimulation and/or suppositories to evacuate each morning on an incontinence pad before doing ADLs may find this to be the most efficient means to achieve program goals. Every effort should be made to individualize the bowel program with regard to positioning, taking care to respect the patient's wishes and abilities, but following guidelines for promoting self-care.

Positioning is also important when considering the administration of enemas or suppositories. The patient should be positioned on the left side (Sims' position) for these procedures as well as for the rectal check for impaction. This puts the bowel in the most anatomically correct position for medications to be effective and aids in retention of the suppository. Of course, various physical constraints may exist that preclude following this guideline, such as a recent left hip fracture. However, positioning should always be considered when undertaking any type of bowel program.

Activity

Activity is a key factor in promoting a great many physical functions, and bowel elimina-

tion is no exception. Because with age the gut slows down and peristalsis occurs in a more sluggish manner, the additional implications posed by immobility have a significant effect on bowel function. Constipation is the most common problem related to inactivity. Those with impaired physical mobility may spend more time in chairs and less time ambulating than before. Considering also the difference in diet that occurs with hospitalization or institutionalization, the digestive system experiences some significant changes.

Activity, particularly ambulation, helps promote digestion and peristalsis. Any type of active (versus passive) exercise should help promote good bowel habits. Those with more severe mobility impairment take increased time to become established in a bowel routine (Munchiando & Kendall, 1993). The fact that persons who experience disabilities such as occur with stroke usually regain bowel control within a couple weeks after onset lends credence to the notion that activity plays an important role in normal bowel function, because exercise and ambulation skills are emphasized during this time in rehabilitation. When general guidelines such as avoiding the use of bedpans and instead ambulating or transferring persons to the toilet are followed, mobility is promoted. This contributes to maintaining and reestablishing appropriate bowel habits.

Functional incontinence is a possibility in bowel elimination, particularly for older adults who may live alone or lack assistance. This type of incontinence is related to a person's inability to make it to a facility (commode or toilet) in order to void or defecate. Sometimes this is the result of physical limitations, such as having to use a walker or wheelchair. Other times it may be because the restroom or toilet facilities are inaccessible to the patient because of distance, clutter, or other barriers. In such cases, the GRN should evaluate the cause of the incontinence and attempt to help the person identify and remove obstacles to continence. This may mean rearranging the furniture, using a bedside commode, or educating the caregiver as to the person's needs.

Medications

There are two main routes of medication used for bowel programs: oral and rectal. Medications come in several different forms, including bulk formers, stool softeners, peristaltic stimulators, lubricants, saline laxatives, and hyperosmotics. Rectal medications come in suppository form, mini-enemas, or enemas. Both classifications are discussed here to help the GRN determine appropriate recommendations.

Oral: There are several further classifications of oral medications, including bulk-forming agents, irritants or stimulants, stool softeners, saline laxatives, lubricants, and hyperosmotics. Stool softeners and bulk formers are treatments of choice, but fluid intake should be between 2500 and 3000 ml/day for maximal effectiveness. Defecation should occur within an hour of the planned time. Laxatives and enemas should be used for emergencies only (Davis et al., 1986).

Bulk-forming agents work by aiding in the absorption of water from the intestines, providing bulk and moisture to the feces. They bind with water to form a gel but need an adequate water supply to be effective. The effect of this type of medication usually occurs within 12 to 24 hours but may take 2 to 3 days for a full effect (Stone, 1991), and it is generally taken once or twice per day. Examples of bulk formers are Metamucil, Fibermed, and FiberCon. Disadvantages of this type of preparation include flatulence and bloating, hardened stools, and possible bowel obstruction if water intake is poor. Bulk-forming medications should be used with caution in individuals with cardiac or renal problems or for those who are under fluid restriction.

Irritants or stimulants are laxatives that alter intestinal mucosal permeability. Many stimulate peristalsis. The onset of action for oral medications of this type may be 6 to 10 hours. Medications that act in this manner include cascara, senna, bisacodyl (Dulcolax), and castor oil. Of these, cascara has a mild laxative effect, whereas bisacodyl and castor oil are considered strong irritants. Bisacodyl is often used in bowel preparation kits prior to medical or diagnostic procedures. The main disadvantages of the stronger irritants are cramping and diarrhea. Over-the-counter preparations are also available, including Ex-Lax and Feen-a-Mint.

Stool softeners are one of the most commonly used oral medications in gerontological rehabilitation. They help prevent constipation by altering the surface tension of the fecal mass to promote water absorption, which results in softer, more easily passed stools. Docusate sodium (Colace) and docusate calcium (Surfak) are examples of this type of laxative. They are generally gentler than some other forms of medications and have fewer side effects. However, it is essential that fluid intake be adequate, at least 2000 ml/day (especially of water), for Colace to be used effectively. For patients who have difficulty with constipation but also tend to have hard stool higher up in the rectum as a result of decreased motility, the GRN may suggest Peri-Colace or Senokot. Peri-Colace combines the stool softener Colace with a peristaltic stimulator that helps move the stool along the intestines and further down into the rectum for expulsion. The nurse can assist the patient and physician in identifying which of these medications would be most helpful.

Saline laxatives contain salts, which attract water, producing the desired effect. They act by increasing osmotic pressure, thereby increasing the water content in the stool to soften it. Saline laxatives should be used with discretion and infrequently, because they produce a watery stool within 3 to 6 hours or less. Use of laxatives can cause electrolyte imbalances as well as a decrease in serum albumin (Pahor, Guralnik, Chrischilles, & Wallace, 1994). The most commonly used hospital laxative of this kind is magnesium citrate (or other magnesium preparations), which is often used as a bowel preparation.

Commercially available products include milk of magnesia and Haley's M-O. These are often used in long-term care. Caution should be exercised to use these only on a short-term, as-needed basis and not for long-term maintenance of a bowel program.

Mineral oil is considered a lubricant and works well for some patients. It lubricates the fecal mass and intestinal mucosa to promote comfort and ease of defecation. Adequate fluid intake is also necessary when taking mineral oil. Because of its consistency, mineral oil should be used with caution in patients who have impaired swallowing and is not a drug of choice for many rehabilitation patients, because aspiration can occur. Additionally, the stool may sometimes become too soft, creating difficulty in moving the stool to the rectum, thus contributing further to constipation.

Hyperosmotics include sorbitol and lactulose. These medications draw water from tissue into the feces by a local irritating action that increases the water content, softening the stools. Laxatives are not needed in addition to these. The main disadvantage is diarrhea, and electrolyte imbalance can occur over time.

Rectal: There are several popular rectal medications used in rehabilitation. These include suppositories such as glycerin, Dulcolax, Ceo-Two, and the Therevac mini-enema. Some notes about administering rectal suppositories may be helpful. Suppositories, by nature of their action, need to be in contact with the rectal mucosa to produce the desired effect. Therefore, they will be ineffective if placed within an impaction. This is one reason why impactions should be removed prior to instituting the bowel program. The suppository needs to be placed above the internal sphincter next to the mucosal lining. Additionally, the GRN should be aware that lubricant used with certain suppositories will inactivate them. This is discussed in the following paragraphs. Suppositories are generally not fast-acting (15 to 60 minutes) in the older population. So the timing of administration should be planned as part of the patient's rehabilitation regimen.

Suppositories should not be used routinely in the bowel program because they do not promote normal bowel activity or self-care and can cause atony of the colon.

The glycerin suppository is considered a mild to moderate agent. It is of waxy consistency and causes localized peristalsis by acting as an osmotic agent. The main adverse effect is rectal discomfort or irritation. Lubricant can be used. This would be a good choice for the patient who just needs a little help in expelling firm stool.

The Ceo-Two suppository works on a different mechanism than most others. It is activated by placing it in a cup of water until it begins to bubble, then inserting it into the rectum. It releases carbon dioxide, which distends the bowel and allows the stool to come down. Using lubricant with this type of suppository will negate its effect. As with the glycerin suppository, this can be used effectively for patients who may have stool lower in the rectum but have trouble expelling it. It can cause bloating and cramping.

The Dulcolax suppository is the strongest of the three discussed here. It irritates the colon and rectal mucosa, resulting in reflex peristalsis. Although it may produce better results, it may cause stronger abdominal cramping and should be used only if other suppositories are not effective. These suppositories are often used in preparation of the bowel prior to tests or surgery because of their strong effect.

The Therevac mini-enema is a good alternative to suppositories for older rehabilitation patients. It comes in a soft plastic ampule that contains about 4 ml of a liquid solution of Colace, glycerin, and softsoap base. Because the medication is already in liquid form, it works more quickly and saves the time waiting for a solid suppository to melt. The medication can come into immediate contact with the rectal mucosa, yielding quicker results. Dunn and Galka (1994) found a significant improvement between results with the Therevac mini-enema over traditional bisacodyl therapy with younger patients with SCI. Therevac mini-enema was originally designed for use by spinal cord patients, and its effectiveness in geriatric patients has yet to be established. However, clinical experience suggests that this is a good alternative for older patients, because the time needed to produce a bowel movement is shorter, usually within 15 minutes. This is less fatiguing to patients and decreases the amount of time spent sitting on the commode or toilet, thereby having possible indirect benefits on decreasing skin breakdown. Also, it eliminates the need for the invasive contact of suppository insertion, because the nurse inserts only the tip of the ampule into the rectum, versus a gloved finger. Another added feature is that these can be purchased with benzocaine added (which helps prevent hyperreflexia in at-risk patients with SCI), which provides a bit of anesthetic for those elders with painful hemorrhoids (a common problem). The main drawbacks to this type of treatment are the expense and particularly the potential trauma caused to the rectum by the edges of the ampule if not inserted carefully. Although the container is soft and pliable, piercing the narrow end with a sharp object is inconvenient. Also, more lubricant is required to prevent trauma to the rectal wall. Twist tops were at one time available and provided rounded edges, which were preferable.

Enemas are available in many different types of preparations, from soapsuds to oil retention. Enemas should be rarely used in rehabilitation; they most often aid in establishing a clean bowel prior to beginning a program. They should never be used routinely. A Fleet Enema, which is smaller and more convenient, is usually sufficient to produce the desired results. Large amounts of solution (more than 1 pint) should never be given to an elderly individual. This stretches the bowel, thereby decreasing the potential for future success with any bowel program. Such use of enemas can also cause fluid and electrolyte imbalances and malabsorption of nutrients. The days are past of 2000-ml soapsuds enemas given to those in nursing homes via long red rubber tubes threaded high into the bowel. Large-bulk enemas can contribute to vasovagal responses, fainting, and even death from cardiac arrest.

Digital Stimulation

This is a technique used to relax the rectal sphincters to allow stool to be expelled. Digital stimulation is frequently used in bowel programs for patients with SCI and has been used with some success in stroke patients (Venn et al., 1992). Digital stimulation involves placing a gloved, lubricated finger into the rectum and stimulating relaxation of the inner sphincter by gently rotating the finger in a clockwise motion. Relaxation of the sphincter should occur within 30 seconds to 2 minutes, and stool should be expelled. For patients with SCI, this technique may replace use of suppositories and is thus preferable. However, those persons susceptible to autonomic hyperreflexia may require use of an additional local medication such as Nupercainal lubricant to decrease stimulation that can trigger an episode. This would refer particularly to patients with lesions above T6.

Several serious considerations should be given if using this approach with elderly patients. Many may find this socially and culturally unacceptable. If so, this would not be a technique to use. It is also more invasive to the patient, both physically and emotionally, than other methods. Additionally, physical problems such as hemorrhoids would make digital stimulation painful. Cardiac conditions could be aggravated by this procedure, and it should be used only with great caution in the elderly.

Evaluation

Evaluation of bowel function is documented on the Functional Independence Measure (FIM) sheet in the chart as well as the nurse's notes. This provides a comparison for determining progress in this area during rehabilitation. Of course, if a scale is not used, the GRN can use other forms of measurement to evaluate the success of the bowel program. If a bowel tree, such as that in Figure 8–1, is used, the GRN is able to evaluate the effectiveness of nursing interventions on a regular basis.

Evaluation should be made in terms of

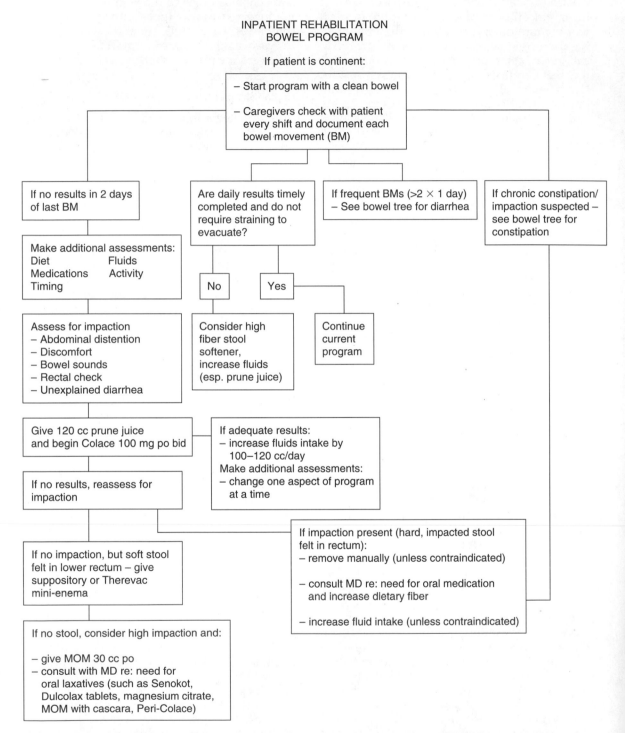

Figure 8–1 Bowel tree for inpatient rehabilitation. (Modified from Nursing Division Care Guidelines, Rehabilitation Institute of Chicago.)

overall goals. Therefore, if a person has established a regular, convenient, affordable, and dependable bowel pattern that fits his or her lifestyle and resources, the main objective has been met.

BLADDER MANAGEMENT

Bladder management for elderly rehabilitation patients is generally a greater challenge. In addition to the estimates that at least half of all older adults in long-term care facilities experience urinary incontinence (Mohide, 1986; National Institutes of Health, 1988; Ouslander, 1986; Palmer, German, & Ouslander, 1991; Simons, 1985; Tunink, 1988), approximately 1.5 million noninstitutionalized adults have incontinence problems (McCormick & Burgio, 1988). All told, urinary control difficulties affect at least 10 million adult Americans and cost about $10.2 billion annually to manage (National Institutes of Health, 1988). This section discusses incontinence and various types of neurogenic bladders.

Incontinence

Urinary incontinence is the major cause of institutionalization and has a negative impact on independence and self-esteem. Many elders consider it a normal part of aging, yet hide their problem from friends, family, and health care providers. Despite its widespread incidence, incontinence is largely a treatable problem that should not be considered a normal part of aging. Such difficulties are complicated when an older person experiences a chronic illness or disease such as stroke and additional neurogenic factors come into play.

The GRN needs to develop keen assessment and interviewing skills to determine whether urinary incontinence existed prior to this recent health alteration so that realistic goals may be set (Colling, 1988; Duffin & Castleden, 1986). Regardless of pre-existing conditions, however, certain guidelines to improve bladder control are helpful. It should also be remembered that urinary incontinence may be one of the first signs of urinary tract infection in the elderly. Thus, a urine culture and sensitivity test should first be done on older adults with unexplained incontinence.

The relationship of age and incontinence is unclear, although the incidence of incontinence does increase with age. However, this may be more a result of immobility and dependency than chronological age, because a majority of patients with bladder incontinence have limited mobility (McCormick & Burgio, 1988; Pires, 1996). Bladder training has been shown to be effective for older women with incontinence (Fantyl et al., 1991). Prompted voiding decreases incontinence episodes among even severely debilitated nursing home patients (Schnell et al., 1989), but scheduled voiding may be more effective (Kaltreider, Teh-Wei, Igou, Lucy, & Craighead, 1990). Urinary incontinence in most elders in rehabilitation can be managed with a combination of habit training, bladder retraining, and positive reinforcement (Burgio & Burgio, 1986). However, more nursing intervention studies with rehabilitation elders are needed to establish the most appropriate treatments for various problems.

Incontinence has been associated with depression in women (National Institutes of Health, 1988) and can result in embarrassment due to odor. These factors can in turn affect socialization and sexuality. In addition to the stigma and emotional problems incontinence can cause, skin breakdown occurs in the form of rashes or infections. Because many incontinence problems are hidden, they go unreported, often until more serious effects have developed.

Types of Incontinence

Incontinence refers to an involuntary loss of urine. The most common means for assessment and categorization of incontinence in long-term care is to use guidelines such as those set forth by the National Institute on Aging (1991). Five types of incontinence are commonly recognized: stress, urge, overflow, functional, and mixed. A variety of factors can contribute to incontinence in gerontological rehabilitation patients. These are presented in Table 8–3.

Stress: Stress incontinence results from leakage of urine that occurs when intra-abdominal pressure exceeds the voluntary inhibiting ability of the sphincters to retain it. This can happen when coughing, sneezing, laughing, or exercising or during other activities that create pressure on the bladder. This most common type of incontinence is found especially in younger females who have born several children, but it also occurs in elderly females as a result of weakened musculature. It is largely treatable and often curable. The GRN may recognize this problem in older women (postmenopausal) using sanitary napkins routinely. Many aged females believe

Table 8–3 POTENTIAL FACTORS CONTRIBUTING TO URINARY INCONTINENCE IN THE OLDER REHABILITATION CLIENT

Immobility, functional impairment
Urinary tract infection
Medications
Neurogenic bladder dysfunction
Poor behavioral adjustment
Cognitive deficits
Decreased bladder capacity
Delirium
Dementia
Rectal impaction
Lack of caregiver support
Environmental barriers
Anxiety
Caffeine or other bladder irritants
Depression

this is a normal part of aging, and because it involves smaller amounts of urine, they resort to using peripads to hide the problem. Because success has been obtained with noninvasive methods, the GRN should urge patients with this difficulty to seek treatment.

Urge: Urge incontinence refers to one's inability to hold the urine long enough to make it to the toilet. Bladder contractions cause such a strong urge to void that if the individual does not reach an appropriate facility quickly, loss of urine can occur. This can be caused by an uninhibited neurogenic bladder, which results in frequent bladder contractions but loss of inhibitory reflexes. Patients with stroke, dementia, Parkinson's disease, and MS often experience this problem. It can also be caused by an enlarged prostate in men or may be an early warning sign of bladder cancer (National Institute on Aging, 1991). Although this type of incontinence does occur in healthy older adults, it is also largely treatable, so should not be ignored.

Overflow: Urine is leaked out of a full bladder with this type of incontinence. The person experiences overfilling and distention resulting in incontinence. This is often the result of an areflexic, or autonomous, neurogenic bladder, such as occurs with SCI or lesions. For elderly men, it could be a result of blockage, such as happens with prostatic enlargement. Diabetic patients may have overflow incontinence as a result of loss of normal bladder contractions.

Functional: When causes are not physiological in nature, the term functional incontinence is used. This refers to persons who would normally have bladder control but are incontinent because of the inability to reach the toilet in time. This might be because of physical limitations, such as hemiplegia or arthritis, or other environmental barriers, such as distance to the facilities. Functional incontinence is also often correctable through environmental modifications and rehabilitation (Wyman, Elswick, Ory, Wilson, & Fantl, 1993).

Mixed: Mixed incontinence is a term sometimes used when an individual displays several factors or symptoms from more than one of the other major categories. An example would include the older multiparous female stroke patient with uninhibited neurogenic bladder who displays urgency (urge incontinence) as well as leakage of urine during therapeutic exercises (stress incontinence).

Mechanism of Micturition

There are several structures that are involved in voiding, or micturition. The bladder, or detrusor, is a reservoir for holding the urine and is made up of layers of smooth muscle. Usual bladder capacity is 350 to 450 ml, with a sensation of fullness occurring at about 300 to 400 ml. The first desire to void may occur around 150 to 200 ml. When the detrusor contracts, the sphincters relax and urine is released, unless complicating factors are present. The internal bladder sphincter is under involuntary control. The external sphincter is made of skeletal muscles and is controlled voluntarily. The pelvic diaphragm, also under voluntary control, can stop and start the urine stream. The pelvic nerve that controls bladder function is located at the S2–S4 level of the spinal cord. Motor fibers here (and at T11–L1 for the bladder neck) innervate, via the pudendal nerve, the external sphincter and pelvic floor muscles. All these mechanisms create a "reflex arc," which, if intact, can be stimulated to produce voiding if needed.

For normal voiding to occur, the coordinated effort of all these structures must work together simultaneously. As stretch receptors in the bladder indicate that it is full, inhibitory reflexes allow a person to wait until appropriate time and facilities are found (a person can voluntarily start and stop the flow of urine). The bladder contracts, and the sphincters relax, allowing the urine to be released and emptying the bladder. However, in the case of a person with neurogenic problems or disease, several obstacles to normal bladder function can occur. These are discussed in the following sections.

Understanding the Effects of a Neurogenic Bladder

Several different types of bladder problems are seen in rehabilitation patients. The kind of bladder function that is present is largely determined by the location of injury within the body. Being familiar with the spinal cord tracts that control function will assist the GRN in understanding why various types of control and sensation may be present. There are three major tracts through which the brain and spinal cord communicate about the bladder: the cortical regulatory, dorsal column, and lateral spinothalamic. The names indicate their location within the nervous system. The cortical regulatory tract in the spinal cord assists with voluntary control. The dorsal column tract signals filling and distention. The lateral spinothalamic tract senses pain and temperature.

Uninhibited

The person with an uninhibited neurogenic bladder may experience sensation but lack voluntary control. The characteristics of this type of bladder function include urgency, frequent bladder contractions, complete emptying (unless other complications are also present), and nocturia. The reflex arc is intact. Persons with this kind of bladder have a lesion somewhere along the cortical regulatory tract. This is common with stroke, head injury, Parkinson's disease, Alzheimer's disease, cerebral palsy, and MS.

Because this is an upper motor neuron disorder, any patients with damage in the brain may experience this type of bladder. The cortical regulatory tract is related to voluntary control; therefore, incontinence would be expected. Bladder capacity is decreased because involuntary voiding occurs before the usual level of fullness is reached. However, nursing treatment including scheduled voiding, monitoring fluid intake, and habit retraining is highly effective. Medications are available to assist with bladder or sphincter control until proper patterns are developed.

Reflexic

Those with reflexic bladders, as with bowels, have an intact reflex arc, which can be stimu-

lated to assist with voiding. A reflex neurogenic bladder (also an upper motor neuron disorder) occurs when there is an interruption of the ascending sensory tract above the S2–S4 level. This can also be referred to as suprasacral, spastic, or central neurogenic bladder. Patients with this problem may include those with SCI, trauma, infection, MS, or tumors above the sacral level.

Persons with this type of bladder lack sensation to void. This causes the classic symptoms of urinary retention and large residual amounts. Incontinence also occurs as a result of lack of cerebral control. Nursing interventions center around emptying the bladder through intermittent catheterization and using suprapubic triggers to stimulate spontaneous voiding via the intact reflex arc.

Areflexic

As the name suggests, in the areflexic, or autonomous, bladder there is damage to the reflex arc. This lower motor neuron disorder produces a flaccid, atonic bladder because of injury to the S2–S4 segments. Peripheral reflexes are absent or diminished. Patients have involuntary voiding, no sensation, and overflow incontinence. This would include persons with sacral SCI (many paraplegics), inflammation of the spinal cord, diabetes (in some cases), intervertebral disk disease, and tumors of the lower spine or other trauma to the cauda equina area. During the period known as "spinal shock," a patient may also show signs of autonomous neurogenic bladder. This occurs after an SCI and may last from a few weeks to 6 months. Outcome of bladder function cannot be determined until this time has passed. Nursing treatment of an areflexic bladder is aimed at avoiding fullness, because reflux can occur and damage the renal structures. The Credé and Valsalva maneuvers are also used, along with intermittent catheterization to empty the bladder.

Other Types

Two other bladder types are noted (Pires, 1996): sensory and motor paralytic. The sensory paralytic bladder involves damage to the sensory side of the micturition arc. Persons with this type of dysfunction can void on their own but may lack sensation of fullness, resulting in increased bladder capacity and distention. Examples are those with diabetic neuropathy, MS, or other trauma to this area. Treatment is to avoid overdistention of the bladder and use scheduled voiding. The motor paralytic bladder involves damage to the motor side of the micturition arc. These individuals have sensation but have impaired voluntary control. This results in large residual amounts of urine and increased bladder capacity. Although fullness, pain, and temperature may be sensed, motor loss can result in decreased bladder tone. Symptoms include straining to void and a poor urine stream. Treatment involves intermittent catheterization and use of the Credé and Valsalva maneuvers. The Credé method is performed by placing the blade of one hand over the area of the bladder, above the symphysis pubis, and pressing gently in and downward to encourage urine expulsion. The Valsalva maneuver is performed by the person by "bearing down" as when having a bowel movement or coughing. By taking a deep breath, closing the glottis, and contracting the abdominal muscles, intra-abdominal pressure is increased and may assist in bladder emptying. This technique may be contraindicated in many older adults, such as those with cardiac problems or those who should avoid increased intracranial pressure.

Assessment

Assessment of an individual's bladder function may present a challenge, particularly if it is not possible, or not feasible, to obtain urodynamic studies. In the acute hospital setting, the physician may order such tests if there is a question as to which type of neurogenic bladder a patient has. However, as the traits of each suggest, unless complicating factors are present, it is often possible to treat the patient based on assessment alone. The GRN's knowledge of the mechanisms and nursing interventions for neurogenic bladders can be crucial in the long-term care setting or community, where financial constraints or inaccessibility of resources makes reliance on diagnostic testing unrealistic (Moore, Griffiths, Latimer, & Merke, 1993).

If diagnostic tests are used, they are helpful in determining the cause of difficulty. Such tests include measurement of blood urea nitrogen (BUN), serum creatinine, and creatinine clearance; blood glucose level; urinalysis and urine cultures; x-rays; urodynamic studies; and ultrasound. Although there are multiple types of studies available to aid in diagnosis, these must be used selectively. A core evaluation can include basic laboratory tests such as urinalysis, measurement of serum creatinine or BUN, and postvoiding residual urine volume (National Institutes of Health, 1988). Many older rehabilitation patients do not require testing beyond a thorough history and physical examination when the cause or predisposing factors are obvious. For example, an older woman with a recent stroke may present with urge incontinence. This would be a common finding. Likewise, if an 83 year old female with eight children experienced stress incontinence, this may not be cause for urodynamic testing prior to treatment.

Urodynamic tests "are designed to evaluate the anatomic and functional status of the bladder" (Pires, 1996, p. 437). Common tests include uroflowmetry to measure the rate of urine flow, cystometry to test detrusor function, and simple cystometry that answers questions about bladder filling and urge to void. Urethral pressure profiles as well as electromyogram to measure electrical activity of the striated urethral sphincter muscle can help diagnose detrusor sphincter dyssynergia when used in combination with cystometrogram, which measures bladder volume and pressure.

A thorough history of the patient's premorbid voiding habits, surgical procedures, toileting habits, and social support is indicated. A voiding diary, which records the times, amounts, episodes of incontinence, and other pertinent information, can assist the GRN in obtaining a more accurate picture of the person's current patterns. This should ideally be done, in the absence of diagnostic tests, before the bladder program is set up.

Physical examination is also required. The person's cognitive status, amount of mobility, motivation, self-care ability, and level of alertness all contribute to a successful bladder program. Impaction should be ruled out as a cause of incontinence. Genital and rectal examination includes observation of skin condition, signs of infection, prostatic enlargement in males, and vaginitis in females. A pinprick test can determine whether perineal sensation is present. The GRN can also test for specific reflexes to obtain a better picture of function. For example, a positive bulbocavernous reflex (anal contraction in response to squeezing of the glans penis or clitoris) indicates an intact sacral reflex arc. Additionally, a simple test for stress incontinence can be done by having the individual with a full bladder perform activities such as coughing forcefully and ascertaining leakage of urine.

The postvoid residual (PVR) is a relatively simple measure of how well a person is emptying the bladder. This can be done by performing straight catheterization immediately after a person has voided to check for residual urine or by using a type of bladder scan device. The bladder scan has the advantage of being noninvasive, yet it provides information as to the amount of urine left in the bladder, preventing unnecessary catheterization. According to the Agency for Health Care Policy and Research (AHCPR) urinary guidelines (Urinary Incontinence Guideline Panel, 1992), no more than 200 ml should remain in the bladder after voiding or this is incomplete emptying. Less than 50 ml indicates complete emptying.

A piece of equipment is currently being used to measure PVR urine without catheterization and can assist in planning bladder programs by providing information about bladder capacity and urge. These bladder scan machines use ultrasound to provide a picture of bladder volume (Fig. 8–2). This is a nursing measure that takes only a few minutes to complete and is less invasive than straight catheterization. This scanning device can be useful for fluid and bladder management and bladder training as well as in the diagnosis and treatment of incontinence. It provides the added benefit of eliminating unnecessary catheterizations.

To use the bladder scan, or bladder volume instrument (BVI), the nurse positions the patient as flat as possible in bed. The patient is told about the procedure and that it causes no pain. It is important to also tell patients that this is not an x-ray, but works with ultrasonic waves. The area above the symphysis pubis is lubricated with ultrasonic transmission gel to promote good contact between the scanner and the skin. The scanhead is initially positioned at about a 45-degree angle, with the contact point facing toward the patient's feet. The button on the handle is pressed when ready to scan, and the machine will read out a picture of the bladder onto the screen, along with data about the amount of urine measured. The objective is to obtain the most accurate scan by being able to view the entire bladder within the colored area on the screen. This often requires the nurse to angle the scanhead in various directions (but always toward the bladder), depending on the patient's size and the amount of urine in the bladder. The scanhead is repositioned, and this procedure repeated until the entire bladder is visualized on the screen, and the maximum amount of urine is read. It may take several tries to obtain the most accurate reading. (The newest models of the BVI are even more simple to use.) Instructions on the machine can then be followed to print out the results, which can be attached to the patient's chart for documentation.

This is an excellent instrument, which provides valuable information to the GRN but is safer and less invasive for the patient. The time needed to complete a scan is much less than for a catheterization, and it is convenient and easy to use. The BVI reads bladder volume ranges from 0 to 1000 ml. The liquid crystal display is easy to visualize. It is highly accurate, although it may be difficult to use in the obese patient. Although the BVI is not inexpensive, the cost is easily justified by the savings in exposure to potential infection, and some facilities have paid for the instrument by charging fees per use, as one would for using a catheterization kit.

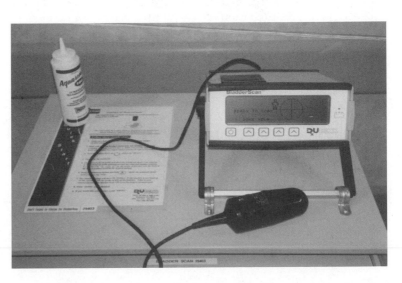

Figure 8–2 Bladder scan device uses diagnostic ultrasound to help establish appropriate bladder programs.

The GRN possesses special knowledge related to the pathophysiological mechanisms that contribute to the incontinence of older adults who have rehabilitation diagnoses. However, a realistic look at the incidence of incontinence within long-term care institutions suggests that a simpler method for classification and treatment of bladder dysfunction may be indicated. These are less physiologically based classifications; dysfunction may be attributed to neurogenic causes in some instances, but could be the result of other pre-existing or concomitant problems in the older adult. This is why an accurate and thorough history and physical is essential.

Complications of Bladder Dysfunction

There are many complications associated with neurogenic bladders, as well as with incontinence due to other causes. Some of these can be life-threatening, and some occur more frequently in the older population.

Detrusor Sphincter Dyssynergia

This type of dysfunction results from asynchrony of the sphincters. As the detrusor contracts, the sphincters do not relax. This results in a poor urine stream, large residual urine amounts, and an increased incidence of urinary tract infections (UTIs). Treatment is most effective with medications such as diazepam (Valium), dantrolene sodium (Dantrium), or baclofen (Lioresal), which decrease the spasticity of skeletal muscles, promoting relaxation of the external urinary sphincter. (Valium should be used only with extreme caution in older adults.) With detrusor sphincter dyssynergia, performance of the Valsalva or Credé maneuvers is contraindicated, because this could cause damaging reflux. Such complications occur commonly with SCI.

Hydronephrosis or Reflux

When obstruction occurs, whether from stricture, congenital malformation, or an overdistended bladder, reflux of urine from the bladder into the kidneys can occur, causing hydronephrosis. This is a complication to which persons with neurogenic bladder must be constantly alert, particularly those prone to overflow. Patients with SCI are particularly at risk. Intake and output should be monitored, and urodynamic studies should be done routinely. Medications such as bethane-

chol (Urecholine) increase bladder tone and contractions of the bladder. Oxybutynin chloride (Ditropan) relaxes smooth muscles through antispasmodic properties.

Urinary Tract Infection

Infections related to bladder dysfunction are common. Approximately 40% of all nosocomial infections are UTIs (Dittmar, 1989). Those with SCI or diabetes and the elderly are at greatest risk. Women are more at risk of UTIs than men because of a shorter urethra. Indwelling catheters are a major source of infection, both from contamination during insertion and from continued exposure of the bladder to bacteria that can come from the catheter. UTIs remain a major cause of death in persons with SCI. Prevention of UTI is of prime concern and can be accomplished largely through adequate fluid intake.

Calculi

Older rehabilitation patients who experience immobility are particularly at risk for development of kidney or bladder stones. With inactivity, calcium leaves the bone and can be displaced elsewhere. Although the majority of stones are passed spontaneously, calculi cause extreme pain and discomfort. Some experts believe that decreasing calcium and phosphorus in the diet reduces the chance of calculi development. Increasing fluids to 3000 ml/day and promoting weight bearing activities should reduce the person's risk.

Signs and symptoms of calculi include pain that appears as dull flank pain or irritation that moves and radiates, depending on the location of the stone. Nausea, vomiting, and elevated pulse and blood pressure can also result. For elders with sensory damage, pain may not be felt, so the GRN must rely on other signs such as sweating, bladder spasms, or blood in the urine to detect this problem. Diagnostic studies can confirm presence and location of calculi. Treatment can center on increasing the acidity of the urine to prevent stone formation, forcing fluids, restricting calcium, surgery, or ultrasonic disintegration.

Autonomic Hyperreflexia (Dysreflexia)

This is an acute medical emergency that requires prompt treatment. Autonomic hyperreflexia is most often seen in persons with cervical SCI, but it occurs in 80% of those with SCI above T6 level (Dittmar, 1989). Usually occurring within the first 6 months after injury, this complication of neurogenic bladder can be seen from 3 weeks to 6 years after injury.

Autonomic hyperreflexia is caused when stimuli sent to the brain via the spinal cord cannot reach the message center. Sensory receptors in the S2–S4 region are stimulated, sending impulses to the brain. Because these are blocked, the stimuli continue and the impulses build, producing a reflex arteriolar spasm through the autonomic nervous system. This leads to arteriole vasoconstriction and elevated blood pressure, with massive vasodilation to the heart and the brain. Once the brain centers have detected an elevation in blood pressure, the brain decreases the heart rate and dilates smaller vessels, in an attempt to compensate. Efferent impulses from the sympathetic ganglia of the spinal cord dilate blood vessels above the lesion, resulting in flushing and sweating and a continued rise in blood pressure. Blood vessels from the lower body are constricted, causing pallor and "goose flesh."

These mechanisms cause the clinical signs and symptoms seen in autonomic hyperreflexia. If unrecognized and allowed to continue, these physiological changes can result in systolic blood pressures as high as 300 mmHg. Stroke and coma or death can occur.

Causes of this disorder center around the S2–S4 sites. The most common cause is a distended bladder, as in cases in which a person with SCI and an areflexic bladder may have skipped a catheterization. A kinked or blocked indwelling catheter in the bladder may also be a common cause. Impaction that distends the rectum, genital stimulation, urological or gynecological procedures, pressure sores, pregnancy, and rapid emptying of an overdistended bladder are other common causes. For the older rehabilitation patient, bladder distention and impaction are the two most likely stimuli.

The GRN should be alert to the signs and symptoms of autonomic hyperreflexia because it is a life-threatening condition (Table 8–4). The patient presents with hypertension, bradycardia, flushing, redness of face, a blotchy neck, and perspiration of the skin above the level of injury. Complaints include a pounding headache and blurred vision.

As with most complications in gerontological rehabilitation, prevention is the best treatment. Bladder fullness must be avoided in patients, especially those with complete le-

sions above the T6 level. A reliable bowel program will help prevent constipation. Treatment is directed at relieving the causing stimuli (Table 8–5) and lowering the blood pressure. There are some immediate actions the nurse can take toward managing the hypertensive crisis. The head of the bed should be raised immediately to take advantage of orthostatic hypotension. The GRN should be aware of the patient's baseline vital signs. The average blood pressure for a quadriplegic is 90/60 mmHg sitting, and not all patients will present with such obvious hypertension in early stages. The aged individual may show less of a rise in blood pressure than a person in his twenties. The physician should be notified. If the patient has a catheter, it should be checked to make sure it is not kinked. If bladder distention is suspected, perform a catheterization to relieve the causative stimuli, allowing the urine to drain slowly. When doing a rectal check or any other such procedure, the anal area or urethra may be locally anesthetized. For example, when inserting a suppository, it is recommended for patients prone to autonomic hyperreflexia that a local anesthetic cream or gel be used. For emergency treatment of dangerous hypertension, intravenous vasodilators such as hydralazine

Table 8–4 SIGNS AND SYMPTOMS OF AUTONOMIC HYPERREFLEXIA

Hypertension (based on baseline blood pressure)
Bradycardia (as low as 20–30 beats per min)
Red face; blotchy skin on face and neck
Flushing and perspiration above the level of injury
Pounding headache
Blurred vision
Pallor below level of lesion
Complaints of anxiety, nervousness
Nausea

Table 8–5 CAUSATIVE FACTORS IN AUTONOMIC HYPERREFLEXIA

Bladder distention or fullness
Kinked or blocked catheter tubing
Impaction or rectal distention
Genital stimulation
Urological or gynecological procedures
Rapid emptying of the bladder
Pressure sores
Pregnancy and delivery

(Apresoline) may be ordered. Sublingual nifedipine (Procardia) is also a common medication used. For those with long-term difficulties, surgical procedures may be an option.

Goals

The goals of any bladder management program are relatively straightforward. Like bowel protocol, the bladder program should be inexpensive, realistic, and effective. The main purpose is to empty the bladder of urine and thus prevent infection or potential complications. Regular emptying of the bladder also contributes to a better detrusor blood supply. Reestablishing independence in voiding or bladder management is of primary importance. To achieve these objectives, a combination of bladder training, behavior modification, and medications may be needed, with the least invasive effective method to be used.

Interventions

Gross (1990) stated that nursing can clearly make the difference in success or failure of bladder management. This strong statement reflects the importance of nursing knowledge put to proper use through the implementation of appropriate nursing interventions. The interventions discussed here are based on recommendations of expert clinicians and the research currently available in the field. Nursing management of older patients with bladder dysfunction continues to evolve as more research is published that tests hypotheses about nursing interventions.

There are several categories of treatment for incontinence. These include behavioral, medical, and surgical interventions. The most desirable and least invasive methods of treatment for older adults are behavioral. However, there are many instances in which a combination of medication and behavior modification is most effective, particularly in the case of a patient with recent neurogenic bladder dysfunction. Behavioral interventions include bladder retraining, pelvic muscle exercises, and biofeedback (Burgio & Burgio, 1986; McDowell, Engberg, Weber, Brodak, & Engberg, 1994; Petrilli, Traughber, & Schnelle, 1988). Some of the terms used in the literature are confusing and may be used interchangeably, such as timed voiding and habit training, prompted and scheduled voiding, and not all sources are in agreement as to what these actually refer to. An attempt is made

here to distinguish between terms and the methods used for particular problems.

Bladder Training

Bladder training is a general term that refers to the training, or more accurately, the retraining, of the bladder. Some experts refer to this method as a separate behavioral intervention (Burgio & Burgio, 1986; Fantyl et al., 1991). However, when GRNs use this term, it most often encompasses other more specific, noninvasive interventions such as scheduled voiding, habit training, timed voiding, and prompted voiding. Table 8–6 lists commonly used terms for bladder training. In this text, it is defined broadly as a behavioral approach to bladder management that involves specific toileting protocol. If bladder training has not been successful within 2 weeks after removal of an indwelling catheter, then drug therapy may be needed (Resnick, 1993). Lower overall FIM scores have been associated with poorer bladder outcomes, and those patients with more bladder and toileting problems on admission may be less likely to achieve continence before discharge (Owen, Getz, & Bulla, 1995).

Some patients may have better outcomes with certain approaches than with others. For example, adults with head injury have been well managed with a combination of fluids, scheduled voiding, and positive reinforcement (Grinspun, 1993). Stroke patients who are alert and oriented may have more success with traditional scheduled voiding than those who have cognitive problems including disorientation and memory loss (Owen et al., 1995). Elderly institutionalized patients seem to experience less incontinence with a prompted voiding approach. Thus, GRNs should be flexible and alert to the unique needs of each patient.

Scheduled Voiding: This term can be used generally to refer to a planned voiding program but more specifically to a protocol that usually increases length of time between voidings. This method of behavior modification requires patient education about scheduled voluntary voiding. Many sources call this bladder training. Bladder training is recommended as an initial step for older women and has been found to decrease incontinence episodes by as much as 57% (Fantyl et al., 1991). Scheduled voiding can also reduce nocturnal voluntary micturition.

Initially, patients may use the bathroom

Table 8–6 SPECIFIC TERMS USED FOR BLADDER TRAINING OR RETRAINING

Term/Type	Traits
Habit training	Toileting is fixed or flexible Patients reminded to void at regular intervals Attempt made to match person's voiding patterns with toileting schedule Effective for those with urge and functional incontinence
Timed voiding	Patient is toileted every 2–3 hr whether or not urge is present Responsibility is on caregiver May be used prior to habit training Purpose is to decrease incontinence episodes
Scheduled voiding	Scheduled time set for voiding whether urge is present or not Begins with short intervals (30–60 min) Patient instructed to resist urge until next scheduled void Length of time between voids gradually increased Positive reinforcement and patient education are important components Used for persons with urge incontinence or neurogenic bladder (especially uninhibited) Purpose is to promote self-care and retrain bladder muscles Often called bladder retraining
Prompted voiding	Scheduled voiding program Regular checks for wetness/dryness Responsibility placed on patient Prompts patient to use toilet Requires consistency, education Used often in long-term care facilities

and empty their bladders every 30 to 60 minutes regardless of urge. This can be increased 30 minutes each week, with a goal of 2½- to 3-hour intervals. Greengold and Ouslander (1986) used the term *scheduled voiding* to refer to toileting every 2 hours while awake, and used *bladder retraining* to mean toileting of self with gradual increase in toileting intervals. Regardless of the term used, interventions related to this type of behavioral modification are highly successful in older patients (Fantyl et al., 1991; McCormick & Burgio, 1988; Pearson & Droessler, 1988).

The interval between voidings is not a magic number, although toileting every 2 hours has been used with success as a standard for managing incontinence. Other methods may be used with effectiveness in the rehabilitation setting. For example, perhaps an initial 60-minute interval is not required to maintain continence for the 65 year old with a mild stroke. By examining the patient's voiding patterns, the nurse may use a combination of habit training and scheduled voiding to plan the most appropriate program for that patient. Similarly, the GRN may initially place the patient on a scheduled voiding program and then progress to a habit training protocol once continence has been reestablished. The amount of time the nurse has to help establish a bladder program before the patient is discharged is also a factor. Obviously, those patients in acute rehabilitation may not have a long enough stay to increase toileting intervals to 3 hours before discharge if using some of the guidelines previously described. Many stroke patients experience success in establishing bladder control and self-management using this scheduled voiding approach.

Several additional factors can affect the success of any bladder training program. As stated previously, if urodynamic studies are available and ordered by the physician, the results can assist in choosing the appropriate protocol. The presence of UTI can cause incontinence and should be ruled out if problems persist. If an indwelling catheter was present, chances are good that the patient has a UTI. Rectal impaction can also cause incontinence. The nurse should also keep in mind that the bladder is a muscle, which can become deconditioned just as other muscles, particularly if an indwelling catheter has been in place for any length of time. Long suggested that "self-induced deconditioning" occurs when a patient is anxious about incontinence and decreases the time between voidings, resulting in a decreased bladder capacity and subsequent incontinence (1985, p. 33).

Habit Training: Habit training differs from scheduled voiding by using the patient's voiding pattern to determine the schedule. This can be fixed or flexible and is adjusted to accommodate the patient's pattern of incontinence (Burgio & Burgio, 1986). The goal is to reduce incontinence and keep the patient dry (Greengold & Ouslander, 1986; Pires, 1996). The term *habit training* is often confused with *scheduled voiding*, as evidenced by its use in research studies. Rewards and positive reinforcement have often been used with habit training. This is one of the most frequently used behavioral methods for management of incontinence among nursing home patients.

Timed Voiding: Although this term is often used interchangeably with habit training, it can be distinguished in gerontological rehabilitation. Timed voiding would refer to a fixed, not flexible, aspect of habit training. An example would be a commonly used method such as "toilet every 2 hours." The patient's patterns are not a factor. This has been used effectively in rehabilitation for years. However, the focus of such a method is to reduce incontinence, not necessarily to retrain the bladder. It is this factor that distinguishes it from both habit training and scheduled voiding.

Prompted Voiding: Prompted voiding is another term that appears in the nursing liter-

ature. This technique also relies on positive reinforcement, but the responsibility for continence is shifted from the caregiver to the patient. Prompted voiding refers to the reminders that staff give to patients regarding toileting. The nurse checks with the patient on a regular basis (usually hourly) to see whether he or she is wet or dry. Prompted voiding helps patients realize incontinent episodes and can significantly decrease the frequency of incontinence, even in severely debilitated nursing home patients (Schnell et al., 1989). However, prompted voiding alone may not be effective in curbing incontinence. In alert women, prompted toileting worked best when combined with positive reinforcement such as praise from the caregiver (Kaltreider et al., 1990).

Intermittent Catheterization

Intermittent catheterization is necessary when a patient cannot voluntarily expel urine from the bladder. This occurs in the case of patients with urinary retention, such as with areflexia, or those with detrusor sphincter dyssynergia. Patients with SCI, stroke, or MS may require intermittent catheterization on a short-term or long-term basis.

The length of time between catheterizations is crucial for a patient who is not voiding at all on his or her own. Waiting more than 8 hours to empty the bladder of a patient whose fluid intake is adequate can result in distention and subsequent infections and complications. The most appropriate way to set the times of catheterizations is by keeping an accurate record of intake and output. If more than 400 ml of urine is obtained at each catheterization, the time in between needs to be decreased. It is not unusual for a patient with SCI to be on a self-catheterization (SC) schedule every 4 hours.

Conversely, if a patient is voiding even a small amount on his or her own and bladder retraining is being practiced, then it is important not to catheterize too often in the absence of distention. This is because the bladder muscle must be retrained and will likely be lazy and not as effective with complete emptying initially as it was premorbidly. If a strict catheterization schedule is adhered to in this case, the patient may never have the opportunity for the bladder to regain its tone. This is particularly true after removal of an indwelling catheter. The GRN must learn to find a balance between the need for bladder emptying to prevent infection and complications and the goal of bladder retraining. This is only accomplished through knowledge, experience, and careful planning.

There are products currently available that require no touching of the catheter. They are self-contained within a long, plastic-type, sterile bag and threaded through the top, which may contain an introducer to the urethral opening. The catheter is threaded into the bladder through the sterile bag, so the person performing the catheterization never touches the catheter. The urine drains into the sealed bag, and the catheter can be removed back into the bag. The drainage bag is marked to assist in measurement of output. This type of product has been shown to decrease the incidence of infection (Charbonneau-Smith, 1993).

For the patient with long-term bladder management problems, self-catheterization should be taught. If the patient is unable to perform this task, a caregiver should be instructed. This requires information, demonstration, practice time with supervision, and return demonstrations. Caregivers often experience a great deal of anxiety around learning this skill, largely due to fear, but also because it involves intimate contact and invasion of privacy. In situations in which the caregiver cannot or will not perform needed intermittent catheterizations, other options, such as an indwelling Foley catheter or a suprapubic catheter, should be explored. Because of the importance of the patient's being able to return home, and the implications that incontinence or urinary retention have on discharge status, all viable options must be considered. The technique chosen for long-term bladder management must fit the patient's needs, abilities, and resources, although it may not be the first choice of the health care professional.

Intermittent catheterization (IC) done within the hospital setting is performed with sterile technique. However, most patients and caregivers use clean technique at home if this is done on a regular basis. This is more practical and certainly more cost-effective for the patient, provided the catheters are properly cleansed and no infection is introduced through carelessness, such as lack of hand-washing. Catheters are reused, cleaning between times with soap and water or a mild bleach solution and a thorough rinsing, then stored in a clean plastic bag between uses. The GRN should instruct the patient to discard catheters that have become cracked or damaged, because they can cause urethral and bladder trauma. Although the incidence of UTIs using clean technique for IC is less than with an indwelling catheter, current research is examining such procedures as microwaving catheters to sterilize them at home.

Indwelling Catheters

Nosocomial infections are often attributed to indwelling urinary catheters. Poor sterile technique on insertion may be partially to blame for this. However, all patients with catheters in place are prone to UTIs. This type of management is used as a last resort, but the situation and resources of the patient must be considered.

Indwelling catheters should be removed as soon as possible in the rehabilitation program. Although many stroke patients have a catheter in acute care, it is one of the main goals of the GRN to begin bladder training and program establishment early in the rehabilitation process. Catheters should be removed early in the morning so that the patient's voiding ability can be monitored throughout the day and toileting can be initiated. In addition, the physician can be notified of any problems before bedtime. Clamping regimens prior to removal have not been shown to affect voiding patterns in stroke patients, so are not recommended practice (Gross, 1990).

If a patient goes home with an indwelling catheter, it should be changed about once per month. The patient or caregiver should cleanse around the tube and meatus daily with warm, soapy water. Some health care providers recommend using a topical antibiotic or Betadine cream around the meatal entry site and top of the tube to help prevent infection. The patient or caregiver needs to be instructed in home management of the catheter, including measuring intake and output, signs and symptoms of UTI, what to do if the catheter become plugged, proper anchoring of the catheter, and the like.

An additional consideration is the impact that the indwelling catheter has on the patient's self-esteem and sexuality. Patients may be hesitant to ask the nurse whether having a catheter in place prohibits sexual intercourse. The GRN should not hesitate to introduce this subject before the patient's discharge so that information and counseling can be given and misinformation dispelled. Too often, this aspect of care is overlooked, and patients and their families are forced to rely on guesswork to solve some of these problems. The presence of a catheter does not automatically mean that a man cannot achieve an erection. Likewise, health care professionals should never assume that because a person is considered elderly that sexuality is no longer a significant issue.

Patients with catheters can indeed have sexual intercourse, but they should receive instructions before discharge. For a man, the catheter can be folded along the penis, and a condom used to cover both the penis and the catheter. For women, the catheter can be taped out of the way, onto the abdomen. The bladder should be emptied as much as possible before this. Both partners need to be sensitive to the changes that have occurred as a result of physical dysfunction, and expectations may need to be adjusted. Those on particular bowel programs should be encouraged to have this completed before engaging in intercourse. Larger rehabilitation facilities have nurses and physicians who specialize in sexual counseling for those with disabilities, including bladder dysfunction and the presence of a urinary catheter. GRNs should make appropriate referrals if a problem is beyond their scope of practice or knowledge. Any GRN, however, can acknowledge patients' sexual needs and desire for intimacy, giving them permission to ask questions or express closeness with their significant other.

Prescribed Fluid Intake

An adequate fluid intake is essential in preventing UTIs. Because UTIs are a significant contributor to incontinence in the older rehabilitation patient, a vicious circle can develop if a balance is not achieved. Therefore, a fluid regimen is necessary for establishing an appropriate bladder program.

The amount of fluid that a person should consume must be balanced with toileting schedules, activities, and resources. An older adult who drinks the recommended 1500 to 2000 ml of fluid per day but has functional incontinence may need to modify the times and amounts consumed. A person should never severely limit fluid intake in order to be able to perform IC less often. Yet, some patients are prone to do this. The GRN must instruct patients and caregivers on the need for balancing intake and output and incorporating adequate fluids into the bladder program. A lack of fluids contributes to UTI, dehydration, and constipation, all common problems for the elderly.

Pelvic Floor Muscle Exercises

Exercises that strengthen the pelvic floor are helpful in reducing incontinence, because they allow the patient to achieve greater control of muscles that prevent leakage. Kegel exercises, named for the doctor who developed them, significantly reduce both urge and stress incontinence when done consistently and correctly (Burgio & Burgio, 1986; Flynn, Cell, & Luisi, 1994; Pearson & Droessler, 1988). The usual reasons for the ineffectiveness of such exercises are related to use of the wrong muscles and inconsistency in performing the exercises. The GRN should give clear instructions both verbally and in writing to patients who are using this technique to decrease incontinence and promote bladder control. Table 8–7 provides some suggestions.

Kegel exercises have several advantages over other interventions such as biofeedback or surgery. They are relatively simple and are noninvasive in nature. Kegel exercises can be done at virtually any time of the day, and without special equipment, once the person has learned the correct technique. Although used more frequently for women with incontinence problems, men may also benefit from strengthening the pelvic floor muscles. These exercises are often prescribed after radical prostatectomy.

The GRN should be certain that the person understands which muscles are to be used in performing these exercises, because using the wrong muscles will have little effect in reducing incontinence. Consistency, practice, and repetitions should be emphasized (see Table 8–7). Biofeedback can be useful in assisting individuals to identify the correct muscles.

Biofeedback

Another successfully used method for bladder retraining and preventing incontinence is biofeedback. A form of behavioral training, biofeedback "aims to reverse incontinence by altering physiologic responses of the bladder and pelvic floor muscles, which mediate incontinence" (Burgio & Burgio, 1986, p. 820). This has been most effective in helping reduce incontinence with a younger female population, but it has also been effective for both older men and women with urge incontinence, even when timed voiding was not effective. Devices that are used to provide biofeedback information to patients, such as bladder or rectal probes, may hinder older

Table 8–7   CLIENT TEACHING: KEGEL EXERCISES

The purpose of these exercises is to help strengthen the muscles that support the bladder and surrounding structures. By exercising them as you would any other muscle group, you can make them stronger and learn to control them voluntarily. Learning how to squeeze the urethra closed by tightening those muscles when needed can help decrease incontinence.

Locate the correct pelvic floor muscles. This is done most easily by sitting on the toilet and beginning to urinate. Stop the stream of urine. Even if you cannot completely stop it, but it slows down, you are using the right muscles. Practice this several times.

The buttocks should not tense when performing these exercises. Your abdomen should not be moving when you do this either. If they do, go back to the toileting exercise and practice locating the correct muscles again.

Do not hold your breath when doing these exercises.

To perform a Kegel exercise, squeeze the pelvic floor muscles and hold for a slow count of 3. Then relax the muscles for a slow count of 3. This is one repetition.

Do this a total of 45 times per day by dividing into 15 repetitions each: lying, sitting, and standing. This helps condition your body to reacting in different positions, as it may feel differently.

If unable to do 15 exercises at a time, do fewer, but more frequently.

These exercises can be done anywhere without anyone noticing you are doing them. At first, it might be best to do them at a regular time each day so you don't forget, such as before or after meals. Gradually incorporate them more often into your daily routine such as riding to work, watching television, and, of course, going to the toilet.

Don't get discouraged. It will take time to develop muscle strength.

You should notice a difference in your ability to prevent incontinence as these muscles get stronger. When the urge is felt to void, use a Kegel exercise to tighten the urethra until you can get to the bathroom. Combining these exercises with the other things mentioned by your nurse, such as habit training and fluid management, should help control your incontinence.

women from further participation in a training program because of their more invasive nature.

Remember that goals should be mutually established and client-centered. Although this technique is useful, if older women are uncomfortable with the use of biofeedback instruments, it is better to choose a program that they will participate in than to "scare them off" of further bladder training. Ascertaining an individual's openness to each technique or method is an important step in establishing the appropriate bladder program.

Evaluation

In addition to using FIM or other scores to evaluate progress in bladder function, the GRN can look at other outcome measures. The number of incontinence episodes should decrease as the bladder program becomes effective. The person may report a greater ability to retain urine in the event of urge or stress incontinence. Those with catheters recently removed should exhibit signs of returning detrusor tone, such as more complete emptying and less frequency or urgency. The bladder volume instrument (BVI) provides feedback in terms of bladder capacity and efficiency of emptying.

If the goal is maintenance, and not independence in bladder function, then it is appropriate to use other outcomes for evaluation. The patient should receive plenty of fluids, be able to balance intake and output, maintain an efficient system to empty the bladder, and remain free from UTI. The patient, family, or caregiver should be instructed in needed skills to meet these objectives and should be able to demonstrate competence in the area of bladder management.

If progress is not evident within 2 weeks of program initiation, the person and program should be reevaluated. Obstacles to success, such as UTIs or other urological difficulties, can develop during the course of bladder retraining, so the GRN must be alert to these potential barriers. Nurses implementing these protocols in the home need to carefully assess the family/caregiver situation as well as possible functional barriers for the patient. Acknowledging the individual's support system, socioeconomic resources, and physical needs will assist in establishing a suitable program. Not all techniques work equally well for each case. Understanding the cause behind neurogenic bladders and the common complications will help the GRN identify appropriate recommendations for establishing a bladder program that best suits each individual client.

REFERENCES

Behm, R. (1985). A special recipe to banish constipation. *Geriatric Nursing, 6*, 216–217.

Brocklehurst, J. C., Andrews, K., Richards, B., & Laycock, P. J. (1985). The incidence and correlates of incontinence in stroke patients. *Journal of the American Geriatrics Society, 33*, 540–542.

Brown, M. K., & Everett, I. (1990). Gentle bowel fitness with fiber. *Geriatric Nursing, 9*(6), 26–27.

Burgio, K. L., & Burgio, L. D. (1986). Behavior therapies for urinary incontinence in the elderly. *Clinics in Geriatric Medicine, 2*, 809–827.

Charbonneau-Smith, R. (1993). No-touch catheterization and infection rates. *Rehabilitation Nursing, 18*, 296–299.

Colling, J. (1988). Educating nurses to care for the incontinent patient. *Nursing Clinics of North America, 23*(1), 279–289.

Davis, A., Nagelhout, M. J., Hoban, M., & Barnard, B. (1986). Bowel management: A quality assurance approach to upgrading programs. *Journal of Gerontological Nursing, 12*(5), 13–17.

Dittmar, S. (1989). *Rehabilitation nursing: Process and application*. St. Louis, MO: C. V. Mosby.

Duffin, H. M., & Castleden, C. M. (1986). The continence nurse adviser's role in the British health care system. *Clinics in Geriatric Medicine, 2*, 841–855.

Dunn, K. L., & Galka, M. L. (1994). A comparison of the effectiveness of Therevac SB and Bisacodyl suppositories in SCI patients' bowel programs. *Rehabilitation Nursing, 19*, 334–338.

Fantyl, J. A., Wyman, J. F., McClish, D. K., Harkins, S. W., Elswick, R. K., Taylor, J. R., & Hadley, E. C. (1991). Efficacy of bladder training in older women with urinary incontinence. *Journal of the American Medical Association, 265*(5), 609–613.

Flynn, L., Cell, P., & Luisi, E. (1994). Effectiveness of pelvic muscle exercises in reducing urge incontinence among community residing elders. *Journal of Gerontological Nursing, 20*(5), 23–27.

Gender, A. R. (1996). Bowel regulation and elimination. In S. Hoeman (Ed.), *Rehabilitation nursing: Process and application* (pp. 452–475). St. Louis, MO: Mosby-Year Book.

Gibson, C. J., Opalka, P. C., Moore, C. A., Brady, R. S., & Mion, L. C. (1995). Effectiveness of bran supplement on the bowel management of elderly rehabilitation patients. *Journal of Gerontological Nursing, 21*(10), 21–30.

Greengold, B. A., & Ouslander, J. G. (1986). Bladder retraining: Program for elderly patients with post-indwelling catheterization. *Journal of Gerontological Nursing, 12*(6), 31–35.

Gresham, G. G., Duncan, P. W., Stason, W. B., et al. (1995). *Post-stroke rehabilitation*. Clinical practice guideline, No. 16 (AHCPR Publication No. 95-0662). Rockville, MD: U.S. Department of Health and Human Services, Public Health Service, Agency for Health Care Policy and Research.

Grinspun, D. (1993). Bladder management for adults following head injury. *Rehabilitation Nursing, 18*, 300–305.

Gross J. C. (1990). Bladder dysfunction after stroke: It's not always inevitable. *Journal of Gerontological Nursing, 16*(4), 20–25.

Kaltreider, D. L., Teh-Wei, H., Igou, J. F., Lucy, C. Y., & Craighead, W. E. (1990). Can reminders curb incontinence? *Geriatric Nursing, 11*(1), 17–19.

Long, M. L. (1985). Incontinence: Defining the nursing role. *Journal of Gerontological Nursing, 11*(1), 30–35.

Lorish, T. R., Sandin, K. J., Roth, E. J., & Noll, S. F. (1994). Stroke rehabilitation. 3. Rehabilitation evaluation and management. *Archives of Physical Medicine and Rehabilitation, 75*, S-47–S-51.

McCormick, K. A., & Burgio, K. L. (1988). Incontinence: An update on nursing care measures. *Nursing Clinics of North America, 23*(1), 231–264.

McDowell, B. J., Engberg, S., Weber, E., Brodak, I., & Engberg, R. (1994). Successful treatment using behavioral interventions of urinary incontinence in homebound older adults. *Geriatric Nursing, 15*, 303–307.

Mohide, E. A. (1986). The prevalence and scope of urinary incontinence. *Clinics in Geriatric Medicine, 2*, 639–655.

Moore, K., Griffiths, D., Latimer, G., & Merke, R. (1993). Twenty-four-hour monitoring of incontinence and bladder function in a community hospital. *Journal of ET Nursing, 20*(4), 163–168.

Munchiando, J. F., & Kendall, K. (1993). Comparison of the effectiveness of two bowel programs for CVA patients. *Rehabilitation Nursing, 18*(3), 168–172.

National Institute on Aging, National Institute of Diabetes and Digestive and Kidney Diseases. (1991). *Age page: Urinary incontinence* [Brochure]. Washington, DC: U.S. Department of Health and Human Services.

National Institutes of Health. (1988). Urinary incontinence in adults. *Consensus Development, Conference Statement, 7*(5), 1–11.

Ouslander, J. G. (1986). Commentary. *Clinics in Geriatric Medicine, 2*, 711–713.

Owen, D. C., Getz, P. A., & Bulla, S. (1995). A comparison of characteristics of patients with completed stroke: Those who achieve continence and those who do not. *Rehabilitation Nursing, 20*(4), 197–203.

Pahor, M., Guralnik, J. M., Chrischilles, E. A., & Wallace, R., B. (1994). Use of laxative medication in older persons and associations with low serum albumin. *Journal of the American Geriatrics Society, 42*(1), 50–56.

Palmer, M. H., German, P. S., & Ouslander, J. G. (1991). Risk factors for urinary incontinence one year after nursing home admission. *Research in Nursing and Health, 14*, 405–412.

Pearson, B. D., & Droessler, D. (1988). Continence through nursing care. *Geriatric Nursing, 9*, 347–349.

Petrilli, C. O., Traughber, B., & Schnelle, J. F. (1988). Behavioral management in the inpatient geriatric population. *Nursing Clinics of North America, 23*(1), 265–277.

Pires, M. (1996). Bladder elimination and continence. In S. P. Hoeman (Ed.), *Rehabilitation nursing: Process and application* (pp. 417–451). St. Louis, MO: Mosby-Year Book.

Resnick, B. (1993, November). Retraining the bladder after catheterization. *American Journal of Nursing*, 46–49.

Schnell, J. F., Traughber, B., Sowell, V. A., Newman, D. R., Petrilli, C. O., & Ory, M. (1989). Prompted voiding treatment of urinary incontinence in nursing home patients: A behavior management approach for nursing home staff. *Journal of the American Geriatrics Society, 37*, 1051–1057.

Simons, J. (1985). Does incontinence affect your client's self-concept? *Journal of Gerontological Nursing, 11*(6), 37–40.

Stone, J. T. (1991). Managing bowel function. In W. C. Chenitz, J. Y. Stone, & S. A. Salisbury (Eds.), *Clinical gerontological nursing: A guide to advanced practice* (pp. 217–232). Philadelphia: W. B. Saunders.

Tunink, P. M. (1988). Alteration in urinary elimination. *Journal of Gerontological Nursing, 14*(4), 25–30, 46–47.

Urinary Incontinence Guideliine Panel. (1992, March). *Urinary incontinence in adults: Clinical practice guideline* (AHCPR Pub. No. 92-0038). Rockville, MD: Agency for Health Care Policy and Research, Public Health Service, U.S. Department of Health and Human Services.

Venn, M. R., Taft, L., Carpentier, B., & Applebaugh, G. (1992). The influence of timing and suppository use on efficiency and effectiveness of bowel training after a stroke. *Rehabilitation Nursing, 17*(3), 116–120.

Wells, T. J. (1988). Research methods, outcomes, and issues. *Journal of Gerontological Nursing, 14*(9), 11–13.

Wyman, J. F., Elswick, R. K., Ory, M. G., Wilson, M. S., & Fantl, J. A. (1993). Influence of functional, urological, and environmental characteristics on urinary incontinence in community-dwelling older women. *Nursing Research, 42*, 270–275.

Chapter 9

Enhancing Cognition, Communication, Sensory Perception, and Learning

The difficulties associated with cognitive and perceptual deficits are often seen in elderly rehabilitation clients. A variety of factors can contribute to impaired perception, whether cognitive or sensory. More than 80% of nursing home patients have dementia, behavior disorders, psychosis, or depression, yet less than 5% of them receive mental health care (Rovner, Steele, Shmuley, & Folstein, 1996). Cognitive deficits that accompany many of the chronic problems seen in gerontological rehabilitation, as well as normal aging changes, can also alter behavior and contribute to a lack of progress in rehabilitation. Many types of deficits in these areas affect the person's capacity, willingness, or readiness to learn. The gerontological rehabilitation nurse (GRN) can foster communication through the use of some basic techniques and can enhance an individual's sensory perception by structuring nursing interventions that consider the patient's unique needs. Visual and auditory problems frequently accompany increased chronological age and can complicate treatment of other medical diagnoses. By incorporating principles of adult teaching and learning into nursing care, understanding may be enhanced and lead to more positive outcomes. Strategies for teaching and learning are discussed in a separate section in this chapter.

The ability to perceive and process sensory input is also related to circulatory status. Poor circulation in the extremities, whether from hemiparesis after a stroke or from peripheral vascular disease, affects sensory perception. For example, elders are more prone to burns from heating pads because of decreased circulation and sensory perception as well as more fragile skin. Peripheral neuropathy related to diabetes is also a common contributor to lack of sensation and can result in wounds without the patient's realization until infection has set in. The issues of mental status or cognition, with resulting communication impairment, and loss of sensory perception of any degree are interrelated factors. These are discussed in this chapter as they relate to each other within the rehabilitation framework. As with any other problems, the initial step is a thorough assessment.

First, it is important to be able to distinguish between the normal aspects of aging and what has occurred as a result of a disease process. Elders will experience a less resilient cardiovascular system than younger individuals. The heart is less able to compensate for increased demands placed on it than in younger years. Other common effects of aging may be a result of cultural norms and different environments. For example, the incidence of coronary artery disease is high in the United States and Canada but lower in Russia, for although they may eat a high-fat diet, the typical Russian's exercise level seems to counteract those negative effects. Although many living in China use tobacco heavily for years, their average life span is over 70, but they eat a diet low in fat and walk or ride bicycles as a main form of transportation. So, when performing any assessment, the GRN should be certain to consider cultural and ethnic variations as well as important environmental variables.

As previously stated, sensory and perceptual function and cognition are affected by changes in circulation. Without proper tissue perfusion, oxygen cannot reach the areas where it is needed. Likewise, without adequate gas exchange, even good circulation will not be sufficient to meet the body's demands. The interrelatedness of these aspects with regard to the ability of the brain to process sensory stimulation and the ability of the rest of the body to carry out appropriate functions are considered here.

IMPORTANCE OF MAINTAINING ADEQUATE CIRCULATION

An adequate blood supply to vital organs is essential in maintaining and promoting health in any individual. As a person's age increases, however, even normal changes that occur with aging can compromise the integrity of the circulatory system. The incidence of hypertension increases with age as vessels become more stiff and less elastic, causing resistance in peripheral vessels to increase. This in turn increases the workload on the heart and can result in cardiac enlargement. Alterations in cardiac system function can occur as a result of arteriosclerosis, atherosclerosis, valvular changes, and other blockages in the circulatory system secondary to disease processes. Other concomitant medical problems such as diabetes, varicose veins, heart murmurs, and respiratory problems are also common in the elderly adult. Such secondary diagnoses can contribute to deterioration of the adequate functioning of the overall circulatory system. Any of these conditions can affect a person's sensory perception and cognition, because adequate circulation is necessary for tissue perfusion to the centers of the brain where communication, memory, and other important functions take place.

Other abnormalities such as fractures, aneurysms, phlebitis, or blood clots can create an emergency situation for the older adult. Although auxiliary blood supplies may develop if larger vessels become blocked over a period of time, the elderly adult has less overall cardiac reserve than a younger person. Thus, added stress put on the heart during a physical crisis may have more disastrous consequences.

The hazards of immobility have serious consequences for the circulatory system. In the hospitalized or immobilized patient particularly, the formation of blood clots can threaten other vital systems even when they occur in the periphery. Asymptomatic deep vein thrombosis (DVT) may be present in many elderly patients (Harrell, 1997), and lack of activity only aggravates this problem. When a DVT is diagnosed, a greater danger may be posed if the clot breaks and travels to a more vital center. This is why rehabilitation patients who develop a DVT may be placed "on hold" for therapy or transferred to a medical unit until the clot is resolved, because continued vigorous exercise may put the patient at extreme risk. Some facilities feel that if the DVT is distal to the popliteal area, the patient may be able to continue therapy; femoral DVTs are considered more dangerous. A clot dislodging from the leg and traveling to the blood supply of the brain can cause stroke; if it travels to the lungs, it can result in pulmonary embolus; and if it travels to the heart, heart attack or cardiac arrest can result. So the entire combination of heart, blood vessels, and other vital organs must be considered when discussing circulation.

There are several nursing diagnoses that fall under the category of alterations in tissue perfusion. These can be divided according to cerebral, peripheral, cardiac, renal, and gastrointestinal (Table 9–1). Before the acceptance of North American Nursing Diagnosis Association (NANDA) diagnoses, the generic term *circulation* was used. The functioning of other organs (such as the lungs) can closely affect what occurs in the circulatory system; therefore, some of the more common primary medical problems seen in gerontological rehabilitation are discussed here in relationship to circulation.

Tissue Perfusion and Cognition

Adequate cerebral circulation is necessary to maintain normal neurological functions, including cognition, communication, and sensory perception. *Alteration in tissue perfusion: cerebral* is the nursing diagnosis used when an interruption in the blood supply to the brain has occurred. Although this is an appropriate diagnosis for the acute stroke patient, many avoid its use in long-term care, stating that it is a former problem and not the emphasis of rehabilitative nursing. This is only partly true. Rehabilitation must emphasize restoration, but restoration cannot occur without maintenance of essential life functions, and that cannot occur if such necessary vital organs such as the brain, heart, kidneys, or intestines are threatened. When circulation to the brain is impaired, whether from a clot,

Table 9–1 ALTERATION IN TISSUE PERFUSION: COMMON RELATED MEDICAL DIAGNOSES IN ELDERLY REHABILITATION PATIENTS

Cerebral

Stroke
Traumatic brain injury
Closed head injury
Brain aneurysm
Subarachnoid hemorrhage
Cerebrovascular diseases

Peripheral

Hypertension
Peripheral vascular disease
Arteriosclerosis
Deep vein thrombosis
Fractures
Postural hypotension
Spinal cord injury
Other neurological disorders

Cardiac

Myocardial infarction
Dysrhythmias
Angina
Ischemic heart disease
Congestive heart failure
Coronary artery disease
Atherosclerosis
Valvular heart disease

Renal

End-stage renal disease (ESRD)
Acute or chronic renal failure/insufficiency
Recurrent urinary tract infections
Autonomic hyperreflexia
Neurogenic bladder
Kidney transplant

Gastrointestinal

Colostomy
Bowel obstruction
Chronic constipation
Peptic ulcer
Hiatal hernia
Diverticular disease
History of gastrointestinal surgery
Abdominal aortic aneurysm

hemorrhage, or obstruction, the brain does not receive adequate amounts of oxygen. Build-up of plaque in the carotid arteries can contribute to transient ischemic attacks (TIAs) and stroke, both of which result in symptoms of impaired levels of consciousness and/or cognition.

Although gerontological rehabilitation nursing focuses on the long-term manage-ment of health alterations, it is necessary that the nurse recognize, and be able to prioritize, the underlying medical problems that have caused the observed symptoms. Table 9–2 lists several common nursing diagnoses that might relate to altered cerebral circulation in elderly rehabilitation patients.

There are some rehabilitation nurses who will undoubtedly disagree that the diagnosis of *alteration in tissue perfusion: cerebral* should be a primary nursing diagnosis for the elderly stroke rehabilitation patient. In fact, the core curriculum for rehabilitation nurses (3rd edi-tion) does not even list this as a nursing diag-nosis frequently associated with stroke (McCourt, 1993). This may be because rehabil-itation clients are generally expected to be medically stable to be admitted to the rehabil-itation program. This is often not the reality. Rehabilitation units are being forced to take patients with increasingly complex medical problems to maintain their census, particu-larly in the wake of the subacute care move-ment. The defining major and minor charac-teristics for altered tissue perfusion include traits commonly seen in rehabilitation pa-tients, and related factors include arterial thrombosis, arteriosclerosis, hypertension, and aneurysm (Carpenito, 1992), all causes of stroke. It must be recalled that the GRN does not solely focus on the rehabilitative prob-lems of the patient, but uses both gerontologi-cal assessment skills as well as rehabilitation expertise to provide quality care. Because stroke is a recurring disease that occurs most frequently in those older than age 65 and is often caused by hypertension (a chronic problem in the elderly), the GRN must not neglect to assess the primary medical prob-lems when performing nursing assessments.

The nursing problem list, or nursing diag-nosis list, should be determined by the ac-tions of the nurse, not vice versa. The nursing care plan should be a reflection of the

Table 9–2 NURSING DIAGNOSES RELATED TO COMMUNICATION, BEHAVIORAL, AND SENSORY DEFICITS

Sensory/perceptual alterations (visual, auditory, kinesthetic, gustatory, tactile, olfactory)
Altered thought process
Unilateral neglect
Self-care deficits
Alteration in comfort
Sensory deficit
Sensory overload

planned, expected nursing interventions for that specific patient and show what interventions are being done. A nurse caring for the elderly stroke patient will surely assess neurological status such as level of consciousness, speech, grip strength, and orientation. This would be a higher priority than first assessing the patient mobility status, because a person can live without ambulation but not without circulation to the brain. Altered tissue perfusion is a problem that we know has existed for the stroke patient and whose origins have most likely not just disappeared now that the patient is in rehabilitation. In addition, there are other team members, such as the physical and occupation therapists, who will address mobility issues, but the assessment of neurological status is a nursing responsibility.

PHYSICAL ASSESSMENT

Cerebral tissue perfusion is assessed by performing a neurological examination. The essential elements of a routine neurological examination for an elderly rehabilitation patient with this nursing diagnosis includes assessment of the following: level of consciousness, memory, orientation, grip strength, speech quality, pupils, general physical and facial observation, and any behavioral changes.

When assessing level of consciousness, the nurse should remember that level of arousal varies with disease process, particularly in patients with a head injury. Scales such as the Glasgow Coma Scale, for low-level functioning, or the Rancho Los Amigos Cognitive Scale may be useful for those patients who are less alert or disoriented. Any decrease in arousal or attention level may indicate a problem. It is also important, however, to consider the time of day at which the assessment is made. Older adults who have experienced a stroke, for example, may be less alert in the evening secondary to the fatigue caused by both the stroke itself and the rigorous therapy schedule. This may sometimes lead to a misinterpretation of cognitive status or level of consciousness. Nurses should compare assessments with those on other shifts and discuss concerns with other team members who may have observed the patient in a different situation or time of day. Environmental factors such as noise and distraction levels can also interfere with such assessments. All factors must be considered before a nursing judgment is made about level of consciousness and response to stimuli.

Orientation and memory can be assessed by simply asking whether the patient knows where he or she is or what day it is. Standardized tools to assess orientation provide more reliable and valid measurements. However, the GRN using such tools needs to choose the instrument carefully and understand its purpose (McConnell & Murphy, 1997). Orientation to time and place must be interpreted with caution, as unfamiliar surroundings can cause temporary confusion in some elderly patients. They may know that they are in the hospital for rehabilitation but not remember whether it is Tuesday or Friday. A more reliable way to assess patients' orientation status may be to ask whether they recall their own name or the names of relatives or visitors who might be present. Small lapses in memory may not be significant. For example, most healthy adults at one time or another have forgotten the name of an acquaintance or where they put the car keys. The most significant memory changes are related to those items that most older adults could reasonably be expected to remember, like their own name, the city they live in, who is the current president, or what is the name of their pet. Being unable to recall these pieces of information may warrant further testing.

Grip strength is an important and useful assessment tool. The patient is instructed to grasp two fingers of the nurse's hands in each of his or her hands and simultaneously squeeze tightly. Grip strength should be relatively equal (with hand dominance considered) to be normal. Those patients with altered cerebral function often experience hemiplegia or hemiparesis. Although not always evident by general observation, assessing the grip strength indicates to the nurse on which side the patient's weakness in the upper extremities lies and is a simple way to compare the left and right sides.

Noting the quality of the patient's speech is also an important indicator of neurological function. Slurred or garbled speech is a warning sign of stroke. Patients who were admitted with clear speech that has since deteriorated may be exhibiting a newly developed, progressing, or completing problem with the cerebrovascular circulation. This can also occur with TIAs, a common precursor to stroke. The speech therapist will document continued assessments during his or her sessions with the patient receiving therapy but cannot be with the patient around the clock as are members of the nursing staff, so this becomes an important nursing responsibility.

Checking *pupils* for *equality* of size, shape

(round), reaction to light, and accommodation (PERRLA) provides a peek into the working of the brain. Patients with head injury or brain damage may demonstrate unequal pupil size or reflexes. Any changes in pupillary response can be significant and should be reported to the physician.

Additional assessment factors would of course include general observation and monitoring of laboratory values. Diagnostic tests such as electroencephalograms, computed tomographic scans, magnetic resonance imaging, or carotid arteriograms can provide more concrete information about occlusions or abnormalities in the cerebrovascular system.

POSSIBLE CONCOMITANT PATHOPHYSIOLOGICAL FACTORS

In order to appreciate the range of problems experienced by elderly rehabilitation patients, it is necessary to be familiar with the normal changes that occur with aging. Likewise, the many common abnormalities that older adults bring with them to the long-term care setting can compound existing rehabilitation diagnoses and make adjustment more difficult. Herein lies both the difficulty and the challenge of gerontological rehabilitation nursing.

Although elderly adults often suffer from acute maladies, they more often live daily with chronic problems. Not only, then, do rehabilitation professionals need to be knowledgeable in the care of persons with disabilities, but they should also be prepared to recognize signs and symptoms of other medical problems that may occur in the aged adult. Because of the normal changes that occur with aging and the complexities presented by multiple system involvement, the older adult often presents an atypical picture that can complicate diagnosis. The concomitant existence of new pathological conditions, such as deep vein thrombosis in a patient with immobility, can hinder rehabilitation progress and may necessitate more acute medical care.

Cardiovascular Changes with Normal Aging

As the body ages, the cardiovascular system experiences some significant changes. The cardiac valves may increase in thickness and blood vessels become less elastic and more stiff. Harrell (1997) summarized the normal cardiovascular changes with aging to include

"a moderate increase in blood pressure, especially systolic blood pressure; prolonged contraction time; a slow ventricular filling rate; and increased stiffness" (p. 226). The incidence of coronary artery disease also increases with age and is the major cause of heart disease and death in older Americans (Cohen & Van Nostrand, 1995). High serum cholesterol levels are a major risk factor for atherosclerosis and cardiovascular disease, compounding conditions that exist with normal aging and making health promotion about low-fat and low-cholesterol diets essential for older adults (Dellasega, Brown, & White, 1995). Despite these disheartening facts, regular vigorous exercise and a prudent diet can help clear the heart of fatty deposits and decrease the risk of heart attack. Older adults should be encouraged to engage in an exercise program, even if activity is limited, because it is beneficial to multiple systems in the body, even in small amounts.

Other cardiac changes include a decreased cardiac output, putting elders at risk when performing strenuous activities that they may not usually engage in, such as shoveling snow, because the heart is less able to respond to the increased demand on it. Diastolic murmurs are common in the elderly. Sometimes a pre-existing murmur becomes more obvious with age but is often left untreated unless the individual is symptomatic. The incidence of premature beats also increases with age, but these are often clinically insignificant. Wenger (1990) stated that supraventricular premature beats are present in nearly all individuals older than 80 years of age, even if no cardiac disease is present. It is important to note, however, that approximately 50% of elderly persons show abnormalities of the resting electrocardiogram, and that the electrocardiogram may often provide evidence of myocardial infarction not suspected from the clinical history alone (Wenger, 1990). Several types of dysrhythmias, but particularly atrial fibrillation (a major contributor to stroke), are more common in the elderly and are treated on an individual basis.

In addition, when assessing the apical pulse of an elderly patient, the point of maximum impulse may be dislocated in comparison with a young adult. This may be due in part to structural skeletal changes that occur with aging. Therefore the diagnostic significance of location of the apex is somewhat confounded by this usual occurrence. However, it is important that the practitioner obtain a baseline assessment to determine normal location of the apex for each individual. Dislocation of the point of maximal impulse can be an indication of cardiac enlargement. The heart rate at rest should not show significant changes with age. Thus, a normal resting pulse for an elderly adult would be similar to that of a younger adult.

Arteriosclerosis, commonly known as hardening of the arteries, seems to be a progressive and age-related disease. The risk of this, too, can be reduced by prudent living, a heart-healthy diet, and regular exercise. Blood pressure tends to rise with age, significantly in the systolic phase and slightly in the diastolic, as a result of the increase in peripheral resistance. The venous system is less affected by normal aging than the arterial system.

Common Cardiovascular Abnormalities

Congestive Heart Failure

Congestive heart failure (CHF) occurs when the heart is unable to pump an adequate supply of blood to meet the needs of the tissues. This can occur as a complication of other abnormal processes such as congenital heart or valve defects, coronary artery disease, or respiratory problems.

Common symptoms of congestive heart failure include shortness of breath, pulmonary congestion, bilateral pedal edema, agitation, restlessness, nausea, dizziness, and weakness. However, the older adult may be asymptomatic until an advanced stage.

The goals of treatment for CHF are to reduce cardiac workload, improve contractility, and reduce sodium and water retention (Ritchie, 1993). This is most often accomplished, for both older adults and middle-aged adults, by a combination of medications, lifestyle modifications, and dietary changes. Pharmacological agents that are commonly used include vasodilators (to decrease workload), digitalis (to increase cardiac output by strengthening force of contractions), and diuretics (to prevent or decrease sodium and water retention). Suggested lifestyle modifications may include weight loss (if obese), an individualized activity program that may involve elimination of strenuous activities (even bedrest), or a routine to promote physical conditioning, depending on the severity of CHF, and dietary restrictions such as lowering the amount of salt used.

Coronary Artery Disease

Coronary artery disease (CAD), or coronary atherosclerotic heart disease, increases in incidence with age. Some texts refer to coronary heart disease (CHD) as a general term for cardiac problems. Approximately 5.4 million people are diagnosed with coronary artery disease each year (Rhodes, Morrissey, & Ward, 1992). More than two thirds of the cardiac deaths among those Americans older than 65 are due to CAD (Wenger, 1990). *Atherosclerosis*, a large contributor to this disease, refers to build-up of plaque within the large vessels coming from the heart. This form of arteriosclerosis results in blockage and hardening of the coronary arteries, leading to increased workload and subsequent cardiovascular abnormalities. In addition, atherosclerotic disease of the aortic arch has been deemed a risk factor for ischemic stroke particularly related to cerebral emboli (Amarenco et al., 1994). Modifiable risk factors for CAD in the elderly are basically the same as for the general population. These include smoking, stress, a high-fat high-cholesterol diet, obesity, hypertension, diabetes, and a sedentary lifestyle. Postmenopausal women are at increased risk for developing CAD. In fact, the number of men and women with coronary problems nears equality around the range of 80 years of age (Wenger, 1990).

Angina pectoris is a symptom of myocardial ischemia. This may present an atypical picture in the older adult, complicated by other concomitant medical problems, making diagnosis difficult. The chest pain described by elderly adults may be less severe and more vague, often confused with a "bad case of indigestion." The nurse should be suspicious of any type of complaint of epigastric or substernal pain (reported as indigestion) from an older adult, even one with no prior cardiac history, particularly if not relieved by antacids within a reasonable time period.

The initial nursing treatment for angina is to stop any physical activity that may have preceded the pain and have the patient rest. This is followed by administering nitroglycerin sublingually (for those patients with known history, under a physician's care), which dilates the coronary arteries to promote oxygenation to the heart muscle. However, because many elderly persons experience severe unstable angina, immediate medical treatment may be necessary if symptoms are not relieved by the usual nitroglycerin therapy. Patient education as to prevention of precipitating factors is an important nursing intervention. The onset of chest pain can be a frightening experience, and one that requires both emotional support for the patient and good assessment skills on the part of the nurse.

Myocardial infarction (MI) is a common problem for older adults. It occurs especially in men with a history of hypertension and arteriosclerosis (Eliopoulos, 1997). The symptoms of an MI (or heart attack, in layman's terms) are chest pain that continues for more than a few minutes, pain that radiates to the jaw or shoulder, complaint of a feeling of tightness or pressure in the chest, or complaint of severe indigestion not relieved by antacids. If a person exhibits any of the aforementioned symptoms, particularly if he or she is elderly, the emergency medical system should be activated immediately. The exception to this rule would be a patient with known angina who is under a doctor's care. However, if anginal pain is not relieved by nitroglycerin, the person should be taken to the nearest emergency medical facility. The chances for survival after an acute MI have improved significantly in recent years, in part as a result of the increased number of people in the community who are trained in cardiopulmonary resuscitation and who activate the emergency response system immediately, as well as the availability of advanced medical interventions. Immediate medical care and/or life support is usually essential for the survival of the victim of acute MI. Nurses should remember, however, that older adults often present with atypical symptoms, including vague, non-specific complaints, or they may even deny complaints of pain, which can preclude immediate diagnosis of these types of conditions. Assessment of other factors such as pale, moist skin, perspiration, dysrhythmias, and change in vital signs is then increasingly important.

Initial treatment includes patient stabilization by decreasing workload on the heart and assessing damage to the myocardium. Medical intervention may include the use of anticoagulants (particularly if the MI was as a result of a clot) and other medications that may increase the regularity and force of myocardial contractions. Surgical intervention may be indicated in the event of occlusion or stenosis. An individual rehabilitation plan will follow and continue after discharge. Nursing in cardiac rehabilitation is a specialty requiring expertise in the areas of cardiac nursing using rehabilitative principles.

Hypertension

Hypertension is a common problem among the elderly. The risk factors for high blood pressure include race (African-Americans more than European-Americans), gender (men more than women), and heredity, as well as smoking, obesity, high-fat diet, lack of exercise, and stress. Hypertension is sometimes called the silent killer, because symptoms may not appear until an advanced stage, particularly in the older adult. When symptoms are present, the individual may complain of a headache or dizziness.

Primary prevention is the best way to combat hypertension. Some risk factors may be reduced or eliminated by lowering cholesterol, cessation of smoking, and maintaining recommended weight. Nurses play an important role in the education of older adults about the effects of hypercholesterolemia and other factors related to hypertension. A meta-analysis of 102 studies by Devine and Reifschneider (1995) to determine the effects of psychoeducational care on blood pressure demonstrated that statistically significant treatment effects were obtained with patient education, medication compliance, and compliance with health care appointments. Each of these areas fall within the nurse's realm for patient teaching.

Not many years ago, hypertension in older adults was often left untreated unless blood pressures were higher than 200/100 mmHg and the individual was symptomatic (Eliopoulos, 1993). Current medical treatment is more aggressive. A diagnosis of hypertension is generally made for an older adult if the average systolic blood pressure on several measurements taken at three consecutive visits is higher than 140 to 160 mmHg and/or the diastolic pressure is higher than or equal to 90 mmHg (Miller, 1995; Roben, 1993). Approximately 35% to 40% of American elders experience hypertension, which, if primary, usually begins before the age of 55 (Chenitz, Stone, & Salisbury, 1991). Isolated systolic hypertension (systolic readings of 160 mmHg with diastolic pressure of less than 90 mmHg) occurs more frequently in the elderly as age increases, particularly in women (Roben, 1993). Systolic-diastolic hypertension (higher than 160/95 mmHg) doubles the risk of death in men and increases mortality in women by two and one-half times (Harrell, 1997).

Because hypertension is the number one risk factor for stroke and can be contributory to the onset of congestive heart failure, cardiovascular disease, and MI, elderly adults should be instructed to have their blood pressure (BP) checked regularly. Harrell stated, "in the elderly, the initial goal of therapy is to reduce the systolic BP to less than 160 mmHg (if the initial systolic BP is >180 mmHg) or to reduce systolic BP by 20 mmHg (if it is between 160 and 179 mmHg)" (1997, p. 229). Those under a physician's or primary health provider's care need to follow their medical regimen closely to prevent complications of hypertension.

Diuretics are the first treatment of choice for the hypertensive older adult. Nurses should be aware that many blood pressure medications are costly, and it is not unusual for an elderly person to be on a combination of antihypertensives or diuretics to achieve a stable outcome. Such factors as lack of financial resources or even forgetfulness on the part of the client can contribute to the elimination of scheduled medications, which can lead to hypertensive crisis and stroke. Many persons will stop taking their medication if they "feel better" or avoid taking a diuretic if they are going out for the day in order to reduce urinary frequency. In addition, occasionally, elders believe that because their blood pressure was within normal limits at a check-up, this means they no longer have a problem. Making the link between the effect of the medication and the controlling of blood pressure, as well as possible side effects, is an important concept for nurses to convey to these clients.

Peripheral Vascular Disease

Peripheral vascular disease (PVD) is a general term for disease processes that affect the extremities. PVD often occurs in various forms and levels of severity in the elderly, in part due to fatty build-up in the vessels over time, but it also may be a result of years of hypertension or diabetes. The lower extremities show more obvious changes, and decreased circulation in the legs and feet may have more serious implications in terms of functional status. Complaints of decreased circulation or sensation in arms and hands may be more of an indication of disease processes than aging.

One of the most important aspects of circulatory assessment for the nurse to make is that of peripheral circulation. The immobilized elderly are at an increased risk of developing clots in the extremities, not only because peripheral circulation is usually decreased with age, but also because of the hazards that come with diminished activity or illness. Using a pulse rating scale helps document a baseline so that comparisons may be made on a regular basis. It should be re-

membered that an older adult may not exhibit the same symptoms or typical signs of severity as a younger adult, making continued evaluation of the patient's circulatory status particularly essential.

The nurse should be certain to ask questions that assess and evaluate circulation and sensation. These should include inquiries such as: Are your feet cold? How many blankets do you sleep with at night? Do you find yourself needing to wear socks to bed in order to keep your feet warm? Do you use a heating pad, electric blanket, or hot water bottle for warmth? Do you have any numbness or tingling in your legs or feet? Do you have any pain in your legs? Patients who do not report any problems, but have bruises, scabs, and other signs of injury, may not be aware of injury owing to decreased sensation or perception. Such practical information may clue the professional to potential or pre-existing problems.

Arteriosclerosis

Arteriosclerosis, also known in lay terms as hardening of the arteries, is especially common in diabetics but is considered an age-related, progressive disease in the United States. This hardening of the small arteries most often affects smaller vessels, and thus may be considered PVD.

One of the particular dangers for the elderly with arteriosclerosis is the narrowing of the arteries that can occur with advanced stages of this disorder. In addition to being a contributing factor to hypertension, carotid artery occlusion, coronary artery disease, aneurysms, and other pathologic conditions, portions of plaques built up in the vessels can break loose and travel to other parts of the body, leading to heart attack, pulmonary emboli, or cerebrovascular accident.

The best treatment for arteriosclerosis is primary prevention. Elders should be encouraged to maintain a healthy, low-fat diet, participate regularly in an exercise program (even if minimal), have their cholesterol level checked yearly, and visit their doctor regularly. Once arteriosclerosis has occurred, some effects may be reversed by prudent living, so elders should be encouraged that even with increased age, a change in lifestyle does make a difference in healthy outcomes. In the event of occlusions due to clots, anticoagulant therapy is indicated. More specific nursing interventions and implications are discussed in later chapters.

Aneurysms

Aneurysms, or a weakening in the wall of a vessel, can occur at any age, and may be related to a variety of controllable or uncontrollable factors. However, in older adults, advanced arteriosclerosis is usually the cause of the development of aneurysms (Eliopoulos, 1997). Abdominal aortic aneurysms (AAAs) most frequently occur in older adults, particularly those with a history of cardiac problems, including congestive heart failure, myocardial infarction, angina, and arteriosclerosis (Eliopoulos, 1993). Aneurysms may occur in various parts of the body including, but not limited to, the brain, aorta, and abdomen. Many aneurysms, if detected early, can be treated successfully with surgery. Again, the nurse must be alert to subtle changes in the patient's status, because the older adult with a leaking or rupturing aneurysm may present with vague symptoms that begin slowly, even over a period of days, then appear to rapidly escalate until the patient goes into shock and becomes restless and disoriented. Even in an emergency situation such as a rupturing AAA, the patient's complaints may be nonspecific, masking the true diagnosis. It is essential that the nurse provide clear and concise documentation of the patient's condition and alert the physician to any suspicious signs or changes in health status.

Varicose Veins

Varicose veins, although often not considered a major health threat, are one of the main circulatory complaints of older adults, with women more often citing this problem than men (Cohen & Van Nostrand, 1995). Causes of varicose veins include lack of exercise, loss of elasticity that can normally occur with aging, and an increased amount of standing. Treatment of varicosities occurring in the legs includes promoting venous return by exercise, particularly walking or bike riding, use of elastic stockings (such as antiembolism hose), and preventing the use of tight clothing or leg-crossing. Tendencies toward varicose veins may be hereditary. Severe problems may be corrected by surgery through ligation and vein stripping.

Respiratory Changes with Normal Aging

Several changes occur in the respiratory system with aging. Generally, the airways and tissues involved in respiration become less elastic, more rigid. There is decreased diffusion due to decreased blood flow to the pulmonary circulation. There is a decrease in maximum breathing capacity, vital capacity, residual volume, and functional capacity, resulting in less available useful oxygen. This can contribute to abnormal sensations and decreased cognition from hypoxia. The power of respiratory accessory muscles and abdominal muscles decreases, with an increase in chest wall rigidity. This, combined with increased airway resistance from less elasticity can lead to increased anterior/posterior diameter of the chest, most obviously seen in those with chronic obstructive pulmonary disease (COPD).

Respiratory problems also affect sensory perception and behavior. A person with COPD will likely have less tolerance to activity. Changes in the extremities such as clubbing of fingers, poor skin turgor, dusky skin color, and decreased capillary refill with nailbed discoloration are all signs of poor gas exchange.

Respiratory diseases are more prevalent in the elderly. Environmental factors can play a key role in the development of respiratory problems. For example, it is estimated that the death rates in those who smoke are four times that of the average non-smoker, but the risk of lung cancer for an elderly smoker is 10 times as great.

The nurse should be aware that the changes of normal aging put the older adult at risk for breathing problems. Pulmonary hygiene for those immobilized in acute care is essential. Promoting adequate hydration and nutrition, exercise, and mobility all help to decrease the risk of respiratory complications. Symptoms of ineffective airway clearance or impaired gas exchange may be more subtle in the elderly, but common general symptoms of respiratory difficulty include shortness of breath, dyspnea at rest or with exertion, pallor, weakness, coughing, and increased sputum production. Hypoxia as a result of these conditions can negatively affect memory and cognitive status.

The GRN should also include as part of the assessment observation of the patient using inhalers. The GRN should watch for correct technique and note whether the patient may be over- or underdosing. Opportunities for patient and family teaching may be taken at this time. Several common respiratory problems are discussed in the following section.

Common Respiratory Abnormalities

The most frequently reported chronic respiratory conditions (based on interviews of the civilian noninstitutionalized population) include chronic bronchitis, asthma, hay fever/allergic rhinitis, chronic sinusitis, emphysema, and malignant neoplasms (Cohen & Van Nostrand, 1995). Several of these conditions are referred to with the term *chronic obstructive pulmonary disease*, meaning long-term respiratory problems.

Chronic Obstructive Pulmonary Disease

This term is used generally to refer to long-term obstructive respiratory problems. Approximately 80% of the elderly experience some degree of COPD, in which carbon dioxide is retained. Some conditions that fall under this category are mentioned later. For all patients with various types of COPD, the nurse should focus care on teaching good breathing techniques, decreasing risk factors, promoting fluids and adequate nutrition, and good body posture.

Asthma

As with the general population, the causes of asthma in the aged are unknown, although hereditary properties seem to play a role. Some individuals develop asthma in later years, but many have lived with this chronic condition for much of their lives.

The usual treatment is similar to that of the younger adult and includes bronchodilators (often managed with inhalers) or theophylline/aminophylline. Emergencies related to asthma attacks are handled similarly to those in the younger population.

Although those individuals who have lived with this condition for years may recognize aggravating factors that precipitate exacerbations, the nurse needs to give additional instruction to newly diagnosed aged patients. In addition, respiratory changes that occur with normal aging may necessitate more careful monitoring of the patient's respiratory status.

Bronchitis

Chronic bronchitis is a frequently reported problem among the elderly. Symptoms may include a productive cough, wheezing, shortness of breath, and recurrent respiratory infections. Increased mucus production from chronic inflammatory processes can obstruct the bronchial tree, leading to carbon dioxide retention and subsequent emphysema.

Medical and nursing treatment is aimed at thinning and removing secretions by adequate hydration and encouraging expectoration. The nurse should provide education about factors that aggravate this condition, including smoking (even when second-hand), and emphasize the importance of proper pulmonary hygiene.

Emphysema

This progressive COPD can be caused by chronic bronchitis and chronic irritation, including environmental factors that may occur in the workplace, or from smoking. Emphysema is typically slow in onset, eventually causing the individual to experience symptoms such as a chronic cough, progressive dyspnea, hypoxia, fatigue, and weight loss. Complications that may result include respiratory infections, CHF, and dysrhythmias. Treatment includes postural drainage, bronchodilators, breathing exercise, and proper body positioning to maximize airflow. Pursed-lip breathing may assist with prevention of collapse of the alveoli, which can occur with decreased ability to expel carbon dioxide. Respiratory problems may cause anxiety in the patient, a condition that may only aggravate the patient's feeling of "lack of air." Anxiety must be addressed and controlled before rehabilitation progress can be expected. Increases in exercise demanded by therapy can trigger episodes of dyspnea. A careful balance must be struck, then, between rehabilitative interventions such as building strength and endurance, and the prevention of respiratory distress.

Pneumonia

Pneumonia is one of the leading causes of death in older adults and remains a frequent reason for hospitalization of the elderly. Despite its occurrence in the aged population, pneumonia is often undetected because the individual may demonstrate atypical symptoms or no symptoms. Pneumonia is common after stroke because of aspiration of food or fluids, particularly if the patient experiences "silent aspiration" or this problem is undiagnosed. Typical signs of pneumonia include shortness of breath, dyspnea, weakness, fever, and productive cough. The elderly may display confusion, fatigue, anorexia, or other confounding conditions. On auscultation, the breath sounds may be diminished and difficult to assess (Chenitz et al., 1991), or reveal the more expected rales and rhonchi.

Treatment includes antibiotic therapy based on the result of culture and sensitivity tests. Nursing measures should focus on proper respiratory hygiene, hydration, nutrition, coughing and deep breathing exercises, suctioning as needed (with particular care to prevent hypoxia), and supplemental oxygen as ordered. The respiratory therapist, in addition to providing necessary treatments to the patient, is a good resource for the nurse with regard to pulmonary care for the older patient.

Tuberculosis

The incidence of tuberculosis (TB) is increasing, particularly among the institutionalized elderly. The symptoms for an older adult may not be typical (fever, night sweats) or may go undetected. The nurse should be aware that many false-negative readings can occur in the elderly. Many physicians and health departments routinely require two negative intradermal Mantoux tests about 1 week apart before a negative result is confirmed (Eliopoulos, 1997). Those with a positive PPD (purified protein derivative) test will always have subsequent positive results and thus should receive a chest x-ray. The nurse should be certain to ask patients whether or not they have ever had a positive reaction to the tuberculin skin test before administering it.

Finkelstein (1996) provides several guidelines for interpreting PPD skin reactions based on information from the Centers for Disease Control and Prevention. An area of induration measuring 5 mm or more is a positive result in some cases, including those with human immunodeficiency virus (HIV) infection, those who have had close recent contact with a person with TB, and those with fibrotic chest x-rays that suggest healed TB. A reaction of 10 mm or larger is considered to be positive if the patient falls into one of the following categories: HIV-negative intravenous drug users, persons with chronic medical conditions that increase the risk of progression from latent infection to active disease, children younger than 4 years of age, persons born in countries with a high prevalence of TB, persons from medically indigent or low socioeconomic areas, institutionalized persons, such as long-term care residents, and others identified by the public health authorities as being at high risk for infection. For persons older than the age of 35 years who do not meet the previously stated criteria, at least a 15-mm induration is required to indi-

cate a positive result. Nurses should be reminded that induration is palpated, not measured by observed redness.

The treatment of TB in the elderly is similar to that for the general population. This includes proper rest, nutrition, hydration, and medications. TB is spread primarily through droplet nuclei or via the respiratory system. The nurse should remember that for many older adults a diagnosis of TB carries a devastatingly negative stigma because of prior experiences in which this was a difficult to treat, institutionalizable disease. The effectiveness and convenience of new treatments, as well as cure rate, should be emphasized.

Lung Cancer

Lung cancer occurs more frequently in elderly men than older women and more often in whites (Cohen & Van Nostrand, 1995). It is the second leading cause of death in the aged (Johnson, 1995). Smoking is one of the most significant risk factors for lung cancer. Symptoms include dyspnea, coughing, chest pain, fatigue, anorexia, and wheezing. Diagnosis is made through examination of sputum, bronchoscopy, and biopsy. Surgical intervention, chemotherapy, and radiation are options for treatment.

Indications for nursing interventions are the same as for other age groups. Particular emphasis should be placed on pulmonary hygiene, breathing exercises, and management of anxiety. Family support and education are essential.

Sensory and Perceptual Deficits Associated with Aging

More often than not, it is the common sensory and perceptual deficits that complicate and interfere with the patient's participation in rehabilitation. Although some patients experience visual deficits such as glaucoma, this is often already controlled and does not necessarily hinder progress in the rehabilitation program. But things such as "normal" hearing loss, opacity of the lens, slower lens accommodation, and slower reflexes can slow the patient's forward progress by contributing to the incidence of falls, miscommunication, or misunderstanding of instructions. Table 9–3 summarizes normal sensory changes that occur with aging.

The most obvious sensory changes that occur with age are related to vision and hearing. Peripheral vision decreases. Lens accommo-

Table 9–3 COMMON SENSORY CHANGES THAT OCCUR WITH AGING

Vision

Peripheral vision decreases
Lens accommodation decreases
Presbyopia
Lens becomes more opaque; more light required to see
Color of eyes fades
Macula degenerates
Cataracts
Tearing decreases
Increased susceptibility to irritation and infection
Retina shows observable vascular changes

Hearing

High-frequency tones are less perceptible (presbycusis)
Lip reading may be used to fill in hearing loss

Touch

Decreased sense of light touch
Increased pain threshold
Paresthesias in extremities due to ischemia

Taste

Taste buds atrophy
Decreased acuity

---

dation also decreases, meaning elders may require more light to see. Many elders do not wish to drive at night, because the darkness and glare of headlights makes them feel unsafe behind the wheel. Cataract formation is common and is considered by some experts to be an "almost normal" part of aging because it occurs so frequently. New and improved treatment for cataracts makes their correction a relatively minor problem and one which is also less likely to impede recovery from a long-term illness. Other visual changes include a decrease in tear production, resulting in greater potential for eye infection and irritation. This is also often easily corrected by the use of artificial tears. The shape of the eyeball also changes over time, with most middle-aged adults developing presbyopia, or farsightedness. This is evident when persons hold the reading material farther away to see it without their corrective lenses. The use of glasses compensates for these problems in most cases.

With aging also comes some predictable hearing loss. High-frequency tones are less perceptible (presbycusis); this can contribute to the appearance of confusion when a person catches only part of what is being said. The whisper test is a good and reliable screening tool for hearing loss. Elders may rely on lip reading to fill in what they cannot hear. This has important implications for GRNs teaching with this age group. Hearing aid technology has helped those with hearing loss. However, hearing aids also amplify extraneous sounds, which can be annoying for the wearer. Many auditoriums or churches now have special devices for the hearing impaired that link into the sound system and thus eliminate the other sounds such as pages rattling and people whispering.

The skin undergoes significant changes, many of which were discussed in Chapter 6. Elders may have cooler skin temperature, with decreased perspiration. They also may have diminished sensation to light touch, even in the absence of disease. Care must be taken to protect delicate skin from extremes in temperature. The use of heating pads and hot water bottles should be discouraged. However, wrapping flannel or terry cloth strips around the affected area uses natural body heat. This is both effective and safer than the use of mechanical equipment for warmth.

Nervous system changes result in a slowing of voluntary reflexes. The ability to respond to multiple stimuli, especially in a crisis situation, is diminished. Sleep changes also occur. Although some elders stay in bed for longer periods of time, they do not spend as much time in restful stage IV sleep and often awaken during the night. This frequent awakening is sometimes related to the need to void. Insomnia is, however, the most frequent sleep disorder in the elderly and can contribute to a poor participation in rehabilitation.

Intelligence is not affected by age. A large number of neurons are lost in the brain over time; however, this does not normally affect one's ability to learn or assimilate new information. Processing of multiple stimuli may take longer in the very old, and a small amount of memory loss is considered usual. However, this should be distinguished from pathological processes such as dementia.

One common ailment that affects many older adults and bears special mention is chronic sinusitis. Although this may seem like a minor complaint, it is named consistently as one of the top 10 chronic illnesses in those older than 65. Chronic sinusitis usually results from multiple, repeated sinus infections. This can cause scarring and eventual narrowing of the opening of the sinuses so that they are often filled with mucus. Contributing factors can include colds, allergies, pollution, polyps, smoking, and hay fever. The symptoms are headaches and pressure in the area around the nose and eyes. Pain increases when the head is bent down. The person may have a runny nose with a yellow-green discharge. All these symptoms can interfere with an older person's ability to participate in rehabilitation, both from sinus headache pain and the blockage of nasal passages.

Antibiotics are used to treat bacterial sinus infections. Saline nasal spray will help cleanse the nasal passages and promote drainage. An anti-inflammatory nasal spray may be prescribed during flare-ups. Gargling with warm salt water also helps dry and cleanse the throat from mucus build-up. Use of a vaporizer or humidifier and an air filter or cleaner may also help alleviate sinusitis. Some persons recommend herb teas as a home remedy for symptomatic relief.

Psychosocial and Other Assessment Factors

A variety of other factors besides physiological can also affect a person's cognitive and perceptual status. These may include but are not limited to the existence of confusion, dementia, depression, pain, sensory deficit, or sensory overload. Major issues relating to assessment of these processes are discussed here.

Delirium, Dementia, or Depression

Recognizing the different between delirium, dementia, and depression will assist the nurse in planning appropriate interventions. Several characteristics of each of these conditions help differentiate between them.

Often elders placed in an unfamiliar setting experience delirium (or acute confusion) early during hospitalization. This is usually transient and improves with time, having a shorter duration than either clinical depression or dementia. Yet, delirium can be caused by a host of other factors, including infection, anemia, electrolyte imbalance, hypoxia, malnutrition, and hypotension. The GRN needs to assess the confused patient for these potential problems. Delirium may be eradicated by simple treatment such as correcting electrolyte imbalance, but it may also be attributed to a combination of more complex problems. The onset of delirium is generally more acute than with dementia or depression. It may be worse at night and in the early morning. The person's level of alertness and orientation may vary. Memory of recent events may be impaired. The individual's thinking skills are often disorganized or distorted, and he or she may suffer from delusions. The score on a Mini-Mental State Examination (MMSE) will be better than that of a person with dementia, but worse than a person with depression, and affect will vary. Although use of safety devices that restrain a person's mobility is generally avoided, they may sometimes be needed for the patient's safety when delirium occurs. It is preferable, however, to have a family member present so that restraints are not used, because this can increase anxiety and irritability often associated with delirium.

Depression can be situational and may be expected to some degree in the rehabilitation setting among those patients grieving a loss. The onset of depression often coincides with life changes, and its course may fluctuate with situations. The person's thinking is usually intact, but the memory will seem selective. Perception of the environment is also intact. Insomnia may accompany depression and result in a disturbed sleep-wake cycle. An electroencephalogram (EEG) will be normal, as will the results of an MMSE. The person also displays a depressed affect. Other signs and symptoms of geriatric depression appear in Table 9–4.

Depression is reversible, unlike most dementias, and can even be brought on by medications. Those medications that might contribute to depression include antihypertensives, hormonal therapy, sedatives, alcohol, cimetidine (Tagamet), and L-dopa. Several medical illnesses can result in secondary depression, such as hypothyroidism, hypoglycemia, neoplasms, nutritional deficits, neurological diseases, inflammatory problems,

Table 9–4 SIGNS AND SYMPTOMS OF GERIATRIC DEPRESSION

Lethargy
Disinterest in activities
Poor appetite
Weight loss
Suicidal thoughts or verbalizations
Depressed mood or affect
Insomnia or hypersomnia
Vague complaints of fatigue or loss of energy
Verbalizations of guilt or worthlessness
Difficulty concentrating or making decisions
Anxiety

and infections. Depression may also be seen in elderly persons as a result of chemical imbalances. The GRN should be aware that a variety of underlying medical problems can contribute to depression and that physical illnesses need to be examined as causal factors.

Dementia, in contrast, is progressive and long-term. The symptoms previously known as senility are now referred to as dementia. Some dementias are more treatable than others, largely depending on the cause. This chronic disorder runs a long course that can last for years. A person with dementia can be alert; orientation and memory may be impaired, although remote memory may be retained longer than recent memory. An EEG shows normal or slow results, and MMSE scores are below average. Some dementias, such as the Alzheimer's type, are progressive and irreversible. Dementia is not a normal part of aging, however, and does not happen to the majority of elderly. It is important to note, however, that depression and dementia can frequently coexist.

Alzheimer's disease (AD) is a severe form of dementia, which can only be definitively confirmed through autopsy, although today's health care professionals are able to make an accurate diagnosis prior to death in the majority of cases. Approximately 50% of elders older than 85 years of age have AD (Lucero, Hutchinson, Leger-Krall, & Wilson, 1993). The signs and symptoms seen in AD result from degeneration of the brain that affects the ability to remember, think, and perform activities of daily living (ADLs). Many of the warning signs of AD (Table 9–5) are seen in stroke patients and those with head injury, multiple sclerosis, or Parkinson's disease. Therefore, a thorough history and physical assessment, as well as laboratory tests, is indicated for any patient whose symptoms seem inconsistent with their medical rehabilitation diagnosis.

Alzheimer's disease is characterized by progressive forgetfulness. This insidious disorder affects more than 4 million Americans, most of whom are cared for by a family member. The disease progresses through early confusion, in which the patient has good and bad days, to late confusion, when the person may get lost in familiar places and forgets appointments. At this time, the recent memory is impaired, with patients forgetting things such as what they had for lunch that day or a social event they had attended. In the early dementia stage, there are fewer "good" days, with the person forgetting names of close relatives, becoming easily frustrated, frequently repeating things, word searching, and wandering. The caregiver is sometimes called the "hidden victim," because the constant supervision required results in a great deal of stress. In the stage of middle dementia, the person cannot safely be left alone and may begin to show more physical signs of disability, such as trouble completing ADLs. The last stages of the disease can leave the person physically and mentally incapacitated and unable to recognize even the closest family members. Many require institutionalization because family members are no longer able to provide care and safety for them at home.

Both causes and cures for AD continue to be studied. Research suggests that medications used for other conditions may be of some benefit. For example, the National Institute on Aging and the National Institutes of Health (U.S. Department of Health and Human Services, 1994) reported that researchers found a lower incidence of AD among people who took anti-inflammatory drugs for arthritis. Additionally, the potential connection between estrogen deficiency in women and the increased incidence of AD is being explored. Other research in AD is examining the possibility of gene mutations, autoimmune reactions, and specific chemical deficiencies as contributors to AD, but a number of studies continue. Some experimental drugs show promise in relieving symptoms, but there is no known cure for the disease.

Table 9–5   CLIENT/FAMILY TEACHING: WARNING SIGNS OF ALZHEIMER'S DISEASE

1. Recent memory loss that affects job skills
2. Difficulty performing familiar tasks
3. Problems with language
4. Disorientation of time and place
5. Poor or decreased judgment
6. Problems with abstract thinking
7. Misplacing things
8. Changes in mood or behavior
9. Changes in personality
10. Loss of initiative

From Alzheimer's Disease and Related Disorders Association (1996). *Is it Alzheimer's? Warning signs you should know.* Chicago: Author. Reprinted with permission from the Alzheimer's Association, 1-800-272-3900, *www.alz.org.*

Characteristics of Cognitive Impairment

Assessment of basic cognitive function should include several factors. Orientation, memory, judgment (especially in real life situations), calculations, and three-stage commands (simple tasks) all are items to be addressed. Some of these are incorporated into a thorough neurological examination, as stated previously. There are also many scales and tools to assist the GRN in determining whether cognitive deficits exist. However, these may be impractical for the staff nurse in long-term care or the community, so other observations, such as those discussed in the following section, may be more practical.

Many traits are commonly associated with cognitive impairment and may provide cues for the nurse about deficits in this area. Of importance to assess is the side and location of brain damage. The GRN will expect to see more subtle cognitive deficits in the person with right brain damage and more obvious sensory and perceptual losses in the individual with left brain injury. However, "right hemisphere damage does affect performance of certain verbal memory tasks" (Welte, 1993, p. 631), such as sequencing and detecting categories. In the case of diffuse brain damage, such as may be caused by trauma, ruptured aneurysm, or blockage of a major artery, a variety of impairments may be noted. An individual with traumatic brain injury may experience a range of problems that vary in severity. These could include memory deficits, poor attention and concentration, impaired judgment, and slowed thought processes (Veltman, VanDongen, Jones, Buechler, & Blostein, 1993). The person with multiple sclerosis may exhibit attentional impairment (Jansen & Cimprich, 1994).

Characteristics that may indicate cognitive impairment include memory loss, poor concentration, trouble with sequencing, short attention span, disorientation, progressive forgetfulness, personality changes, lethargy, anger or hostility, inability to make decisions, difficulty processing multi-step (more than two steps) instructions, agitation, and inability to correct personal mistakes. More specific outward indications of cognitive deficits would include patients applying lipstick crooked, missing buttons when buttoning a shirt, not being able to write a letter, or expressing that they no longer enjoy reading since their illness.

Pain

Alteration in comfort is often related to pain in the older rehabilitation client. Discomfort may be the result of a variety of conditions.

The majority of individuals older than 65 years of age experience arthritis, which may cause pain when engaging in physical or occupational therapy. The rigors of the inpatient rehabilitation program itself can cause muscle and joint discomfort because it usually represents a drastic increase from the person's previous exercise regimen. An increase in immobility can result in discomfort from more time in bed and less activity.

Pain may also be present as a result of the problem for which the patient is receiving rehabilitation. For example, the person with a hip fracture or hip replacement may have postsurgical pain. The elder who suffered trauma as a result of a fall or other accident may have multiple bruises. The stroke patient often complains of pain after shoulder subluxation, which sometimes occurs. Those with spinal cord injuries or multiple sclerosis may have uncomfortable muscle spasticity. The person with an amputation can experience phantom limb pain as well as pain in the stump area after surgery. In addition, the use of braces or ankle-foot orthoses (AFOs) can create discomfort.

Patients older than 80 years of age have been shown to be at higher risk for pain when hospitalized for hip fracture, other types of fractures, infection, or depression. Amount of pain reported during hospitalization was associated with pain 2 months after discharge, suggesting that discomfort in the acute care setting may increase risk of experiencing pain later and at home (Desbien, Meuller-Rizner, Connors, Homel, & Wenger, 1997).

Signs and symptoms of pain or discomfort in the elderly adult are similar to those of the general population but may be less pronounced. Often, elders with chronic problems become so accustomed to having daily pain, such as that with arthritis, that they become somewhat desensitized to pain, or perhaps sensitized to others' reactions to their complaint of pain. It is, therefore, particularly important that the nurse listen carefully to any complaints of the patient with regard to discomfort. Sometimes cultural or gender influences cause a person not to report pain to the nurse until it becomes intolerable. The GRN must be observant for typical physical signs of pain (related to possible infection) such as redness, swelling, warmth, tenderness, or fever. Other indications from the patient may be moaning, groaning, grimacing, flinching, rocking, guarding, and rubbing or protecting the painful area. The GRN should ask patients to rate their pain on a scale (0 to 10 is a common scale) on a regular basis for several reasons. First, even if pain is not present, it gives patients permission to express their pain and encourages them to think about whether or not they have discomfort. It also shows that the nurse considers their comfort important and an essential part of the healing process. Some patients, who would otherwise be reluctant to voice complaints of pain, may feel more at ease if this is part of the daily expectations. Another important benefit to having patients rate their pain on a standard scale is that it provides a means of documentation, as well as comparison, giving the nurse a baseline from which to view subsequent complaints. Pain medications or other forms of treatment should be supplied promptly to alleviate the patient's pain and reinforce prompt reporting of discomfort.

A debate continues about when pain is considered acute and when it is chronic. Although definitions that give time guidelines are useful, it is questionable whether something such as back pain is acute on day 60 and chronic on day 61. The dilemma is evident. The general rule that GRNs should remember is that pain is whatever the person says it is. This means that only the patient can tell you what pain is for himself or herself.

GRNs should evaluate their own attitudes toward pain management. A patient who is in constant, severe pain will not be able to effectively participate in the rehabilitation process. Thus, the patient should be included in the team discussion about pain relief whenever possible. The basic need of comfort must be met before expectations that demand physical strength and energy from the patient.

Sensory Deficit

Many, if not most, older rehabilitation patients have some degree of sensory deficit. The people most commonly affected are the elderly, those with physical limitations, the mentally retarded, those with psychoses, the homebound, and those who are depressed. The elderly are at particular risk because of the sensory and perceptual changes that occur with aging, such as impaired hearing and visual deficits. Other situations that can put a patient even more at risk are a restricted environment, isolation precautions, impaired communication, brain damage to the sensory center, and sensory impairments such as blindness and deafness. Disease processes such as diabetic retinopathy or glaucoma can result in blindness. Diabetic retinopathy has resulted in blindness in more than 6% of those older than age 75 (Cleary, 1996). Glaucoma is also a leading cause of blindness and is frequently seen in older adults, although the age of onset is generally between 40 and 65 years (Eliopoulos, 1997).

There are several indications that a person may be experiencing sensory deficit. The symptoms to which GRNs should be alert are anxiety, irritability, drowsiness, disorganized thinking, depression, lethargy, disorientation, and hallucinations. Assessment of the person who is at risk is the first step in preventing sensory deficit.

Sensory Overload

Sensory overload occurs when individuals are unable to process the amount of stimuli from their environment. Some older adults can experience this even in the absence of disease. For example, in order to process multiple stimuli, the older adult may require a longer period of time. If this time is not available, sensory overload can result. Case Study 9.1 gives an illustration of this.

CASE STUDY 9.1

Mr. Tillis, a 77 year old man in good health, was driving his Cadillac on an icy road. Passengers in the car included his elderly wife and three of his grade-school-aged grandchildren. When the traffic light in front of him turned yellow, Mr. Tillis put on his brakes, but his car slid into the middle of the busy intersection and stopped directly beneath the light, blocking traffic in all directions. People from each way began to honk their horns, Mrs. Tillis was hollering at her husband to move the car, and the three children in the back seat were saying, "Grandpa, you're blocking all the cars! Back up!" Mr. Tillis seemed unable to take any action for quite some time, and just kept saying, "What?! What?!" Finally realizing how he needed to correct the situation, Mr. Tillis backed his car up to allow traffic to flow again, but not without expressing great frustration. The problem was not just the icy road, but his inability to quickly correct his error because of multiple distracting stimuli from the environment.

Sensory overload may be seen in older rehabilitation patients with respiratory or renal insufficiency, head injury, end-stage renal disease, or the spinal cord–injured person on a ventilator. Sensory overload results in inaccurate interpretation of stimuli (Carpenito, 1992).

Other physical processes can contribute to sensory and perceptual alterations such as overload. These may include fluid and electrolyte imbalances, poor oxygenation or circulation, and any sensory organ alterations. A stressful environment or sleeplessness can also contribute to sensory overload. Signs of a lack of quality sleep include restlessness, lethargy, listlessness, ptosis of the eyelids, irritability, unkempt appearance, feelings of fatigue, hand tremors, inability to make decisions, and increased disorientation.

GOALS

Many goals are appropriate for patients with cognitive and perceptual disturbances or communication deficits. (Nursing diagnoses related to these problems are listed in Table 9–2). Goals depend on the nature of the problem. The nurse will target interventions toward assisting the patient in using effective means of communication, improving memory problems, increasing sensory awareness, and preventing injury.

For example, the primary overall goal for an elderly patient with altered cerebral tissue perfusion is to maintain adequate circulation to the brain. This can be facilitated by aiming nursing interventions at short-term goals that promote the primary objective. Short-term goals would include the patient's being free of symptoms such as blurred vision, headaches, and slurred speech. It is desirable that the patient be alert and oriented, respond appropriately to questions, and be able to participate in therapy. Long-term goals could include an improvement in cognitive status such as memory or the attainment of a more alert state. Seeing that short-term goals are met will ultimately promote long-term goal attainment.

Goals for the patient related to sensory perception may include increased orientation to reality, improvement in memory, increased participation in therapeutic activities, and remaining free from injury. Other desired outcomes may be to arrange for a hearing evaluation or fitting with a hearing device. Communication boards may need to be developed in conjunction with the speech therapist to facilitate communication goals.

If impaired memory is a problem, goals would relate to improvement in concentration and attention span, as well as reality orientation. Goals for a person with alteration in perception of self-concept (such as unilateral neglect) are that the patient learn compensatory techniques such as scanning, respond to verbal or tactile cues, and remain free from injury.

INTERVENTIONS

Nursing interventions are planned to accomplish stated goals. These would include those aimed at assessment, behavior modification, and environmental changes. A review of several problems associated with cognitive and perceptual deficits appears in Table 9–6. This discussion is divided into categories in which the GRN may be likely to implement interventions.

The GRN should be aware that the results of neuropsychological testing can assist in the development of appropriate nursing care plans and goals (Bondy, 1994). If a neuropsychologist is part of the rehabilitation team, the results of his or her assessments can help analyze relationships between the brain and the client's behavior. The neuropsychologist may perform testing in cognitive domains such as attention, executive functions, sensation and perception, memory, language, intelligence, and motor performance. Of course, these areas are often evaluated by other rehabilitation team members as well, such as the neurologist or speech therapist, but can be used by the nurse as diagnostic tools to assist in developing a holistic plan of care tailored to the individual with cognitive deficits.

Teaching and Learning

Although a significant loss of neurons in the brain normally occurs with aging, ability to learn, or intelligence, is not significantly affected. However, several effects of aging do influence the older adult's capacity to recall newly acquired information (Oldaker, 1992). Changes in vision, hearing, and memory (see Tables 9–2 and 9–3) can influence learning capacity and potential. Likewise, physical changes can interfere with the capacity to perform certain tasks (such as arthritis interfering with the ability to give oneself an insulin injection).

Older adults may benefit more from cer-

Table 9–6 PROBLEMS ASSOCIATED WITH COGNITIVE AND PERCEPTUAL DEFICITS

Term	Characteristics
Wernicke's aphasia	Fluent, unmeaningful speech; receptive aphasia
Broca's aphasia	Broken but meaningful speech; expressive aphasia
Global aphasia	Combination of receptive and expressive aphasia; poor prognosis; most difficult to treat
Apraxia	Difficulty using objects or doing tasks appropriately due to lack of memory of how to perform
Somatognosia	Lack of recognition of body parts as one's own; can lead to neglect
Anosognosia	Not acknowledging one's body part as one's own; a severe form of neglect
Right/left indiscrimination	Inability to distinguish right from left; need tactile or gesture cues to follow right/left commands
Neglect	Lack of awareness of part of the body; usually one-sided; may be related to visual deficits
Homonymous hemianopia	Loss of vision in the same half of each eye (temporal half of one and nasal half of the other)

tain approaches to learning new tasks. For example, one nurse educator stated that although teaching aids were a valuable tool in promoting health, "there can be no substitute for time spent with the client on a one-to-one basis" (Manship, 1994, p. 291). Teaching and learning should be a mutual process between the GRN and the client. The GRN should allow the person to be part of the process. That is, goals should be negotiated and mutually established.

The GRN should also remember some general principles in teaching older clients, which consider the common physical limitations associated with aging. This would include simple things such as avoiding glare, making handouts larger, and seating those hard of hearing closer to the speaker. Table 9–7 summarizes some of these reminders.

GRNs can use some specific strategies to enhance learning. First, readiness to learn should be assessed. There are better times for teaching than others. Have specific tasks to teach. Repetition and time for practice are important. Vary the modalities for teaching, when teaching in a group setting, because persons may learn better by one means rather than another (for example, sight versus hearing). Limit the amount of information provided at each session, and focus on teaching what is essential. Remember that "the goal of patient education is not only to gain the older adult's cooperation (compliance), but also to encourage the older adult to change behavior (adherence)" (Oldaker, 1992, p. 55). "In general, effectively teaching the elderly requires a little more time, a need to point out the relevance of the task, adapting teaching methods to accommodate aging changes, and providing practice in the desired behavior" (Weinrich, Weinrich, Boyd, Atwood, & Cervenka, 1994, p. 500).

Promoting Sensory Perception and Processing of Stimuli

Some basic interventions can assist the older adult with sensory perception. The nurse should remind the patient to use appropriate devices that increase sensory perception. For example, hearing aids and glasses (as appropriate) should be worn during the rehabilitation program. Although the patient may find them cumbersome or forget to apply them in the morning, much better comprehension of instruction is usually obtained when these devices are used. The GRN should also not overlook the obvious when it comes to sensory problems. Case Study 9.2 presents the instance of an elderly man who was nearly labeled as confused and combative, and almost dismissed from the rehabilitation unit, until a simple, correctable cause (decreased hearing due to cerumen impaction) for his problems was found. Cerumen impaction is easily diagnosed via otoscopic examination (Meador, 1995) but may be overlooked as a cause for apparent confusion or noncompliance.

Table 9–7 REMINDERS FOR TEACHING THE ELDERLY CLIENT

Visual
Use bright, direct lighting, unless contraindicated owing to visual disturbances (such as recent cataract surgery).
Do not stand by a window—avoid glare.
When using visual aids, use large, well spaced letters—black on white is best.
Keep clients close to the speaker, or if in a large room, be certain that the audience can see and hear the speaker.
For individual teaching, make sure that the client's glasses are clean.

Auditory
Limit distractions: eliminate extraneous noise, close doors, turn off televisions or radios, limit interruptions.
Face the audience. Speak directly to the individual in a one-to-one setting.
Never cover your mouth when speaking (many elders rely on lip reading to compensate for hearing deficits).
Speak slowly and clearly.
If appropriate, wearing bright colors of lipstick may help elders who use lip reading.
Before proceeding, ask if they can hear you.
Use assistive devices (make certain hearing aids and microphones are turned on) as needed.

General Teaching and Learning Suggestions
Keep teaching sessions short and to the point.
Handouts should be simple and clear.
Relate relevance of the topic to adult experiences within the group.
Use the principles of adult learning when planning an educational session.
Pace the presentation to reflect the unique needs and understanding of the group or individual.
Avoid the temptation to overload with too much information.
Remember that adults need a motivation to learn.
Provide immediate feedback to questions and comments.
Give an overview of the material to be covered and explain its relevance.
Keep information simple and specific—avoid technical jargon.
Use a variety of teaching modalities such as videotapes, hands-on experiences, samples of products, group discussion, overheads, pamphlets, and handouts.
Emphasize the patient's learning responsibility.
Be enthusiastic about your subject. If the teacher isn't, the learner will not be.
Summarize important points.
Teach a procedure close to the time it will take place.
When teaching skills, allow time for practice, return demonstrations, questions, and review sessions.
Stick to the essentials needed to maintain life and prevent complications, but be prepared to address additional questions.
Keep the environment conducive to learning. For group sessions, the room temperature should be comfortable for the majority; potentially noxious stimuli (such as cigarette smoke) should be avoided; seats must be easily accessible.
Use a sufficiently large room to accommodate those with wheelchairs, walkers, and other assistive devices; make certain exits are not blocked; have additional nursing personnel available should needs arise (such as toileting).
Be thoroughly familiar with resources available within the community and the individual facility.

CASE STUDY 9.2

Mr. Busk was admitted to an inpatient rehabilitation unit of a large midwestern hospital after having a stroke. The nurse who performed his pre-admission evaluation considered him an appropriate candidate for the unit, but shortly after arrival, Mr. Busk seemed confused. He did not follow directions well, although his physical and cognitive limitations seemed to be minimal. He was angry and belligerent at times. At the weekly team meeting, the staff expressed frustration that Mr. Busk was not cooperating with them and was not meeting his goals. If no improvement was shown soon, he would have to be discharged. The rehabilitation physician sought to rule out other physical problems that may have been contributing to Mr. Busk's behavior. On examination of the patient's ears, a large amount of impacted wax was discovered. The doctor ordered Debrox treatment with irrigation. The next day, Mr. Busk seemed like a new man. He was cheerful and excited about participating in the rehabilitation program. He told the nurse, "I haven't heard this well in years!" What could have been labeled as delirium or combative behavior was simply due to impacted earwax! Because Mr. Busk was only catching small portions of the staff's directions, he seemed uncooperative. The rehabilitation setting required him to work with many different people and process multiple stimuli, which he found difficult and frustrating because he could not hear. Mr. Busk went on to achieve all his goals and was discharged home in less than 2 weeks.

──────

After the GRN has assessed the areas and potential areas in which the person may experience problems with perception, interventions can become more specific. Those persons with sensory alterations may experience deficits or overloads. For the person with sensory deficits, the GRN should aim interventions at decreasing anxiety and providing familiar sights, sounds, and smells as well as objects with tactile familiarity.

If the person has visual deficits, the nurse should continually help orient him or her to the time of day and scheduled activities. When working with a patient who is blind, nurses and all other caregivers should identify themselves each time upon entering the room and prior to doing any treatments. All procedures should be carefully explained. Because many team members may work with the client throughout the day, all should be aware of the patient's limitations and provide consistent treatment.

Patients with difficulty hearing, but who have not had a prior hearing evaluation, can take advantage of the availability of the audiologist, who may be an adjunct team member at many facilities. Hearing evaluations can assist the physician in diagnosing any disease processes or in ordering hearing devices that can assist the person's comprehension of auditory stimuli. The nurse should also be certain to face the older person when speaking, to facilitate hearing and understanding.

The patient with sensory overload requires some additional interventions. The GRN may need to provide for quiet activities. A calm environment is essential. This may necessitate turning off the television or radio, limiting visitors, closing the patient's door, and planning for sleeping time. Carefully explaining all procedures helps avoid additional overload, and orientation to the environment should also continue.

The patient with traumatic brain injury rated as level IV on the Rancho Los Amigos Cognitive Scale provides an excellent example of reasons to avoid or control sensory overload. Patients in this phase of recovery are easily agitated and can become combative, aggressive, or even violent. Sometimes a seemingly insignificant occurrence such as too many visitors in the room can cause a behavioral outburst precipitated by too much sensory stimulation. In a case such as this, the patient may give early signs of agitation through body language, such as clenching the fists, or express anxiety or suspicion. The GRN should talk in slow, quiet tones and immediately remove the causing stimulus once it is identified. Communication with all team members and the family is important to avoid future episodes of overstimulation. If the patient does become violent, the nurse should approach him or her out of reach, look directly at the patient, and use a soft but commanding voice. The GRN should also remember, however, that direct eye contact has different cultural meanings and is considered offensive in some cultures. It is often helpful, and sometimes necessary, for female nurses to have to ask for help from male personnel, including security guards, to control a violent patient. The presence of a male authority figure often helps calm the patient and avoids the use of restraints when the combative patient becomes a danger to himself or herself or others. When caring for a patient who tends to become violent, the nurse should always have an exit from the room, avoid bending over the patient if hitting or biting is a problem, keep the environment free from items that could be used as weapons, protect the patient from hurting himself, and learn what events precipitate behavioral outbursts and uncontrolled behavior. Nearly half of all rehabilitation nurses have experienced some type of injury at the hands of patients. It is therefore important to recognize signs that indicate potential for violence and take appropriate actions.

Enhancing Memory and Cognition

For the person with impaired memory, several interventions may help. It is important to realize that when elders suffer severe memory loss, particularly recent memory, it places a great deal of responsibility on the caregiver and family members. When the caregiver is a family member, frustration and anger can result at having to constantly repeat what was said just minutes before. The GRN will need to emphasize to caregivers that patients do not wish to forget things, but this is beyond their control. Interventions are aimed at assisting the patient and the caregiver or family members in working together so the patient can be managed at home.

Establishing a routine is important. Doing things at the same each day helps the patient develop patterns. Repetition is essential and should be done with patience. "Practice in a supportive environment can facilitate memory of the older person" (Green & Gildemeister, 1994). Devices such as maps, lists, books, and journals can be used. The patient should record plans and daily activities in the journal. Family members can then refer to this when providing memory cues. An audio or video cassette tape can be used to walk patients through certain tasks they might forget, such as taking medications (Cook & Thigpen, 1993).

During the off-shifts, GRNs can also incorporate the patient's memory aids, such as a journal, into nursing care. This provides an ideal teaching situation. Family members may be instructed to write all activities of the evening in the journal. This would include such things as the names of people who visited, what the patient ate for dinner, how far the person walked, and what time they went to bed. Before visiting hours end, the GRN can use this tool to review the evening's activities with the patient and family, reminding the patient of what occurred. The journal will likely also be used the next day in therapy to help cue the person's memory of recent past events.

Simple questions about memory function can alert GRNs and staff to memory problems in older adults. Research suggested that elderly persons' complaints about memory loss may be a new promising indicator of memory impairment and that follow-up should be undertaken whenever subjective complaints are noted (Jonker, Launer, Hooijer, & Lindeboom, 1996). GRNs should ask direct questions about older adults' perceptions regarding their own memory.

Reality orientation is a priority. Having large, readable clocks on the wall assists the patient in maintaining orientation to the time of day. Calendars are useful when kept current. The type that need to be changed daily are fine, but only when they are accurate. Some nursing homes and hospitals announce the day of the week each morning, along with what activities are planned. Likewise, families can remind patients each morning at breakfast what day it is and what will be done. It may be helpful to plan certain activities, such as shopping or going to the bank, for the same day each week and record this in the patient's journal or on the calendar as a reminder. Consistency of routine is important to reality orientation.

When communicating with the person with impaired memory, keep sentences short and to the point. Provide immediate feedback to questions. Be certain that aids such as glasses or hearing aids are in place prior to conversations. Use multiple modalities when teaching, such as those that stimulate several senses (sight, touch, and hearing). Case Study 9.3 provides an example of the challenge families may face in dealing with an elder with memory impairment.

CASE STUDY 9.3

Mrs. Lesley was a 68 year old widow in good physical health who lived alone in a small town. Her son and his family lived about 30 minutes away and visited her regularly. One day, Mrs. Lesley called her daughter-in-law to say that someone had broken into her house and stolen her purse. Mrs. Lesley's son and daughter-in-law knew that sometimes she was forgetful, but they rushed to her house to make sure she was all right. On arrival, they found Mrs. Lesley agitated and confused, saying many of her things were missing. She had also called the police. The house seemed in order, so the search for the purse began. It was found in the oven, where Mrs. Lesley had apparently put it and forgotten. Based on this and many other similar incidents demonstrating increasing forgetfulness and the inability to care for herself, Mrs. Lesley was diagnosed with Alzheimer's disease. The decision was made that Mrs. Lesley required constant supervision, and she went to live with her son.

When the GRN is working with a patient experiencing cognitive deficits, some additional interventions may be indicated. The environment should be well controlled. Group instruction would not be ideal in most cases. Allow the individual more time to process what is being said to them. Use simple sentences and avoid multi-step instructions. Break tasks down into smaller steps.

Nursing interventions can be tailored to the individual, using knowledge related to the person's diagnosis. For example, when nurses reinforce the techniques taught to head-injured clients in therapy, continuity of care and treatment, ongoing feedback, and better family involvement are promoted (Grinspun, 1987). For those with left brain damage, demonstration may work better than verbal instruction. For those with right brain damage, verbal cues may suffice. A variety of modalities may be tried and then teaching tailored to the unique learning abilities of each person. Art therapy may help decrease isolation (Sterritt & Pokorny, 1994). Pet therapy or horticulture therapy can also give patients or residents a sense of purpose and help hinder physical debility.

It must be noted that in some cases there will be progressive loss of memory and cognitive function. This is particularly frustrating to the alert patient and the caregiver. When no treatment can be found to prevent this deterioration, then maintenance interventions are indicated. Although the suggestions previously detailed should still be implemented, expectations of improved outcomes should be realistic to reflect the situation. The 89-year-old with a failing memory is not likely to greatly benefit from medical therapy, and even if this was the case, the benefits may not outweigh the risks. In this case, patience on the part of the caregiver will be of the utmost importance in assisting the person in maintaining a positive self-image in the face of memory loss. Caregivers will likely need to share and vent their frustrations, and this is often best done in a group setting with other caregivers who are experiencing similar difficulties. A good example of such a support group are those for family members of Alzheimer's patients. Additionally, family members should plan to have respite time and should be made to feel this is necessary, without guilt, to providing long-term care for anyone with a progressive memory loss.

Working with Persons with Aphasia

Some general guidelines for working with persons with aphasia should be followed. More specific interventions are used depending on the type of aphasia present.

Speak in slow, simple sentences, allowing time for processing. Do not raise your voice, unless the person is also hard of hearing. Aphasia does not mean deafness. Do not assume that a slow response or no response means the patient did not understand the question. Ask whether he or she did. If it is necessary to repeat a question, do not change the wording. Allow at least a minute to pass for the person to process the question. Realize, however, that the patient's nodding the head appropriately in response to questions must be assessed for accuracy. In early stages, aphasics often confuse head nods when meaning "yes" or "no."

Extreme patience must be used. The patient is already likely highly frustrated, often feeling trapped inside the body with a lot to say but no way to communicate it. Loss of language can be devastating. The GRN should acknowledge that the patient may feel frustrated, angry, and helpless, but inspire hope that speech may soon return with help of rehabilitation professionals and determination on the part of the patient. If others are observing speech therapy sessions or communicative encounters, their number should be limited. The patient must be treated with dignity and his or her privacy respected. Avoid unnecessary questions, so that the person's energy can be saved for important tasks.

Continue to talk to the patient even if he or she does not answer. Encourage family members to do this also. Any form of communication the patient tries to use should be encouraged, whether verbal, gesturing, or with a communication board. A communication board with pictures is often effective before speech returns, in order to help the person communicate basic needs. Pictures commonly used might include a toilet, a glass, food, a bed, a face with a grimace indicating the need for pain medication, and the words "yes" or "no." All members of the interdisciplinary team should learn how to relate to those using a communication board or other such device.

Even simple approaches to treatment can be effective in helping the aphasic stroke patient regain the use of words (Loughrey, 1992). If swear words or other inappropriate terms are all that the patient can say, supply the correct word and ask the patient to repeat it, but do not discourage use of language. Family members will need explanation about the patient's changed vocabulary if only one or two words return at first. Case Study 9.4 presents a situation in which the patient's only verbal communication was swear words and how the family and staff managed this situation.

CASE STUDY 9.4

Mrs. Davis, a 65 year old grandmother, was admitted to the rehabilitation unit with left-sided stroke, right hemiplegia, and expressive aphasia. Her only verbalizations were swear words, which she used regularly. Mrs. Davis' husband and grown children were visibly distressed at her use of language. This was a strong Catholic family, and the daughter expressed her dismay to the nurse, saying that Mrs. Davis had never sworn in her life and was a deeply religious person. The nurse provided the family with information about aphasia and encouraged them to meet with the speech therapist. Together, the team members were able to help the family understand that their mother was not meaning to curse at everyone, but this was the only form of language that had returned. The nurse spent a great deal of time working with the family members and the speech therapist to provide a consistent approach to care and deal with the family's concerns. By supplying the correct words to Mrs. Davis, she did have most of her normal speech patterns return, but this took intensive speech therapy and the patience of her family.

Pain Management

Alteration in comfort is common in the geriatric rehabilitation setting. Nursing treatment is aimed at relieving pain and discomfort as well as teaching patients to manage chronic pain. A variety of treatment modalities can be used for pain relief. Heat and cold applications are often used by physical therapists as they work with the functionally disabled. The transcutaneous electrical nerve stimulator (TENS) is a device that "distracts" the pain transmission thereby decreasing painful sensations through electrical impulses. GRNs should be familiar with this equipment if the patient is wearing it on the unit or at home so that questions from the family can be answered.

Nurses should use palliative pain relieving measures when possible for those with chronic pain. Techniques such as relaxation therapy, subdued lighting, back massages, therapeutic touch, or music therapy can decrease the need for medications. Diversion can be effective for mild to moderate pain but is generally of little help with severe pain. Additionally, many patients will have lived with chronic pain for many years and have home remedies that they have found effective. GRNs should be open to cultural traditions that have been passed down through generations as a potential source of pain relief for the patient. Persons may be reluctant to share these with the nurse unless they feel their ethnic and cultural beliefs will be accepted. Chapter 13 further discusses how nurses can become more culturally sensitive.

Other obvious pain relieving interventions are proper positioning, repositioning, and turning schedules. Often discomfort is caused by pressure areas, whether from immobility, laying in bed, or sitting in an uncomfortable position. Devices to pad and cushion bony prominences should be used as necessary. Hemiplegic arms should never be left dangling during transfers or when ambulating, but should be supported with a lapboard when in the chair or with a hemi-sling. Nurses need to reinforce the patient's self-care abilities in doing wheelchair lifts and leans as well as skin checks. Pain can also be caused by ill-fitting braces or AFOs. The patient should be instructed to promptly report any discomfort related to adaptive equipment.

Pain medications should be used appropriately. Having a standard pain rating scale will assist the nurse in selecting the most appropriate medication from those ordered. Rehabilitation patients who have recently undergone orthopedic surgery, such as hip or knee replacement, may initially take narcotic medications for pain control. For other patients, over-the-counter medications such as acetaminophen (Tylenol) are often effective enough to provide relief. Nurses should expect patients to express some muscle soreness or stiffness as they begin the intense hours of therapy required in many settings. Pain medication is most effective when given at least 30 minutes before therapy sessions. This should be written into the patient care plan or Kardex and on the medication sheet to promote consistency and quality of care. Nurses should not hesitate to offer analgesics to patients who are in need of them, remembering that optimal participation in the rehabilitation program cannot occur when the individual is in too much discomfort.

One specific type of pain category is worth noting here. Amputees often experience different types of pain sensations, including phantom pain and sensation and stump pain. Phantom sensation is described as feelings of pressure, cold, wetness, tingling, prickling, or the like in a body part that has been removed and for which there is no effective treatment. Amputees describe the sensation as being so real that the body part still seems present. A large number of persons with complete spinal cord injury (no motor movement below the level of injury) experience paresthesia in their paralyzed parts. Phantom pain is a painful sensation in the missing or paralyzed body part. For many years this was believed to be a psychogenic type of pain, so much so that amputees were afraid to tell their physicians for fear of being labeled mentally ill (Davis, 1993). Researchers now feel that phantom pain occurs with such frequency among amputees that it is a physiological anomaly and unrelated to psychological characteristics in most cases. Treatment of phantom limb pain includes using one's prosthesis, stroking or stimulating the stump, heat, electrical stimulation, and distraction (Davis, 1993). Stump pain is a less common complaint than phantom limb pain. It can be related to a variety of causes, but the most common is an improperly fitting prosthesis (Davis, 1993). Nurses need to be especially alert to any indications that suggest that the person's prosthesis needs to be adjusted. This should be promptly reported to the physician and prosthetist. Persons with amputation may also have severe stump pain during the rehabilitation process after surgery as a result of incisional pain, poor circulation, and/or infection. The cause and nature of the person's pain should be explored in each situation.

Managing Behaviors That Interfere with Rehabilitation

Most patients on inpatient acute rehabilitation units do not have such severe behavioral deficits that they cannot participate in rehabilitation. Otherwise, such lack of attention may prohibit their admittance to this type of intense therapy. The obvious exception to this rule is the person with head injury, who, as he or she recovers, is likely to exhibit many inappropriate social and cognitive behaviors. However, this rather predictable process is in contrast to the elderly patient with progressive deterioration of mental status, or the person who is suffering from acute confusion or delirium. Those GRNs working in long-term care settings must often deal with residents who are withdrawn, disoriented, confused, demanding, combative, or demented. General guidelines can help the nurse effectively assist the person to a higher level of personal control or self-care.

Clear expectations should be given of what is acceptable and unacceptable behavior. The GRN can significantly influence positive outcomes by controlling the environment. This can be done by providing a calm and quiet setting for recovery. Good communication between patients and team members allows sharing of problems and effective treatments. Acknowledging the patient's feelings but using a warm, yet firm, consistent approach to managing behavior that interferes with rehabilitation is essential. Maintaining a sense of humor can help patients or residents and staff cope with awkward situations and relieve tension.

More specific interventions are related to individual behavior, as discussed in the following sections.

Wandering

Some patients with cognitive impairments or dementia will wander. This is often seen in nursing home patients. It is important for the GRN to ascertain the context of the behavior and its meaning for the patient. The following factors have been related to wandering: mental impairment, confusion, unfamiliar environment, stress, anxiety, boredom, lack of control, lack of exercise, diseases of the central nervous system, and cardiac decompensation (Lucero et al., 1993).

Staff should be alert to individuals who tend to wander. The reason for this behavior should be explored with the patient. Perhaps the person walks and wanders because he or she is afraid, unfamiliar with the environment, or having feelings of insecurity, or he or she may not be able to express a reason. Distraction is helpful at times, as is providing a familiar routine and increased security in their particular setting. Providing structured time for these patients may decrease the incidence of wandering behavior (Lucero et al., 1993). Walking may be a coping mechanism for patients and could be used to their benefit.

When wandering behavior is not modifiable, alerting devices can be used, such as bed alarms that warn staff when the person has left the bed or chair. For those who seek to leave the facility, environmental changes may provide assistance. These could include painting door knobs the same color as the walls, using mirrors to disguise doors, or using certain optical patterns that do not reveal exits. Having volunteer escorts and posting STOP signs may also help. These strategies may allow the person to wander in a safe area under the supervision of the staff and avoids the use of restraints, which often aggravates the problem.

Withdrawal

Older persons may withdraw socially and emotionally from others. This occurs more commonly in the institutionalized, depressed aged. Physical causes should be explored. If clinical depression is suspected as the cause, the physician should be notified, because medications could be of significant benefit. Other causes could include sensory deprivation from aphasia, poor vision, or deafness. Patients may display a negative attitude toward life and speak of giving up. The GRN should encourage the patient to verbalize his or her feelings, using rehabilitation principles to emphasize the patient's strengths.

Disorientation

This type of behavior is best dealt with by providing frequent, brief contacts throughout the day. At each contact, communication should be encouraged and reality orientation given. Interventions are aimed at bringing the person back to reality. The nurse should not participate in any fantasy or hallucinogenic conversation. Giving persons tasks to help them remain occupied or encouraging their participation in hobbies may help. Additionally, in a group setting, the person may benefit from reality orientation that can occur from peers, but confrontation should be avoided.

Combativeness

For the patient with a tendency toward violence or combativeness, the nurse can follow several safety guidelines: Stop any activity. Get help if needed.

Remove the patient from the situation and try to calm him or her. Distraction will at times avert a dangerous situation, but it is not always effective. Angry outbursts from the person should not be taken personally.

Often the person is unable to control the behavior once it is triggered.

The nurse should identify stress-producing stimuli and attempt to control them. The nurse should also avoid physical injury to himself or herself. This can be done by identifying patients who tend toward violent behavior and taking the necessary steps to avoid situations that could escalate or put the nurse in danger. For patients who become agitated, preventive strategies such as activity tables with non-removable parts or sketch pads to allow for expression through art may be helpful. Combative patients should not be left alone and may need one-to-one supervision to avoid the use of physical restraints (Temple, 1994).

Demanding Behavior

Demanding patients require special attention from the nurse. The motive behind the patient's demands is the key to understanding this behavior. Often, older patients feel helpless and powerless. They may unconsciously compensate for this by demanding more time and attention from the staff, seeking some control over the situation. Individual attention often allays demands, but it can also contribute to unrealistic expectations from the patient or resident that his or her every desire will be immediately met. Limits should be set and expectations explored. Discussing demanding behavior with the patient can assist in the setting of realistic goals. Requests by the patient should be repeated and clarified. Mutual communication is important in establishing appropriate roles for both the patient and the nurse.

Promoting a Positive Self-image

Because depression is so prevalent among the elderly, even in the absence of chronic disease or illness, GRNs should take special steps to try to combat the tendency toward depression (see Table 9–4). Patients in rehabilitation are trying to adjust to life-altering changes and thus are particularly susceptible to the onset of depression. Up to half of elderly stroke patients suffer from depression (Clothier & Grotta, 1991). Bruckbauer (1991) stated that stroke survivors with anterior cerebral lesions (left more often than right) were at greater risk for mood disorders. The institutionalized elderly have a high incidence of depression as well, which can contribute to many other problems. For instance, researchers have shown that depressed residents in nursing homes were more likely to complain of pain, whether or not they had cognitive impairment (Cohen-Mansfield & Marx, 1993).

GRNs should not neglect to perform thorough assessments to detect the presence of depression or other cognitive disorders such as delirium. Nurses may not be comfortable in assessing areas such as perceptual disturbances or delirium, but such skills are essential for proper treatment (Morency, Levkoff, & Dick, 1994). Careful documentation and discussion of the patient's situation with the physician can assist in more appropriate pharmacological treatment. Medications are effective in treating depression for many elders in rehabilitation. However, the GRN should be aware that the therapeutic effect of the drug may not be noted until weeks after treatment is initiated, as in the case of maprotiline (Ludiomil).

Older adults with functional limitations may be dealing with difficult self-esteem issues. Feelings of inadequacy, loss of control, and powerlessness can lead to depression, withdrawal, and even thoughts of suicide. Common rehabilitation problems that might alert GRNs to the potential for a negative self-image include physical changes such as colostomy, amputation, hemiplegia, paralysis, burns, facial palsy, obesity, and the like.

The nurse should assist the patient with good grooming and personal hygiene. Individuals should be encouraged to wear their own clothes and not hospital gowns. Privacy should be provided to acknowledge the sexuality of the person. Positive feedback should be provided to the person. They should not be treated like invalids. Emphasize strengths and acceptance of limitations. Demonstrate acceptance of the individual and encourage family members to do the same. Educate the person and partner that sexuality is closely related to self-esteem and involves more than just physical intimacy. Opening the door to discussion of issues related to sexuality and self-image gives the patient permission to ask questions and acknowledges the person's needs for intimacy despite physical limitations.

Nurses can also create an environment that is warm and accepting. Many conversations between nurses and clients center around personal care or custodial needs (Coulson, 1993). GRNs need to take time to get to know patients and their families on a more personal level so that conversations can be meaningful and therapeutic. The admission assessment provides an excellent time to discover what is meaningful and important to the patient. The physical layout of the facility is also of importance. Hallways should be well lit, as well as restrooms and other walkways. Walls should be painted or papered in cheery, soft colors, because this promotes a comforting, relaxing look. Glare, as occurs with high-gloss finishes, should be avoided. Consistent staff assignments can also help improve the tone of the unit. Nurses are generally more satisfied when they feel a sense of ownership over their team. Some benefits to hiring full-time staff to act as primary nurses or case managers are the improvement in consistency of care, increased involvement and knowledge of the patients and families, and greater satisfaction on the part of clients as a result.

EVALUATION

Nurses can evaluate the effectiveness of nursing interventions through examining outcomes related to sensory perception, cognitive status, and communication. Persons with several sensory and perceptual deficits such as hemianopia, hemiplegia, neglect, and presbyopia are attaining important goals when they are able to function in their daily roles and perform self-care. Although they may experience a number of deficits from both normal aging and a disease process, maximal independence level should be strived for. When this is achieved, practical goals have been met.

Evaluation of sensory perception must be ongoing. Concomitant factors related to cardiovascular and respiratory problems should be documented and addressed. Positive outcomes related to improved cognitive status would include improvement in memory, increased ability to perform tasks and follow multi-step instructions, and maintaining an alert mental state.

Patients are meeting goals when effective two-way communication, whether verbal or non-verbal, is taking place. When the person is able to notify the staff of needs, whether through the use of speech, gestures, or a communication board, desirable outcomes are being accomplished.

For those with behavioral problems that interfere with the rehabilitation process, establishing some personal control over these behaviors is one indication of goals being met. Another outcome measure is knowledge and ability on the part of the caregiver to manage behavioral difficulties in a variety of situations. Positive outcomes related to reducing the incidence of injury would include a decreased number of falls, a decrease in the use of restraints, and a decrease in the need for medications to control or modify problems with behavior.

REFERENCES

Amarenco, P., Cohen, A., Tzourio, C., Bertrand, B., Hommel, M., Besson, G., Chauvel, C., Touboul, P. J., & Bousser, M. G. (1994). Atherosclerotic disease of the aortic arch and the risk of ischemic stroke. *New England Journal of Medicine, 331,* 1474–1479.

Bondy, K. N. (1994). Assessing cognitive function: A guide to neuropsychological testing. *Rehabilitation Nursing, 19*(1), 24–30, 36.

Bruckbauer, E. A. (1991). Recognizing poststroke depression. *Rehabilitation Nursing, 16*(10), 34–36.

Carpenito, L. J. (1992). *Nursing diagnosis: Application to clinical practice.* Philadelphia: J. B. Lippincott.

Chenitz, W. C., Stone, J. T., & Salisbury, S. A. (1991). *Clinical gerontological nursing: A guide to advanced practice.* Philadelphia: W. B. Saunders.

Cleary, B. L. (1996). Age-related changes in the special senses. In M. A. Matteson, E. S. McConnell, & A. D. Linton (Eds.), *Gerontological nursing: Concepts and practice* (pp. 386–405). Philadelphia: W. B. Saunders.

Clothier, J., & Grotta, J. (1991). Recognition and management of poststroke depression in the elderly. *Clinics in Geriatric Medicine, 7,* 493–506.

Cohen, R. A., & Van Nostrand, J. F. (1995). Trends in the health of older Americans: United States, 1994. National Center for Health Statistics. *Vital and Health Statistics, 3*(30).

Cohen-Mansfield, J., & Marx, M. S. (1993). Pain and depression in the nursing home: Corroborating results. *Journal of Gerontology: Psychological Sciences, 48*(2), 96–97.

Cook, E. A., & Thigpen, R. (1993). Identification and management of cognitive and perceptual deficits in the rehabilitation patient. *Rehabilitation Nursing, 18*(5), 310–313.

Coulson, I. (1993, May/June). The impact of the total environment in the care and management of dementia. *The American Journal of Alzheimer's Care and Related Disorders and Research,* 18–25.

Davis, R. W. (1993). Phantom sensation, phantom pain, and stump pain. *Archives of Physical Medicine and Rehabilitation, 74,* 79–85.

Dellasega, C., Brown, R., & White, A. (1995). Cholesterol-related health behaviors in rural elderly persons. *Journal of Gerontological Nursing, 21*(5), 6–12.

Desbien, N. A., Meuller-Rizner, N., Connors, A. F., Homel, M. D., & Wenger, N. S. (1997). Pain in the oldest-old during hospitalization and up to one year later. *Journal of the American Geriatrics Society, 45,* 1167–1172.

Devine, E. C., & Reifschneider, E. (1995). A meta-analysis of the effects of psychoeducational care in adults with hypertension. *Nursing Research, 44,* 237–244.

Eliopoulos, C. (1993). *Gerontological nursing.* Philadelphia: J. B. Lippincott.

Eliopoulos, C. (1997). *Gerontological nursing.* Philadelphia: J. B. Lippincott.

Finkelstein, L. E. (1996). TB or not TB? How to interpret a skin test. *American Journal of Nursing, 96*(12), 12–13.

Green, P. M., & Gildemeister, J. E. (1994). Memory aging research and memory support in the elderly. *Journal of Neuroscience Nursing, 26,* 241–244.

Grinspun, D. R. (1987). Nursing intervention in cognitive retraining of the traumatic brain injury client. *Rehabilitation Nursing, 12,* 323–330.

Harrell, J. S. (1997). Age-related changes in the cardiovascular system. In M. A. Matteson & E. S. McConnell (Eds.), *Gerontological nursing: Concepts and practice.* Philadelphia: W. B. Saunders.

Jansen, D. A., & Cimprich, B. (1994). Attentional impairment in persons with multiple sclerosis. *Journal of Neuroscience Nursing, 26,* 95–101.

Johnson, A. P. (1995). The pulmonary system and its problems in the elderly. In M. Stanley & P. Beare (Eds.), *Gerontological nursing* (pp. 201–209). Philadelphia: F. A. Davis.

Jonker, C., Launer, L. J., Hooijer, C., & Lindeboom, J. (1996). Memory complaints and memory impairment in older individuals. *Journal of the American Geriatrics Society, 44,* 7–13.

Loughrey, L. (1992). The effects of two teaching techniques on recognition and use of function words by aphasic stroke patients. *Rehabilitation Nursing, 17*(3), 134–137.

Lucero, M., Hutchinson, S., Leger-Krall, S., & Wilson, H. S. (1993). Wandering in Alzheimer's dementia patients. *Clinical Nursing Research, 2,* 160–174.

Manship, A. (1994). Treatment of hypertension in the elderly. *British Journal of Nursing, 3,* 287–291.

McConnell, E. S., & Murphy, A. T. (1997). Nursing diagnoses related to physiological alterations. In M. A. Matteson & E. S. McConnell (Eds.), *Gerontological nursing: Concepts and practice* (2nd ed., pp. 222–255). Philadelphia: W. B. Saunders.

McCourt, A. (Ed.). (1993). *The specialty practice of rehabilitation nursing: A core curriculum.* Skokie, IL: Rehabilitation Nursing Foundation.

Meador, J. A. (1995). Cerumen impaction in the elderly. *Journal of Gerontological Nursing, 21*(12), 43–45.

Miller, C. A. (1995). *Nursing care of the older adult: Theory and practice.* Philadelphia: J. B. Lippincott.

Morency, C. R., Levkoff, S., & Dick, K. (1994). Research considerations: Delirium in hospitalized elders. *Journal of Gerontological Nursing, 20*(8), 24–30.

Oldaker, S. M. (1992). Live and learn: Patient education for the elderly orthopaedic client. *Orthopaedic Nursing, 11*(3), 51–56.

Rhodes, R., Morrissey, M. J., & Ward, A. (1992, March/April). Self-motivation: A driving force for elders in cardiac rehabilitation. *Geriatric Nursing*, 94–98.

Ritchie, D. (1993). Cardiovascular problems. In D. L. Carnevali & M. Patrick (Eds.), *Nursing management for the elderly* (3rd ed., pp. 423–451). Philadelphia: J. B. Lippincott.

Roben, N. (1993). Hypertension. In D. L. Carnevali & M. Patrick (Eds.), *Nursing management for the elderly* (3rd ed., pp. 529–542). Philadelphia: J. B. Lippincott.

Rovner, B. W., Steele, C. D., Shmuley, Y., & Folstein, M. F. (1996). A randomized trial of dementia care in nursing homes. *Journal of the American Geriatrics Society, 44*, 7–13.

Sterritt, P. F., & Pokorny, M. E. (1994). Art activities for patients with Alzheimer's and related disorders. *Geriatric Nursing, 15*(3), 155–159.

Temple, C. M. (1994). Managing physical assault in a health care setting. *Rehabilitation Nursing, 19*(5), 281–286.

U.S. Department of Health and Human Services, Public Health Service, National Institutes of Health, National Institute on Aging. (1994). Research is the key to unlocking the mysteries of Alzheimer's disease. In *Progress report on Alzheimer's disease* (NIH Publication No. 94-3885).

Veltman, R. H., VanDongen, S., Jones, S., Buechler, C. M., & Blostein, P. (1993). Cognitive screening in mild brain injury. *Journal of Neuroscience Nursing, 25*, 367–371.

Weinrich, S. P., Weinrich, M. C., Boyd, M. D., Atwood, J., & Cervenka, B. (1994). Teaching older adults by adapting for aging changes. *Cancer Nursing, 17*, 494–500.

Welte, P. O. (1993). Indices of verbal learning and memory deficits after right hemisphere stroke. *Archives of Physical Medicine and Rehabilitation, 74*, 631–636.

Wenger, N. K. (1990). Cardiovascular disease. In C. K. Cassel, D. E. Riesenberg, L. B. Sorensen, & J. R. Walsh (Eds.), *Geriatric medicine* (pp. 152–163). New York: Springer-Verlag.

Part III

Nursing Implications in the Care of Older Adults with Specific Rehabilitative Health Alterations

■

Chapter 10

Stroke

Stroke is the leading cause of disability in older adults and the third leading cause of death behind heart disease and cancer (National Stroke Association [NSA], 1995). According to the NSA (1995), more than half a million people each year in the United States have a stroke. Hypertension is the number one risk factor for stroke and is known to be a major chronic health problem for those older than the age of 65 years. Two thirds of those who have strokes are older than 65. High blood pressure also occurs more frequently in certain ethnic groups than in others, such as those of African and Hispanic descent, placing them at greater risk for stroke and at a younger age. Generally, men are at greater risk of stroke than women. However, after menopause women's risk for stroke approximates that of men. Of those who experience a stroke, approximately one third die. Those surviving may be left with permanent disabilities that affect their capacity for self-care.

Stroke is a recurring disease that can have lifelong effects on the person and the family. One in four hospital admissions for stroke is for recurrence, and those who have had a stroke are five times as likely to have another (Goldberg & Berger, 1988). Stroke can be simply defined as an interruption in the blood supply to the brain, but its effects are in no way so simple. The medical term for stroke is cerebrovascular accident (CVA), implying that it is an event characterized by a rather sudden onset of symptoms that relate to the circulation in the brain. It has been likened to a heart attack and is sometimes referred to as a "brain attack" by stroke authorities in explaining the process to laypersons.

Stroke poses many complications for the older adult. It is the number one diagnosis for hospital discharge to a nursing home or skilled care facility, evidenced by the fact that 35% of all long-term care residents have had a stroke (NSA, 1995). The effects of stroke affect the entire family in every area of life.

REVIEW OF BRAIN STRUCTURES AND FUNCTION

The two main arterial systems that supply the brain are the carotids and the vertebrobasilar arteries. The circle of Willis is a ring of arteries formed by the convergence of these major blood vessels that supply the cerebrum. The major vessels that supply the cerebrum are actually located distally to the circle of Willis and include the right and left internal carotids and the right and left vertebral arteries. The vertebral arteries enter the skull to form the basilar arteries. Other main branches within the brain are the anterior, middle, and posterior cerebral arteries, as well as the anterior and posterior communicating arteries.

There are four major lobes of the brain, each serving a special function. These include the frontal, temporal, parietal, and occipital lobes. All parts of the brain work together, but each area serves a unique function.

The frontal lobe regulates behavior, emotions, and some motor function. Damage to the frontal lobe can result in personality changes, poor judgment, lack of concentration, impaired problem solving abilities, Broca's aphasia, and inappropriate social behavior. Voluntary movements may be impaired. Focal seizures, emotional lability, and a flat affect are also common.

The temporal lobe affects the ability to hear and interpret sound as well as smell and taste. Interruption to the blood supply in this area can cause receptive aphasia, irritability, behavioral changes, and auditory deficits as well as hallucinations.

The parietal lobe controls sensory and perceptual functions, including peripheral sensation. If this area is damaged by stroke, it can result in apraxia, neglect, astereognosis, and loss of ability to discriminate between left and right.

When the occipital lobe is affected, visual disturbances occur. If this primary visual area sustains injury, hemianopia and other visual deficits may result.

A large area of the brain affects one's speech. The speech center is located in the left hemisphere, particularly the frontal and temporal lobes, even in left-handed people. So those with damage to the left side of the brain often experience more severe verbal communication deficits.

WARNING SIGNS OF STROKE

At least 10% of all strokes are preceded by a transient ischemic attack (TIA). This is an acute episode with neurological deficits (such as loss of consciousness; blurred vision; loss of feeling in the legs, arms, or face; or slurred speech) that pass without leaving residual deficits, lasting several minutes to several hours (usually less than 24 hours). Those who have a TIA are 10 times more likely to have a stroke. Such an episode should be viewed as a the body's way of signaling a possible impending cerebrovascular event. Reversible ischemic neurological deficit (RIND) is similar to TIA but lasts 24 to 48 hours without residual effects (Bronstein, Popovich, & Stewart-Amidei, 1991; Caplan, 1988).

Gerontological rehabilitation nurses (GRNs) should educate their older clients and family members or significant others to recognize the classic signs and symptoms of stroke. The NSA (1994) lists seven warning signs: numbness and/or tingling, speech difficulties, headache, blurred vision, dizziness, loss of consciousness, and the sudden inability to speak or move. These signs should never be ignored or dismissed, particularly in the older adult. Some of the warning signs of strokes are similar to symptoms of other problems, but in the population that is at risk (those older than 65), any of these symptoms should be reported to a physician or primary care provider immediately.

TYPES OF STROKE

Three main classifications, or types, of stroke are noted here: thrombotic, embolic, and hemorrhagic. When an infarction occurs in the brain, it is caused by either a thrombus or an embolus. Strokes caused by embolism or hemorrhage usually give little or no warning signs, but persons with thrombotic CVA often first exhibit TIAs and other warning signs of stroke. However, because the origin of stroke cannot always be determined, the term *thromboembolic stroke* is often preferred by physicians (Sandin & Mason, 1996). For the purposes of this discussion, the three major types of stroke will be distinguished.

The most common type of stroke is *thrombotic*, meaning a blockage originating in the brain. This is caused by atherosclerosis and narrowing of the arterial lumen, which can also be referred to as stenosis. These causes are associated with modifiable risk factors that are discussed later in this chapter. Approximately 75% of strokes are the result of local thrombotic occlusion of the carotid or cerebral arteries, resulting in brain infarction in the areas supplied by those vessels (Roth, 1988). Sixty percent of thrombotic strokes occur during sleep.

An *embolic* stroke is often the result of heart disease. Those persons with atrial fibrillation or flutter are more likely to experience a stroke. When no other cause of stroke is immediately apparent, the patient's cardiac history should be suspected. With atrial fibrillation, the heart does not maintain a normal sinus rhythm, allowing tiny clots to form. These may break off and travel to the brain as emboli, resulting in stroke. Other causes of embolic stroke include fat or tumor cells, sepsis, endocarditis, and deep vein thrombosis.

Hemorrhagic stroke occurs when a blood vessel in the brain leaks or bursts. A ruptured or leaking aneurysm, congenital (A-V) malformation, or hypertension can be causal factors. This type of stroke usually occurs without usual warning signs, but the person may present with a sudden onset of severe headache, followed quickly by symptoms of stroke. Hypertension is considered the number one risk factor for stroke; over time it weakens the vessel walls, making the person more likely to experience stroke of this kind.

RISK FACTORS FOR STROKE

There are many known risk factors for stroke. These can be categorized as controllable or uncontrollable: some factors are pre-existing and beyond intervention; other influences can be modified or changed. Medical and nursing treatment focuses on a person's controllable factors.

Uncontrollable risk factors include age, gender, race, and heredity. Those older than age 65 are at greater risk for stroke. Men tend to experience stroke more often than women until menopause, after which both genders are nearly equal in incidence. African-Americans have a higher rate of stroke because of hypertension and may experience this at an earlier age. Hereditary properties such as the tendency toward hypertension and stroke in the family are also beyond the control of health professionals.

The risk factors that are targeted for modification in the older adult to reduce the likelihood of stroke include hypertension, high cholesterol, heart disease, smoking, obesity, stress, and diabetes. High blood pressure was formerly often not diagnosed in the older adult, because most older people remain asymptomatic until the later stages of hypertension. Research on the relationship between hypertension and stroke has influenced health care professionals to screen people more closely, particularly those thought to be at greater risk for hypertension. Early prevention and treatment measures (such as blood pressure screening or lowering sodium intake) are now recommended for everyone.

Adults are becoming more conscious of the need to control their high blood pressure as a means of preventing other health problems. Even treatment of mild hypertension can significantly reduce the risk of stroke. Thus, blood pressure screening in older adults takes on increased importance. GRNs need to be aware that this is an area in which education of the person and the family should be addressed. This is discussed later in this chapter.

A diet low in saturated fats can help reduce cholesterol levels—a contributing factor in the development of atherosclerosis and arteriosclerosis, which increase stroke risk. Regular exercise also helps to clear fatty deposits from the heart. The GRN should reinforce to the older adult that it is never too late to begin an exercise program, and the benefits are many. In addition to reducing cholesterol and triglyceride levels, weight loss and muscle toning occur, and a feeling of well-being is increased. Cardiac and respiratory function can be enhanced, and with this comes increased stamina. Even obese adults can change their lifestyle with proper exercise and nutrition. However, this may require counseling and the guidance of health care professionals. Fad diets that promise quick results should be avoided, because rapid weight loss in the older person can be extremely detrimental to health and promote a false sense of accomplishment that further erodes self-esteem when he or she is no longer able to maintain a rigorous dietary schedule. A wise guideline is to increase activity and decrease caloric intake by eating heart-healthy foods. This should result in a more gradual weight reduction of 1 to 2 pounds per week. Those with obesity should consult a health care professional for supervision of their weight loss or cholesterol reduction program. It should be noted here that some individuals have a hereditary predisposition to higher cholesterol levels, even when in peak physical condition. Some of these persons will require medications to help reduce their cholesterol levels to a safer range. The potential side effects of these medications should be discussed with the patient and family.

Heart disease is another controllable risk factor. Those with heart disease are five times more likely to have a stroke than those without (Goldberg & Berger, 1988). As a secondary complication, cardiac deaths account for 10% to 20% of mortality associated with CVA (Brott, 1991). Persons can reduce their risk of heart disease, and thus their risk of stroke, by following dietary guidelines such as those set forth by the American Heart Association (see Chapter 5) and maintaining a regular exercise program. For the older adult, walking is one of the best and least expensive forms of activity. In many parts of the country, indoor shopping malls open their doors early to elders who wish to walk inside, so that inclement weather need not prohibit them from exercising. The large open hallways that connect the shops make a long, smooth track on which to walk. Adults who take advantage of this service often make time to socialize and visit with others doing the same. Programs of this kind thus provide many benefits besides the physical. This type of support from the community is commendable. In areas where this service is not yet available, the GRN can act as an advocate or mediator by arranging for it to be offered when there is a need.

The risk of heart disease and stroke can also be reduced by a person's quitting smoking. For the older adult, smoking is an extreme hazard. It contributes greatly to the chance of lung cancer, respiratory difficulties, heart disease, and stroke. Some adults may be under the false impression that some forms of tobacco are safer than others. GRNs can assist the person and family in reducing the risk of stroke by providing accurate information about facts associated with smoking. The American Lung Association (ALA) stated that all tobacco products are harmful to a person's health. This includes cigarettes, pipes, cigars, and chewing tobacco or snuff. Secondhand smoke also contains harmful chemicals and can contribute to chronic bronchitis and asthma. Nicotine is present in all forms of tobacco and is an addictive substance. The ALA (1992) also holds the position that using lower tar and nicotine products does not reduce the risks caused by smoking. Smokeless tobacco in the form of snuff also increases the risk of heart disease and stroke by elevating heart rate and blood pressure, increasing the workload of the heart. However, even an older person who has smoked for years and quits can reduce or eliminate many of the effects of smoking on the lungs. It should be emphasized that it is not too late to quit smoking, even at an advanced age.

Reducing a person's stress level is also desirable when considering stroke prevention. This is also true of heart disease, although the additional factor of hostility is now thought to be the emerging critical factor related to heart disease in those with type A personality characteristics. An increased level of stress over time can contribute to hypertension, if left unchecked. Once again, activity and exercise can help control stress, and eating proper amounts of foods containing essential vitamins and minerals will help the body combat the effects of stress. Modifications in lifestyle may also be needed. For example, a 65-year old woman caring for her frail 85-year-old mother at home may require a helper at home or periods of respite in order to avoid the negative effects that the caregiving burden can place on her. GRNs can intervene in such instances by linking the family with community resources that can help meet their needs. Educating the family about caregiver burnout and related factors can also help prevent the extreme stress associated with these circumstances. Lack of finances can be a source of stress that can contribute to stroke incidence in lower socioeconomic groups. Nurses need to be aware of community services, clinics, church groups, and the like that can help meet the unique needs of those without insurance, transportation, or other resources.

Adults with diabetes are at greater risk for stroke because of the cardiovascular changes that occur with the progression of this disease. Adults with diabetes run twice the risk of stroke from atherothrombolytic brain injury (Goldberg & Berger, 1988). Elevated blood glucose levels over time also cause vessels to become stiff and less elastic, contributing to hypertension and thus increased stroke risk.

Stroke in younger adults may be more likely due to congenital malformations or cocaine abuse than to other risk factors. Although these risk factors are seen less often in the older population, the GRN should be aware that drug and alcohol abuse as well as physical anomalies can possibly be the source of stroke.

SECONDARY COMPLICATIONS OF STROKE

Physical complications from stroke abound. Physicians have commonly recognized several secondary complications that may occur after stroke: pneumonia, pulmonary embolism, cardiac problems, urinary tract infection, decubitus, contractures, and nutritional deficits.

For those who do survive the initial insult of stroke, death can occur later from respiratory or other complications. Twenty-nine percent of deaths are related to pneumonia, and 13% are from pulmonary embolism (Caplan, 1991). Stroke patients are at risk for nutritional deficits (Buelow & Jamieson, 1990) and thus the complications that arise from this. The hazards of immobility such as skin breakdown and contractures are not uncommon. Emotional swings may occur, and depression affects approximately half of stroke patients within the first 2 years (Caplan, 1991; Friedland & McColl, 1992). Table 10–1 summarizes common secondary complications of stroke.

Coronary artery disease (CAD) is often associated with stroke in the older patient. In one study, 46% of stroke patients in the sample had a history of CAD (Roth, Mueller, & Green, 1988). Congestive heart failure (CHF) has been found to adversely influence a person's overall functioning and mobility level

Table 10–1   SECONDARY COMPLICATIONS OF STROKE

Respiratory difficulties
  Pneumonia
  Pulmonary emboli
Cardiac problems
  Congestive heart failure
  Myocardial infarction
  Other cardiac diseases
Urinary tract infection
Decubitus
Contractures
Nutritional deficits
  Low protein (low albumin)
  Anemia
  Weight loss
Pain
  Related to shoulder subluxation
  Joint immobility
  Muscle atrophy
  Spasticity
Decreased range of motion
Edema
Swallowing disorders
Deep vein thrombosis
Affective disorders

related to task performance. Additionally, those survivors with both CAD and CHF had three times as many cardiac complications as those without.

Medical treatment is aimed at reducing complications associated with stroke and improving functional outcomes. Gerontological rehabilitation nursing also has these goals but emphasizes teaching of the patient, family, and caregiver in order to prepare them for a smooth transition to the home environment and to life with what may have resulted in chronic disability.

REHABILITATION AFTER STROKE

Stroke rehabilitation, and the setting in which it occurs, varies between regions in the same country, as well as between countries. Stages for assessment for post-stroke rehabilitation from the clinical practice guidelines of the U.S. Department of Health and Human Services appear in Figure 10–1. The needs, resources, and abilities of the patient will help determine the most appropriate setting for rehabilitation. Figure 10–2 provides a flow chart for directing persons toward appropriate services.

The focus of stroke rehabilitation includes mobility training, activities of daily living (ADLs), communication, nutrition, behavior, continence, social support, and sexual function (Dobkin, 1991; Estol & Caplan, 1990). Blood pressure management, respiratory care, cardiac care, and skin preservation are also important considerations. All of these are areas in which the GRN makes assessments, assists patients toward independence, and provides education to families and caregivers.

There is clinical research that supports the notion that rehabilitation leads to improved outcomes (Davidoff, Keren, Ring, & Solzi, 1991). Reding and McDowell (1989) demonstrated that participation in focused stroke rehabilitation programs resulted in improved mobility function and the ability to perform ADLs. Dobkin (1991) argued that generally those admitted with higher functional scores were discharged with higher scores. Advanced age, however, is a complicating factor in stroke rehabilitation. Adults 75 years of age or older who participated in inpatient rehabilitation were shown to have comparable cognitive function but poorer motor function than those younger than 75 (Falconer, Naughton, Strasser, & Sinacore, 1994). Older adults also generally have poorer motor function at discharge and may be more likely to be placed in a nursing home.

Controversial techniques used by some physicians to promote positive functional outcomes include prolonged restraint of the unaffected upper extremity in order to improve function in the affected limb. Taub et al. (1993) found that this approach was effective in restoring substantial motor function in stroke patients who had chronic motor impairments. These approaches violate much of traditional medical treatment and have serious implications for the emotional well-being of stroke survivors. Another source of controversy in medical treatment is the use of dantrolene sodium (Dantrium) to improve muscle tone and response. A study by Katrak, Cole, Poulos, and McCauley (1992) showed that 200 mg/day of Dantrium had no effect on tone or functional outcome for stroke patients, contrary to popular belief. The GRN should be aware that stroke care is constantly evolving, and new techniques to improve function are being explored. Knowledge of current medical strategies will assist the nurse in providing informed care to patients and families.

The benefit of formal rehabilitation after stroke has been the target of much criticism. Unfortunately, the number of statistically sound studies that use refined measurements

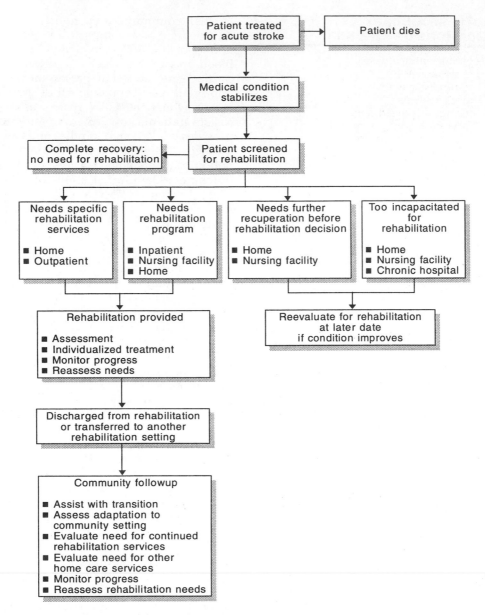

Figure 10–1 Stages of assessment for post-stroke rehabilitation. (From Gresham GE, Duncan PW, Stason WB, et al. (1995, May). *Post-stroke rehabilitation*. Clinical Practice Guideline, No. 16 (AHCPR Publication No. 95-0662). Rockville, MD: U.S. Department of Health and Human Services, Public Health Service, Agency for Health Care Policy and Research.)

to assess outcomes have been limited (Dobkin, 1991). However, the majority of research, as well as conventional wisdom, lends strong support to the need for activity and mobility after stroke. This fact is not in dispute. Yet, it is unclear whether positive outcomes are due to participation in a rehabilitation program or to other extraneous or intrinsic variables. Stroke recovery or adaptation seems to be a highly individual experience. Indeed, some

stroke survivors have suggested that physical therapy was a hindrance, stating, for instance, "I was able to get off the treadmill to despair, which was where physical therapy had been leading me" (Cohn, 1994, p. 18). Other stroke survivors have suggested that persons must find their own way to get well (Josephs, 1992; Veith, 1988). Other survivors feel that rehabilitation caused them to achieve much greater levels of independence. More nursing re-

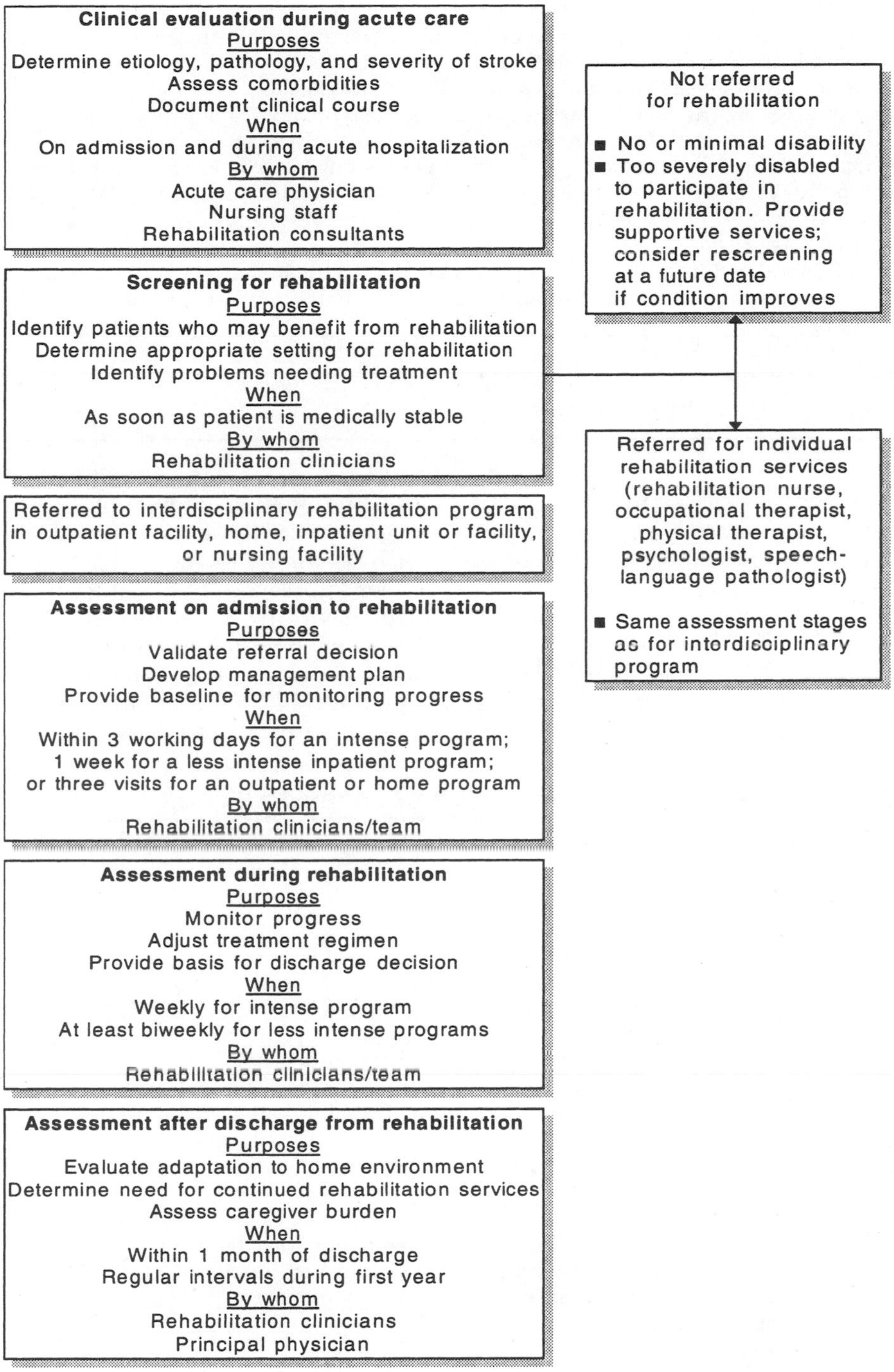

Clinical evaluation during acute care
Purposes
Determine etiology, pathology, and severity of stroke
Assess comorbidities
Document clinical course
When
On admission and during acute hospitalization
By whom
Acute care physician
Nursing staff
Rehabilitation consultants

**Not referred
for rehabilitation**

■ No or minimal disability
■ Too severely disabled
to participate in
rehabilitation. Provide
supportive services;
consider rescreening
at a future date
if condition improves

Screening for rehabilitation
Purposes
Identify patients who may benefit from rehabilitation
Determine appropriate setting for rehabilitation
Identify problems needing treatment
When
As soon as patient is medically stable
By whom
Rehabilitation clinicians

**Referred for individual
rehabilitation services**
(rehabilitation nurse,
occupational therapist,
physical therapist,
psychologist, speech-
language pathologist)

■ Same assessment stages
as for interdisciplinary
program

Referred to interdisciplinary rehabilitation program
in outpatient facility, home, inpatient unit or facility,
or nursing facility

Assessment on admission to rehabilitation
Purposes
Validate referral decision
Develop management plan
Provide baseline for monitoring progress
When
Within 3 working days for an intense program;
1 week for a less intense inpatient program;
or three visits for an outpatient or home program
By whom
Rehabilitation clinicians/team

Assessment during rehabilitation
Purposes
Monitor progress
Adjust treatment regimen
Provide basis for discharge decision
When
Weekly for intense program
At least biweekly for less intense programs
By whom
Rehabilitation clinicians/team

Assessment after discharge from rehabilitation
Purposes
Evaluate adaptation to home environment
Determine need for continued rehabilitation services
Assess caregiver burden
When
Within 1 month of discharge
Regular intervals during first year
By whom
Rehabilitation clinicians
Principal physician

Figure 10–2 Clinical flow diagram for stroke rehabilitation. (From Gresham GE, Duncan PW, Stason WB, et al. (1995, May). *Post-stroke rehabilitation*. Clinical Practice Guideline, No. 16 (AHCPR Publication No. 95-0662). Rockville, MD: U.S. Department of Health and Human Services, Public Health Service, Agency for Health Care Policy and Research.)

Table 10–2 GENERAL APPROACHES TO TRADITIONAL NURSING CARE OF THE STROKE PATIENT

- When working with the patient, encourage use of the affected side to reduce neglect.
- When the person is alone, place items (such as the call light, tissues, and other personal effects) on the unaffected side to promote self-care and safety and to avoid isolation.
- Use a variety of teaching modalities during educational sessions to promote learning.
- Minimize distractions during educational times. Keep sessions short and relevant.
- Use terms such as "affected/unaffected" side or "weak/strong" side instead of "good/bad."
- Use a critical pathway to promote consistency of care, but remember that each patient is unique, and adapt nursing care accordingly.
- Alternate rest and activity.
- Build endurance slowly. Remember, a stroke is exhausting to the patient.
- Include the person and the family in the plan of care.
- Assist the patient and family in setting reasonable goals.
- Make early referrals to stroke services.
- Connect the family with a stroke support group or club.
- Use a discharge follow-up plan.

search is needed to explore the process of post-stroke adaptation, so that nursing interventions can be planned more effectively to meet patient and family needs.

EFFECTS OF STROKE AND APPROACHES TO NURSING CARE

The principles discussed in Part II, Promoting Wellness and Self-Care, provide the basis for effective nursing interventions in care of the stroke patient. General approaches to care such as those in Table 10–2 are indicated. Other approaches to nursing should be modified according to each individual patient. Nursing diagnoses commonly associated with stroke are listed in Table 10–3. Moore stated it well: "Excellent nursing care is essential whenever caring for a stroke patient—to

Table 10–3 COMMON NURSING DIAGNOSES RELATED TO STROKE

Impaired physical mobility
Unilateral neglect
Impaired swallowing
Ineffective airway clearance
Impaired gas exchange
Alteration in tissue perfusion: cerebral
Alteration in tissue perfusion: peripheral
High risk for injury
Alteration in nutrition: less than body requirements
Altered sensory perception
Self-care deficits (related to toileting, dressing, eating, bathing)
Impaired communication
High risk for impaired skin integrity
Activity intolerance
Decreased endurance
Alteration in bowel elimination (constipation, diarrhea)
Alteration in urinary elimination (incontinence, retention)
Altered role performance
Spiritual distress
Hopelessness
Powerlessness
Pain
Self-esteem disturbance
Social isolation
Sleep pattern disturbance
Impaired home maintenance management
Discharge planning needs
Knowledge deficit
Fear/anxiety
Grieving

prevent potentially fatal complications, promptly detect problems, and intervene if they arise. Your role is crucial, too, in getting your patient started on the long road to rehabilitation and recovery" (1994, p. 50). The GRN goes beyond the acute care phase and assists the patient on the road to recovery. Understanding the common characteristics of patients with left or right hemisphere stroke is one of the keys to providing more specific, effective care (Hart, 1990; Williams, 1992). Table 10–4 summarizes important aspects of stroke care.

Controversy still remains about which treatment approach in nursing is better. Many rehabilitation units use the Bobath approach, which emphasizes the use of both sides of the body continuously, whereas others prefer traditional nursing. Lewis (1986) found that when the Bobath technique (or neurodevelopment treatment [NDT]) was used consistently by nurses, the patients (especially left hemiplegics) showed greater functional gains and had greater functional improvements than when traditional approaches were used. Conversely, Salter, Camp, Pierce, and Mion (1991) did not find the NDT approach to be superior to traditional nursing care. Thus the debate continues.

Regardless of the overall approach used to care, there are several areas that deserve special notice. Teaching in each of these areas is particularly essential in promoting optimum outcomes for the patient. Physical rehabilitative care of the stroke patient involves several important areas of nursing assessment and interventions. These include monitoring vital signs, nutritional status, bowel and bladder function, sensory perception, medications, behavior, skin integrity, physical and emotional changes, and activity and endurance levels; discharge planning; and providing patient and family teaching.

The effects seen with stroke depend on the location of insult within the brain and which nerve cells have been damaged or destroyed. Oxygen deprivation destroys brain cells that cannot repair themselves. Each stroke is different, and it has been said that each stroke has its own personality. However, certain deficits are common with stroke (Table 10–5), and the knowledge of these can help the GRN to plan effective nursing care. The stroke affects the entire family, not just the patient, so the nurse must be prepared to devote a substantial amount of time to focused teaching both for the stroke survivor and the caregiver.

Motor Deficits

Certain motor deficits are common as a result of stroke. When the damage occurs in one side of the brain, weakness or paralysis is seen on the opposite side of the body. So, a right CVA results in left hemiplegia or hemiparesis. *Hemiplegia* refers to a lack of functional movement, or paralysis, on one side of the body. *Hemiparesis* means weakness on one side. There is some degree of inconsistency of the use of this vocabulary. For instance, a physical therapist may consider the person to

Table 10–4   SPECIAL INDICATIONS IN CARE OF RIGHT AND LEFT HEMISPHERE STROKE SURVIVORS

Right Hemisphere Stroke
Foster a calm and unrushed environment.
Move slowly around the person.
Break tasks into simple steps.
Protect the patient from injury.
Be alert to deficits that may not be overt.

Left Hemisphere Stroke
Speak slowly and distinctly.
Use simple sentences.
Encourage all forms of communication.
Use a variety of communication techniques: gesturing, cues, pointing, writing, communications boards, yes/no questions (if appropriate). Find what is most effective for each person.
Allow time for the person to respond.
Provide teaching in a quiet, structured environment.
Monitor the patient for swallowing difficulties.
Promote a positive self-image by attention to good grooming, personal hygiene, and positive reinforcement.

Table 10–5 COMMON DEFICITS CAUSED BY STROKE

Common Characteristics Associated with Stroke of Either Side
Emotional lability
Some memory impairment
Depression
Weakness/paralysis
Sensory deprivation or alteration
Social isolation
Fatigue
Insomnia

Right Hemisphere Stroke
Left hemiparesis or hemiplegia
Left homonymous hemianopia
Difficulty with spatial-perceptual tasks
Difficulty with sequencing
Difficulty following multi-step directions
Difficulty writing
May not acknowledge or accept limitations
May overestimate abilities
Impulsive
Quick and often careless movements
Anosognosia or other forms of left-sided neglect
Socially indifferent
Sometimes euphoric, with inappropriately low anxiety
Higher risk for falls because of lack of safety awareness
Deficits less easily recognized by others
Memory deficits related to performance

Left Hemisphere Stroke
Right hemiparesis or hemiplegia
Right homonymous hemianopia
Aphasia (especially expressive)
Reading/writing problems
Dysarthria
Dysphagia
Anxious when trying new tasks
Tends to fret and worry
Slow, cautious behavior
Easily frustrated
Memory deficits related to language

have a hemiplegic arm if he or she is unable to lift it for functional use, whereas the nurse may call it hemiparesis if there is some shoulder movement, because he or she does not consider it paralysis.

Hemiplegia may be difficult for the family to understand. One particularly effective teaching strategy to assist the family and caregiver with sensing the effects of upper extremity paralysis is the use of a simulated "hemiplegic arm." This consists of a sleeve of material that is weighted with sand to the poundage of a flaccid arm. The family member can don this apparatus, which fits over the arm like a shirt sleeve and attaches to the body much like a sling. The person is then asked to walk around and perform other activities with the device on but not using that arm. This gives others a better feeling of what it is like for the patient after stroke to try to balance and attempt activities with what feels like "dead weight" pulling on the shoulder. Such types of exercises give family members and caregivers a more realistic and memorable sensation of what it is like to have hemiplegia, and they are more apt to remember and be sensitive to that deficit and support the affected limb at home (preventing possible shoulder subluxation or other injury).

A common "language" should also be agreed on between team members within each facility. Table 10–6 lists commonly ac-

Table 10–6 TERMS USED IN STROKE REHABILITATION

Ankle-foot orthosis (AFO): a short leg brace that fits inside the shoe to provide support for the lower extremity; helps prevent dragging of the foot during ambulation

Activities of daily living (ADLs): activities associated with everyday routines, including dressing, bathing, grooming, and other bodily self-care

Instrumental activities of daily living (IADLs): activities other than ADLs that include meal preparation, shopping, money management, housework, and using the telephone

Community reentry (CRE): reintegration of a person into social activities and functions within the community

Cerebrovascular accident (CVA): impairment of blood supply to the brain; stroke

Functional: use of skills for purposeful and meaningful activities in a reasonable time frame

Transient ischemic attack (TIA): acute symptoms of brain anoxia that are resolved within 24 hours, leaving no residual effects

Hemiplegia: functional loss of the use of half of the body

Hemiparesis: weakness in half of the body

Aphasia: difficulty in using or understanding language

Apraxia: difficulty using familiar objects appropriately, secondary to loss of memory of how to perform the activity rather than loss of motor function

Ataxia: uncoordination, or impaired balance, especially when ambulating

Perseveration: involuntary, inappropriate repetition of words or actions

Anomia: inability to recall names of people or items

Emotional lability: apparent emotional fluctuations, or highs and lows, resulting from a chemical imbalance in the brain after stroke; can result in crying jags that are unconnected to actual emotions

Dysphagia: trouble with eating or swallowing

Dysarthria: impairments in the muscles associated with speech

Homonymous hemianopia: visual loss in the nasal half of one eye and the temporal half of the other

Anosognosia: a severe form of neglect in which the person does not acknowledge a body part as their own

Proprioception: awareness of one's body parts in space

Field cut: loss of vision in a portion of the visual field

Cues: verbal, tactile, or gesturing communication used as prompts to direct or clue an individual in appropriately performing activities

Gait training: ambulatory training and strengthening of the lower extremities for the purpose of walking

Cognition: mental functions including orientation, judgment, memory, reasoning, and sensory perception

Flaccid: total lack of muscle tone; floppy; total paralysis

Range of motion (ROM): the range or degree of movement of a joint

Somatognosia: lack of awareness of body parts

Spasticity: an involuntary increase in muscle tone that can result in stiffness, spasms, or pain

cepted definitions for terms used in rehabilitation of stroke survivors. The GRN should take care to properly use and document these terms. The use of terms on the patient care plan or record (Kardex) such as "right hemi" or "left hemi" are confusing, because they do not make clear whether this refers to the stroke, weakness, or paralysis. Complete wording such as "right CVA with left hemiplegia" is much more clear. Dysarthria (dysfunction of muscles used in speech) and dysphagia (impaired swallowing mechanism) are also common with stroke. These are often associated with aphasia, or difficulty with the use of language.

Balance problems are common after stroke, often due to altered proprioception, hemiplegia, hemiparesis, or unilateral neglect. Ataxia, or uncoordinated movement, can also interfere with the person's ability to ambulate, eat, and perform other self-care tasks.

Sensory Deficits

Many sensory problems can result from stroke. Damage in the brain may cause visual deficits, tactile alterations, impaired proprioception, and several other perceptual deficits related to body schema. These are complicated by normal sensory changes that have occurred with advancing age, making rehabilitation more challenging. These difficulties are discussed briefly here.

Vision

Older adults frequently experience impaired vision as a normal part of aging, particularly with regard to lens accommodation and opacity. Cataracts can further diminish vision, but they are generally treatable through surgical interventions. The individual with stroke may have other visual problems that are complicated by pre-existing cataracts or untreated visual disturbances that occurred before the stroke. Physicians, nurses, and therapists who work with mature adults should be alert to the effects of aging on vision, as well as other common deficits caused by the stroke itself. *Homonomyous hemianopia* is one visual deficit associated with stroke. This refers to a loss of vision in half of the visual field on the same side. In other words, the person experiences loss of sight in the temporal half of one eye and the nasal half of the other.

The GRN may help the family or caregiver better understand the phenomenon of homonymous hemianopia, and the confusing effects it may have on the patient, through a simple educational exercise. A pair of glasses with tape covering the parts where vision is lost can be made to simulate what the patient sees. The GRN can guide family members wearing the glasses through a set of instructions, such as picking up a utensil and trying to feed themselves or transferring objects from one surface to another. This demonstration allows the family to see how much all of us rely on our sight to guide our activities. When vision is impaired, it can result in confusion and disorientation, leading to an impairment in the ability to function in usual daily roles. Actual participatory activities such as this often work better to facilitate the family's understanding of the patient's condition than just lecture or discussion, although these are certainly used in conjunction with physical participation.

Double vision, or *diplopia*, and decreased visual acuity are also common results of stroke. The GRN assesses for these conditions (see Chapter 9) by screening vision in the total visual field, testing acuity, peripheral vision, and accommodation. The nurse should note comments that might indicate visual deficits, such as, "I just don't read the paper anymore," or "I used to enjoy reading, but it hurts my eyes now." Other indications could include lipstick put on crookedly, shaving only parts of the face, or only half of the food on the plate being eaten because the other half was not seen. In any cases of visual disturbances, the GRN should teach the patient scanning techniques. Scanning involves turning the head slowly from side to side (and up and down) so that the entire normal field of vision is seen. This is a means of compensating for loss in portions of the visual field. The physician will generally refer the patient to a specialist if corrective lenses or other apparatus could be of assistance. However, these deficits are largely untreatable medically, so compensatory techniques should be emphasized.

Sensation and Perception

With advanced age, the ability to perceive light or superficial touch in the form of pressure, pain, or temperature changes is diminished. When stroke has occurred, the response to such tactile stimuli may also be absent or diminished. The combination of these deficits results in serious safety implications for the older adult.

The skin of an older person is more fragile and prone to breakdown. Thus, prolonged exposure to extremes in temperature can result in more extensive tissue damage than in the healthy younger person. Hemiparesis and hemiplegia resulting from stroke do not affect only motor function, but sensory perception as well. Individuals may not even perceive a body part as their own. The term *agnosia* indicates the inability to recognize or identify things in the environment by use of the senses. *Somatagnosia* and *anosognosia* are two types of perceptual disturbances that involve lack of awareness or neglect of body parts (see definitions in Table 10–6). Health care professionals can assist persons with these problems by helping them become more aware of the neglected part while promoting safety measures to protect them from harm.

The patient's awareness of his or her neglected body part can be enhanced by several measures. The nurse can demonstrate recognition of the person's neglected limbs by touching the affected arm or leg, using appropriate terms (not "bad" side) in describing it, and reminding the person to observe where the extremity is at all times. The patient should be encouraged to move and exercise the affected extremity using the stronger limbs as needed. Individuals can perform passive range of motion by themselves on immobile fingers and wrists. A weaker leg can be lifted with the stronger leg underneath it. All these strategies help increase a person's awareness that the affected body part is still important and is their responsibility to care for and protect.

Apraxia may also be a result of stroke. The GRN can recognize apraxia when a patient is unable to use familiar objects appropriately. For example, the nurse provides the patient with a washcloth for use in morning care and the person uses it to "brush" his or her hair. Or the patient is given a toothbrush and puts it under the arms as if applying deodorant. These examples of apraxia result from a loss of memory of how to use these objects or the inability to relearn, not from motor deficits or the inability to perform the tasks. The problem is thought to be an interruption in the connection between the site where motor acts are formed and the motor association areas responsible for the action. The GRN may need to give frequent cues and reminders during performance of ADLs. The occupational therapist and GRN can work together to determine which cues work best for each patient in assisting them to perform self-care.

Trouble discriminating left and right is also common with stroke. In these situations, the GRN must use other cue besides "left" or "right," such as pointing to or touching the affected extremity. This can be particularly problematic during transfers when trying to cue the patient to move. The GRN can try statements such as "pick up the leg that is next to me" as he or she assists during transfers if other cues are not effective.

Language Deficits

Difficulty in using or understanding language is common after stroke. Several conditions are possible, but major deficits are discussed briefly here. Language deficits may take the form of *expressive aphasia*, if there is damage to Broca's area of the brain. This results in trouble transforming sound into understandable speech. Affected individuals may understand what is being said to them but be unable to give a verbal response. This is extremely frustrating for both the patient and family. When speech does return, it may be broken, nonfluent. The patient may search for words or be unable to find the correct word. The nurse may need to supply the patient with the correct word and should encourage all verbalizations. Nursing implications for working with patients with aphasia is further discussed in Chapter 9.

Another condition is called *receptive aphasia*. This is when the person is able to speak with fluency, rhythm, and normal sounding speech but uses words incorrectly so that it is basically meaningless. The individual may not be aware of these errors and may have difficulty understanding what is said to them or interpreting the spoken word. This is also called Wernicke's aphasia.

Global aphasia is the most devastating deficit, because it involves a combination of expressive and receptive aphasia. The person is unable to communicate on any level, and the prognosis for recovery is poor. Alexia, the inability to understand the written word, and agraphia, the inability to express ideas in writing, are other language problems associated with stroke.

GRNs should be aware of which specific types of sensory/perceptual deficits the patient has in order to provide competent care. For instance, nursing treatment of the person with expressive aphasia may include having him or her write requests on paper, yet this would not be appropriate if the person had agraphia.

Psychosocial and Emotional Changes

Cognition

Intellectual deficits may also be a result of stroke. These include memory loss (usually in relation to performance or language), a shorter attention span, tendency toward distraction, poor judgment, inability to transfer learning from one situation to another, and the inability to calculate, reason, sequence, or engage in abstract thought processes. Team members work on an individual basis with stroke survivors who have these problems. The speech therapist will design an individualized program with structured therapy to help retrain these thought processes. The GRN should consult with the speech therapist to obtain feedback as to what techniques are being used so that care on the unit can be consistent. If no speech therapist is available, nurses can assist long-term care patients with these problems by engaging them in simple exercises that allow them to practice sequencing, reasoning, and making decisions in a calm, structured, controlled environment. The nurse should allow the person plenty of time to respond and be prepared to give cues as needed. Suggestions of games and activities that help promote these types of cognitive exercises are given in Appendix 10A under Discharge Planning.

Emotions

Emotional changes also occur with stroke. Mood swings are common. *Emotional lability* refers to the easy expression of emotions that may be inappropriate to the situation. Crying jags can be frequent if the person has emotional lability. Generally, it is best to ignore the crying or provide distraction if it has been determined that the emotional outburst is unrelated to the person's true feelings.

Stroke survivors also experience feelings of powerlessness, loss of control, and helplessness. They may have a reduced tolerance to stressful situations and have to develop new coping skills. Other extreme emotions are common, such as fear, hostility, anger, frustration, withdrawal, and depression. Persons may feel isolated and express feelings of despair and loneliness. Body-image disturbances may occur if paralysis is present or the individual has adaptive equipment or uses a wheelchair or walker. The reaction of others can largely influence a stroke survivor's perception of self.

GRNs can assist persons feeling powerless to identify power resources in their life. Power components or sources suggested by Orem (1995) and Miller (1992) are sometimes factors that the patient cannot change at the time, such as educational level. However, the nurse can assist the person to enhance those power sources that do exist, such as the ability to make decisions about care of self, the ability to acquire knowledge, and the ability to order self-care actions. These are certainly incorporated into rehabilitative nursing care. According to Orem's theory (1995), these types of power components promote self-care agency, or the capacity for self-care, a major goal of gerontological rehabilitation nursing.

Miller (1992) listed seven power sources: physical strength and reserve, psychological stamina and social support, positive self-concept (self-esteem), energy, knowledge, motivation, and belief system (hope). According to her developing concept of powerlessness, nurses can help patients combat this feeling by assisting them in recognizing, maximizing, and utilizing their resources. The GRN can do this with almost all of the power sources identified by Miller.

Physical strength and reserve is built up by therapy and endurance training. The entire rehabilitation program contributes to this. Psychological stamina and social support are often linked. The GRN can assist persons with this by providing relevant, informative teaching about what the patient and family needs to know. (Examples appear in Table 10–8 and Appendix 10A.) Social support systems such as family, caregivers, friends, and spiritual leaders should become part of the rehabilitation nursing care plan. A positive self-concept can be enhanced through attention to good grooming, personal hygiene, and promotion of decision-making, as well as opening the door for questions about sexuality after stroke. Energy levels should increase with therapeutic activities and endurance building. Motivation and belief systems are more intrinsic and influenced by a variety of factors, most of which are beyond the GRN's control. However, helping the patient and family to set and meet realistic goals is one way to promote motivation. Many stroke survivors have one or two special events that they have been looking forward to (such as a wedding anniversary or birth of a grandchild), and this can provide motivation for recovery. The nurse can use these events to structure therapeutic activities. For example, helping the patient learn to hold a weighted doll in practice for holding the new baby in the family provides practical experience and opportunities for conversation. Belief systems will have been formed long before the onset of stroke, but hope is a recurring coping mechanism used by most stroke survivors (Bronstein, 1991). Although the need to be realistic is always present in post-stroke rehabilitation nursing, the GRN must always foster hope, for it is this quality that often allows the person to achieve outcomes far beyond what traditional predictions would suggest.

Roles Changes

Changes or strain within a person's roles almost always occur after stroke. The husband who was the breadwinner now trades places with the wife, who must get a job to meet the medical expenses incurred. The wife who was the caregiver of the family must now be cared for. Adult children are caring for aging, disabled parents. These are adjustments that are not always easy for families to make. Some patients may be unable to accept their new self-image and role changes and therefore withdraw or choose not to perform self-care. By assisting the patient and family in examining their respective roles prior to the stroke and discussing changes that will be made, the GRN can open up areas for exchange between staff and families. GRNs should remember that although the goal of all rehabilitation is to promote the patient's maximum self-care, total self-care is often not possible or realistic. Thus, nurses and caregivers must be flexible and help the entire family to find the best way for them to adapt and cope with the changes brought on by stroke.

Nurses need to promote a positive self-image by encouraging the person to pay attention to personal hygiene and good grooming. Many fears can be allayed by education of the patient and family about what to expect after stroke. Depression is such a common problem after stroke that some units require all patients admitted with this diagnosis to have a consultation with the unit psychologist. Some family members may feel as though their loved one has died and a stranger has taken his or her place. GRNs need to be able to assist families in working through the grieving process. This is best done through consistent teaching from a knowledgeable nursing professional.

Depression

Because depression is such a common occurrence after stroke, particular attention should be paid to the prevention or assessment of it. Depression also occurs more frequently in the older population, so it is not surprising that stroke survivors should experience it. Friedland and McColl (1992) stated that an increase in depressive symptoms could occur between 4 and 6 months after stroke. This is about the time most patients have severed the final ties with any outpatient therapy or home care services. The incidence of depression may peak between 7 months and 1 year after stroke and then decline after 1 year. Easton, Rawl, Zemen, Kwiatkowski, & Burczyk (1995) believed that the 4-month period is crucial in stroke recovery, because this seemed to be when patients and families felt they were totally on their own. This time period may be shortened in today's new health care system, where patients may receive less follow-up care.

Almost half of stroke patients experience depression within the first 2 years after onset (Caplan, 1991). Depression can cause a significant decrease in social activities (Bronstein, 1991). The depressed stroke survivor also has a negative view that affects the entire perception of self, his or her surroundings, and his or her future (Hibbard, Grober, Gordon, Aletta, & Freeman, 1990). This can certainly inhibit progress toward self-care. There has been some speculation that persons with left brain damage experience depression more frequently than those with right brain injury, but Gordon et al. (1991) found no significant relationship between the side of brain injury and depression. Their study did confirm well-documented research that post-stroke depression was common among all stroke patients (but it was independent of side).

Depression within long-term care residents is also common, but it is often left undiagnosed. Clinical depression can result from chemical imbalances in stroke and is treatable with medication. However, some medications may take weeks to achieve a therapeutic level in the body, making them seem ineffective. Also, side effects and drug interactions from such medications must be carefully considered. A diagnosis of clinical depression should not be made or taken lightly. It must be distinguished between situational depression, which is also common after stroke or institutionalization, as one grieves losses. A holistic approach must be taken to the person's environment and socioeconomic resources before they are labeled with clinical depression.

Insomnia

Sleep disorders are not rare among the healthy aged, so it is not surprising that insomnia would be a complaint after stroke. Older adults get less quality sleep than younger persons, and results of stroke may increase the inability to sleep. Factors such as uncomfortable positioning, pain, muscle spasticity or cramps, and skin irritations can affect sleep.

All other interventions should be initiated before giving medications for sleep. These include promoting a calm and quiet environment for rest, providing a bedtime snack if desired, backrubs, music, or reading material. The patient's nighttime habits before sleep (even before illness) should be examined and used when possible. Patients should be educated that a bed is for sleeping, so if they are unable to sleep, they should get out of bed, try some other activity, then go back to bed. Keeping a diary of sleep-wake patterns may help determine problem areas. The effects of therapy, visitors, and the environment should be considered. If these efforts fail, medications should be given judiciously and not too much past midnight, because sleeping pills given during the night often cause the older person to be lethargic until noon the next day. Such effects preclude involvement in therapy and alter normal wake-sleep cycles, causing even further disruption in sleep patterns.

Care should be taken when administering sleeping aids to older adults. Medications are absorbed more slowly but stay in the body longer with advanced age. This can lead to altered performance of sleeping medications for these patients. Triazolam (Halcion), 0.125 mg p.o. at bedtime, was formerly prescribed by physicians for this problem. It was thought to have fewer "hangover" effects the next day for those who are participating in therapy. However, this medication can give a euphoric feeling to patients, something that can aggravate the problems seen, especially with right-sided stroke patients. It is infrequently prescribed now because of adverse affects. Diphenhydramine (Benadryl) 25 mg p.o. at bedtime is used in some long-term care facilities to promote sleep; it seems to work well for many patients, with few side effects. This avoids the sleepy effects seen the next morning with some other medications.

Coping, Social Support, and Adaptation for Patients and Families

The psychosocial and educational arenas are the areas in post-stroke care where documentation for nursing has made the most impact. Easton et al. (1995) found that rehabilitation patients who received follow-up from a rehabilitation nurse used more positive coping strategies that those who did not. Maintaining control is a recurring coping strategy among these patients.

Nursing research in the area of the post-stroke rehabilitation process is scarce. Stress and coping models, as well as others developed from psychological and sociological theories, are most often used as frameworks for research in this area. Alterations in behaviors and socialization after stroke (Farzan, 1991; Friedland & McColl, 1992), depression (Hibbard et al., 1990), and coping strategies (Easton et al., 1995) are areas in which theories from other disciplines have guided research. Some of these cases resulted in the development of practice models. For example, Roy's adaptation model has been used to frame results of the spouse's positive effect on the stroke patient's recovery (Baker, 1993). Corbin and Strauss developed nursing strategies related to management of chronic illness. However, their "chronic illness trajectory" is more a framework than a theory, because the relationships between concepts are not well defined (Woog, 1992). Nursing's focus is often on acute care, and because stroke recovery is a long-term, variable process, the expense and physical constraints of research in this area may have prohibited further studies and theory development.

The mechanism and process of recovery or adaptation after stroke is poorly understood. Little research has been done with stroke survivors themselves. One of the few qualitative studies in post-stroke rehabilitation nursing was done by Folden (1994), using a grounded theory approach to describe how stroke survivors managed multiple functional deficits produced by stroke. The process was labeled as "ensuring forward progress" (1994, p. 81). Her results indicated that each person defined recovery "as the accomplishment of personal goals" (1994, p. 81). In another study, Folden (1993) used Orem's theory of nursing systems and the self-care deficit theory of nursing to test the effect of a supportive-educative nursing intervention on older adults' perceptions of self-care after stroke. Results of this research helped confirm Orem's belief that these types of nursing interventions can increase a person's self-care ability.

Representative writings of stroke survivors have suggested that there may be a process unique to stroke recovery and rehabilitation. Some authors have intimated that each person finds his or her own way to adjust, and that this is a journey that each goes through individually (Josephs, 1992; Moss, 1972). Yet individuals with stroke seem to share a common bond and experience similar emotions. One stroke survivor listed challenges he faced: aphasia, feeding himself, toileting and incontinence, traveling, emotional swings, changes in jobs and roles, working in the kitchen, and dealing with plateaus in recovery. These are also areas in which the GRN can educate patients and families, link them with community resources, and prepare them for the home environment by good discharge planning and follow-up. Future nursing research needs to be done to explore the journey that persons undertake after stroke in order to adjust to life with the changes that ensue and how nurses can best assist patients with this process.

Caregivers of stroke patients have received attention in the literature as well (McLean, Roper-Hall, Mayer, & Main, 1991; Rosenthal, Pituch, Greninger, & Metress, 1993; Watson, 1986). They can have either a positive or negative influence on the adaptation of the stroke survivor. Baker (1993) found that the average Barthel Index score was significantly higher for stroke survivors who had a spouse. This supports the popular theory that social support acts as a buffer against stress. Ragsdale, Yarbrough, and Lasher (1993) suggested that nurses who support the family relationship (according to social support theory) will help stroke patients "heal" more successfully. However, there is conflicting evidence about this idea also. Friedland and McColl's (1992) findings did not support the theory that social support interventions would affect psychosocial outcomes related to depression. However, the intervention was not given during the "crisis period," and this may have affected the results.

Caregivers can also have a negative impact on stroke recovery. Evans, Bishop, and Haselkorn (1991) found that caregiver-related problems had a negative effect on rehabilitation outcomes. Their findings indicated that those persons at risk for less than optimal care at home had caregivers who shared four major factors: were more likely to be depressed, less likely to be married to the patient, had a less than average knowledge of stroke care, and had higher family dysfunction. These factors have tremendous implications for the practice of rehabilitation nursing of the stroke patient. Nursing treatment should focus on increasing the family's and caregiver's knowledge about stroke and caring for the person with stroke and strategies to reduce depression and dysfunction.

Bowel and Bladder Dysfunction

Alterations of various kinds may be present after stroke with regard to bowel and bladder function. The most common problems are constipation and urinary incontinence. Uninhibited neurogenic bowel and bladder are the most frequent classification.

Although diarrhea and bowel incontinence may occur after stroke (31% of patients), this is usually easily managed before discharge, and control often returns naturally during the hospital stay (Lorish, Sandin, Roth, & Noll, 1994). Constipation, however, is a more persistent problem and is linked to the normal aging process, in which this is also common. Inactivity, change in diet and fluid intake, swallowing problems, and other factors found in long-term care add to the stresses on the gastrointestinal system that occur after stroke (Munchiando & Kendall, 1993). Constipation is as much or more a result of the secondary effects of stroke than of the brain damage itself. Thus, managing factors such as those discussed in Chapter 8 is the best way to combat constipation.

Lorish et al. (1994) stated that urinary incontinence among stroke survivors is highest (50%–70%) during the first month after stroke and decreases over time. Sandin and Mason (1996) suggested that although not all stroke survivors achieve bladder continence, the incidence of incontinence at 3 months after stroke is about 14%, close to that of the general elderly population. Gross (1990) cited the most common voiding problems after stroke: urgency, frequency, incontinence, and urinary retention. Owen, Getz, and Bulla (1995) found that some stroke patients remained incontinent even after bladder management programs in rehabilitation. Those who did not achieve continence after stroke were more likely to have cognitive deficits, especially difficulty with orientation to time, memory, and problem solving. However, even those with cognitive alterations and dementia have shown improvements in bladder continence with training.

Urinary incontinence after stroke is a serious problem that can cause the person to be admitted to a nursing home or other long-term care facility instead of being discharged home. It is, therefore, an important consideration for GRNs in planning nursing care. Most stroke patients have an indwelling Foley catheter to the bladder during the acute hospital stay. This is removed based on several criteria, including the patient's functional status, the family's wishes, the person's urological status, and the ability to participate in bladder training. Nurses in rehabilitation generally prefer the catheter to be removed as early as possible in the program so that bladder retraining can begin. Contrary to some previously held beliefs, Sandin and Mason stated that "alternate periods of clamping and draining an indwelling catheter does not train a post-stroke bladder and has no role in stroke rehabilitation" (1996, p. 30). This was supported by nursing research and clinical practice guidelines for post-stroke rehabilitation (Gresham et al., 1995; Gross, 1990). The best time to remove the catheter is early in the morning, so that if the patient experiences difficult voiding, the physician can be notified during daytime hours and orders received so that appropriate interventions are carried out in a timely manner. This also allows the staff to begin a bladder retraining program during the day and does not interfere with the person's needed rest at night. A minimum of 1500 ml of fluid per day should be encouraged. Although increasing fluids is known to decrease the incidence of urinary tract infections, expecting an intake of more than 2000 ml/day for an older adult may be unrealistic and cause fluid overload in some patients.

Behavior modification is the nursing treatment of choice in bladder retraining. Techniques such as scheduled, timed, or prompted voiding should be used. Biofeedback and Kegel exercises are also helpful with many patients. These treatments are discussed at length in Chapter 8. Scheduled voiding is often the most effective method, although the specific approach selected is based on a thorough assessment. With scheduled voiding, the person is initially assisted with toileting every 2 hours regardless of the urge to void. This should help prevent incontinent episodes. The amount of time between voidings is eventually slowly lengthened by half-hour increments to 4 hours if no incontinence has occurred. Any medical or complicating factors (such as fecal impaction or urinary tract infection) that could contribute to the patient's incontinence should be addressed.

Some stroke survivors experience urinary retention. In addition to behavior modification, intermittent catheterization may be necessary. The goals of bladder management are to have complete emptying, prevent urinary tract infection, and choose a method that fits the patient's lifestyle and resources. The GRN may need to provide instructions on intermittent catheterization to the family, caregiver, or patient.

Medications may be needed to help with bladder dysfunction after stroke. Some commonly used medications for bladder management after stroke are listed in Table 10–7. The GRN should be familiar with the purpose and effect of these medications so appropriate treatment can be identified for the patient's particular problems. Several of these medications, such as diazepam, dantrolene sodium, and baclofen, are mainly used for treatment of other problems related to muscle spasticity

and should not be used for long-term management of bladder problems. Such pharmaceutical interventions are used only when other treatments are unsuccessful and should be given with caution to older adults because of potential side effects on the cardiac, respiratory, and hepatic systems. However, they are prescribed by some rehabilitation physicians for temporary assistance with bladder management with success.

Seizures

Seizures occur in between 4% and 15% of stroke survivors (Asconape & Penry, 1991). Approximately half of these seizures occur within 24 hours of the stroke (Sandin & Mason, 1996). A seizure is an abnormal electrical firing of neurons in the brain that can result in an alteration in consciousness, abnormal body movements, and inappropriate behavior. Early seizure activity can occur within 2 weeks and may be isolated, without recurrence. Rehabilitation professionals may be the first to witness a person's seizure, because it may be more likely to occur with increased stress and fatigue (Sandin & Mason, 1996). In some patients, stroke can cause chronic epilepsy. This is more common with lobar hematoma and subarachnoid hemorrhage (Asconape & Penry, 1991).

There are three basic types of seizures: partial, generalized, and status epilepticus. The GRN should recognize the signs of each type of seizure so that accurate reports may be

Table 10–7 MEDICATIONS COMMONLY USED FOR BLADDER DYSFUNCTION AFTER STROKE

Medication	Effect/Use
Propantheline bromide (Pro-Banthine)	Suppresses detrusor hyperactivity
Oxybutynin (Ditropan)	Relaxes smooth muscle (detrusor and internal sphincter); used when frequent bladder contractions or spasms are present; helps control urge incontinence
Imipramine (Tofranil)	Increases internal sphincter tone; decreases bladder contractility; used to help control incontinence
Bethanechol (Urecholine)	Increases bladder muscle tone and efficiency of bladder contractions; used when emptying is incomplete (such as with atonic bladder)
Terazosin (Hytrin)	Decreases bladder tone; used in outlet obstruction or dysfunction of external sphincter
Dantrolene sodium (Dantrium)	Relaxes smooth muscle; antispasmodic; used for detrusor sphincter dyssynergia (DSD)
Diazepam (Valium) Baclofen (Lioresal)	Decreases spasticity of skeletal muscles such as external sphincter, used for DSD

documented to ensure proper medical and nursing care.

Partial seizures are the most common and usually result from a specific focal point or scar on the cortex. Two subcategories of partial seizures are noted: simple and complex. Those persons with simple seizures may exhibit stiffening, jerking movements, and tingling, but without loss of consciousness. Those with complex activity demonstrate lip smacking, decreased memory afterward, and fumbling.

Generalized seizures involve both sides of the brain and are also referred to as tonic, clonic, tonic-clonic (grand mal), or petit mal (Sandin & Mason, 1996). There is a loss of consciousness, stiffness, and jerking. The jaw is clamped and respirations can cease. These symptoms may last for 1 to 2 minutes.

The most severe and serious type of seizure is status epilepticus, but this is less common after stroke than generalized and partial types. This is seizure activity that lasts for 30 minutes or more and is life-threatening. It constitutes a medical emergency and requires immediate treatment with intravenous medications (such as diazepam [Valium] to relax and phenytoin [Dilantin] to combat the seizures), suctioning, and oxygen therapy.

Strokes are the most common cause of epilepsy in the elderly. The usual diagnostic test for seizure activity is an electroencephalogram (EEG). This may be fatiguing for the older patient, because the preparation for the test requires sleep deprivation. The test itself involves exposure to a variety of environmental stimuli such as light and other manipulations in order to detect any abnormal brain patterns. The EEG procedure lasts about 45 minutes and involves placement of electrodes on the scalp surface to monitor brain activity. However, an EEG is not always helpful in detecting abnormal brain wave patterns in the stroke survivor because epileptiform activity is often low in these patients (Asconape & Penry, 1991). Neurological testing and careful observation of the patient are also indicated. Magnetic resonance imaging (MRI) or computed tomography (CT) scans also help visualize areas of damage in the brain from stroke. The CT scan is used to differentiate hemorrhagic from ischemic stroke (Moore & Trifiletti, 1994), but MRI will reveal evidence of an ischemic stroke sooner than CT.

Medical treatment for seizure after stroke varies by physician and institution. Early isolated seizures may not be treated with prolonged medication regimens unless they occur later than 2 weeks after stroke. Some physicians prescribe antiseizure medication for stroke patients even if no seizure activity is present, but this is controversial and is not recommended in current clinical practice guidelines (Gresham et al., 1995). Seizures can be controlled in the vast majority of cases with medications such as phenytoin (Dilantin), phenobarbital, or carbamazepine (Tegretol). Surgical advances have made it possible for physicians to map areas of the brain that fire abnormally to cause seizures and then surgically alter the brain to prevent this.

Nursing care for the person with seizures includes padding the side rails, monitoring for any evidence of seizure activity, and checking laboratory values (such as phenytoin [Dilantin] level) to monitor for therapeutic range or toxicity. If the nurse witnesses seizure activity, it is important to describe it carefully to the physician and also to note what activity precipitated it and whether or not the patient had an aura (an unnatural feeling or sensation occurring prior to the seizure). In addition to giving the appropriate medications as ordered, the GRN may need to teach the patient and family about seizure disorders in stroke and the importance of medications in preventing further incidents. Reviewing what should be done if the person experiences a seizure at home will also help to allay fears because a plan has been made.

Circulatory and Respiratory Care

Although many stroke patients do not present with immediate respiratory complications, this is an area of primary concern for the GRN. A person's PaO_2 level (amount of oxygen that lungs deliver to the blood) often decreases with age, and hemiplegic persons have additional problems. Respiratory drive and intercostal muscle function are adversely affected by paralysis after stroke. Brott (1991) recommends 2 to 4 L/min per nasal cannula be used, particularly during activities, stating that physicians have used this regimen for a number of years in his rehabilitation facility without adverse risks for the patient. Mobile oxygen tanks are available on many units and have become increasingly light weight and portable, facilitating the use of supplemental oxygen for older stroke patients.

Pneumonia and pulmonary embolism are common complications that can lead to death after stroke. Careful assessment of the lung fields should be done on each shift to detect any early changes. Turning, coughing, and deep breathing, in addition to increased physical activity in therapies and on the unit, help ventilate the lungs and reduce respiratory hazards from immobility. This is particularly essential for the older adult whose vital capacity and useful oxygen is decreased.

Many of the complications of pneumonia are due to aspiration and bacteria (Brott, 1991). Aspiration can largely be prevented by careful assessment of swallowing abilities. A speech therapy consult should be initiated when there is any doubt. For those GRNs working in nursing homes where this is not feasible, aspiration pneumonia is a particular hazard, especially in the frail elderly. Even though a patient admitted to a long-term care facility with a diagnosis of stroke does not evidence any swallowing problems on admission, a lack of activity and common changes associated with increased age can cause this to occur at a later time. Chapter 5 provides suggestions for improving swallowing function.

Approximately 40% of stroke patients are silent aspirators (Caplan, 1991). This means they may present no symptoms such as choking or coughing although material goes into the lungs. A particular challenge is the person with a nasogastric feeding tube, which is both a source of bacteria and a contributor to aspiration. Correct placement should be confirmed before anything is put down the tube. If a person's swallowing function has not improved significantly within 3 to 4 weeks after stroke, a gastrostomy tube should be considered. With any person receiving tube feeding, even via a G-tube, the head of the bed should be kept elevated, because aspiration can still occur. Case Study 10.1 gives an example of what can happen if this is not maintained.

CASE STUDY 10.1

Mr. Jamison was a 70 year old man who was admitted to an inpatient rehabilitation unit with a diagnosis of left stroke with right hemiplegia, aphasia, and dysphagia. Because of several post-stroke complications, his length of stay was longer than usual. He also had intermittent periods of confusion. When his swallowing ability had not improved after 3 weeks of intensive speech therapy, a G-tube was placed to ensure proper nutrition and hydration and to prevent aspiration. During the night, while his tube feeding was running, Mr. Jamison became disoriented and used the bed controls inappropriately, placing himself in the Trendelenburg position, with the head of the bed lower than the feet. He suffered aspiration and subsequent pneumonia as a result of this incident. Although he eventually made significant progress in all areas of the rehabilitation, the complications nearly resulted in death and meant a much longer stay in the hospital as well as tremendous stress on the patient and family.

Many physicians prescribe prophylactic heparin (often 5000 units every 12 hours subcutaneously) to prevent complications due to clots such as pulmonary embolism. Low-molecular-weight heparin derivatives (such as Lovenox) have become increasingly popular for several reasons, including that less monitoring is needed and they come in premeasured dosages. The GRN should remember that anticoagulant therapy is indicated only in the case of stroke from thrombus or embolus, but obviously not in hemorrhagic stroke. Laboratory results should be monitored; physicians often prefer to keep the prothrombin time within higher than normal levels to prevent clotting. Thus, the patient should be cautioned against the use of razors, use extra padding in the wheelchair to prevent bruising, and take particular care when using adaptive equipment. The nurse should teach the person and family the signs of bleeding, such as bruising, tarry stools, bleeding gums, headache, coffee-ground emesis, and the like.

In addition to respiratory care, monitoring cardiac and circulatory status is also important. The apical and other pulses should be carefully assessed each shift. To detect a carotid block, the stethoscope is placed over the carotid artery, and it is evaluated for the sound of a bruit (a swishing or whooshing sound). This will be heard when the internal diameter of the artery has decreased to 3 mm or less. Narrowing to smaller than 1 mm is critical and usually indicates the need for surgery (Kistler, 1989). Transient ischemic attacks (TIAs) are another indication of impaired carotid circulation. Doppler studies can also provide information. Evaluation by cerebral angiography is risky in the older patient, because this can cause an embolus or tear the artery; and carotid endarterectomy is also controversial, because it may result in serious complications.

Cardiac deaths account for 10% of 20% mortality from stroke (Brott, 1991). Circulatory status is medically evaluated through many different tests, including CT scan, MRI, lumbar puncture, cerebral arteriogram, and Doppler studies, which provide information about the cause of stroke. The GRN should be alert to results of these diagnostic tests. Treatment for blood clots typically includes warfarin and aspirin (the latter primarily for maintenance), depending on the severity. Even mild hypertension should be treated, and the person should be taught about the importance of keeping the blood pressure under control.

Teaching with regard to hypertension and blood pressure monitoring is a frequent need in post-stroke care. Some older adults may think that if they check their blood pressure at home and it is 120/80 mmHg that they no longer have a problem. The connection between the effects of the antihypertensive medication and the blood pressure reading is not always made. A teaching tool such as the one in Figure 10–3 can be used to promote continuity of care among nursing staff in teaching skills such as taking a blood pressure to family members. Before the development of this guide, techniques for teaching and taking blood pressures on one rehabilitation unit varied somewhat and were confusing to patients. A tool such as this can be developed according to specific needs of each facility and unit for each skill that is frequently taught. Once such an instrument has been developed (a task for the advanced practice nurse [APN] or more experienced nurse if no APN is available), nursing staff is given inservice training on its use so consistency and continuity are ensured. The spaces provided on the tool let staff know that demonstration and repeated return demonstrations are expected. The person learning the skill also receives a copy for reference. The nurse can take the step-by-step instructions to the bedside for use in teaching. Family members feel more confident with repeated opportunities for supervised instruction. This also provides a means of more thorough and concise documentation that communicates problems in teaching or learning with other staff members.

Activity

The benefit of early mobility cannot be overemphasized in nursing care of the stroke patient. Passive joint range of motion should begin in acute care as soon as possible, with physical and occupational therapy being initiated even before admission to a formal rehabilitation program. This helps prevent contractures and decreased joint mobility, which can quickly occur without active movement. Based on results of studies such as the Copenhagen Stroke Study (Nakayama, Jorgensen, Raaschou, & Olsen, 1994), one would conclude that rehabilitation is most crucial during the first 3 months after stroke, during which time most significant gains are made. Thus, nurses who work in long-term care, whose patients may not have had the opportunity for intensive rehabilitation, will need to bear more responsibility for the person's functional activity.

The amount of therapy received by a resident in a large long-term care facility will not be adequate to ensure optimum outcomes if not supported by nursing personnel throughout the rest of that resident's care. Proper transfer techniques that promote self-care and cuing the person to perform appropriate movements (see Chapter 7) should be reviewed.

Activities that are meaningful and purposeful to the individual's performance of ADLs and instrumental activities of daily living (IADLs), as well as hobbies and personal goals, should be emphasized. The principles of adult learning support the idea that such activities will be undertaken with greater interest and motivation by the person if they are congruent with his or her own goals. The ability to ambulate independently is almost always a primary desire of stroke survivors. Any therapeutic recreation or exercises that promote this ability should be pointed out to the patient in relation to his or her objectives.

Activity intolerance is common in the geriatric stroke patient (Mol & Baker, 1991). Dyspnea, weakness, and changes in vital signs can signal activity intolerance. Of particular note in a study by Mol and Baker (1991) is that activity intolerance occurred in about half of their sample. These authors suggested that low-risk rehabilitation exercise programs need to be developed for stroke patients to avoid the risk of another stroke and meet the goal of increased activity.

Pain may be a hindrance to movement and mobility. Some pain will likely be present when a new exercise program or therapy has begun. Other sources of pain may be edema in the affected extremities, shoulder subluxation, or skin breakdown. Measures of prevention should be taken early to prevent these

The patient or significant other _____ will:

	Date Initiated	Reviewed	Completed
1. Receive written and verbal instruction on taking blood pressure. _____ _____ _____			
2. Apply BP cuff with arrow over brachial artery.			
3. Make sure BP cuff is snugly applied to upper arm, sleeve up, arm straight, palm up (will use arm recommended by nursing staff in the event of contraindications of the use of one arm).			
4. Apply bell of stethoscope to area of brachial artery.			
5. Put earpieces of stethoscope into ears.			
6. Tighten pressure control valve on rubber hand bulb.			
7. Inflate cuff to _____ mmHg.			
8. Slowly release cuff pressure by loosening pressure control valve.			
9. Accurately read systolic* and diastolic* BP (to be checked by nurse with double stethoscope).			
10. Completely release air in cuff.			
11. Remove stethoscope and BP cuff.			
12. Purchase appropriate BP equipment as suggested by nursing staff (see below).			

COMMENTS: _____

_____

_____

NOTE: It is the procedure of this Unit to encourage the use a manual BP cuff (versus digital) unless the patient/significant other who is taking the BP has a hearing problem, arthritis, or any other difficulty which would prevent accurate use of such a cuff. A good manual brand to recommend is by Marshall, found at Osco Drugs or Walgreens, cost approximately _____. Digital cuffs have been found to be unreliable in some cases and should be checked against a Unit machine for accuracy and reliability prior to use.

DEFINITIONS: *Systolic—mmHg at which pulsing sound is initially heard.
*Diastolic—mmHg at which pulsing sound disappears (versus muffled).

Revised 9/90

Figure 10–3 Easton/Zemen (E/Z) blood pressure teaching tool. (Used with permission of Kris Easton and Donna Zemen.)

occurrences. A stretch glove (such as Iso-toner) may be worn to promote venous return in a hemiplegic hand. An arm trough can keep the affected hand elevated when sitting up. Elastic hose help promote venous return but must be applied before the person rises in the morning to be effective in decreasing edema. Elevation of the lower limbs in the wheelchair is not generally very effective, but sequential compression devices in combination with thromboembolitic deterrent stockings have been shown to help decrease the likelihood of deep vein thrombosis and edema.

GRNs need to schedule pain medications to be given at least 30 minutes before therapeutic activities when needed. Waiting until pain has reached a moderate to severe level is unwise and results in less participation in activities as a result of discomfort of the patient.

Nutrition

Stroke patients are at particular risk of altered nutrition. Nutritional needs may increase, yet "the patient's status demands nutritional intake that the patient's disabilities prohibit" (Buelow & Jamieson, 1990, p. 260). Older adults also commonly experience iron deficiency anemia, and this is complicated when a stroke affects the ability to eat or swallow. Serum albumin level is an accurate predictor of general nutritional health and may help predict overall stroke outcomes. The close link between nutritional status and morbidity and mortality is discussed in Chapter 5. Nursing interventions appropriate to the stroke patient are also discussed in that chapter.

For the person who is able to swallow safely, foods should be made available that stimulate the appetite. The GRN can work with the dietitian to offer choices to patients with limited options secondary to restrictions. Those persons on diabetic or renal diets have fewer selections from which to choose, and adhering to the prescribed diet may be challenging. A greater challenge, however, is assisting the older person who can drink only thickened liquids to achieve a daily intake of 1500 ml. The GRN must make a concerted effort to plan specific amounts of liquid throughout the day to meet this goal.

Many stroke survivors experience dysphagia and require the use of a feeding tube. The GRN needs to calculate the necessary water per day and disperse this throughout the tube feeding schedule to ensure adequate hydra-tion. It should be remembered that although many tube feedings are high in fiber, there must be adequate water intake as well for this to be effective in preventing constipation. The amount of water used to flush the tube between feedings and medications is not usually adequate, so a specific plan should be documented on the Kardex and care record.

Skin Integrity

Skin breakdown after stroke is common, because the changes with normal aging combined with the effects of immobility provide suitable grounds for pressure sore development. Nutritional deficiencies compound these effects and result in slow wound healing, further complicating the process. An additional consideration is the presence of adaptive equipment that can cause friction and skin irritation. The coccyx and heels are essential areas to protect, because these are often the first sites of breakdown.

Prevention is the key to maintaining skin integrity. Nursing interventions such as those discussed in Chapter 6 should be implemented. These measures should begin the minute the patient is admitted to the facility and should be focused on those at highest risk. Common sense will alert the nurse to which patients are at greatest risk, although the use of risk scales are helpful for a more objective assessment. Care should be taken, however, to remember that each older person is at some risk for impaired skin integrity because normal changes associated with advanced age. The stroke not only exacerbates pre-existing tendencies but also adds confounding factors.

CRITICAL PATHWAYS

Using a critical pathway such as that shown in Figure 10–4 can help promote consistency and quality of care. The emergence of critical pathways may have resulted from the need for cost-containment and cost-effective care within hospitals, but their use can have many benefits for both patients and staff. The development of critical (or clinical) pathways in gerontological rehabilitation requires specialized knowledge of the patients for whom they are written and provides an opportunity for advanced practice nurses (APNs) to become involved in the determination of patient care regimens.

Romito (1990) lists several benefits of critical paths for stroke patients. These include

Continuum of Care Pathway
DRG 14/Stroke
Phase V
Rehab Focus-SNF, Rehab Unit

Saint Margaret Mercy
Healthcare Centers

Addressograph

[M] = Moderate [S] = Severe

Time Frame	V-1 Rehab 24°–48° SNF 24°–72° Dates	V-2 Rehab 2–5 days SNF 3–7 days Dates	V-3 Rehab 5–14 days SNF 7–14 days Dates	V-4 Rehab 14–21 days SNF 14–21 days Dates	V-5 Rehab 21 days–discharge SNF 21 days–discharge Dates
Consults	Primary Care M.D. Rehab M.D. PT, OT, CD, CM Nutritional Consult Activity Assessment [TCC/SCC]	Rehab: Psychology consult Audiology	[M] Recreation Therapy Rehab reevaluation for SNF	[S] Recreational Therapy	Home with: HHC ___ OP ___ ECF ___ Other ___
Diagnostics	Rehab: 1. Admission from outside facility: SMA, CBC, U/A SNF PPD—if not done prior to admission 2. Swallow evaluation per CD 3. Protime where appropriate for all admissions	1. Abnormal labs secondary to diagnosis 2. [S] Modified barium swallow if indicated 3. Calorie count if appropriate	1. Weekly Protime 2. TCC/SNF and PPD on 14th day	→ →	Outpatient setup as ordered →
Treatments	Nutritional evaluation Therapy evaluations: Nursing Psychosocial TED Hose/SCD	1. Swallow protocol 2. Foley discontinued; bowel program initiated	1. Patient/Family teaching initiated by nursing: ___	→ →	→ →

	V-1	V-2	V-3	V-4	V-5
Meds/IVs	Anticoagulant treatment as appropriate / Continue medications	→		→	→
Diet	Continue diet as ordered	[M] Tolerating adequate nutritional intake →	→	[S] Initiate p.o. feeding as appropriate	→
Activity	PT, OT, CD protocol	[S] Tolerating altered consistency/tube feeding without aspiration, diarrhea [M] Attending 100% of therapy W/C up to 3° at a time [S] Attending 50–75% of therapy W/C 1½° at a time	[M] ADL evaluation [S] Attending 100% of therapy W/C 2° increments	[S] ADL evaluation	→ →
Assessment Intervention	DVT Skin Bowel/Bladder Functional status Fall Risk Assessment DC plan	Rehab: 1. Therapy assessments completed in 48°; SN= 72° 2. Psychosocial evaluation 3. Post Foley/bladder training	Signs/Symptoms: UTI Skin breakdown Aspiration	Functional gains	→ →
Timeframe	V-1 Rehab 24°–48° SNF 24°–72°	V-2 Rehab 2–5 days SNF 3–7 days	V-3 Rehab 5–14 days SNF 7–14 days	V-4 Rehab 14–21 days SNF 14–21 days	V-5 Rehab 14 days–discharge SNF 14 days–discharge
Teaching/ Discharge Planning	Patient/family instructed on levels of care	DC plan initiated Therapeutic treatment plan initiated [PT, OT, CD]	Patient instructed re: Mobility precautions, home environmental barriers Patient/family conference	DME's ordered as appropriate. Family instructed re: Special precautions and home needs.	Patient/family instructed re: post D/C office visit and follow up

Figure 10–4 Critical pathway for stroke patients in inpatient rehabilitation. (Used with permission of Sheila Kwiatkowski.)

Illustration continued on following page

Expected Outcomes A = achieved N = not achieved [note variance]				
Patient/famly verbalize understanding of pathway progression and outcomes ———. Variance:	Absence of: Infection, skin breakdown, DVT, aspiration ———. Variance: [M] Patient attending 100% of therapy sessions ———. Variance: Adequate nutritional intake and hydration ———. Variance: [S] Patient attending 50–75% of therapy sessions ———. Variance: Return to preadmission bowel/bladder status ———. Variance:	1. In/out of bed, minimum assist to ——— C.G.A. ———. Variance: 2. On/off toilet/chair, minimum assist/C.G.A. assist ———. Variance: 3. Ambulates minimum 50 ft with standard walker and minimum assist to C.G.A. of one. Variance: 4. ADL activities with minimum assist of one ———. Variance: 5. Able to identify purpose and dosage of meds ———. Variance:	1. Family attended therapy training ———. Variance: Rehab: 2. Patient successfully accomplished apartment stay goal/home pass ———. Variance: 3. Patient able to identify S/S of infection, DVT, safety and mobility precautions ———. Variance:	1. Patient/family aware of follow-up visits ———. Variance: 2. DME's delivered to home/placement ———. Variance:

Clinical pathways are guidelines and must be individualized for each patient's needs.

Table 10–8 AREAS FOR TEACHING IN STROKE REHABILITATION

Definitions of stroke
Risk factors and warning signs of stroke
Rehabilitation after stroke
Hypertension
Nutritional needs
Bowel and bladder management
Skin care
Sexuality and self-image
Communication
Emotional changes
Medication management
Safety and the home environment
Community resources

improved functional outcomes, better inter-disciplinary communication, establishment of a forum for collaborative practice between doctors and nurses, promotion of patient understanding of the stroke recovery process, decreased length of stay, better discharge planning, more relevant documentation, and better communication with insurance companies.

STROKE EDUCATION

There are several ways to ensure that patients and families receive the information needed to cope and adjust with the changes that occur after stroke. It is unwise to think that families will be able to successfully master the skills and knowledge required without some assistance, whether formal or informal. Most stroke survivors or their family members and caregivers will seek out information, if for no other reason than to become more comfortable with certain tasks or the new role of caregiver. The fear and anxiety experienced by both the survivor and the family may be paralyzing at times. The GRN's job is to give these persons the information they need and want (Table 10–8) to successfully and comfortably adjust to the changes that occur after stroke. (See Case Studies 10.2 and 10.3 for examples.)

CASE STUDY 10.2
The Patient with Right Hemisphere Stroke

Reverend Leonard was an articulate, well-educated man, age 60, who experienced a right hemisphere thrombotic stroke secondary to hypertension. As a result of the stroke, Rev. Leonard had moderate hemiparesis of the left upper and lower extremities. He had no other significant health problems, but he had poorly managed his high blood pressure. Rev. Leonard's major goals for post-stroke rehabilitation were to ambulate independently and return to work in his roles as a church leader and father of his large family. Rev. Leonard's job was highly stressful, involving his supervision of a large number of churches and traveling to different parts of the country. Because his functional and motor deficits were relatively minimal and he exhibited no difficulties with speaking or swallowing, Rev. Leonard's recovery initially seemed to progress quickly. He was able to verbally express himself eloquently and appropriately, having many years of experience as a minister. At first, the nursing staff thought that his progress would be fast and he would recover with minimal deficits. However, the speech therapist expressed concerns about Rev. Leonard's cognitive status. During therapy sessions, it became apparent that Rev. Leonard had severe deficits in processing and sequencing information, as well as writing difficulties. Similar to many patients with right hemisphere stroke, the patient denied these deficits and spoke of driving as soon as he was discharged, although he was unable to correctly put three steps together in logical order (such as when parking a car). Although the nurses and therapists worked together to assist Rev. Leonard in accepting his limitations and working to compensate for them, he refused to acknowledge his limitations. Because his cognitive deficits were so well hidden, the family had difficulty believing what was told them by the staff, until they saw specific examples of his lack of cognitive processing in the speech therapy sessions. This included observation by Rev. Leonard's wife and adult children of his inability to follow multi-step commands, put three pictures in a logical sequence, or write sermon notes. When given an assignment to write out his thoughts about a certain passage of scripture (the staff used principles of adult learning by incorporating the patient's previous roles and skills into tasks for rehabilitation), several other thought processing problems became evident. Some visual neglect was noted also by the location of words on the page. Additionally, Rev. Leonard was at high risk for falls because he had poor safety awareness and mild spatial-perceptual deficits. Safety precautions were maintained with the least restraint possible, although the patient felt he did not need any extra safety precautions. This patient represented a particular challenge for the nursing staff because his most severe limitations were cognitive, yet this was not apparent when carrying on a conversation with him. Extensive teaching by the GRN had to be done with the family to facilitate their understanding of what happens during stroke and the deficits that can result. The importance of monitoring blood pressure and taking prescribed medications for control of hypertension and prevention of another stroke was emphasized by the GRNs. Additionally, at least two family members were shown how to take Rev. Leonard's blood pressure and performed accurate return demonstrations. A further complication was that this patient would be expected to be at risk for spiritual distress, but he exhibited an almost euphoric view of his situation. Throughout his rehabilitation stay, Rev. Leonard continued to feel that he would return immediately to his prior job and former activities, but his wife realized this was an unrealistic expectation. Together, the team and family attempted to help the patient realize his deficits. This was done through videotaping of the patient giving a sermon, helping him examine his writing, encouraging self-correction, and assisting him in seeing errors in judgment. By discharge, the patient still hoped to return to his job with modification of the amount of traveling, although the family now had more realistic expectations. This case study illustrates some of the common problems in dealing with patients with right hemisphere stroke.

CASE STUDY 10.3
The Patient with Left Hemisphere Stroke

Mrs. Shelby was a 66 year old woman with a left CVA and right hemiplegia. She had a history a rheumatic heart disease, atrial fibrillation, and dysrhythmias, as well as atrial insufficiency with left ventricular failure. On admission to inpatient rehabilitation, Mrs. Shelby required moderate assistance of two people to transfer; she had facial droop and slurred speech and a Foley catheter for bladder incontinence; and she was on a mechanical soft diet owing to minimal dysphagia. Daily prothrombin times were called to the physician, who ordered warfarin (Coumadin)

accordingly. The patient was also taking Lanoxin for her cardiac condition. Nursing care focused on physical assessment for possible complications, prevention of skin breakdown, education of the patient and family, promotion of activity, discharge planning, and bladder training. Daily physical assessments were performed, including vital signs. Proper diet was maintained, and a swallowing protocol set up by the speech pathologist was followed. An arm trough was used when Mrs. Shelby was up in the wheelchair, and a hemisling was used for transfers and ambulation. The Foley catheter was discontinued and toilet training begun with scheduled voiding. Intake and output was recorded. Individual education was given to the patient and the family regarding medications, pulse-taking, and side effects of Coumadin therapy. They also attended six sessions of the unit's stroke education series, which facilitated discussion and questions about stroke risk factors, the rehabilitation process, skin care, sexuality after stroke, emotional changes, bowel and bladder regulation, safety in the home, and re-entering the community. By discharge, Mrs. Shelby's speech had become more clear, and although she had permanent hemiplegia of the right upper extremity, no pain or shoulder subluxation had occurred. Her skin remained intact. She was continent of bowel and bladder, and she had questions answered about sexual changes after stroke. Mrs. Shelby was able to recognize her medications and state their purpose as well as times she took them. A medication box was used successfully. She seemed accepting of returning home with some supervision, modification, and adaptive equipment, which allowed her to resume many of her previous role tasks. Mrs. Shelby and her husband planned to continue participation in the stroke support group offered by the hospital.

One-to-one teaching is usually an ideal situation, yet not always practical or cost-efficient, depending on the number and type of units where care is given. Within the community, this type of teaching is done in the home. Still, the benefits of group learning, discussion, and interaction after stroke have more intangible benefits, such as social support and decreasing anxiety. Individualized teaching should always be part of discharge planning and preparation. No educational group or session can take the place of direct and one-to-one nurse-patient interaction. Family members need the opportunity to observe, practice, and demonstrate skills that they will be expected to perform alone at home. Tasks such as administering tube feedings, performing intermittent catheterization, giving medications, or even putting on an external catheter can be extremely anxiety producing, particularly for an elderly caregiver. For example, the wife of an older stroke survivor may be reluctant to apply an external catheter to her husband, because this requires a different level of intimacy and interaction than she is comfortable with or accustomed to. Teaching must be tailored to meet the patient and caregiver at their current level of understanding and with the emotional, coping, and financial resources they presently have.

Another excellent way to ensure that most patients or residents receive the basic information about stroke is to develop and implement an educational series. Easton, Zemen, and Kwiatkowski (1994) found that such a program was well received in a rehabilitation setting, and patients who had been discharged stated that it was very helpful to them. Other nurses have reported similar outcomes, as well as positive changes within the nursing department as a result (Kernich & Robb, 1988).

The clinical nurse specialist (CNS), if available, is the ideal person to develop this program. Experienced GRNs could also initiate and/or teach in such a group. Easton et al. (1994) further describe how to develop and implement a stroke education series if the reader wishes more specific information.

The leader of the group should be enthusiastic and dynamic, with solid group facilitation skills. The location of the sessions should be easily accessible and ensure a calm and quiet environment conducive to learning and sharing. Attendance should be documented. A follow-up plan including evaluation of the course should be in place.

Sessions should be kept to under one hour, with content being limited to 20 to 30 minutes and time allowed for questions and discussion. Information given should reflect the needed knowledge for discharge to the home environment, if this is the destination of most participants. Visual aids, videos, handouts, and other written information should be provided and should coordinate with the topic for the day. The instructor should avoid jargon and use terms that the audience can relate to and understand. Appendix 10A illus-trates the wording chosen and the content presented in one series as an example. The reader will note that most of the content is kept simple and to the point. Having the lecture material for the sessions (as well as the supplies needed) in writing helps promote continuity in teaching and provides security for newer nurses wishing to get involved in educational sessions. Those nurses wishing to develop such a program within the community or long-term care facility may modify the content to fit the needs of their clients. It should be clearly defined whether the primary goal of the program is education or social support. Each can and should exist with the other, but the focus will determine the direction of the sessions. The example given was set up as a stroke education program for patients and families in an acute rehabilitation setting (Appendix 10A).

One of the most important aspects of a stroke education group is the psychosocial support it provides (Pasquarello, 1990). All the knowledge about stroke that GRNs can give to patients cannot take the place of the camaraderie and support gained through interaction with others who are experiencing the same process and problems. Time for questions, discussion, and sharing should always be incorporated, because this is essential to any group learning.

If the focus of the group needs to be more social than educational, a stroke club or support group should be started. Hospitals often offer such a group for survivors and their families after discharge. This is discussed in the following section.

STROKE CLUBS AND SUPPORT GROUPS

The purpose of a stroke club or support group is to provide a safe environment in which those who participate can feel free to express feelings, frustrations, conflicts, and solutions (Pierce & Salter, 1988). Validation of self-worth and helpful problem solving can take place. A feeling of understanding is present between the members who share the effects of stroke on their families. Often, life-long friendships are made between survivors of stroke and their families within the hospital. A post-discharge stroke club allows these people to remain in contact and provide further support to each other. This networking can mean the difference between positive coping and the use of negative adaptive strategies.

Table 10-9 EXAMPLE OF ITEMS SUBMITTED FROM A REHABILITATION UNIT TO A DAILY HOSPITAL NEWSLETTER FOR ONE WEEK DURING NATIONAL STROKE AWARENESS MONTH

Day 1

May is National Stroke Awareness Month. The staff of Inpatient Rehabilitation would like to take this opportunity to remind everyone of some of the startling statistics from the National Stroke Association (1995):

- Each year: 500,000 people experience a stroke
  150,000 people die from stroke
  Stroke costs our nation $25 billion
- Stroke is the third leading cause of death in the United States.
- At least 3 million stroke survivors today live with some degree of disability.
- Stroke is a major reason for people going to a nursing home.
- Stroke is largely preventable.

Day 2

Do you know the warning signs of stroke? The majority of people do not. By recognizing these signs and taking action, you may be able to prevent a stroke, or at least reduce its severity if one does occur:

- Blurred vision or decreased vision in one or both eyes
- Numbness, tingling, or weakness in the face, arms, or legs
- Difficulty speaking or understanding
- Dizziness, loss of balance, any loss of consciousness
- Trouble swallowing
- Headache (usually severe and with an abrupt onset)

Day 3

Do you know the risk factors for stroke? If you have any of these risk factors, be sure to consult with your primary health care provider and follow your individually prescribed program to lower your risk of stroke.

Those that can be changed:

- High blood pressure
- High cholesterol
- Heart disease
- Smoking
- Using excessive amounts of alcohol
- Obesity

Those that cannot be changed:

- Age older than 65 years
- Gender (men more than women until menopause, then about equal)
- Race (blacks have higher incidence than whites)
- Family history of stroke
- Diabetes

Day 4

Guidelines for stroke prevention: Modify your lifestyle to reduce risk factors—control high blood pressure, high blood sugar (with diabetes), or pre-existing heart conditions per your physician's recommendations. Do not ignore the warning signs of stroke, and get medical follow-up immediately if they do occur. Stop smoking. Limit alcohol use. Keep weight and cholesterol levels within recommended limits. Follow a regular exercise regimen. Eat heart-healthy foods low in saturated fats. Be aware of your local health care resources should the need arise.

Day 5

The staff of the inpatient rehabilitation unit at this hospital specializes in comprehensive inpatient stroke rehabilitation using a team approach. A weekly educational series is offered each Thursday from 4–5 P.M. in the rehabilitation gym for patients and families who would like to learn more about stroke prevention and post-stroke treatment. A stroke support group also meets monthly for educational and social activities. The entire rehabilitation team along with the National Stroke Association would like to encourage everyone to "Be Stroke Smart." For further information, please contact Kris, our clinical nurse specialist, at extension 4919.

Some support groups meet on a monthly basis, some more frequently. Meetings may have an educational theme for the day or involve a light-hearted discussion with refreshments. Groups may plan outings or trips in which arrangements are made for a bus that accommodates those with adaptive equipment such as wheelchairs and walkers. The group coordinator can make arrangements with facilities, restaurants, theaters, or hotels for special accommodations based on the unique needs of the group. Having a nurse along adds a sense of security. Traveling with a group who has special needs also makes one feel less alone or different. Stroke survivors often say they feel a kinship to other survivors that is unique, and sometimes closer than that felt for those even in their own family. This mutual understanding fosters bonds that can buoy the survivors' positive outlook to life after stroke.

COMMUNITY CARE

One of the ways in which GRNs can get involved in post-stroke rehabilitation is to promote recognition of the problems of stroke within the community. In 1992, the National Stroke Association (NSA) waged a nationwide campaign to increase awareness of the public about stroke. A survey had revealed that 97% of Americans did not know the warning signs. Thousands of facilities, agencies, and schools participated in this effort. Information and educational materials for preparation and disbursement were provided, largely as a result of a generous grant from a large corporation. Table 10–9 shows how one nurse manager supported National Stroke Awareness Month and dispersed knowledge of stroke from the NSA to her own facility. This was accomplished by putting announcements in the daily hospital newsletter read by the employees, staff, families, and visitors. Large posters were set up in the lobbies, and blood pressure screening was offered. The rehabilitation unit displayed pictures and brochures describing their services. A page was taken in the large local newspaper to alert readers to the warning signs of stroke, as well as where treatment, services, and resources could be obtained. These activities serve as an example of how GRNs can have an impact on the health of their communities through prevention and screening.

The NSA welcomes the formation of chapters in all parts of the country. This active organization provides informative materials for the public as well as health professionals. The goals of the NSA are "to reduce the incidence and severity of stroke through: prevention, medical treatment, rehabilitation, family support and research" (1991, p. 1). A complete list of materials (some offered free of charge) can be obtained, as well as information on starting a local stroke chapter through the NSA, by calling 1-800-STROKES.

Nurses can also become involved in efforts to prevent stroke by providing volunteer educational sessions at local churches, senior centers, schools, and community meetings. GRNs can participate in career days at grade and high schools to promote awareness of resources for those with disabilities. Additionally, many communities have clinics for those who are without insurance or who cannot afford health care in traditional settings. These facilities generally welcome nursing volunteers.

Nurses often think of other creative ways in which to alert the public about prevention of stroke. Hospitals, colleges of nursing, and nursing organizations can combine to put on an "aging fair" for adults in the region. Student nurse organizations can participate in walk-a-thons or other fund-raisers to raise money for stroke research. Nurses may lead exercise groups for the aged in long-term care facilities or start their own stroke club. The opportunities for involvement within the community with regard to disease prevention are plentiful, but efforts may need to be initiated by GRNs who are concerned with the health of the older adults in their own communities.

REFERENCES

American Lung Association (of Northern Indiana). (1992). *Facts about second-hand smoke.* South Bend, IN: Author.

Asconape, J. J., & Penry, J. F. (1991). Poststroke seizures in the elderly. *Clinics in Geriatric Medicine, 7,* 483–492.

Baker, A. C. (1993). The spouse's positive effect on the stroke patient's recovery. *Rehabilitation Nursing, 18*(10), 30–33.

Bronstein, K. S. (1991). Psychosocial components in stroke: Implications for adaptation. *Nursing Clinics of North America, 26,* 1007–1015.

Bronstein, K. S., Popovich, J. M., & Stewart-Amidei, C. (1991). *Promoting stroke recovery.* St. Louis: Mosby–Year Book.

Brott, T. (1991). Prevention and management of medical complications of the hospitalized elderly stroke patient. *Clinics in Geriatric Medicine, 7,* 475–490.

Buelow, J. M., & Jamieson, D. (1990). Potential for altered nutritional status in the stroke patient. *Rehabilitation Nursing, 15*, 260–263.

Caplan, L. R. (1988). TIAs: We need to return to the question, 'What is wrong with Mr. Jones?'. *Neurology, 38*, 791–793.

Caplan, L. R. (1991). Diagnosis and treatment of ischemic stroke. *Journal of the American Medical Association, 266*, 2413–2419.

Cohn, S. (1994). Reinventing myself. *Be Stroke Smart, 11*(3 & 4), 17–18.

Davidoff, G. N., Keren, O., Ring, H., & Solzi, P. (1991). Acute stroke patients: Long-term effects of rehabilitation and maintenance of gains. *Archives of Physical Medicine and Rehabilitation, 72*, 869–873.

Dobkin, B. H. (1991). The rehabilitation of elderly stroke patients. *Clinics in Geriatric Medicine, 7*, 507–523.

Easton, K. L., Rawl, S., Zemen, D. M., Kwiatkowski, S., & Burczyk, B. (1995). The effects of nursing follow-up on the coping strategies used by rehabilitation patients after discharge. *Rehabilitation Nursing, 4*(4), 119–126.

Easton, K. L., Zemen, D. M., & Kwiatkowski, S. (1994). Developing and implementing a stroke education series for patients and families. *Rehabilitation Nursing, 19*, 348–350.

Estol, C., & Caplan, L. R. (1990). Therapy of acute stroke. *Clinical Neuropharmacology, 13*(2), 91–120.

Evans, R. L., Bishop, D. S., & Haselkorn, J. K. (1991). Factors predicting satisfactory home care after stroke. *Archives of Physical Medicine and Rehabilitation, 72*, 144–147.

Falconer, J. A., Naughton, B. J., Strasser, D. C., & Sinacore, J. M. (1994). Stroke inpatient rehabilitation: A comparison across age groups. *Journal of the American Geriatrics Society, 42*(1), 39–44.

Farzan, D. T. (1991). Reintegration for stroke survivors: Home and community considerations. *Nursing Clinics of North America, 26*, 1037–1048.

Folden, S. L. (1993). Effect of a supportive-educative nursing intervention on older adults' perceptions of self-care after a stroke. *Rehabilitation Nursing, 18*(3), 162–167.

Folden, S. L. (1994, Fall). Managing the effects of a stroke: The first months. *Rehabilitation Nursing Research*, 79–84.

Friedland, J. F., & McColl, M. A. (1992). Social support intervention after stroke: Results of a randomized trial. *Archives of Physical Medicine and Rehabilitation, 73*, 573–581.

Goldberg, G., & Berger, G. G. (1988). Secondary prevention in stroke: A primary rehabilitation concern. *Archives of Physical Medicine and Rehabilitation, 69*, 32–40.

Gordon, W. A., Hibbard, M. R., Egelko, S., Riley, E., Simon, D., Diller, L., Ross, E. D., & Lieberman, A. (1991). Issues in the diagnosis of post-stroke depression. *Rehabilitation Psychology, 36*(2), 71–87.

Gresham, G. E., Duncan, P. W., Stason, W. B., et al. (1995). *Post-stroke rehabilitation*. Clinical practice guideline, No. 16. (AHCPR Publication No. 95-0662). Rockville, MD: U.S. Department of Health and Human Services, Public Health Service, Agency for Health Care Policy and Research.

Gross, J. C. (1990). Bladder dysfunction after stroke: It's not always inevitable. *Journal of Gerontological Nursing, 16*(4), 20–25.

Hart, G. (1990, March/April). Strokes causing left vs. right hemiplegia: Different effects and nursing implications. *Geriatric Nursing*, 67–70.

Hibbard, M. R., Grober, S. E., Gordon, W. A., Aletta, E. G., & Freeman, A. (1990). Cognitive therapy and the treatment of poststroke depression. *Topic in Geriatric Rehabilitation, 5*(3), 43–55.

Josephs, A. (1992). *Stroke: An owner's manual: The invaluable guide to life after stroke*. Long Beach, CA: Amadeus Press.

Katrak, P. H., Cole, A. M. D., Poulos, C. J., & McCauley, J. C. K. (1992). Objective assessment of spasticity, strength, and function with early exhibition of dantrolene sodium after cerebrovascular accident: A randomized double-blind study. *Archives of Physical Medicine and Rehabilitation, 73*, 4–9.

Kernich, C. A., & Robb, G. (1988). Development of a stroke family support and education program. *Journal of Neuroscience Nursing, 20*, 193–197.

Kistler, P. (1989, August). How can we prevent strokes? *Harvard Medical School Health Letter*, 1–5.

Kübler-Ross, E. (1969). *On death and dying*. New York: Macmillan.

Lewis, N. A. (1986). Functional gains in CVA patients: A nursing approach. *Rehabilitation Nursing, 11*(2), 25–27.

Lorish, T. R., Sandin, K. J., Roth, E. J., & Noll, S. F. (1994). Stroke rehabilitation. 3. Rehabilitation evaluation and management. *Archives of Physical Medicine and Rehabilitation, 75*, S-47–S-51.

McLean, J., Roper-Hall, A., Mayer, P., & Main, A. (1991). Service needs of stroke survivors and their informal carers: A pilot study. *Journal of Advanced Nursing, 16*, 559–564.

Miller, J. F. (1992). *Coping with chronic illness: Overcoming powerlessness*. Philadelphia: F. A. Davis.

Mol, V. J., & Baker, C. A. (1991). Activity intolerance in the geriatric stroke patient. *Rehabilitation Nursing, 16*, 337–343.

Moore, K. (1994, March). Stroke: The long road back. *RN*, 50–54.

Moore, K., & Trifiletti, E. (1994, February). Stroke: The first critical days. *RN*, 22–27.

Moss, C. S. (1972). *Recovery with aphasia: The aftermath of my stroke*. Urbana, IL: University of Illinois Press.

Munchiando, J. F., & Kendall, K. (1993). Comparison of the effectiveness of two bowel programs for CVA patients. *Rehabilitation Nursing, 18*, 168–172.

Nakayama, H., Jorgensen, H. S., Raaschou, H. O., & Olsen, T. S. (1994). Recovery of upper extremity function in stroke patients: The Copenhagen Stroke Study. *Archives of Physical Medicine and Rehabilitation, 75*, 394–398.

National Stroke Association. (1991). *Be stroke smart* [Newsletter]. Englewood, CO: Author.

National Stroke Association. (1994). *Be stroke smart* [Brochure]. Englewood, CO: Author.

National Stroke Association. (1995). *Be stroke smart* [Newsletter]. Englewood, CO: Author.

Orem, D. (1995). *Nursing: Concepts and practice.* St. Louis: Mosby.

Owen, D. C., Getz, P. A., & Bulla, S. (1995). A comparison of characteristics of patients with completed stroke: Those who achieve continence and those who do not. *Rehabilitation Nursing, 20,* 197–203.

Pasquerello, M. A. (1990). Developing, implementing, and evaluating a stroke recovery group. *Rehabilitation Nursing, 15,* 26–29.

Pierce, L. L., & Salter, J. P. (1988). Stroke support group: A reality. *Rehabilitation Nursing, 13,* 189–190, 197.

Ragsdale, D., Yarbrough, S., & Lasher, A. T. (1993). Using social support theory to care for CVA patients. *Rehabilitation Nursing, 18,* 154–161, 172.

Reding, M. J., & McDowell, F. H. (1989). Focused stroke rehabilitation programs improve outcome. *Archives of Neurology, 46,* 700–701.

Romito, D. (1990). A critical path for CVA patients. *Rehabilitation Nursing, 15,* 153–156.

Rosenthal, S. G., Pituch, M. J., Greninger, L. O., & Metress, E. S. (1993). Perceived needs of wives of stroke patients. *Rehabilitation Nursing, 18,* 148–153, 167.

Roth, E. J. (1988). The elderly stroke patient: Principles and practices of rehabilitation management. *Topics in Geriatric Rehabilitation, 3*(4), 27–61.

Roth, E. J., Meuller, K., & Green, D. (1988). Stroke rehabilitation outcome: Impact of coronary artery disease. *Stroke, 19*(1), 42–47.

Salter, J., Camp, Y., Pierce, L. L., & Mion, L. C. (1991). Rehabilitation nursing approaches to cerebrovascular accident: A comparison of two approaches. *Rehabilitation Nursing, 16*(2), 62–65.

Sandin, K. J., & Mason, K. D. (1996). *Manual of stroke rehabilitation.* Boston: Butterworth-Heinemann.

Taub, E., Miller, N. E., Novak, T. A., Cook, E. W., Fleming, W. C., Nepomuceno, C. S., Connell, J. S., & Crago, J. A. (1993). Technique to improve chronic motor deficit after stroke. *Archives of Physical Medicine and Rehabilitation, 74,* 347–354.

Veith, I. (1988). *Can you hear the clapping of one hand?: Learning to live with a stroke.* Berkeley, CA: University of California Press.

Watson, P. G. (1986). Stroke in the family: Theoretical considerations. *Rehabilitation Nursing, 11*(5), 15–17.

Williams, A. M. (1992). Self-report of indifference and anxiety among persons with right hemisphere stroke. *Research in Nursing and Health, 15,* 343–347.

Woog, P. (Ed.). (1992). *The chronic illness trajectory framework: The Corbin and Strauss Nursing Model.* New York: Springer.

Appendix 10A

Example of a Stroke Education Program for Patients and Families

Developed by Kris Easton, Donna Zemen, and Sheila Kwiatkowski

■

Session 1

TOPICS

What is a stroke?
Hypertension

AUDIOVISUAL AIDS AND EQUIPMENT

Videotape and videocassette recorder (VCR), educational pamphlets, information sheet, posters (circulation, symptoms of high blood pressure, complications of high blood pressure, guidelines for high blood pressure, quiz on hypertension), blood pressure cuff, and stethoscope.

LECTURE/DISCUSSION

I. What is a stroke?
Background statistics (from the National Stroke Association, 1995) tell us that 500,000 to 600,000 people in the United States have a stroke each year. One third (145,000) of these people die. Hypertension is the number one risk factor for stroke. Although the death rate due to stroke is decreasing, the incidence of stroke remains high. Two thirds of those who have strokes are older than the age of 65 years. (Show videotape on living with stroke.)
   A. Definition
      A stroke is an interruption of the blood supply to the brain. This is also called a cerebrovascular accident (CVA).

   B. Types
      We will discuss two main types of strokes: those caused by a clot or those caused by a hemorrhage.
      1. *Clot.* A clot results in blockage of the blood supply. A clot that originates in the brain is called a thrombus. A clot that originates in another part of the body is called an embolus. You may have heard your doctor use these terms to describe the cause of your stroke. An embolus may form in another part of the body such as the leg (as in deep vein thrombosis [DVT]) or the heart (as with heart conditions like atrial fibrillation). If undetected or untreated, these clots can break off and float to the brain, resulting in blockage and stroke.
      2. *Hemorrhage.* A hemorrhage occurs when a diseased artery leaks or bursts and damages brain tissues. High blood pressure can weaken blood vessels and thus needs to be controlled to help prevent this type of stroke. An aneurysm is a weak spot in the blood vessel wall that can occur in people of any age. Such weak spots may also leak or rupture, causing damage to surrounding tissues.
   C. Risk factors
      1. Controllable
         a. Hypertension is number one
         b. Others include high cholesterol, heart disease, TIAs (explain),

diabetes, atherosclerosis, smoking, obesity, stress, heavy drinking, and thick blood
2. Uncontrollable
   a. Age (older than 65 years)
   b. Gender (men more than women)
   c. Race (blacks more than whites)
   d. Heredity
D. Warning signs
Numbness, tingling, speech difficulties, blurred vision, headache, dizziness, loss of consciousness, sudden inability to speak or move
E. Effects of stroke
May be mild or severe, temporary or permanent
   1. Paralysis or weakness on one side, with loss of feeling or sensation
   2. Aphasia—difficulty in understanding and/or using language
   3. Apraxia—not knowing what to do with an ordinary, everyday object
   4. Memory loss, confusion
   5. Bowel/bladder changes
   6. Eating problems, swallowing difficulties
   7. Visual deficits
   8. Skin breakdown
   9. Emotional changes such as feelings of grief, anger, loneliness, helplessness, crying, apathy, depression, mood swings
F. Treatment
Rehabilitation—retraining, relearning
   Therapies (physical, occupational, speech), nursing, social work. (Explain role of each team member.*)
II. What is hypertension?
   A. Definition—Hypertension does not mean high stress or tension, but high blood pressure.
   B. Causes
   Atherosclerosis, arteriosclerosis (fatty build-up and clogging of arteries), high salt intake, hereditary properties Occurs more often in blacks than whites, with black men at special risk.
   C. Treatments
   Watch sodium levels (may be on sodium-restricted diet), exercise, maintain a recommended weight, reduce cholesterol, take medications as ordered, monitor blood pressure, visit health care provider regularly.

---

*The patient is the most important member of the rehabilitation team.

D. Measuring blood pressure
Define top and bottom numbers: systolic is measuring heart at work; diastolic measures the heart at rest. Blood pressure higher than 140/90 is considered high (show poster), but a diagnosis is made based on several visits to the doctor or health care provider, and repeated elevated readings.
   (Demonstrate how to take a blood pressure. Allow family members to try if they wish, with nurse's supervision, at end of session.)

Session 2

(Taught by pharmacist)
Outline of content
I. Role of the pharmacist
II. Explain actions, side effects, and precautions of medication groups:
   A. Antihypertensives
   B. Antibiotics
   C. Oral hypoglycemics
   D. Laxatives
   E. Blood thinners
   F. Sleeping pills
   G. Over-the-counter medications
III. Explain symptoms of allergic reactions, side effects, and food interactions.
IV. Answer commonly asked questions:
   A. What does before and after a meal mean?
   B. What if I miss a pill?
   C. What about the medicines I was on before I came to the hospital?
   D. What if I'm ill one day and unable to take my medicine?
   E. Should I stop taking my medications when I feel better?
   F. What if my medicine is not making me better or isn't doing what it is supposed to do?
   G. Is it okay to take all my pills at the same time?
   H. Why do I bruise with some medications?
   I. Can I save some of my antibiotics if I'm better before they run out?
V. Answer specific patient/family questions.

Session 3

TOPICS

Skin care, bowel and bladder management
I. Skin care

AUDIOVISUAL AIDS AND EQUIPMENT

Pamphlets about pressure sores, foot care; posters on causes of pressure sores and pressure points; Granulex spray.

LECTURE/DISCUSSION

A. Pathophysiology (show poster)
   When we talk about skin care, we are talking not only about the outer layer of skin but the underlying tissue as well. Watching and caring for your skin is especially important after having a stroke or other condition that makes you less mobile than before. Circulation is decreased to certain body areas, along with changes in sensation. You may have some feeling in your stroke side or none at all. That, along with constant pressure from lying or sitting for long periods, can make you prone to skin breakdown and bedsores. Many of you probably already have had some reddened areas or breakdown. After only a few minutes of constant pressure, the skin and underlying tissues start to deteriorate. Other causes of breakdown include shearing force, friction, and chemical irritation.

B. Pressure points (show poster)
   Common areas of skin breakdown from being in bed or immobilized include the ears, shoulders, elbows, buttocks, coccyx, hips, and heels. The most common areas for our patients to have problems are the coccyx and heels, so we need to check these thoroughly and frequently. Also watch for redness or soreness under splints, shoulder slings, ankle-foot orthoses (AFOs), and the like.

C. Treatment and prevention
   It is much easier to prevent a bedsore than to treat a bedsore.
   1. Special mattresses—Foam or air for the bed; wheelchair pads like waffle cushions or ROHO. Take home the foam or air mattresses. You can also buy special mattresses and wheelchair pads at a medical supply store.
   2. Special appliances—Spenco boots (with foam inside), heel and elbow pads. It is important to wear these items if needed. Also take them home to wear.
   3. Turning and pressure relief—Change your position at least every 2 hours. Lie down and get out of the wheelchair 1–2 times per day. Even if you are not tired, it is important to relieve the pressure on your bottom. In the wheel-chair—if you have function of both arms, do wheelchair push-ups (demonstrate). If you have use of only one arm, do weight shifts (demonstrate). Do these every 15–30 minutes. If you are watching TV, do them with every commercial. This allows circulation to be maintained to the coccyx and buttocks. While in bed, keep your head as low as is comfortable. If you raise up the head of the bed, it creates a shearing effect that can tear the skin on your bottom.
   4. Skin care—Keep skin clean and dry. Tell someone if you've had an accident of bowels or urine. If you have a problem with incontinence at night and need to wear adult undergarments (such as Depends), be sure to protect the skin with a cream or ointment. Make sure that your nurse or doctor knows whether you are having incontinence problems. Do not assume this is because you are getting old or that everyone who has a stroke will be incontinent. This is discussed further later in this session. Some skin care products that we use for pressure areas to prevent or treat sores are:
      a. Granulex or Granulderm spray—Use on pressure areas. If you use this at home, you need a prescription for a refill. Also, be careful, because it may stain your bedclothes or sheets.
      b. Aloe Vesta ointment—This protects the skin from moisture. You can buy this without a prescription.
      c. Others—Skin protective dressings like DuoDerm may be used when sores already have developed. Your doctor or our skin care nurse specialist will prescribe an individualized treatment for you if you have breakdown. This might include dressing changes, special ointments, or whirlpool treatments.

5. Diet
   a. Fluids—Drink 1½–2 quarts of fluid per day. If you are dehydrated, your skin loses its protective cushion and will deteriorate.
   b. Protein—You need a high-protein diet. When you are admitted, we do a measure of your protein. The level will be low for most of you because of changes in your health status. Your doctor or dietitian may order a supplement like milkshakes or Ensure, which will give you extra protein, vitamins, and minerals that you need for healing. Be sure to drink these. If you don't like the taste, let us know. We can change it or flavor it.
6. Examination—Learn to check all skin areas daily. You can use a mirror for hard to see areas if you can't have your family member do it. Remember it is much easier to prevent than to heal a sore.

D. Edema
Edema, or swelling, is excess fluid that develops in the arms or legs. This can occur in your stroke side because of decreased circulation and sensation. You may also develop swelling in your legs because, as you get older, the valves break down in your veins, allowing the fluid to leak into the tissues. Edema also makes you more prone to skin breakdown.
   Treatment for edema:
1. Support hose—Wear them day and night. These help decrease swelling by pushing fluid back toward the head. This also helps prevent blood clots by not allowing the fluid to pool in the lower legs.
2. Keep your feet and arms up during the day as much as possible. Put the foot of the bed up slightly at night. Elevate the affected arm on a pillow.
3. Isotoner glove (for hand edema)—Same purpose as support hose for the feet and legs.

E. Foot care
Taking special care of the feet is particularly important for those with diabetes and poor circulation. Improper care can lead to sores and even amputa-tions. Please read our booklet on foot care. Some of the highlights include:
1. Check your feet daily. Check the soles also. Have a family member do it if you cannot.
2. Wear properly fitting shoes. Make them large enough to prevent blisters.
3. Cut toenails straight across to prevent ingrown toenails. Soak feet before trimming to soften the nails. If there is any problem, see a podiatrist. Do not trim calluses or corns yourself.
4. Be careful of hot water. Always test the water with the elbow of your unaffected arm to prevent burns due to lack of sensation.

II. Bowel and bladder management
A. Bladder management

AUDIOVISUAL AIDS AND EQUIPMENT

Foley catheter and tray, blue Chux, poster on treatment of incontinence, pamphlets on incontinence.

LECTURE/DISCUSSION

Incontinence is defined as an unintentional leakage or total loss of urine or stool from the body. The most common problem associated with urination is incontinence. This is *not* necessarily a normal result of aging.
1. Background—The kidneys filter the blood by removing waste products, resulting in the formation of urine. Urine passes from the kidneys through small tubes, called the ureters, into the bladder. The bladder is a storage place for the urine. It is important to know that the bladder is actually a muscle that becomes out of shape when it is not used, such as when you have a catheter in place. Also, when you have a stroke, some of the messages sent by your body to the brain may not get through. The brain controls the contraction of the bladder muscle and opening and closing of the sphincters that let the urine pass out of the bladder via the urethra into the toilet. After a stroke, these things do not always work together or the right signals may not be received. The urethra in females is shorter than in males, and therefore women are more prone to bladder

infections from bacteria. Bladder infections can also cause incontinence.

2. Feelings—Incontinence is often embarrassing and is associated with such emotions as anger, fear of rejection, depression, and frustration. It is important to be patient and talk about these feelings with your family member and nurse.

3. Types of urinary incontinence

   a. Stress—Leakage occurs with laughing, coughing, sneezing, or other activities that increase your abdominal pressure. This has nothing to do with "feeling lots of stress." This type of incontinence happens more often in women who have had several children, because the pelvic floor muscles have weakened.

   b. Urge—This occurs when you have the urge to go, but can't quite make it to the bathroom in time.

   c. Overflow—Leakage that results from an overflow of too much urine in the bladder. You may have trouble releasing the urine.

   d. Total—Constant and usually complete loss of urine.

4. Treatments (show poster)

   a. Kegel exercises—Especially for women, to increase pelvic muscle tone and strength.

   b. Bladder training—The goal is to empty the bladder regularly and completely. Toilet every 2 hours when the catheter is first removed. The nursing staff will probably remind you to try even if you don't feel the urge.

   c. Urinary catheter—Used to drain urine from the bladder into a bag (show and explain how the balloon works, etc.).

   d. External collection devices (show external male catheter)—Especially for men. This fits over the penis like a condom and does not go inside the bladder. It collects urine in a bag through a tube and is often worn at night by men who have leaking and cannot sleep because of incontinence.

   e. Medications—Many different kinds. Your nurse can explain

which pills you are taking, if any, to help your bladder recover.

   f. Other—Biofeedback is often helpful but not available at this facility; surgery is sometimes indicated, but this is rare for our patients.

Conclusion: The caregiver should provide reassurance, assist with and encourage bladder training, reinforce positive behavior, and be patient and understanding. Good skin care and prevention of bladder infections are also essential when incontinence is a problem.

   B. Bowel management

EQUIPMENT

Suppositories, Colace, Therevac mini-enema; cup with 100 ml of water; graduated cylinder with 1000 ml of water.

LECTURE/DISCUSSION

A good bowel program should have the following three goals:

- Predictable—occurring at relatively the same time each day and not making the patient prone to accidents
- Convenient—generally, the simplest effective program is best
- Least expensive—avoid costly suppositories and medications if at all possible

1. Uncontrollable factors related to bowel control

   a. Bowel diseases
   b. Previous bowel surgery
   c. Family history
   d. Effects of disability such as a stroke

2. Controllable facts of a bowel program

   a. Diet—Eat a diet high in fiber. Some foods that are high in fiber include nuts, popcorn, bran, and fruits such as apples, oranges, and prunes.

   b. Fluids—Drink at least 1–2 quarts per day (show container). This amounts to 100 ml (show cup with that amount) every couple of hours during the day until 8 P.M. in addition to liquids you usually drink with your meals. Water is the best fluid to drink.

   c. Timing—Try to have a bowel

movement after meals, especially after breakfast when you body's natural reflexes are helping with peristalsis (the moving of fecal material through the intestines and into the rectum). Try to establish a habitual time for a bowel movement.

d. Activity—Become as active as your condition permits. Increased movement and walking helps prevent constipation.

e. Medications—There are many different medications to aid in the prevention of constipation and the maintenance of a good bowel program. You may need some of these as your body is reacting to the effects of your stroke. However, all the measures mentioned previously should be worked with first, before using medications. Relying on enemas and suppositories is strongly discouraged and will not promote a reliable bowel program for most people with stroke. Most stroke survivors can establish and maintain good bowel function, avoiding constipation, without the regular use of suppositories, laxatives, or enemas.

3. Common medications used right after stroke

a. Oral medications
   i. Bulk formers—Metamucil, Fibermed (show examples)
   ii. Stool softeners—Colace (show capsule) used most commonly; need to drink plenty of water to be most effective
   iii. Peristaltic stimulators—Senokot, Peri-Colace; also help move stool along in the intestines by stimulating peristalsis (in addition to softening stool)

b. Rectal medications (show example of each as explaining)
   i. Glycerin suppository—causes local peristalsis
   ii. Bisacodyl (Dulcolax) suppository—stimulant; irritates the rectal mucosa to expel stool; a stronger type and is often used in preparation for surgery or tests involving the lower gastrointestinal tract
   iii. Ceo-Two suppository — releases carbon dioxide in the rectum to stretch it and let stool be released
   iv. Therevac mini-enema—combination of melted glycerin, soap, and Colace. The tip of the plastic container is cut off and the liquid is squeezed into the rectum. This usually works in 2–15 minutes (faster than solid suppositories) and has shown very good results with our older stroke patients.

Conclusion: Remember that bowel habits are often changed after a stroke. A change in activity level or diet, decreased amounts of fluids taken, and an altered schedule all contribute to constipation. Please try to work with your nurse to establish a satisfactory bowel routine before you are discharged.

Session 4

TOPICS

Self-image, feelings, emotions, communication, sexuality

AUDIOVISUAL AIDS AND EQUIPMENT

Blackboard, chalk, nasogastric tube poster, videotapes (Stroke: Focus on Feelings; Stroke: Focus on the Family), television, VCR, pamphlets (Sexuality After Your Stroke, Sexuality and People with Disabilities, Living with Stroke, Aphasia)

I. The grieving process (use blackboard to sketch Kubler-Ross' stages of grief)
   The definition of grief is a normal reaction to loss, which can be physical (tangible) or symbolic (psychosocial). Some examples of things over which a person might grieve include loss of a child or spouse, loss of independence, loss of a job, loss of a limb, loss of the ability to walk. Grieving is a normal response to loss.
   Health is present when there is a feeling of wellness and stability. It is interrupted by a significant change or event that is seen as a crisis. An example of such an event would be a stroke, amputa-

tion, or diagnosis of a terminal illness.

The stages of grief according to Kubler-Ross (1969) are widely accepted and can be identified in any individual who has suffered a loss. It is important to note that there are no time boundaries during each stage and one may move back and forth between stages at different times. The goal of nursing care during this process is to assist you and your family toward acceptance and increased self-reliance. Both family members and patients may go through a similar process. Try to see whether you can identify with these stages and where you may see yourself right now.

A. Denial—Denial or shock is the first stage of grief. It involves an unacceptance or disbelief of what has happened. You may have felt like "This couldn't have happened to me" or "My husband has always been so healthy. He couldn't be having a stroke."

B. Anger—This second stage of grief results from loneliness, internal conflict, guilt, and a feeling of meaninglessness. This is a time of great emotion that often is expressed in angry words or actions directed at others. It is important for family members and friends of a grieving person to remember not to take angry outbursts personally, but to allow the individual to express frustration in a loving and supportive environment.

C. Bargaining—During this stage, the grieving person often tries to make bargains with God or a higher power in order to change the circumstances that surround the crisis. A gradual realization of the real consequences of the situation leads the person to the next stage—depression.

D. Depression—This stage can often be the longest and most difficult to work through. A patient will often display no emotion and an apathetic attitude toward life. Some individuals need antidepressant medication, which is prescribed by the physician. The family members of a stroke patient also go through feelings of depression, and they may stay in this phase even longer than the patient. If you are a family member who is battling feelings of depression, your nurses and the rest of the rehabilitation team is here to help you. Your situation is not hopeless. There is life after stroke, and our trained staff can help you cope and adjust to these changes.

E. Acceptance—This final stage of the grieving process involves the person's movement toward increased self-awareness and contact with others. The person experiencing the loss learns to cope and adapt to the changes that have taken place. This involves identification and explanation of the loss. This process results in an increased self-reliance and the gradual assumption of a "new" identity.

II. Communication/Swallowing
   A. Aphasia
   Aphasia is defined as problems with understanding and using language. Not all stroke survivors have aphasia. There are many different kinds of aphasia. Your speech therapist will work closely with you if this is one of your problems. Some difficulties commonly associated with aphasia include:

- Inability to form words
- Difficulty eating caused by poor muscle control
- Behavioral changes
- Language and memory changes
- May understand what is said but not be able to speak
- May not understand what is said
- May have speech, but it is not meaningful or understandable

   To a person with severe aphasia, our words may seem like a foreign language. Other kinds of ways to communicate may be needed. Some suggestions for relating to persons with aphasia include:

- Speak slowly
- Be patient
- Encourage the person's attempts to talk
- Give praise for attempts to communicate
- Use gestures, boards, pointing, pictures, and writing if the person cannot communicate by speaking
- Encourage participation in speech therapy sessions

   B. Tube feedings (show poster)
   Often, individuals have difficulty swallowing after a stroke. These per-

sons also often have aphasia from the weakened musculature required to talk and eat. A tube (either a nasogastric tube, which goes through the nose, or a gastrostomy tube, which goes right into the stomach) may be inserted to provide the patient with proper nutrition while he or she is recovering the use of muscles needed to eat without aspirating (choking) food or liquids into the lungs. (Show physical structures on poster, and point out location of feeding tubes, airway, and esophagus.)

The speech therapist and radiologist determine how well a person swallows by looking at the swallowing during what we call a "cookie swallow." During this test, the person is asked to eat or drink different forms of barium and this process is watched through special x-rays. This helps the doctor decide the exact problem and what kind of food that person could safely eat or whether a tube needs to be placed. Most feeding tubes are temporary. The nurse will be happy to answer individual questions for those who would like more information about this.

III. Improving self-image
   A. Emotional changes
      There are many common emotions associated with a loss. Some reactions to loss include feelings of denial, guilt, anguish, sadness, longing, depression, despair, irritability, anxiety, and tension. Often these emotions coincide with physiological reactions such as crying, weight loss, weakness, shortness of breath, nervousness, restlessness, sleeplessness, loss of sexual desire, a tendency to sigh, physical exhaustion, and heart palpitations.
   B. Sexuality
      Sexuality involves how you feel about yourself. Some stroke patients say they don't feel like the same person; some family members say that their loved one is not the same. Remember that things are *not* the same. A crisis has occurred that has changed your lives. However, the goal of rehabilitation is to help you and your family adapt to the changes that have occurred and to move on from here.
   C. Promoting a positive self-image
      There are many ways to help the pa-

tient feel better about himself or herself. The following are some suggestions to promote a positive self-image:
1. Good grooming—A neat appearance tends to make one feel better. Wearing your own clothes instead of a hospital gown or pajamas encourages readiness to face the day. Cleanliness of hair and nails, and morning shaving for men, are encouraged. Women should wear jewelry and apply makeup as they did before. Family members can help a lot in this area.
2. Bowel/bladder training—Encouraging a patient to use the toilet instead of wearing absorbent devices helps promote a positive self-image. Incontinence is a common problem and was discussed in Session 3.
3. Provide privacy—This demonstrates concern and respect for the individual. Close doors and pull curtains as needed. Treat others as you would like to be treated.
4. Be understanding—Allow the patient to vent frustrations. Realize that all individuals need to have some sense of control over their life. Encourage the individual to make simple choices. Above all, exercise patience.
5. Express your own feelings—Closeness can be achieved in many ways. There are many other forms of physical closeness in addition to sexual intercourse. Give each other permission to be a sexual being. Having a disability does not mean that previous feelings and desires are gone. The staff is happy to answer any specific questions you may have on an individual basis.
6. Use your support systems—Families and patients are encouraged to remain strong in their faith and/or previous religious practices. Don't be afraid to ask help of friends, family, and pastors or priests. Utilize your social clubs, committees, and "church family" as before to give you support during this difficult time.

Conclusion: Your relationship may change, but it doesn't have to be in a negative way. People often say that trials have brought them closer together.

IV. Sexuality after stroke
  A. Definition
    Sexuality is that part of our personality through which we express our sexual selves—our maleness or femaleness. It is influenced by our emotions and feelings, instincts and intellect, past experiences, and hope for the future.

    Sexuality does not necessarily mean intercourse. It means sharing warmth and communication. It takes place through touching, talking, hugging, kissing, or just holding hands. It has to do with love, respect, and companionship, which everyone needs. Warmth, caring, and closeness need not end because you have had a stroke or other disability.
  B. Guidelines
    You may feel unattractive or even unloved right now. It is, of course, normal to have these feelings at times. Eventually, you need to accept yourself as you are. Make the most of yourself. You are a worthy person. Your spouse or friend must remember that this is the same person he or she loved before this trauma. Each of you still has the capability to love and be loved. Communication is an important key. Talk to each other about your feelings. Family members—do not treat your loved one like an invalid or infant. Encourage social activities and get them interested in things they enjoyed before. Support their feelings. Spend as much time together as possible, even in the hospital. Do not let the person withdraw. Help him or her with personal hygiene. Use every opportunity to encourage independence.
  C. Fears about resuming sexual activities
    As you think about resuming sexual activities with your partner, you may have several fears:
    1. Fear of having another stroke or even dying during intercourse
      Suggestions: Make sure your blood pressure is under control. There is no documented evidence that intercourse will cause a stroke if the blood pressure is under control. Once your blood pressure is normal for you or controlled with medication, there is no restriction to physical activity. If you have severe heart or lung disease, take a less active role. Wait 6 weeks after cerebral hemorrhage to resume sexual activities. Check with your doctor if you have reservations about resuming.
    2. Fear of not being able to perform.
      Suggestions: There are changes following a stroke. There are also changes due to normal aging and medications. Read our booklet on these changes. Take your time and be patient with each other.
    3. Fear: How can I do anything with my side paralyzed?
      Suggestions: There are alternative positions and aids. These are discussed and demonstrated in the booklet on sexual activities after stroke.
    4. Fear of hurting your spouse or vice versa.
      Suggestions: Once again, good communication is important here. You might have to experiment on what works best for you both. Using pillows for comfort may be helpful.

Remember, the rehabilitation process may be slow. Resuming sexual activity may also take some time. If you or your spouse have any questions, please ask your nurse, social worker, or doctor. We are very open here. We don't want to offend anyone by being overly explicit in our talk today, so please take our booklet, which provides more specific suggestions, and feel free to ask questions at any time.

Session 5

(Talk given by dietitian)

TOPIC

Nutritional management and food selection

AUDIOVISUAL AIDS AND EQUIPMENT

Pamphlets (Eating Right, Climb to a Healthier Heart—from the American Heart Association)
  I. Nutritional management
 II. The truth about fats
    A. Good fats? Bad fats?
    B. Worse fats
III. Cholesterol
 IV. Menu choices
    A. Foods to avoid
    B. Foods to include
    C. Foods to use sparingly

Session 6

TOPICS

Safety, fall prevention, discharge planning, community resources

AUDIOVISUAL AIDS AND EQUIPMENT

Handouts (Home Safety Checklist, Safety and the Older Person, list of local home health agencies and transportation, Senior Wellness Program brochure)

I. Introduction to safety

Falls are one of the leading causes of death in people older than the age of 60. If not fatal, they can cause broken bones, especially hips and arms, head injuries, and of course, lengthier hospitalization. Falls are one of the main reasons our patients have to be readmitted to the hospital. Falls also cause decreased confidence, related to the fear of falling again, and increased dependence on others. This dependence can lead to institutionalization or admission to a nursing home, which we try to prevent.

II. Risk factors for falls

A. Age older than 60—This is the result of slower reflexes, decreased muscle tone, and gait changes associated with normal aging. If you are an older adult, you need to be especially careful to prevent falls, because you are more likely to suffer a broken bone or other serious injury and also take longer to heal than a younger person.

B. Previous history of falls—Determine what caused you to fall before, so that you can try to prevent it from happening again. Research shows that those who have fallen once are more likely to fall again.

C. Seizures—Having a seizure can cause a fall. About 10% of stroke patients have seizures. If you have this problem, you may be taking medication to prevent seizures. Be sure to follow your doctor and nurse's instructions to control this problem.

D. Balancing problems—This is common after stroke and other disabilities. Get up slowly and make sure you have your balance before rising.

E. Sensation—Lack of sensation or feeling in the stroke side can contribute to falls.

F. Weakness or paralysis—This can cause poor balance.

G. Decreased endurance—Being tired can make one more prone to falls.

H. Inability to understand or follow directions.

I. Impulsiveness—This is a problem after stroke, especially with left-sided weakness. Those with right-sided stroke (left weakness) may always be in a hurry with little regard for safety. Persons may overestimate their ability to walk alone.

J. Impaired memory or judgment—Some persons may have poor judgment or be forgetful of safety precautions.

K. Lack of familiarity to surroundings—People fall more often when the room is changed or they are put in the hospital or nursing home.

L. Dizziness—This may be related to heart problems or postural hypotension. This occurs especially in people taking blood pressure medications or after prolonged bedrest. It happens when you get up from a lying position, become dizzy, and may pass out. Always get up slowly and sit on the edge of the bed before standing.

M. Afraid to call for help—Some people do not use the call light because they are hesitant to ask for or accept help. Remember the staff is here for that purpose—to help you until you are able again to help yourself.

N. Medications—Medications may affect the balance of fluid in your body. Pills for water retention, laxatives, those for high blood pressure, and sleeping pills can make you drowsy or dizzy and cause a fall.

Falls are often associated with using the bathroom. In fact, many people fall in a hurry to get to the bathroom. Be careful at night not to trip over things. Put a commode next to the bed if needed. Most falls occur right in your own home, so you need to modify your environment for safety. Normal aging changes, disease changes, medications, and hazards in the environment all can cause falls.

III. Hospital safety

In the hospital, we try to control falls by:

A. Always locking the wheelchair—The brakes must be locked before any transfer. Learn how to lock your chair and make a habit of doing it every time you move from the chair or transfer. Also, don't try to tip your wheelchair.

B. Gait belt—We use the gait belt to assist you with walking and transferring. This gives us something to grip if you start to fall. You can take the gait belt home with you and use it there also as needed.

C. Side rails—We put up the rails on your bed when needed, because this is an unfamiliar place, and this may help remind you to call for assistance if you need to get up during the night. At home you probably won't need them, but you might want to put your bed against the wall toward your weaker side for increased safety.

D. Call light—We have a call button for you to push to call the nurse. At home you may need some method to call for help (such as a bell, a monitor, of lifeline if you are living alone).

E. Night light—We have a night light in the room and cubicle. Older adults need more light to see, so you need to always have some type of night light on at home to prevent accidents.

IV. Home safety

We talked about locking your wheelchair and having a system to call for help. Remember to always rise slowly. Also, wear well-fitting shoes to aid in walking and prevent falls. Keep cords out of the way, and be careful not to trip over pets or children.

A. Stairs—Probably the most notorious for causing falls. There are several ways to make stairs more safe:

  1. Put handrails on both sides. Extend them out 12 inches beyond the step. Paint the handrails and stairs contrasting colors from the walls. Warm colors such as red, yellow, and orange are easier to see.

  2. Have good lighting on the stairs. It's helpful to put a night light at the top and bottom of the stairs.

  3. Use nonskid rubber strips parallel to the edge of the stair. Nonskid rubber strips come in tape form and are available at most large hardware and home improvement centers.

  4. Put light switches at the top and bottom of steps. The switches should be a contrasting color from the walls.

B. Carpet and floors

  1. Thick pile carpet is more likely to cause a fall. Uncut low pile is best.

  2. Make sure all carpet is secure with no fringed edges.

  3. Get rid of all throw rugs. If you must have a throw rug, anchor it to the floor with double-sided adhesive tape.

  4. Put indoor/outdoor carpet in the bathroom and/or kitchen if not using tile. It absorbs water and will help cushion a fall.

  5. Make sure floors are not wet or slick. Take extra care on waxed or ceramic floors.

  6. Put nonskid strips along all doorways and thresholds.

C. Bathroom

The disabled person will tend to hang on to slippery sinks and the wall for support. The bathroom may be too small for the wheelchair or walker, and a fall can result. Some suggestions for making the bathroom safer follow:

  1. Use contrasting colored grab bars wherever needed. Put nonskid colored tape on bars. Put bars in convenient places (by the toilet and tub). Put bars on the strong side for a person with a stroke.

  2. Put nonskid tape along the sink and top of toilet. It provides a nonskid surface and easy visibility.

  3. Use a raised toilet seat.

  4. Use liquid soap dispensers that hang or attach to the wall. This can prevent a fall caused by bending over to look for the soap or slipping on soapy residue.

  5. Use a hand-held shower head, shower or tub chair, or other equipment to make showering or bathing more safe.

D. Kitchen and other rooms

  1. Chairs should have arm rests on both sides for leverage.

  2. Shelves should be between eye and hip level, unless they need to be at wheelchair level.

  3. Use a reacher for high places.

  4. Tables should have straight legs, no wheels. Push or lean against it to check stability.

E. Family support

  1. Walk around your home and look carefully at what could cause harm to your family member who has a

physical impairment. Use a checklist, and correct things to make the house more safe.

2. Observe your family member in action. Don't just ask him or her what they need.

Fall prevention is very important. Considering the consequences, it is much easier to make some changes now than to suffer later.

V. Discharge planning and community resources

A. Discharge planning

Discharge planning begins at admission. The nurse, social worker, and therapists will participate in family conferences. Attendance at these meetings is important. Be sure to write down any questions before the meeting that you may want to ask.

Before discharge, the staff will conduct a home visit to determine what equipment will be needed and to make sure the environment is accommodating to any special needs. The patient and one guest will also receive a graduation supper and diploma.

Set realistic goals. Perhaps trying to get out of the house once a week for the first month for socialization. Have a plan and at least one back-up plan. For example, if your caregiver becomes ill, who will assist you? Ask questions at any time while you are in rehabilitation; feel free to call the unit after you are discharged if other questions arise.

After discharge, try to get involved in life again. Don't just sit at home, although this may seem much easier. It takes courage to reintegrate into the community, but it will be worth it.

Be prepared. Plan ahead. Check out the situation before you go anywhere. Where are the bathrooms? Are they wheelchair/walker accessible? Are there ramps? How many stairs? Will the restaurant prepare the food to your specifications?

B. Community resources

You may return for outpatient therapy or have home health care. This hospital has a variety of services to meet your needs. (Discuss the brochures included with the Senior Wellness Program and explain the services that your hospital offers.) The stroke club meets monthly. Your nurse can give you information about upcoming meetings.

If you have to spend a lot of time at home, there are some games that can be therapeutic in several areas. These include Battleship, checkers, chess, video game systems (such as Nintendo, Sega Genesis, and the like), Scrabble, Mastermind, Yahtzee, Perfection, and card games. These games are good for eye-hand and motor coordination as well as promoting good thinking and memory skills.

Chapter 11

Promoting Independence in Persons with Neurological Disorders

■

Of particular importance to note when considering the material in this chapter is that the literature about aging in persons with some of the neurological conditions presented (such as spinal cord injury [SCI] or multiple sclerosis [MS]) or with functional limitations resulting from these conditions is sparse. The limited number of studies is due in part to the fact that until recently, people often did not live to a full average life span if such problems were incurred at a younger age. However, with the vast strides made in medical treatment and nursing care, a person with SCI, for example, may live to the normal life expectancy of an able-bodied adult (Maness, 1995). This change in life expectancy has serious implications for the health care industry in terms of the amount and quality of care that will be needed for these individuals throughout their life span and into old age. Discussions, case studies, and research data regarding those who have lived much of their lives with chronic illness and functional disabilities are sorely needed and will surely be forthcoming. The purpose of this chapter is to give gerontological rehabilitation nurses (GRNs) the necessary information to provide assistance in maintaining independence and quality of life to those who have experienced the onset of common neurological disorders or injuries later in life or who have lived many years with the deficits left by such conditions.

Many neurologically based disorders affect older adults. Although stroke could be placed into this category, the significant numbers of cerebral vascular accident survivors seen in gerontological rehabilitation warranted a separate chapter. However, in this section, several specific problems will be discussed: SCI, Parkinson's disease (PD), MS, Guillain-Barré syndrome (GBS), lupus, and traumatic brain injury (TBI). Although some of these disorders are not problems that usually originate in old age, those who experience them are now living to achieve old age because of better medical care, as well as technological advances. The discovery of improved and more effective medications has been another factor enhancing both quality and length of life for those in whom these conditions are diagnosed. Yet, as life is prolonged, complications arise from the combination of aging and functional impairments or disabilities.

For nurses working strictly with an older population, discussion of SCI may seem irrelevant. Yet more and more persons with SCI are being cared for in long-term care facilities. Also of importance is that elders are remaining more active than in previous decades and engaging in a variety of activities that put them at increased risk for injury. It is not unusual to see those over age 60 riding motorcycles, flying small airplanes, horseback riding, driving race cars, snowmobiling, driving all-terrain vehicles, scuba diving, skiing, or participating in other hobbies that could be potentially harmful. The number of elders involved in motor vehicle accidents suggests that traumatic injury from even usual daily activities is likely to require GRNs to deal with problems previously thought to be mainly confined to the younger population.

Other causes of spinal injury among the

elderly may include spinal tumors or spinal cord infarction. Paraplegia may also be due to transverse myelitis or be secondary to surgery such as abdominal aneurysm repair. Various degrees of paralysis may also been seen from spinal degeneration or stenosis or as a complication after laminectomies or other back operations. The signs and symptoms seen in such cases may be similar, but with a more variable prognosis than seen in individuals with complete cord transection. As the population ages, these various causes of SCI may become more prevalent.

As a review and update, major signs, symptoms, and treatments will be discussed here. Additionally, nursing interventions and implications will be presented in the context of aging, along with the disabilities that may be caused by each disorder.

SPINAL CORD INJURY

SCI results in the loss of many motor and sensory functions and thus leads to a decrease in the ability to care for oneself. The most common cause of SCI is trauma, including car accidents, falls, and diving accidents. Young adults and those in their late teens are the group most often seen with SCI. For individuals under age 50, the most common cause of SCI is an automobile accident, but for those over 50, falls are more frequently to blame. Elders who survive SCI are more likely to suffer incomplete injuries, especially injury to the cervical spine (Gokbudak, 1985; McGlinchey-Berroth, Morrow, Ahlquist, Sarkarati, & Minaker, 1995).

Two general issues are important to consider when discussing nursing treatment of SCI in older adults: the time passed since the injury and the effects of aging related to the effects of the injury. For an older adult who experiences SCI as an elder, little research discussing differences in adaptation or adjustment has been performed inasmuch as studies on SCI have focused largely on younger adults and teens. However, some recent research includes a study by Pentland, McColl, and Rosenthal (1995) on the effect of aging and the duration of disability on long-term health outcomes after SCI. These researchers found that with increasing age, persons with SCI experienced more fatigue, decreased activity, and greater overall life satisfaction. The duration of SCI had a significantly negative effect on subjects' feelings of financial security and the number of illnesses experienced. The effects of age and the duration of SCI interact

such that advanced age and longer time since injury increase the perception of financial insecurity and threats to health.

Krause and Crewe (1991) concluded that the relationship between aging and adjustment to SCI was complex and influenced by multiple factors associated with aging. These researchers found that activity was strongly correlated with chronological age but that medical stability was more strongly related to the time since injury, with both of these measures being correlated with aspects of life satisfaction. DeVivo, Stover, and Black (1992) found that age was a prognostic factor for long-term survival after SCI (in addition to other factors such as the level of the lesion and completeness of injury). That is, adults age 50 and older with complete quadriplegia had the highest mortality rates among those with spinal injuries.

Trauma to the spinal cord results in damage that can be permanent or temporary, depending on the type of injury sustained. SCI has a devastating impact on the person and family. Permanent paralysis and dependence on others cause the person to deal with self-esteem issues, in addition to many physical problems, and to use coping mechanisms that may be poorly developed with respect to adjusting to this life-altering event. When the person is unable to perform the actual activities needed to sustain life and yet has intact cognitive function, skills will still need to be learned but will emphasize the person's ability to *direct* care. That is, although such individuals may not be able to perform the functional movements needed to meet many of their physical needs, they use their knowledge and expertise to instruct others on how to best assist them. The ability to direct their own care requires that they be taught, an important part of the GRN's role in working with the spinal cord–injured population.

Elders and younger adults who sustain spinal injury will require similar knowledge about home management, but elders might be more likely to be discharged to an extended care facility, depending on their support system and resources. The amount of care required for a person with a complete cervical injury, for example, could overwhelm an elderly caregiver spouse.

An elder has already begun to adjust to the aging process, so the recovery process after SCI will take precedence in teaching. However, an elder generally has less respiratory and cardiac reserve capacity, as well as decreased muscle strength, and may have pre-existing chronic problems such as arthritis with limitations on joint mobility, which generally makes recovery slower and more difficult. Loss of muscle mass, decreased ability to build new muscle secondary to decreased hormone production, and loss of relative upper body strength are additional complicating factors for elderly adults with SCI. Indeed, older adults with SCI have been found to commonly experience several conditions, including carpal tunnel syndrome, chronic obstructive pulmonary disease, myocardial infarction, hypertension, diabetes, kidney stones, and pressure ulcers, with the last three complications most directly related to aging with SCI instead of aging as an isolated factor (McGlinchey-Berroth et al., 1995).

If a person sustains an SCI as a teenager and lives to old age, many years are available to adjust to the effects of the injury, and such longevity testifies to successful adaptation. The emphasis on nursing care will then be on teaching about the effects of aging. The presence of spinal cord damage may "add years" to the body from the excess wear and tear that would otherwise not normally be present, and thus such individuals might seem to age more rapidly. These individuals, then, may be adjusting more to the effects of aging than to the previous injury. Table 11–1 presents areas that will be particularly affected by the combination of aging and SCI for either of the aforementioned situations.

Currently, medical research is examining prevention of secondary damage caused by trauma to the spinal cord through the use of new medications. Methylprednisolone, if given within 8 hours of injury, results in significant improvement at 6 months and 1 year postinjury and is considered standard treatment (Werner, 1997). However, many other medications that show promise in minimizing the negative results of secondary central nervous system (CSN) damage are being examined. Ideally, such medications would be given at the scene of the accident or incident as soon as possible after injury inasmuch as a major purpose of these medications is to limit the extent and severity of the damage caused by trauma. More advanced use of medications by emergency personnel on the accident scene is a possibility in the near future. Researchers will also continue to investigate regrowth of the CNS, functional improvement of partially injured areas of the CNS, and bypass of sites of injury or the use of electrical therapy to stimulate the spinal cord or peripheral nerves (Werner, 1997).

Anatomy and Physiology

The CNS is composed of the brain and spinal cord. The peripheral nervous system has 12 pairs of cranial nerves and 31 pairs of spinal nerves. Each spinal nerve has a dorsal and ventral root. The dorsal (afferent) root controls sensory stimuli and proceeds out of the spinal cord nearer the back of the spinous process. The ventral (efferent) root coordinates motor impulses and originates out of the cord more proximally. At the end of the spinal cord, the lumbar and sacral spinal nerves develop long roots. Together these roots are called the cauda equina (meaning horse's tail because of its resemblance).

The spinal cord system is the mechanism by which impulses are transmitted from the body to the brain. The spinal cord is a clustering of spinal nerves encased in and protected by 33 vertebrae that run from the base of the brain to the tip of the sacrum. These vertebrae are divided into five sections: cervical (7), thoracic (12), lumbar (5), sacral (5), and coccygeal (4).

Several cerebral spinal tracts are also present, each with a specialized function. Knowledge of these tracts aids in understanding the variations of sensory and motor function seen in SCI. The corticospinal tract is associated with voluntary motor function. The spinothalamic tract carries pain and temperature sensations. The dorsal columns and posterior tract relay position, vibration, deep touch, and proprioception.

The autonomic nervous system is activated mainly by centers in the spinal cord, brain stem, and hypothalamus and has two divisions: sympathetic and parasympathetic. These two branches have an antagonistic relationship that is necessary to maintain the balance of bodily functions. The sympathetic system (thoracolumbar) is activated by the stress response and helps in "flight or fight" situations. Sympathetic nerve fibers come from the spinal cord to join the sympathetic chain in the thoracic and lumbar areas. The parasympathetic (craniosacral) system regulates the activities of involuntary muscles and has a more homeostatic function that focuses on conservation, restoration, and maintenance. Fibers in this system leave the spinal cord with cranial nerves III (oculomotor), VII (facial), IX (glossopharyngeal), and X (vagus).

The signs and symptoms seen in SCI occur from damage to the spinal cord. Impulses that were previously relayed from the body through the spinal cord to the brain have

Table 11–1   AREAS PARTICULARLY AFFECTED BY THE COMBINATION OF AGING AND SPINAL CORD INJURY

System	Effects
Skin integrity	Loss of subcutaneous fat with age and decreased perspiration associated with vessel atrophy; increased bony prominences; pooling of fluid in tissues; more fragile dermis leading to an increased susceptibility to pressure sores, especially with paralysis
Temperature control	Elders often experience intolerance to temperature extremes; may have PVD with advanced age; persons with SCI also have an interruption in relay of messages to the brain—may burn more easily, intolerant of extremes in temperature
Range of motion	Joints become more stiff with age and ROM may decrease; SCI may further limit ROM or produce paralysis in already compromised extremities
Muscle and bone mass	Some muscle atrophy with age; females lose bone mass because of osteoarthritis; with SCI, additional loss of calcium from bone because of non–weight bearing; may have muscle atrophy from disuse
Gastric motility	Decreased motility with age; further slowing with immobility after SCI
Sensory perception	Visual acuity and hearing losses all common with aging; may have impaired sensation to light touch; complete SCI may result in no sensory function below the level of the lesion; incomplete SCI varies in sensory deficit
Bowel and bladder function	Elders are often constipated and may have increased urinary frequency or incontinence; SCI results in neurogenic bowel/bladder dysfunction: constipation, alterations in perception of bladder fullness, lack of voluntary control, inability to empty completely, incontinence
Cardiopulmonary function	Cardiac output decreases with age and peripheral resistance increases; less efficient respiration with age (decreased O_2 and increased CO_2); with SCI, blood pressure often decreases, venous stasis can lead to DVTs; subsequent effects on respiratory muscles lead to a further decrease in tidal volume and an inability to cough effectively or manage pulmonary secretions
Nutritional requirements/ metabolism	Metabolism slows with age, as well as with inactivity as in SCI; nutritional requirements are similar: high protein, high roughage/ fiber; plenty of fluids, vitamins, minerals
Renal function	Decreased number of functioning nephrons and decreased glomerular filtration rate with age; those with SCI need frequent renal studies because a neurogenic bladder can lead to hydronephrosis, calculi, reflux
Sexuality/sexual function	Frequency of sexual activity may decrease with advanced age; males with SCI are affected more than females because the ability to achieve an erection varies according to the level and extent of injury; may have total or partial sensory loss after SCI
Self-image/self-esteem	Often poor in the elderly, especially those with depression, or the institutionalized aged; SCI contributes to feelings of dependency, helplessness, depression

PVD, peripheral vascular disease; SCI, spinal cord injury; ROM, range of motion; DVT, deep venous thrombosis.

been interrupted. Prognosis and functional recovery are related to a variety of factors that are discussed in the following sections.

Complete Versus Incomplete Injuries

Three factors are of primary importance for the GRN to note on admission and before the initiation of any activities for persons with SCI. These factors include the completeness of injury, the level of injury, and whether the spine is stabilized. Each of these issues will be discussed in further detail here.

The first question GRNs should ask themselves when working with an elder with SCI is whether the lesion is complete or incomplete. Complete SCI means that the spinal cord is completely transected, destroyed, or irreversibly damaged. Such injury results in permanent motor and sensory loss below the level of injury. Increased age combined with complete quadriplegia results in greater mortality rates, thus suggesting that the prognosis is poor for older persons with complete SCI (DeVivo et al., 1992; McGlinchey-Berroth et al., 1995). At the time of this writing, no reversal or cure for complete SCI is known.

An incomplete injury means that some of the spinal cord has been spared. The end result cannot be predicted as easily because of the minuteness of the nerves and difficulty in determining the extent of trauma. Recovery may even be total with no residual effects, depending on the location and degree of damage and whether treatment is instituted quickly and efficiently. Great variation in motor and sensory function can be seen in individuals with incomplete injuries, and functional outcomes are more difficult to predict, although the prognosis is more hopeful than with complete injuries.

Recognizing the Level of Injury

Levels of injury are determined by the location in the spinal cord. Abbreviations are used for each of the five areas of the spinal cord, and the area involved is assigned a number. The GRN should realize that although only one level may be attributed to a person's injury, functional abilities may relate to adjacent levels. For example, if a person has a C4 injury, some movement may still be noted that a person with C5 injury typically might have. Physicians may diagnose a C4–C5 injury, which captures a better picture of the patient's functional status. Of course, functional status also depends on the nature and

cause of the injury. Table 11–2 gives an overview of the types of functions expected at different levels of SCI.

The Frankel Scale was frequently used to indicate the presence or absence of motor and sensory activity below the level of the injury. A modification of the Frankel Scale is the American Spinal Injury Association Impairment Scale. Function is graded into five categories labeled A through E (Table 11–3). Physicians may use this tool to help specify the diagnosis, so GRNs should be alert to the meanings of each category. Table 11–4 provides definitions of clinical syndromes involving the spinal cord.

Spinal shock is a period immediately after SCI in which the body becomes flaccid, largely because of the immediate effects of trauma, including swelling. Thus, even those with incomplete injuries may seem to be paralyzed below the level of the injury in the first days after the trauma. The bladder and bowels may be flaccid. Once swelling of the cord has subsided, which can take from hours to weeks, a clearer picture of the functional prognosis can be obtained for those with incomplete injuries. Reflex activity generally returns more quickly in individuals with incomplete lesions (Pires, 1996).

It is necessary to assume, upon initial trauma, that the spine needs to be stabilized to prevent further injury. Nurses will recall that emergency medical personnel always apply a cervical collar when head or neck injury is even remotely suspected. This practice provides temporary stabilization to the spine so that further trauma does not occur. The collar will remain in place until diagnostic testing is completed.

Maintaining Spinal Stability

Again, it is essential that the GRN be informed about the completeness or incompleteness of the injury. A person with a confirmed complete injury who is entering the post-acute treatment phase will probably not have a brace. Someone with an incomplete injury should most definitely have a brace or some other type of immobilizer to stabilize the spine. Failure to immobilize an incomplete fracture of the spinal cord can create a complete lesion and subsequent total paralysis.

The GRN should be aware that good communication between the facility from which the person is transferring and the admitting facility must be maintained. Some patients

Table 11-2 FUNCTIONAL LEVELS ASSOCIATED WITH THE LEVEL OF INJURY

Level (Neural)	Muscle Control	Functional Goals	Attendant Care
C1–C3	Limited neck control	Respiratory function dependent on mechanical ventilation or phrenic nerve stimulators. Limited wheelchair mobility in Sipp 'N Puff chair, mouthstick activities, page turner, environmental controls, typewriter, computer	Requires full-time, 24-hr care
C4	Neck control, scapular elevators, diaphragm, trapezius	Wheelchair mobility with Sipp 'N Puff chair. Limited feeding possible with ball bearing feeders, mouthstick activities, page turner, typewriter, computer, environmental controls	Requires 8–12 hr of attendant care
C5	Deltoids, fair to good shoulders, biceps, elbow flexion	Manual wheelchair with quad tips for short smooth surfaces, electric wheelchair for outside or long distances. Needs assist with transfers. May be able to do weight shifts. Self-feeding with splints; operates typewriter, telephone, computer, etc., with assistive devices	Requires 6–8 hr, probably in the morning and evening
C6	Dorsiflexion, wrist extension	Able to propel wheelchair with quad tips, may need electric wheelchair for long distances, sliding board transfers with or without assist. Able to feed self with assistive device, bathe and dress upper extremities. May need assist with lower extremities. May drive with hand controls. Able to write with splints	May need 2–4 hr of attendant care

Level	Muscles	Functional goals	Attendant care
C7–C8	Weak shoulder depression; weak triceps, elbow extension, finger flexion, extension, and abduction	Independent with transfers, feeding, bathing, dressing, and bowel and bladder care. May need assistance with floor-to-chair transfers. Able to drive with hand controls	Probably will not need attendant care
T1–T2	Intrinsics	Fine motor skills involving fingers	No attendant care unless limiting factors are present
T3–T10	Intact upper extremities. Partial to good trunk balance	Independent wheelchair skills, including ramps and curbs. Independent in all transfers. Able to drive with hand controls	
T12–L2	Hip flexors	Emergency ambulation: able to ambulate a few steps with long leg orthoses and crutches. May ambulate short distances in home with long leg orthoses and crutches	
L2–L4	Hip abductors	Total ambulation with short leg orthoses, with or without crutches	
L5–S3	Movement of ankle and toes	Total ambulation without assistive devices	
S2–S4	Perineal musculature, bowel, bladder, sex organs. Movement of large toe	Management of elimination through specific bowel and bladder programs	

Every injury is different; therefore, these functional goals should be viewed only as general guidelines.

Matthews, P., & Carlson, C. (Eds.) (1987). *Spinal cord injury: Rehabilitation Institute of Chicago procedure manual* (Chap. 5). Rockville, MD: Aspen. © 1987 Aspen Publishers Inc.

Table 11-3 THE AMERICAN SPINAL INJURY ASSOCIATION IMPAIRMENT SCALE

A = Complete. No sensory or motor function is preserved in the sacral segments S4–S5.

B = Incomplete. Sensory but not motor function is preserved below the neurological level and includes the sacral segments S4–S5.

C = Incomplete. Motor function is preserved below the neurological level, and more than half of key muscles below the neurological level have a muscle grade less than 3.

D = Incomplete. Motor function is preserved below the neurological level, and at least half of key muscles below the neurological level have a muscle grade greater than or equal to 3.

E = Normal. Sensory and motor function is normal.

From American Spinal Injury Association. (1996 revision). *International standards for neurological classification of spinal cord injury* (pp. 18–19). Chicago: Author.

will not understand the necessity of the brace and will tell the nurses that it is only needed at certain times of the day. The exact physician orders and rationale for any immobilizer should be included on the transfer form. Stabilization of an incomplete injury is extremely important inasmuch as an incomplete injury can become complete if stability is not maintained. Maintaining spinal stability can mean the difference between a person being able to walk again or being wheelchair-bound for life. Removable braces are generally worn constantly except when lying flat in bed. They should not be taken off to shower, nor should clothing be worn underneath them, except for a T-shirt, to avoid altering the fit and function of the device. These orthotic devices are custom-fit for each person by a certified orthotist.

The length of time that the brace is worn is determined by the physician but often lasts a period of 3 months.

Several means of spinal immobilization can be used for a person with SCI. First, all movements of the patient in bed with which the nurse assists should be done by using the logrolling method. That is, the person should be turned as a unit, without twisting, and the spine, head, and neck kept in alignment. This maneuver will initially require the assistance of additional staff members. Once the patient is up and about with the appropriate spinal stabilizer in place, the nurse should still remember to use principles of body mechanics when assisting with transfers and make sure that all orthotic equipment is properly applied and fitted.

Table 11-4 CLINICAL SYNDROMES OF THE SPINAL CORD

Central cord syndrome
    A lesion occurring almost exclusively in the cervical region that produces sacral sensory sparing and greater weakness in the upper limbs than in the lower limbs

Brown-Sequard syndrome
    A lesion that produces relatively greater ipsilateral proprioceptive and motor loss and contralateral loss of sensitivity to pain and temperature

Anterior cord syndrome
    A lesion that produces variable loss of motor function and sensitivity to pain and temperature while preserving proprioception

Conus medullaris syndrome
    Injury of the sacral cord (conus) and lumbar nerve roots within the spinal canal usually resulting in an areflexic bladder, bowel, and lower limbs. Sacral segments may occasionally show preserved reflexes, e.g., bulbocavernosus and micturition reflexes

Cauda equina syndrome
    Injury to the lumbosacral nerve roots within the neural canal resulting in an areflexic bladder, bowel, and lower limbs

From American Spinal Injury Association. (1996 revision.) *International standards for neurological classification of spinal cord injury* (pp. 19, 21). Chicago: Author.

Immobilization of the head and neck is needed when a cervical fracture occurs, especially a high lesion. Such immobilization requires *skeletal traction* to achieve stabilization and reduce the risk of further injury. Several means of achieving this end are possible and vary with the type of injury. The person may require cervical tongs, which are points placed in the temporal bone with weights applied to maintain steady traction. This treatment will necessitate complete bedrest, and the person will be dependent on the nurse or other caregiver for all basic needs because of the immobilization. The *halo device* also provides skeletal fixation to the cervical region. The halo brace can now be incorporated with a body vest or jacket so that many persons can be discharged from acute care and ambulate. However, the head is completely immobilized, so the person would be unable to drive a car or perform many other activities of daily living (ADLs). Even this limited mobility decreases the likelihood of complications from immobility. Preventing infection of the hardware insertion sites is of primary importance because this hardware goes directly into the skull bone. This brace may need to be worn as long as 3 months, so nursing teaching will be essential, and the importance of keeping follow-up appointments with the physician should be emphasized.

Braces of other kinds are also used. Hard and soft cervical collars are sometimes applied for less serious injuries to the neck area or for postsurgical stability. Two other types of braces are commonly used: the sternal occipital mandibular immobilizer (SOMI) and the thoracic lumbar sacral orthosis (TLSO).

The SOMI brace is indicated for stabilization of the cervical spine, usually for injuries that are lower than those needing a halo brace or cervical traction. The person may have undergone surgery to stabilize the spine when bones and ligaments surrounding the spinal cord have been torn or damaged. The SOMI brace, whose name describes the structures it involves, supports the neck so that healing can take place, which usually occurs in about 3 months. Supporting the head in this position relieves pressure on the spine, but the brace must be properly fitted to achieve this goal. If the person is able to turn the head or neck, the brace should be refitted. Figure 11–1 provides a picture of the brace and an example of what information should be emphasized to patients and families when per-forming discharge or home teaching about the SOMI brace.

The TLSO brace, called by some the "turtle shell" because of its appearance (Fig. 11–2), supports those with injury (or postsurgical wounds) between T6 and the sacrum. It keeps the middle to lower portion of the back immobile by preventing bending or twisting. The front and back pieces fasten at the side with Velcro-type closures or straps. The TLSO is also usually worn for about 3 months. The caregiver or a family member will have to assist the patient to help put the brace on and take it off. The brace should only be taken off to wash underneath or change the T-shirt, which must be done with the patient lying flat in bed and turning with the logrolling technique. Some physicians will allow the person to shower with the brace on, but the caregiver will have to help dry thoroughly underneath the brace afterward to avoid skin irritation and breakdown. Figure 11–2 provides an example of teaching that should be done with the patient and family.

Should it become necessary to perform cardiopulmonary resuscitation on a person with SCI who is wearing a brace, the basic principles of life sustenance continue to apply. Opening the airway, however, should be done with the jaw lift maneuver instead of a head tilt or chin lift to avoid flexing the neck. In the case of a person in skeletal traction, the brace may not interfere with chest compressions. If the person with a halo brace is mobile, however, a portion of the chest apparatus may need to be removed. The hardware for removal should always be kept close to the bedside. With the SOMI and TLSO braces, a portion of the brace may need to be removed to perform chest compressions. The top portion of the TLSO brace could be removed while leaving the bottom portion intact. Generally, the rescuers should make every attempt to maintain spinal stability while performing cardiopulmonary resuscitation.

Understanding Functional/Mobility Outcomes

For someone with an incomplete SCI, spinal stability is one of the most important measures to promote later mobility (Case Study 11.1). Such a person may regain complete range of motion and ambulatory function. When an individual has a complete SCI, however, certain functional outcomes can reasonably be expected from the level of injury and muscle control. These outcomes are summa-

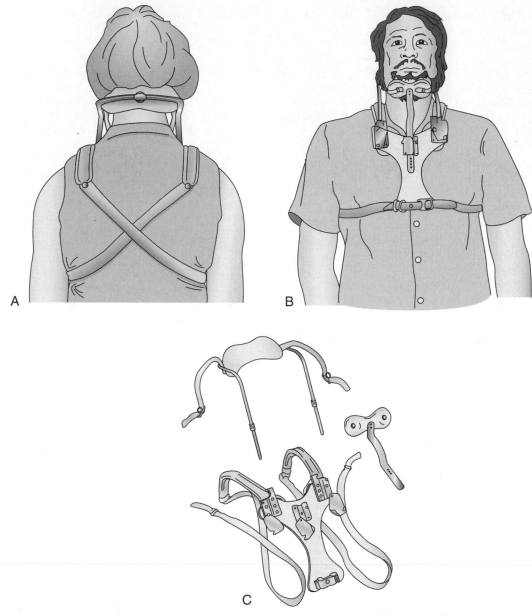

- The *only* clothing you are allowed to wear under your brace is a T-shirt. **Do not** pad your brace with towels or other articles.
- Never place a pillow under your head when you are lying flat. Pillows will move your head forward into a position that may alter the stability of the cervical spine. This will cause your head to tilt forward, resulting in pressure on the chin. You may use the flat cushion given to you at the hospital.
- Remove your brace only to bathe. *You must be lying completely flat in bed to remove your brace.*
- Before your discharge, a nurse will teach you and a family member how to apply and remove the brace. Please feel free to ask for help as needed so that you feel comfortable using the brace.
- Do not drive until the brace is removed. While in the brace, you will not be able to fully turn your head from side to side.
- Do not attempt to bend or lift objects more than 10 pounds.
- Lakeshore Orthotics and Prosthetics will fit you in your brace during your hospital stay. The cost of the brace will be added to your hospital bill.

Figure 11–1 Sternal occipital mandibular immobilizer (SOMI) brace instructions. (Used with permission of Northwestern Memorial Hospital Home Care Department, Chicago, IL.)

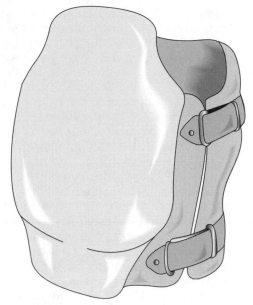

- Always wear your TLSO, even at night. This is very important!
- Wear only a T-shirt or body shirt (made for you) under your TLSO.
- Your brace is custom-molded by a certified orthotist. This ensures that your TLSO fits snugly.
- Remove your TLSO only to wash underneath or change your T-shirt. You must lie flat in bed to remove the brace. Keep your back flat and straight, and turn in a log roll fashion.
- Your brace may get wet. If your doctor allows it, you may shower in your TLSO. *Remember to dry thoroughly under your brace.*
- If your brace is rubbing against your skin and causing redness or irritation, or if you lose weight, the brace may need to be adjusted. Call your orthotist.
- Do not attempt to bend or lift objects more than 10 pounds.
- The cost of your TLSO will be added to your hospital bill.

Figure 11–2 Thoracic lumbar sacral orthosis (TLSO) brace and instructions. (Used with permission of Northwestern Memorial Hospital Home Care Department, Chicago, IL.)

rized in Table 11–2. Every injury and person is unique, so functional goals may vary somewhat, and the information given here should be used only as a guideline.

CASE STUDY 11.1
The Elder with Spinal Cord Injury

James Smith was a 75 year old retired carpenter who fell off a step ladder while repairing the gutters on his house. He sustained an incomplete C5–C6 spinal cord injury and a fractured left wrist, which was put in a cast. His medical history included secondary diagnoses of arthritis, mild hypertension controlled with diet, emphysema, nocturia, and bilateral cataract surgery 2 years previously. Mr. Smith was in the acute care hospital for 10 days before transferring to rehabilitation for more intensive therapy. His spine was stabilized with a SOMI brace. Mr. Smith's support system included his wife Norma, age 72, and two adult daughters who lived nearby. Complicating his recovery were problems with shortness of breath and dizziness, as well as Mr. Smith's refusal to call for help at night for assistance with toileting. His arthritis also made ambulating painful at times and increased his risk for falls. On the rehabilitation unit his blood pressure was found to be elevated, so diuretic therapy was started, which further increased his risk of falls related to safety and toileting needs. The GRN's assessment of Mr. Smith's situation revealed his high value of independence and his pride in being able to take care of things by himself. The GRN identified key areas for teaching such as maintaining spinal stability, preventing injury, alternating rest and activity, recognizing medication effects, and identifying how Mr. Smith's would meet his self-care requisites. The nurse also determined that Mr. Smith had an internal locus of control and displayed characteristics of hardiness. Nursing care and teaching were planned with this point in mind. The GRN instructed the wife, daughters, and Mr. Smith about the importance of preventing further injury to the spine, which could even result in paralysis. The GRN presented this aspect of care as a challenge and one for which Mr. Smith could be in control. Once Mr. Smith understood that his brace was there for his protection and what could happen if he fell again or compromised his spinal stability, Mr. Smith seemed more accepting of assistance and assumed control of preserving his spinal function. He began to use the call light more often and relied on his wife and daughters for help, saying, "This is only temporary." The effect of the diuretic on the bladder and Mr. Smith's desire to get up alone to use the bathroom were remedied by his agreement to use the urinal at night in bed when he went home so that his wife could get a good night's rest. His shortness of breath seemed to improve after diuretic therapy was started. The nurse helped his daughters arrange a schedule of providing respite care for their mother to do shopping or attend her church ladies group. They also volunteered to keep their parents' house clean. Women from the Smiths' church arranged to help with meals for the first week after Mr. Smith's discharge home. Mr. Smith was able to be discharged home within 2 weeks of admission to the rehabilitation unit and completed his recovery at home.

The terms *quadriplegia* and *paraplegia* are frequently used to describe function after SCI. Tetraplegia is often used synonymously with quadriplegia. According to *The New Webster's Medical Dictionary* (1992), quadriplegia is generally described as "paralysis affecting all four limbs" (p. 202). Paraplegia is defined as "paralysis of the lower trunk and the lower limbs" (p. 175). Some liberality should be applied to these terms. A layperson may consider a quadriplegic to be someone who is paralyzed from the neck down. Yet many quadriplegics have some upper extremity movement (see Table 11–2) but not full functional use. The *Core Curriculum* (third edition) from the Rehabilitation Nursing Foundation (Fried, 1993) makes the definitions more explicit. Quadriplegia in this book is described as usually occurring "as a result of injuries at T1 or above." When cervical segments are damaged, loss of motor and sensory function results in impairment in function of the arms, trunk, legs, and reproductive organs in the pelvis. Paraplegia results from injuries at T2 and below, which causes sensory and functional impairment of the trunk and lower half of the body. So one could generalize that those with injuries at C1 to T1 may be described as quadriplegics. Those with injuries at T2 and below are paraplegics.

For all persons recovering from or adapting to SCI, the principles of promoting mobility and functional independence as discussed in Chapter 7 should be practiced. Logrolling should still be used for turning the person in bed. Wheelchair leans and pushups should be taught by the GRN and then practiced regularly by the patient. A trapeze is often used for those with upper extremity strength and function to help with bed mobility.

Several problems complicated by increasing age are common after SCI. Musculoskeletal changes take place from immobility. Bones may lose calcium, and muscles of paralyzed limbs become atrophied. Skeletal malalignment can occur. Joints may be stiffened and muscles weakened. These changes sound similar to those that occur with aging. Consider, however, that a person may have lived with this condition for decades and now the body has begun normal aging changes in addition. This situation would seem to put a paralyzed elder at double risk of complications.

Spasticity is a frequent complaint of persons with SCI. Spasms of the muscles, particularly in the lower extremities, are common. They can be an incapacitating complication of quadriplegia or paraplegia (Toth, 1983). Often aggravated by activity, muscle spasms can interfere with therapy. Sometimes spasticity of the muscles is severe enough that contractures can begin and necessitate casting or splinting. It will be important for the GRN to teach the family that the person cannot control these spasms. It may be disturbing for the family to observe uncontrollable spasms in the lower portion of the person's leg, but they should be informed that medications are frequently helpful in managing spasticity. The application of cold/heat, use of relaxation techniques and biofeedback, or electrical stimulation has been used with some success. The most common medications used include benzodiazepines, especially diazepam (Valium), dantrolene sodium (Dantrium), and baclofen (Lioresal) (Toth, 1983).

Contractures pose another impediment to functional independence after SCI. Because normal motor function has been altered, the normal flexor and extensor actions are not kept in check. When the muscle is inactive, flexors will tend to pull the body inward because they are stronger than the extensors, and contractures result. This type of curling up of the muscles and joints occurs frequently in the hands, arms, and feet. If left unchecked, an immobile person would eventually draw up into a fetal position. The nurse combats these effects by using splints, performing range-of-motion exercises, assisting with proper positioning, and promoting activity.

It is essential that the GRN implement measures to prevent contractures in a person with SCI for several reasons. First, contractures result in loss of function and thus contribute to the inability to dress, self-feed, transfer, or ambulate. Pain is also associated with contractures, as is skin breakdown. Loss of self-esteem follows such interruptions in an already compromised person's capacity for self-care. Activity must be maintained to avoid these complications after SCI.

Promoting Adequate Respiration

One of the major causes of death in those with SCI is respiratory complications. It is important to remember that for any older person with SCI above the T12 level, respiratory care will be of primary concern. Generally, the higher the level of the lesion, the greater the respiratory compromise (Gausch, Linder, Williams, & Ryan, 1991). GRNs must remember that in an older adult, the amount of useful oxygen is already decreased and the strength of accessory breathing muscles is generally weakened, so SCI puts them at extreme risk for respiratory problems, especially pneumonia.

Many of these individuals would not have survived the initial trauma of their injuries were it not for immediate life-saving interventions. With greater numbers of persons in the community being certified in cardiopulmonary resuscitation techniques and activation of the emergency medical system, more people with serious injuries are being saved. Because such was not the case decades ago, the issue of aging with severe functional limitations did not warrant as much attention as it does today.

Table 11–2 also summarizes some respiratory implications resulting from SCI. For those with cervical injury between C1 and C3, mechanical ventilation is required. The person will have a tracheotomy and be dependent on a ventilator. Decreased chest movement and lower volumes of air exchange will be the rule. If the phrenic nerve remains intact, the person may be a candidate for a phrenic nerve stimulator. This device acts much like a pacemaker does: diaphragmatic movement is stimulated to achieve a certain number of breaths per minute. Electrodes are surgically implanted over the phrenic nerve along with an activator. The transmitter device is inserted under the skin similar to a pacemaker, yet it serves the same function as a ventilator so that the person can be free of the ventilator for varying amounts of time. Gradual tolerance must be built up to use the pacer for a long length of time, although some individuals use it full-time by alternating the stimulation of phrenic nerves to give each nerve the required rest period after use (Larson, Johnson, & Angst, 1996). Batteries in the phrenic nerve stimulator should be changed daily, and a backup plan in case of failure of the pacer should be specified.

The GRN should remember that although the person may be maintained on a ventilator, communication in the form of speech is still often possible. However, instead of speaking during expiration as would usually occur, a person on a ventilator talks during inspiration; the air pushed into the lungs over the vocal cords by the ventilator allows speech to be produced. In speaking with a ventilator-dependent person, time must be allowed for responses during the conversation. Remember that the individual may receive only a set amount of breaths per minute (say 10 to 12) from the machine, so pauses should be expected within sentences while the patient waits for the next breath. Talking contributes to a sense of normalcy, which is greatly needed by persons who have no other control over their bodily functions. It also lets them make their needs and wishes known. The role of the speech therapist will be particularly important in the care plan of a person learning to speak while maintained on the ventilator. GRNs should encourage the development of speaking techniques for those who are ventilator dependent but be aware that these techniques may be exhausting for such patients, so periods of rest should be incorporated as they practice and learn what works best for them. Augmentative devices for communication should also be considered for persons with tetraplegia.

For persons with C4–C5 SCI, a tracheotomy will be needed at first. The diaphragm is functional, but other major muscles that assist with respiration are involved (Gausch et al., 1991). The patient will not have a strong cough and thus will have difficulty clearing the lungs. Assistance will be needed with coughing and deep breathing. Respiratory treatments will be needed daily.

Patients with a C6–T1 injury will also have a decreased ability to cough and deep-breathe but will not need a tracheotomy. However, because of the lack of a strong cough in addition to weak accessory muscles, the risk for respiratory infection remains high, and daily treatments should continue.

The T2 to T8 level controls the motor function of the intercostal and thoracic muscles, great determinants of proper respiratory function. Those with thoracic injuries between T2 and T5 are at increased risk for respiratory compromise but are more independent and probably require no attendant care unless other limiting factors are present (Matthews & Carlson, 1987). It will be particularly important for the GRN to teach these individuals the importance of respiratory care because the absence of a caregiver to remind or supervise them may put them at risk for subsequent hospitalizations related to respiratory problems. Devices such as incentive spirometers can be sent home with the person at discharge, and use on a regular basis is encouraged.

Persons with injuries at T6 to T12 have the major muscles of breathing intact, including the abdominal and accessory muscles, and do not require daily respiratory programs. However, a strong cough reflex is still not present, so the risk of infection remains high.

In addition to the services of the respiratory therapist, the GRN will need to promote good pulmonary hygiene habits for the period after discharge or for stay in a long-term care facility. Respiratory care may include the need for suctioning and postural drainage. Breathing exercises such as those used with an incentive spirometer should be encouraged for all SCI patients. Assisted cough is indicated for those with higher-level injuries and is achieved by placing the hands on the abdomen below the ribs but above the umbilicus. As the patient attempts to cough, the nurse assists by pushing gently inward and upward to facilitate the compression movement of the diaphragm. Similarly, with assisted deep breathing, the nurse can use the same position to perform what looks like a slow-motion Heimlich maneuver, or the hands can be carefully placed on the outer portion of the rib cage and gentle pressure applied on exhalation to assist with fuller expiration. This latter method should be used with caution in an older adult because the brittleness of bones from osteoporosis could cause fractures, even with small amounts of pressure. A recent method to produce cough is electrical stimulation of the abdominal muscles. In one study this technique was found to be about as effective as manually assisted coughs (Jaeger, Turba, Yarkony, & Roth, 1993). However, long-term studies are needed to further evaluate the practicality and efficacy of this technique in the SCI population.

Another technique that can be used for those not requiring mechanical ventilation but at risk for respiratory complications is to teach the person to recognize normal movements of the diaphragm and related structures. Such recognition is best learned with the person lying flat in bed. The person's hand is placed on the abdomen below the ribs, but above the umbilicus. As the person inhales, the abdomen should rise. Upon exhalation, the abdomen should go back down. Likewise, the rib cage can be felt to expand and contract. Teaching awareness of these movements is a technique used by vocal coaches and teachers to promote proper abdominal breathing and results in better breath control. If a person does these exercises faithfully and concentrates on working the muscles to achieve a full and deep inspiration, the breathing muscles can be significantly strengthened. It should be noted, however, that the person must have adequate sensory and motor function to learn and perform the exercise described here.

Cardiovascular Considerations

The hazards of immobility significantly affect the cardiovascular system. Two major considerations with spinal cord–injured elders are deep vein thrombosis and orthostatic hypotension. Although these conditions are common to persons of all ages with SCI, an aged individual is at additional risk because of decreased cardiac output, atherosclerosis and arteriosclerosis, and venous stasis. Deep venous thrombosis accounts for at least 12.8% of unplanned hospitalizations of persons with SCI (Ivie & DeVivo, 1994). Additionally, pulmonary emboli develop in some patients, usually within the first few months after injury. Blood clots are so common after SCI that many physicians order prophylactic subcutaneous heparin or a low-molecular-weight heparin such as Lovenox. Heparin is often given at a dose of 5000 U subcutaneously every 12 hours. Lovenox is a more recent option and comes in a premeasured syringe of 30 mg usually given subcutaneously twice per day for the same purpose.

Other nursing measures that the GRN can expect to institute include passive range-of-motion exercises, thigh-high elastic stockings or antiembolism hose such as thromboembolic deterrent (TED) hose, leg exercises, and elevation of the lower extremities. Sequential compression devices are often used in conjunction with antiembolism hose to prevent deep venous thrombosis.

The GRN should recognize the signs and symptoms of deep venous thrombosis and must teach the client and caregiver to also be alert for them, particularly when the person may have no sensation in the lower limbs. Observation of redness, swelling, streaking, warmth, or a positive Homans' sign or palpation of hardness within the leg should be noted. More reliable measures such as calf circumference should be done in the health care facility. Treatment of a clot generally requires hospitalization and a regimen of heparin through intravenous drip. For adults without compromised sensation, a heating pad is sometimes placed under the leg, which is kept elevated, and the person will be kept on bedrest. This practice should not be used on a paralyzed individual or an older adult with impaired sensation and fragile skin. The GRN may recall from previous chapters that one of the greatest dangers of continuing therapy when a clot is present is that the clot might become dislodged, travel to another part of the body, and cause potentially fatal results (such as pulmonary embolism, myocardial infarction, stroke).

Orthostatic hypotension is also common after SCI, especially in those with injuries above T7. Patients with higher injuries may experience a significant drop in blood pressure because of the interruption in vasopressor and cardiac reflexes. Blood pooling in the lower extremities and lack of physical activity, combined with the hazards of immobility, are contributors to orthostatic hypotension. The GRN should carefully monitor blood pressure with the person in lying, standing, and sitting positions. Position changes should be made slowly. A tilt table is often used to gradually build tolerance to the upright position. TED hose may assist with promotion of circulation and prevention of venous pooling. Additionally, elastic bandage wraps, abdominal binders, or corsets may be used to decrease orthostatic hypotension. Vasopressor medications may also be given to constrict vessels and deter orthostatic hypotensive episodes.

It may be difficult to distinguish between the side effects of antihypertensive or cardiac medications and the effect of SCI on blood pressure. The average blood pressure of a quadriplegic may be about 90/50. It is common that changes in position will not be well tolerated, especially initially after injury, and will result in postural hypotension. Position changes should be made slowly, with time to dangle before rising. For an elder who is hypertensive and has an SCI, adjustments in medications may need to be made. The hypotensive effects of both the injury and the medication require frequent monitoring.

Establishing Appropriate Bowel and Bladder Programs

Elimination is a basic human need. SCI not only alters the motor and sensory stimulation needed for control of elimination but also impairs the motor function necessary to be able to engage in an alternative method of management. For example, even if a quadriplegic has an intact reflex for defecation, the hand function to insert a suppository or perform digital stimulation may be absent. This duty may fall to the caregiver, although all types of adaptive devices will be tried in attempts to promote the maximal level of self-care possible.

With the additional factor of age, other elements such as ethnic and cultural beliefs, pre-existing range-of-motion limitations, or social stigma may inhibit the person from desiring or being able to perform independent bowel evacuation. The GRN will need to complete a thorough assessment such as was discussed in Chapter 8. The bowel or bladder program chosen must fit the person's abilities, goals, and lifestyle. If the GRN formulates a program without patient input, it is likely to fail. It is good to remember here that the patient is the most important part of the rehabilitation team.

Bowel Program

The basic effect of SCI on bowel function is that the person is unable to initiate or inhibit a bowel movement. The most common complication in this area post-SCI is constipation, but diarrhea, impaction, and hemorrhoids are also frequent.

Persons with quadriplegia or those with SCI above T12–L1 (high thoracic paraplegia) have an intact reflex arc (which is contained at the S2–S4 segment of the spinal cord). This level of injury allows reflex defecation, and sphincter tone is preserved. Management of reflex neurogenic bowel is discussed in Chapter 8. Because the sphincter still has tone, digital stimulation, with or without suppositories, is often the method of choice for bowel management in these patients.

The functional ability of the person to carry out the bowel program will be an important factor to consider. Those with C4 injuries and above can direct their own program but are dependent on others to carry it out. They may also be unable to sit on a toilet chair unassisted, so evacuation may be routinely done in bed. Those with C6–C8 injuries have more trunk control and may be able to perform the bowel program with adaptive equipment such as a digital stimulator or suppository inserter. Evacuation may still be easier to accomplish in bed than on the toilet, but this decision is determined by considering each individual's abilities, situation, and resources.

Many persons with SCI manage their bowel program quite well at home by balancing fluids and fiber in the diet, along with suppositories, stool softeners as needed, and digital stimulation each morning to evacuate before the day's activities. The reader will recall from Chapter 8 that it is particularly important for the bowel program to be convenient, inexpensive, and reliable, especially for an older person with SCI. Additionally, constipation occurs often in older adults, so those with SCI need to balance controllable factors carefully. Because the benefit of active exercise is not available for many quadriplegics, other factors must be relied on to help with bowel control. The GRN can expect that older adults with SCI will probably require the use of stool softeners and suppositories more often than other persons with functional limitations, such as those with stroke.

The more difficult type of bowel to manage is in those with SCI below T12–L1 (autonomous neurogenic). When damage to the sacral segments occurs, the reflex for defecation is lost. Thus, an individual with paraplegia may have a more difficult time establishing a bowel program than someone with quadriplegia, although these individuals have the benefit of some upper extremity control. One of the major considerations is that the stool cannot be too loose or too soft because sphincter tone may be impaired and stool tends to leak from the rectum. A morning routine is probably preferred for emptying the bowel before activity that could increase intra-abdominal pressure and cause incontinence. Manual extraction of the stool may be necessary inasmuch as the reflex arc for defecation is not intact.

The GRN may expect a longer period to be needed to establish a bowel program for a paraplegic with this type of lower motor neuron bowel function. However, these persons should not need adaptive equipment for the bowel program except perhaps for a special toilet chair. Assessment will need to be made about whether the program is more effective or easier when done in the bed or over the toilet in the chair—remembering that emptying is facilitated by gravity—but the program must be convenient and practical to be successful.

Hemorrhoids, also a frequent complaint among the healthy elderly, are common after SCI. So for an older adult with SCI, this area may be cause for concern. Irritation and trauma to the rectal mucosa can be caused by constipation and straining, multiple suppositories or enemas, or other types of treatments that can aggravate pre-existing hemorrhoidal tissue. Additional suppositories or creams may help soothe the pain and discomfort of hemorrhoids, although those with complete paralysis may not be aware of this condition because of a lack of sensation. The rectal area must be kept clean and dry, free from fecal matter. The nurse should avoid cleansing with rough cloths and may need to opt for using an irrigating bottle externally for cleansing or cotton balls to reduce irritation of tissues. Weight shifts should also be encouraged to reduce pressure on inflamed areas. Inflatable rings should not be used because they increase pressure on vulnerable points, thus also contributing to skin breakdown.

Bladder Program

Two basic types of neurogenic bladder function are noted here: reflexic and autonomous. The basic principles of bladder management as discussed in Chapter 8 should be reviewed. The patient and/or caregiver will need to balance fluid intake and urinary output. The bladder should not be allowed to become distended. Allowing urine to sit in the bladder for any length of time can cause infection. Reflux into the ureters and kidneys can result from just one instance of an overfull bladder and can cause permanent renal damage.

Reflexic: Injuries above the S2–S4 segments leave the reflex arc intact, so reflex voiding can be triggered. The symptoms seen include bladder spasticity, incontinence, and an inability to sense fullness. Treatment will include intermittent catheterization every 4 to 6 hours with suprapubic triggers such as anal stimulation, squeezing the clitoris or glans penis, tapping over the suprapubic area, pinching the thigh, or pulling the pubic hair in an attempt to stimulate voiding before intermittent catheterization. These methods are not equally effective with all patients, but different triggers should be tried. External catheters can help keep the skin clean and dry. Padding may also be needed until a pattern can be established. Medications may be used to decrease spasticity of the sphincter muscles if detrusor-sphincter dyssynergia is a problem.

Autonomous: With an autonomous bladder, the reflex arc is damaged and the bladder is left flaccid. This combination results in urinary overflow and no sensation of fullness. High residual urine volumes are common. Treatment entails use of the Credé or Valsalva maneuver in combination with intermittent catheterization to avoid fullness. A bladder scan, or catheterization, can be done to check postvoiding residuals. Although for some individuals with SCI an indwelling Foley catheter is a more viable option, intermittent catheterization is the preferred treatment. Clean-technique intermittent catheterization has been used with success by many SCI patients, although incontinent episodes may still continue. A combination of medications and intermittent catheterization has been used to increase bladder control (Gray, Rayone, & Anson, 1995).

However, with older persons, it is better that they be able to return home with an indwelling catheter than to have to go to an extended care facility because their spouse or other caregiver is unable or unwilling to assist with catheterization. An intermittent catheterization program takes a long-lasting commitment from the person and family to be successful.

Complications: Prevention of urinary tract infection (UTI) is crucial inasmuch as UTI is a major cause of death in those with SCI. Because the bladder is a frequent site of infection, the amount of time between application of intermittent catheterization should be arranged so that no more than 400 cc of urine is obtained each time. Sterile technique is still the preferred method for intermittent catheterization by staff in health care facilities to prevent nosocomial infection. At home, the person will use clean technique and should be taught to cleanse the catheter with soap and water. Catheters should be stored in a bag in a clean place. No-touch catheterization is another option that has shown a 44.5% reduction in UTIs among a small sample of persons with SCI (Charbonneau-Smith, 1993). Although this method may be more costly than clean technique, it can also be used in the hospital by nursing staff instead of a sterile catheterization kit. The closed sterile system available with no-touch catheters is thought to reduce the possibility of infection being introduced by the person performing the catheterization. Good records of intake and output should be kept, as well as records of incontinent episodes. Signs and symptoms of UTI should be promptly reported to the physician.

In addition to incontinence, incomplete emptying, and reflux, other bladder complications include renal calculi, detrusor-sphincter dyssynergia, and autonomic hyperreflexia. The formation of kidney stones can often be prevented by adequate fluid intake. Many urologists recommend at least 3000 cc of water or other fluid per day for those prone to stones. Such intake may be unrealistic for an elderly adult, so 1500 to 2000 cc may be a better goal. Detrusor-sphincter dyssynergia can be treated with medication to relax the external sphincter and allow urine to be released when the bladder contracts.

Autonomic hyperreflexia occurs in the majority of those with lesions above T6. Causative factors include bladder distention, rectal impaction, genital stimulation, urological or gynecological procedures, or pressure sores (Latham, 1994). (Note that each of these factors is in the sacral areas where the reflex arc for voiding is located.) The person will have headache, hypertension (related to baseline), bradycardia, and flushing and perspiration above the level of the lesion. This medical emergency requires immediate treatment. The head of the bed should be raised to take advantage of orthostatic hypotensive effects. The etiologic stimulus should be identified and relieved. Intravenous medications may be needed to lower blood pressure, but prevention of autonomic hyperreflexia is the best treatment. This topic is further discussed in Chapter 8.

Medical evaluation of bladder and kidney function may involve a variety of tests. Most commonly, individuals with SCI will have an intravenous pyelogram at least once per year (and more often if necessary) to observe function and rule out stones or stenosis. Other common tests include renal ultrasonography, which could be used in place of intravenous pyelography if needed, cystourethrography to check bladder capacity and sensation, and urodynamic studies to diagnose detrusor-sphincter dyssynergia. Laboratory tests include serum creatinine and blood urea nitrogen. A urinalysis with culture and sensitivity studies will help determine the presence of UTI and the type of medication needed to treat the bacteria. The importance of follow-up with regard to renal function and testing (even baseline data) cannot be overemphasized to the client and family inasmuch as UTIs are a major cause of death after SCI.

Generally, those with injuries at C8 or below can probably manage their own bladder program independently. Those with SCI at

C6–C7 may need help emptying leg bags or doing catheter care. Those with injury at C5 and above will require additional assistance.

Promoting Proper Nutrition

Dietary considerations are especially important for an older adult with SCI. A diet high in protein, including eggs, meat, and cheese, is usually recommended. During the acute and rehabilitative phase, double portions of meat may be required. However, elderly adults may have sodium and cholesterol restrictions that limit food choices. Because many experience hypertension, foods with low salt yet high protein may be selected. Similarly, elders on renal diets will probably have sodium and potassium restrictions, with a specified amount of protein. This dietary restriction will present a challenge to GRNs, who should work with the dietitian to ensure essentials of a diet that provides nutrients to the body but avoids items that are restricted. Roughage is needed to prevent constipation. Foods such as whole wheat bread, miller's bran, bran cereal, apples, prunes, lettuce, and other root vegetables or pulpy fruits should be used in plenty. Enough fluids are needed to prevent renal calculi formation. The GRN will recall that if weight bearing is not possible and the body needs calcium, it will take it from bone. This situation causes further complications for the older adult who already combats osteoporosis. A healthy diet goes a long way in preserving and maintaining skin integrity, establishing elimination programs, preventing complications, and promoting general health and a feeling of well-being in spite of functional limitations.

Preserving Skin Integrity

For a person with no sensation below the level of the injury, inspection of the skin on a regular basis is essential to prevent breakdown. Because the person will not feel when breakdown is occurring, sensations cannot be relied upon. Individuals with SCI are particularly prone to pressure ulcers on the sacrum and heels. The skin of a paralyzed older adult may tolerate lesser amounts of pressure and for shorter periods before beginning to break down. So prevention is increasingly essential to preserve skin integrity.

Skin checks should be done by the person or caregiver two to three times per day. Suggestions for times to inspect the skin include before rising from bed in the morning, once during the day (preferably when lying down for pressure relief), and before sleeping at night. A mirror can assist persons in checking their own skin, but such self-examination is still difficult when it comes to positioning and examining the heels. Having a caregiver or family member also inspect the skin daily is a good idea. Areas where braces, stockings, or other equipment has been in contact with the skin must be carefully examined. Additionally, parts of the body in contact with the wheelchair such as calves, heels, elbows, and the entire buttocks represent high-risk areas to be inspected.

The GRN should teach the patient and family to avoid activities or habits that could cause skin damage, including elimination of the use of heating pads, water bottles, or electric blankets. The skin of a person with SCI is more susceptible to burns as a result of altered thermoregulation, and because sensation is lost, no warning signals of damage are perceived until after extensive trauma may have occurred. This situation will be even more true with an older adult, who perspires less, is also less tolerant of temperature extremes, and may have impaired circulation to the extremities because of arteriosclerosis or peripheral vascular disease. Older adults with SCI should not be in direct sunlight for prolonged periods and should wear a strong sun blocker when out. If a burn occurs, proper treatment should be instituted (applying ice for a minor burn or applying a sterile bandage and calling the physician if it is blistered). The GRN may need to dispel myths about treatment involving folk practices in some cultures, such as putting butter on a wound or breaking a blister to heal it.

Rashes, dermatitis, acne, and cellulitis are additional problems associated with the skin of a person with SCI. Groin rashes are common and are best treated by leaving the area open to air and keeping it clean and dry. More severe rashes should be treated by a health care professional because secondary infections can develop. Thickening of the skin and nail hypertrophy of the lower extremities are other complications associated with SCI. Those with higher-level injuries have been found to have a higher incidence of skin thickening because of denervation to the integumentary system (Stover, Hale, & Buell, 1994).

A person with SCI should be taught about regulating sitting times, sometimes called sitting tolerance. Sitting tolerance will vary among individuals. The two most importance places for persons to check after sitting are the coccyx and the ischium (sitting bones). An individual can gradually increase sitting time and lying time by small increments such as 30 minutes in each position, as long as redness is not occurring. Temple (1987) stated that if the visible hyperemic response (redness and heat) resolved in a 15-minute interval, the exposure to pressure was within safe limits. This observation can be used as a guideline to increase sitting or lying times. If a person lies on the side for any amount of time and the bony prominence is red, lying on that side should be avoided until the redness is gone. If an open sore develops, the person must not lie or sit on it. Thus, if a pressure sore develops on the coccyx or ischium, the patient should lie prone or in a side-lying position until it is healed. The GRN must emphasize the importance of preventing breakdown of the sitting bones and coccyx in particular inasmuch as these areas are particularly difficult to heal and cause great inconvenience for the person when unable to sit while waiting for healing. The person can sit on the area again only after it is covered with a scar. However, the skin will be fragile even when it appears to be healed, so sitting times may need to be decreased (to no more than 30 minutes) for a period even after the scar has formed (Temple, 1987).

Other areas of teaching include pressure relief aids and pressure relief techniques. Discharge planning should include ordering of supplies that will pad the skin, especially bony prominences. Such items include sheepskins, special mattresses for the bed (foam, gel, water, air), gel or air cushions for the wheelchair, and heel and elbow protectors. Relief of pressure can be achieved by performing wheelchair pushups and wheelchair leans. These exercises should be done every 15 to 20 minutes throughout the day. If watching television, they can be done at each commercial. A table summarizing how to teach the patient to perform these pressure relief techniques is found in Chapter 6 (see Table 6–2).

Changes in Sexual Function

One of the most devastating changes after complete SCI may be alterations in sexual function. However, for a postmenopausal woman, the changes are less than for a man; for those women of childbearing age, reproductive ability is not affected regardless of the level of SCI. Both genders have no sensation below the level of injury. For females with injuries to T11 and above, orgasm is rare, but few other changes occur (Greco, 1996).

For the male, significant changes in sexual function occur, although the effects of aging may have produced some similar effects already. Generally, males may experience erectile dysfunction, poor sperm counts, or an inability to ejaculate (Emick-Herring, 1993). Two basic types of erection can occur after SCI: reflexogenic and psychogenic. For those with T11 injuries and above, reflex erections occur because the sacral segments regulating this function are intact. No psychogenic erections occur at these upper levels of injury because the sympathetic pathways have been disrupted (Greco, 1996). For males with injuries between T12 and S1, psychogenic and/or reflexogenic erections can occur but may be of poor quality. No orgasmic or ejaculatory sensations are felt even though these processes may occur. For those with injuries to the sacral segments (S2–S4), only psychogenic erections are possible from sympathetic activity. However, erections may not be adequate for intercourse. Devices are available, however, to enable some men with SCI to achieve and maintain an erection long enough to engage in sexual intercourse.

The implications that a combination of aging changes and SCI has on sexuality and sexual function are far-reaching. However, some elders may have already established patterns such as fewer episodes of sexual activity or the use of other forms of expression that may ease the transition better than if they were of a younger age. For those who have aged with an SCI, the changes of aging may be less notable because of the deficits that already exist.

Men with SCI have been found to be more concerned about sexual function than women with SCI. Additionally, age, age at time of injury, and time since the injury have been found to be related to the sexual behavior of women with SCI. That is, younger women were more likely to engage in sexual activity, as were those who were injured at a younger age. Women also expressed more concern over bowel and bladder accidents than men did (White, Rintala, Hart, & Fuhrer, 1994).

The GRN should open the doors of communication about sexuality and sexual function after SCI before the person's discharge because the implications are serious not just for the patient but for the partner as well (DeVivo, Hawkins, Richards, & Go, 1995).

Nurses should be sensitive to the person's cultural or religious background, however, which may discourage or prohibit discussion of subjects considered intimate. Written information and phone numbers that can be called for follow-up or counseling should be provided.

Pain

Although it may be tempting to think that those with complete SCI do not experience pain because "they don't feel anything," such is not the case. First, sensation is present above the level of injury. Second, even those with complete injuries have expressed the experience of unpleasant sensations in parts of the body. Particularly at the level of injury, the person may complain of mild to severe tingling or burning sensations or intractable pain (Sie, Waters, Adkins, & Gellman, 1992). The cause of such sensation is unclear but could be due to scar tissue formation or nerve root irritation. For those with paraplegia, pain may be increased in the upper extremities because of excessive workload of the arms and trunk to perform weight shifts, transfers, and ADLs. Such stress put on non–weight bearing joints over a period of years can lead to an early onset of arthritis or other degenerative joint disorders. Medications for pain or inflammation may help ease symptoms.

In cases of intractable pain, the services of a physician and hospital-based clinic specializing in chronic pain management may be indicated. Transcutaneous electrical nerve stimulation, epidural injection, an intrathecal pump, or nerve root blocks are possible treatments. Additionally, intentional destruction of the nerve root for management of pain or intractable spasms may be considered.

Additional Psychosocial Issues

Although research related to issues surrounding aging with an SCI is scarce, a few common themes have emerged on the subjects of social support, quality of life, and caregiver burden. These issues will be discussed further here.

Social Support

It has long been believed that persons with SCI recover better when placed in an environment with other individuals with SCI. Payne (1993) found that contact with other SCI patients was important to rehabilitation for

sharing, peer support, and decreasing feelings of isolation. Group encounters also enhanced learning and contributed to feelings of adjustment among patients and family members. Blake (1995) identified several factors contributing to social isolation in a small sample of younger males with quadriplegia. The subjects in the study identified factors such as needing increased time to do things, self-care and security issues, lack of money or financial worries, accessibility to buildings, and job and educational options as contributing to feelings of isolation. Such factors are more likely to occur in an elderly person with SCI. Bozzacco (1993) found that although persons with SCI had many restrictions, they thought that they were not especially lonely and did report having friends, relationships with significant others, and community involvement. Mobility and position restrictions were reported to interfere with or delay the establishment of close relationships, as well as the development of a career. All these findings suggest that social support may act as a buffer against stress and promote adjustment to life after SCI. As persons lived longer with SCI, they reported feeling less financially secure, as well as having an increase in symptoms and illnesses (Pentland et al., 1995).

Quality of Life

Studies on quality of life after SCI are limited and generally do not use an older adult sample. Decreased quality-of-life ratings have been associated with greater severity of disabilities (Clayton & Chubon, 1994). Factors associated with an *increased* perceived quality of life were a higher educational level, being employed, and being active in a greater number of social activities (Clayton & Chubon, 1994; Krause, 1992). Factors reported through focus group sessions with quadriplegics (mean age of subjects, 28.15 years) indicated that quality of life was influenced by inner strength/survival, finances, relationships, employment, health, level of activity, assertiveness, and independence level (Bach & McDaniel, 1993).

Ivie and DeVivo (1994) tried to establish a model for predicting unplanned hospitalizations for people with SCI. About 60% of the variance in their study was explained by the following factors: lack of college education, indwelling urethral catheters, complete motor injury, dependency in self-care, and dependence in ambulation. These findings suggest that GRNs could assist patients in preventing hospitalization through nursing education interventions, particularly with regard to bladder management, ambulation, and the performance of self-care activities.

French and Phillips (1991) suggested that persons move through four phases of body image recovery: impact (recognizing the change), retreat (withdrawing from the loss), acknowledgment (facing the change), and reconstruction (living with the reality). These phases are similar to those suggested by Gokbudak (1985), who also gave some indication of the time periods of each phase for older adults with SCI: (1) shock (3–4 weeks), (2) defensive treatment (3–4 months; feelings of denial, anger, indifference), (3) acknowledgment (3–12 months; expressing bitterness, depression), and (4) adaptation and change (12–14 months; increased self-esteem and independence).

GRNs should be aware that the process of adaptation to life after SCI may be long and is affected by multiple factors. Older adults with SCI are likely to experience depression, particularly in the first 3 to 12 months after injury. GRNs should assess the person's uncertainty and vulnerability and structure teaching to allay fears and promote well-being (Wineman, Durand, & Steiner, 1994).

Although persons with SCI may report a decreased perceived quality of life, some interventions have been shown to help combat related depression. A study by Craig, Hancock, Dickson, and Chang (1997) examined the effects of cognitive behavior therapy on those with SCI. A skill-based intervention that taught tasks associated with community reentry via small groups was run over a 10-week period. The researchers concluded that not all persons with SCI need cognitive behavior therapy and that the interventions did not significantly influence the person's self-esteem, self-concept, or anxiety level. However, in subjects reporting an increased depressive mood, cognitive behavior therapy was found to have a long-term effect on decreasing depression (as measured 1 year after injury).

Sports clubs and teams for those with SCI may offer an additional buffer to depression. Wheelchair basketball and bowling are receiving increasing attention and participation. Wheelchair dancing is available in some areas. Archery or other sports such as skiing or fishing can, with proper adaptive equipment, allow seniors with SCI to remain active, thus promoting a sense of normalcy and well-being that contributes to a high quality of life.

Caregiver Burden

Even healthy spouses who are primary caregivers for a person with a long-term disability are at risk for "numerous physical, mental emotional, social, and financial problems of their own" (Holicky, 1996, p. 247). Caregivers commonly experience a wide variety of emotions, including anger, fear, loneliness, resentment, bitterness, isolation, and guilt (Holicky, 1996). Family members may be called on to assume roles that are unfamiliar and uncomfortable for them.

The role of caregiver can be overwhelming to even a healthy younger adult but may at times seem impossible to an older spouse caregiver. The GRN should focus interventions on reducing role fatigue by enhancing the family, increasing social support networks, and linking caregivers to resources that may assist with respite care. Providing information needed (as in Table 11–5), fostering a sense of control to decrease feelings of powerlessness, and identifying support groups are all helpful interventions.

One often overlooked area from which GRNs may arrange for help for families is the local church. If the patient or family has been involved or associated with a church, parish, or synagogue, this tie should be explored as a means of providing assistance to the family. Generally, Christian and other organizations have a mission and ministry within the local community that fuels their desire to provide service to others in need. Given the reports of caregivers who say that their burden would have been lessened if some help were given with household chores or routine tasks, the local church is in an ideal position to provide such assistance.

Caregiver stress has been associated with abuse and mistreatment of elders. Older adults with SCI are often dependent on a caregiver for their basic physical needs, which places them at increased risk for mistreatment and neglect. This observation is particularly true if the caregiver does not have adequate coping abilities, has limited resources, has a history of substance abuse, and experiences emotional, mental, or psychological problems (Campbell & Humphreys, 1993; Decalmer & Glendenning, 1993; Pritchard, 1995; Wilson, 1992). It will thus be especially important for the GRN to thoroughly assess the abilities and resources of caregivers and weigh these qualities against the demands that a home caregiving situation will place on them. In certain situations, placement in a long-term

Table 11-5   CLIENT/FAMILY TEACHING: ESSENTIAL AREAS OF INSTRUCTION NEEDED BEFORE DISCHARGE HOME AFTER SPINAL CORD INJURY

Essential teaching areas

Signs and symptoms of UTI, DVT, respiratory infection, skin breakdown
Intermittent catheterization
Foley irrigation and care
Skin care and treatment of simple groin rash
Prevention of skin breakdown, pressure ulcers
Pressure relief techniques, performing skin checks
Bowel program: diet, suppository, digital stimulation
Respiratory care and pulmonary hygiene
Equipment use and maintenance
Transportation
Wheelchair use and maintenance
Health visits for follow-up care
Sexuality changes
Pain management
Medication schedule
Relaxation techniques
Community resources, support groups

Outcomes: Client (and family/caregiver) will be able to state action to take if

Running a temperature
A blister or pressure sore develops
A blood clot is suspected
UTI is suspected
Residual urine is higher than normal (over 150 cc)
The balloon in the indwelling catheter will not deflate
Any cuts or swelling of the penis are present from catheter use
Autonomic hyperreflexia develops
Rectal impaction is suspected
A groin rash develops

UTI, urinary tract infection; DVT, deep venous thrombosis.

care facility may be more beneficial and healthy for an older person with SCI than returning to the home with an overwhelmed caregiver. Chapter 14 further discusses ways in which GRNs can recognize and prevent mistreatment of elders by caregivers, as well as the notion of caregiver burden.

PARKINSON'S DISEASE

PD affects 10% of those over the age of 65, with the usual age of onset between 55 and 60 years of age (Fitzsimmons & Bunting, 1993; Lannon, Thomas, Bratton, Jost, & Lockhart-Pretti, 1986). More than 1 million Americans have PD, which makes it one of the most common neurological diseases (Chisholm, 1996; Fitzsimmons & Bunting, 1993; Weekly, 1995). One in every 100 persons will have PD by age 55. This incidence rate has remained relatively constant over time (National Parkinson Foundation, 1994). PD affects more males than females (about a 60:40 ratio) and is seen less often in those of African descent (Sprinzeles, 1993).

Characteristics of Parkinson's Disease

PD was first described by James Parkinson as "the shaking palsy" (Lannon et al., 1986). Three major symptoms characterize this disease: bradykinesia, rigidity, and tremor. Bradykinesia is a slowness of movement, especially initiating movement. Rigidity in PD is called *cogwheel rigidity* because movements are ratchet-like and not smooth, with stops and starts giving a jerky appearance (Weekly, 1995). Two thirds of those with PD experience resting tremor. These three main characteristics are used to diagnose the disorder, but many other signs and symptoms are presented in Table 11-6.

Several classifications of PD are noted, but the largest and most frequent type is idiopathic (sometimes called primary parkinsonism). A family history is seen in about 15% of cases (Luis, 1997). Environmental factors may also play a role. Although the etiology is unknown, symptoms result from destruction of neurons in the substantia nigra located deep in the cerebral hemisphere of the brain. The

Table 11–6 SIGNS AND SYMPTOMS OF PARKINSON'S DISEASE

Bradykinesia
Tremor
Rigidity
Listlessness
Frequent, unexplained falls
Micrographia
Shuffling gait, arms stiff at sides, no arm
  swinging
Postural instability
"Freezing" of movements
Mask-like expression
Depression
Slow, monotonous voice
Pill-rolling of the fingers
Drooling
Deficits in judgment
Emotional lability
Decreased attention span
Difficulty concentrating
Altered sleep patterns with frequent awakening
Impaired swallowing
Uninhibited neurogenic bladder
Dementia
Sexual dysfunction

basal ganglia, via production of the neurotransmitter dopamine, facilitates control of fine motor movements, integration of sensory input, and emotional behavior. A lack of dopamine leads to the typical signs and symptoms seen in PD.

The course of PD is variable and the progression slow. Some persons worsen quickly, whereas severe symptoms never develop in others. The diagnosis of PD is based on the person's history and the presence of at least two of the cardinal symptoms. Quality of life is greatly affected by PD, but the disease does not usually alter life expectancy (Sprinzeles, 1993; Washington, 1993). PD is difficult to diagnose in the early stages because symptoms can be indicative of other problems such as adverse drug reactions, orthostatic hypotension, or psychiatric disorders (Calne, 1995).

Treatment of the disorder is primarily medical, and nursing treatment is supportive-educative. The most promising new treatments include pharmacological interventions and neurosurgery. Fetal tissue transplantation into critical areas of the brain striatum have been performed in attempts to reinnervate the basal ganglia to synthesize and release dopamine by stimulated neuron growth (Chisholm, 1996). Although early clinical trials suggest some improvement in motor function

among those with severe idiopathic PD, this technique remains under investigation inasmuch as many ethical and practical issues still need to be addressed. Pallidotomy is another surgical technique that targets a specific area of the brain. This procedure has demonstrated some success in that lesions in the globus pallidus depress abnormal brain activity caused by the depletion of dopamine and thereby alleviate dyskinesia (Calne, 1995). Although pallidotomy was developed in the 1950s, this procedure has received more attention recently for the potential of relieving rigidity and akinesia (Gilbert, Counsell, & Snively, 1996). Thalamotomy is generally chosen to help those with uncontrollable tremors that prohibit functional independence (Krames Communications, 1996). This operation involves placing a "freezing probe" in a specific part of the thalamus to achieve relief of tremor and rigidity (Lieberman, Gopinathan, Neophytides, & Goldstein, 1996, p. 26). Surgical risks may be especially high for older adults, and thalamotomy does not usually eliminate the need for medication entirely, although symptoms may be somewhat relieved.

A person with PD should be distinguished from those with *parkinsonism*, which is identified as "anyone whose movements are impaired by rigidity, tremor, and bradykinesia" (Washington, 1993, p. 2). Parkinsonism can be caused by a host of other problems besides a deficiency of dopamine in the brain (listed in Table 11–7).

The signs and symptoms of PD can be many and may result in impaired physical mobility, cognitive-perceptual deficits, sleep disorders, poor nutrition, alteration in bladder elimination, fatigue, and emotional changes. Whereas medical treatment is pallia-

Table 11–7 POSSIBLE CAUSES OF PARKINSONIAN SYMPTOMS (NOT PARKINSON'S DISEASE)

Overexposure to or ingestion of manganese and
  aluminum ore
Exposure to toxins such as carbon monoxide and
  carbon disulfide
Brain disorders such as progressive nuclear palsy
Other brain trauma
Influenza virus
Encephalitis
Drugs used to treat other illnesses, such as
  methyldopa (for hypertension) or
  phenothiazine (for mental illness)

tive and aimed at symptom management, nursing treatment is aimed at providing support, education, and preservation of strength.

Nursing Implications

Because no cure for Parkinson's disease is known at this time, nursing management will be long term. In addition to the general nursing strategies discussed in previous chapters of this text, several specific areas in which GRN interventions can facilitate independence and adaptation to PD for the person and family are discussed here (Case Study 11.2). Nursing diagnoses related to care of a person with PD appear in Table 11–8. The progressive nature of PD suggests that persons will become increasingly dependent on others if rehabilitation interventions are not instituted throughout the course of the disease. As one nurse educator stated, "Preventing contractures, helping with weight control, promoting adequate bowel function, and keeping the patient physically and psychologically independent requires ceaseless effort on the part of the caregiver. The patient's greatest challenge is to remain self-reliant" (Hurwitz, 1986). Nursing interven-

Table 11–8 POSSIBLE NURSING DIAGNOSES RELATED TO CARE OF PERSONS WITH PARKINSON'S DISEASE

Impaired physical mobility
Self-care deficit
Impaired verbal and written communication
Alteration in sensory perception
Impaired swallowing
Alteration in nutritional status: less than body
  requirements
High risk for injury: falls
Anxiety
Depression
Alteration in bowel elimination: constipation
Alteration in bladder elimination: urge
  incontinence
Knowledge deficit (related to medications, disease
  process)
Alteration in home health maintenance
Powerlessness
Sleep pattern disturbance
Attention deficit
Social isolation
Self-concept disturbance
Ineffective coping
Fatigue
Altered self-esteem
Altered thought processes

tions are mainly related to helping promote self-care and independence.

CASE STUDY 11.2
Parkinson's Disease

Mr. Abrams was a 69 year old bachelor who lived by himself in a third-floor apartment. He was a former music teacher and had continued to direct a small church choir after his retirement. His passions were playing the organ, singing, and listening to opera. Mr. Abrams had suffered from idiopathic PD since the age of 66. Also in his medical history were diabetes, well-controlled with insulin once each morning, hardness of hearing, and obesity. He had been able to take care of himself for the past 3 years but began to have difficulty with his ADLs and maintaining his usual routine in the past year because of increased stiffness and tremors. He was worried that his vocal quality had changed, and this concern bothered him most when he sang. Mr. Abrams' neighbor was a home health nurse, and he sought her advice on how he could remain independent at home. Because the nurse was already familiar with his situation, having known him for some time, she realized that Mr. Abrams' only relative who would be available to assist with his care was an elderly sister who was in poor health. This situation underscored his need to remain self-sufficient. The nurse provided informal suggestions to Mr. Abrams, such as considering moving to a first-floor apartment and engaging in a regular exercise program under the supervision of his physician. She also provided him with several pamphlets, including pamphlets demonstrating exercises for people with PD and a handbook for those with PD. The nurse encouraged Mr. Abrams to discuss his concerns with his doctor and see whether any changes in medication might help alleviate his worsening symptoms. She also praised him for continuing to be active in the community through his church and advised him to consult with his parish leaders if it became necessary to have some help with home maintenance. Mr. Abrams' church congregation, as well as his sister and her grown children, were his main support systems. Mr. Abrams was able to follow the nurse's suggestions. He entered the hospital for a drug holiday and participated in a rehabilitation program, where an exercise program was developed for him. Later, Mr. Abrams was able to have better relief of his stiffness and tremors with a different combination of medications at a lower dose. This adaptation allowed him to retain his independence for a longer period.

Mobility, Functional Independence, and Safety

Resting tremors, which can be aggravated by fatigue, stress, excitement, or frustration, can interfere with the ability to perform ADLs. Spasticity, ataxia, and incoordination also impair mobility and ambulatory status. Falls are a common problem because of these factors.

Exercise has been found beneficial as an adjunct to medication therapy. "Regular physical activity is the most important treatment for Parkinson's disease" (Lannon et al., 1986, p. 129). Palmer, Mortimer, Webster, Bistevins, and Dickinson (1986) demonstrated that both a traditional exercise program and one that incorporated upper body karate training showed similar positive outcomes related to increased function. These positive outcomes included improvements in gait, tremor, grip strength, and fine motor coordination tasks. Mitchell, Mertz, and Catanzaro (1987) similarly found that functional mobility was improved when persons with PD participated in a nurse-run aerobic flexibility program. These authors also stated that the participant's perception of social support was improved as a result. Gauthier, Dalziel, and Gauthier (1987) studied the effects of group occupational therapy on a small sample of patients with idiopathic PD. The researchers, using treatment and control groups, demonstrated that with 20 hours of occupational therapy in addition to a medication regimen, patients with PD maintained functional status over 1 year, including a decrease in bradykinesia at 6 months. The control group showed a decrease in independence and perceived the progression of their disease to be more severe than did the group who received occupational therapy rehabilitation. These findings support the theory that exercise, in various forms, is beneficial to patients with PD.

The American Parkinson Disease Association suggests that persons with PD should engage in regular exercise to help improve mobility (Wichmann, 1990). Exercises can be incorporated into the person's daily routine (such as during ADLs) but may be most beneficial when the person is rested and medica-

tions are allowing more freedom of movement. Adequate rest periods should be planned, and exercises should be smooth and not bouncing. Walking and swimming are two additional forms of activity that help improve the cardiovascular system as well as promote joint and muscle function.

Fall prevention, as seen in Chapter 7, can be enhanced by exercise programs such as those discussed earlier. Because a person with PD has multiple functional and cognitive deficits, safety will be an important nursing consideration.

Patients with PD "tend to fall backward very easily with only a light push" (Kitamura et al., 1993), which places them at high risk for falls. Persons with PD may also experience "freezing," where movement just stops. Besides the usual nursing interventions related to safety that were discussed in previous chapters, an additional consideration should be noted for persons with PD. Kitamura and colleagues found that visual information was an important factor in helping patients with PD maintain an upright posture. With eyes closed, patients were more likely to shift their body weight backward than was a control group. Patients with PD may have an unstable posture and be unable to correct their body tilt. This tendency was even more exaggerated when the person could not use visual information to help correct changes in body position. The researchers concluded that "PD patients are using visual information as a sort of adjustment mechanism for maintaining the upright posture to shift the CCP (center of contact pressure) position forward, probably to prevent falling backward" (p. 1111). Given the results of this study, GRNs should make certain that adequate lighting is provided to patients who may get up during the night so that visual information can be processed. Glasses, if used, should be worn at all times when ambulating. The person should have routine eye examinations to detect any changes in vision and update prescriptions. Screening should also be done at this time for such conditions as glaucoma or cataracts, which can be treated. The importance of visual input should be emphasized to the family and appropriate measures taken.

Independence in Eating and Swallowing

A person with PD is at risk of swallowing difficulties. The effects of the disease can result in increased esophageal transit time and delayed swallowing. Athlin, Norberg, Axelsson, Moller, and Nordstrom (1989) found that most patients with PD also had a decreased sense of smell. Incoordination of motor function, including inappropriate hand position and movement, can result in difficulty with self-feeding. Patients with PD may also need to concentrate while eating because of oral apraxia and high distractibility. Choking is a potential problem.

The GRN can assist persons with PD in self-feeding activities by minimizing distractions and providing frequent cues. Placing the person with others who may have swallowing difficulties may be of benefit for monitoring but could also prove distracting. Having one single caregiver help assist with or direct the meal may be a more desirable approach. This issue could certainly be an area for family teaching and involvement. Adaptive utensils such as plate guards or built-up handles may assist in managing the food. The occupational therapist can provide additional suggestions for equipment that could be helpful. Many patients will spill their food because of tremors. The GRN may need to steady the hand and help guide it to the mouth. Deficits in eye-hand coordination may interfere with the person getting food into the mouth, and the person may also have trouble manipulating food in the mouth because of impaired tongue control. Trying different head positions and placement of food in the mouth may help. A different type of diet or consistency might also make self-feeding easier in some cases.

Meeting nutritional requirements is difficult for patients with PD. Not only do effects of aging such as taste bud atrophy make food seem less palatable sometimes, but a decrease in the sense of smell can also contribute to poor appetite. Many patients with PD experience depression, which can also suppress appetite. Some may have nausea or other side effects from medications. Additionally, although a diet high in protein is desirable for healing and adequate nutrition, it may interfere with the effectiveness of levodopa therapy. Finding a balance between all these factors while promoting proper nutrition will be a team challenge.

Eating is a also social phenomenon, and cognitive-perceptual as well as emotional changes may alter the person's ability to engage in usual eating behavior. Generally, GRNs should be aware that patients with PD are likely to have eating and swallowing difficulties. The speech therapist's evaluation will be of help in determining an appropriate diet and related nursing interventions.

Medication Management and Drug Holidays

Table 11–9 lists medications commonly used in the treatment of PD. Four major types of drug therapy are noted: anticholinergics, levodopa, monoamine oxidase (MAO) B inhibitors, and dopamine agonists. For most of a person's illness, a combined regimen of levodopa or levodopa/carbidopa (Sinemet) and a dopamine agonist is used. According to Calne (1995), the standard pharmacological treatment is to begin with levodopa and then add bromocriptine or pergolide when the levodopa dose "reaches 600 to 800 mg/day of a standard preparation or 800 to 1,000 mg/day of a controlled-release preparation" (p. 84). This practice allows for lower doses of two medications to be given versus higher doses of one in an attempt to decrease side effects and potential toxicity. The use of pergolide as an adjunct to Sinemet resulted in antiparkinson benefits, improved "on" time, and a reduction in the dose of levodopa (Sanchez-Ramos, 1994). The major side effects of drug therapy in PD are depression, urinary incontinence, nausea, orthostatic hypotension, dyskinesia, on-off effects, confusion, and hallucinations.

Anticholinergics reduce the increase in cholinergic influence resulting from decreased dopamine. The major effect of these types of drug in PD is to reduce resting tremor and rigidity, but they have little effect on akinesia or action tremor and are thus usually best administered in the earlier stages of the disease (Swonger & Burbank, 1995).

Levodopa is used like a replacement therapy for dopamine, much like insulin is used to treat diabetes. Dopamine does not cross the blood-brain barrier, so levodopa is used. A precursor to dopamine, levodopa helps most in alleviating the muscle weakness and action tremors seen in patients with PD. Levodopa decreases bradykinesia and rigidity. It may be used in combination with anticholinergics for those with advanced parkinsonism. Levodopa is best used in continuous rather than intermittent therapy to promote its beneficial effect of alleviating motor fluctuations (Chase, Engber, & Mouradian, 1994). A major problem in treatment with levodopa is that absorption of the drug is variable. Regular and predictable absorption enhances treatment and is most often altered by diet (Nutt, 1994). Additionally, fluctuations may

Table 11–9   DRUG THERAPY IN PARKINSON'S DISEASE

Medication	Effects	Side Effects

Anticholinergics*
  Atropine
  Benztropine (Cogentin)
  Biperiden (Akineton)
  Diphenhydramine (Benadryl)
  Ethopropazine (Parsidol)
  Orphenadrine (Disipal)
  Procyclidine (Kemadrin)
  Trihexyphenidyl (Artane)
	Reduces resting tremor and rigidity	Tachycardia, palpitations, flushing, orthostatic hypotension gastrointestinal problems, ocular disturbances, confusion, agitation, depression, dry mouth, constipation

Levodopa† (L-dopa)
  Levodopa/carbidopa
    (Sinemet)
	Alleviates akinesia and action tremors	Nausea, vomiting, decreased appetite, dry mouth, constipation, visual disturbances, orthostatic hypotension, cardiac dysrhythmias, confusion, anxiety, depression, insomnia, hallucinations, fatigue, dyskinesias

Dopamine agonists‡
  Amantadine (Symmetrel)
  Bromocriptine (Parlodel)
  Pergolide (Permax)
	Similar to levodopa, but sustained longer to reduce end-of-dose failure	Fatigue, depression, insomnia, hallucinations, confusion, ataxia, dizziness, seizures, slurred speech, dyskinesias, edema, CHF, visual problems, urinary incontinence

MAO B inhibitors§ Selegiline	Addition to levodopa/carbidopa therapy: allows for dose reduction and longer responsiveness; reduces dyskinesias induced by levodopa	Nausea, abdominal pain, cardiovascular effects, skin reactions, visual disturbances, sexual dysfunction, confusion, hallucinations, vivid dreams, dyskinesias

CHF, congestive heart failure; MAO, monoamine oxidase.
*Take with meals to avoid gastric upset, avoid use in those with glaucoma, and promote fluid and fiber to prevent constipation effects. Anticholinergics may add to pre-existing depression, and Parsidol has additional side effects, including seizures and hematological reactions.
†The initial dose should be low, with gradual increments added; oral doses of vitamin B_6 can inhibit uptake, so the patient should avoid excess vitamins with pyridoxine. Watch the additive effects of other medications that contribute to orthostatic hypotension. Regular eye examinations should be arranged. Levodopa can aggravate pre-existing psychosis. The response time varies after initiation from a few weeks to 3 to 4 months. It is harder to regulate the dosage in obese elders. The peak action of levodopa is achieved after 30 minutes to 2 hours, and it is absorbed best with decreased protein in the diet. Levodopa is often used with carbidopa to form Sinemet, which promotes uptake.
‡Take with meals to avoid gastric irritation. Dopamine agonists are often used in combination with levodopa; similar benefits are produced while allowing smaller dosages to be taken. Bromocriptine and pergolide provide actions similar to those of levodopa but require higher dosages and thus lead to adverse reactions. Amantadine can be used for drug-induced parkinsonism.
§Should be used with levodopa/carbidopa therapy. Theoretically MAO B inhibitors could help prevent progression of disease, but this benefit is under testing.

cause a wearing-off effect from too little drug in the system to dyskinesias from an excess of levodopa.

Selegiline (deprenyl) is a more recent selective MAO B inhibitor and thus avoids many of the food and drug interactions present with nonselective MAO inhibitors. Theoretically, selegiline is thought to have a neuroprotective effect. It is presently used in conjunction with levodopa/carbidopa and can help reduce the dosages needed, as well as prolong responsiveness. Selegiline does not, however, decrease the long-term problem of dyskinesia (Hely & Morris, 1996).

Dopamine agonists improve the signs and symptoms of parkinsonism. The three most widely used in clinical practice are amantadine (Symmetrel), bromocriptine (Parlodel), and pergolide (Permax). These drugs are usually administered as adjuncts to levodopa and/or anticholinergic therapy and improve some symptoms by acting as a substitute for dopamine in the brain (Krames Communications, 1996). They act quickly and can be used to reduce end-of-dose failure of levodopa (Swonger & Burbank, 1995). Their benefits are similar to those of levodopa, but side effects may be more pronounced and include confusion and hallucinations (Calne, 1995).

Long-term drug therapy has several disadvantages, including side effects, periods of lack of drug action, and a wearing-off effect. Long-term use of levodopa and other anticholinergics may result in toxicity with symptoms such as confusion, hallucinations, nightmares, dyskinesias, and sleeplessness. Levodopa's effectiveness can also wear off in 2 to 5 years (Lannon et al., 1986; Lieberman, 1994) and result in decreased periods of symptom relief for the patient. Lower-protein diets help decrease response fluctuations but must be used with care inasmuch as reducing protein in an already compromised elderly patient could have serious consequences (Lieberman, 1994). Redistributing protein intake so that protein is reduced during the day when functional mobility is most important is one strategy used (Sprinzeles, 1993). The GRN should work with each individual to balance maximum drug effectiveness with adequate protein in the diet and avoidance of nausea from medication.

Complete withdrawal of medication after a period of long-term therapy may be necessary to regain the benefits of the drugs without chronic side effects. Older patients were often admitted to inpatient rehabilitation for a drug holiday, although this practice may not be paid for by Medicare and is thus seen less frequently in rehabilitation. A drug holiday is a period of usually 3 to 14 days in which carbidopa/levodopa is no longer given to a person with PD (Lieberman et al., 1996). It is used with success in patients who have progressed to higher levels of the medication for control of symptoms and have generally been taking the drug for at least 2 years. Because the person may experience adverse effects from drug withdrawal, this process is usually done in the hospital, often on the rehabilitation unit. Although not all patients benefit from a drug holiday, improvement afterward can last from days to months (Lieberman et al., 1996). After a successful drug holiday, the person can usually obtain relief of symptoms at a lower dose than before. Time away from the medication is thought to reset and resensitize dopamine receptors.

Promoting Sleep

Sleep pattern disturbances are common in persons with PD. Dreams or hallucinations and anxiety may contribute to insomnia. The GRN's goal will be to promote the establishment of adequate sleep patterns, which can be achieved by providing a quiet environment, as well as turning and positioning the body for comfort. Relaxation strategies should be tried while keeping in mind that persons with PD may have attention deficits and difficulty concentrating. Music therapy or back rubs may help ease tension and promote relaxation. Sleeping medications may be needed. The person should be kept busy and active during the day so that dozing does not interfere with night sleep. If muscle rigidity interferes with sleep, range-of-motion exercises and increased activity during the daytime may help.

Supportive-Educative Interventions for the Patient and Family

Many areas will need to be addressed by the GRN when teaching the patient and family about PD. Assessment of learning abilities and needs is the first step in this process. The principles of adult learning should be applied, with the nurse acknowledging that the person needs motivation to learn and may only be ready to deal with the basics of care, depending on a variety of factors, not the least of which are the course and severity of the illness. A follow-up program is ideal to address issues that will arise in long-term management. Home health care nurses should be prepared to educate the patient and family about progression of the disease and changes in medication effects that may occur in later stages of the illness. Areas for teaching include bowel and bladder management (see principles in Chapter 8), the medication regimen, nutrition, activity, promoting ambulation, encouraging sleep, communication deficits, and progress of the disease. Table 11–10 summarizes some key areas for teaching of the family and person with PD.

Table 11–10   CLIENT/FAMILY TEACHING: KEY AREAS IN PARKINSON'S DISEASE

Essential teaching areas

Medication therapy: dosages, indications for use, side effects, wearing-off effects, on-off effects, drug holidays, promoting absorption

Fall prevention: making the home safe, effects of disease on balance and muscle tone

Disease progression: slow, variable, expectations of each stage

Effects of disease on mobility, bowel and bladder function, sleep, eating and swallowing, attention span, self-care ability, roles of patient and family members, communication abilities

Nutritional needs: fluids, fiber, maintaining adequate caloric intake, weekly weights, protein per physician's order, effect of diet on medication uptake

Swallowing problems: preventing choking and drooling, following speech therapist's instructions, maintaining proper consistency of food ordered, sitting upright for meals, giving cues and assistance with self-feeding

Roles of the rehabilitation team members in assisting the person with PD

Promoting self-care: arranging living space to maximize performance, allowing plenty of time to complete A.M. care and ADLs, using the OT as a consultant, acknowledging physical limitations, encouraging daily activity

Promoting sleep and relaxation: providing nonstressful, quiet environment; increasing daytime activities; judicious use of sleeping aids, relaxation techniques; alternating rest and activity

Communication: related to dysarthria and changes in vocal quality

Outcomes: Client (and family/caregiver) will

Recognize the role of medications in controlling symptoms such as rigidity, tremors, and dyskinesias

Identify side effects of medications

Describe benefits of a drug holiday

List ways to improve home safety

Prepare a proper diet with adequate fluids, fiber, and protein

Describe the effects of PD on the person

Follow the speech therapist's recommendations for diet consistency and safe swallowing

Report signs and symptoms of impaired swallowing

Engage in relaxation activities that decrease anxiety and promote sleep

Use alternative methods of communication when verbalizations are not sufficient

List several community resources and a local support group that could be of service

PD, Parkinson's disease; ADLs, activities of daily living; OT, occupational therapist.

Habermann (1996), in a study of persons with PD in middle life, found several common demands of day-to-day maintenance, including demands of the illness such as acknowledging initial symptoms of the illness and seeking help, balancing responses to diagnosis, coping with body image changes, gaining knowledge (both formal and practical), and dealing with unpredictability. Changing roles and relationships, as well as a sense of one's own identity, were also common issues. Subjects in this study expressed the importance of medication management in relation to their ability to function. For men, this point was particularly important when it had an impact on the ability to work at a job, remain employed, or drive a car (Nijhof, 1995).

Because PD may run a long and variable course, care for the caregiver will be especially important. Caregivers and family members should be encouraged to remain in-volved in their own activities and hobbies. They will need to be taught that communication problems may occur in the patient. Speech may be slow and slurred or difficult to hear. The person will require more time to respond, but this change does not necessarily indicate cognitive deterioration. The GRN can make referrals to the speech pathologist as needed throughout the course of the illness. Explanations of any changes in the physician's orders and treatments should be given to the caregiver. Persons with PD do not usually require institutionalization, so the long-term burden on the home caregiver is great. However, dementia may develop in 40% of people with advanced stages of parkinsonism (Sprinzeles, 1993). Urinary incontinence becomes another problem for many persons. Changes in sexual patterns may occur secondary to an inability to engage in traditional sexual functions because of physical or sensory losses. Feelings of powerlessness may arise. Guilt, anger, and frustration may be felt on the part of the person and partner. The GRN can help the family and patient with these emotional changes by being a good listener and providing connections with resources, support groups, and community services. Nursing interventions should empower the person and family to maintain independence and stability.

MULTIPLE SCLEROSIS

MS is a chronic, progressive, degenerative disease affecting nearly a quarter of a million people in the United States (Hainsworth, 1994; Miller & Hens, 1993). Years ago, this disorder was sometimes characterized as the 7 plus 7 plus 7 disease. This description was a means to help identify stages in progression in that diagnosis was made during the first period of 7 years when symptoms were mild, the second 7 years would bring moderate problems and adjustments to lifestyle, and the last 7 were characterized by increasing difficulties and eventual death. Thus, a person's life expectancy after diagnosis was generally thought to be no longer than about 21 years. Although this sequence was a helpful way to remember the potential clinical course of the disorder at that time, much has changed in the medical treatment of MS in the past decade. Because of the introduction of new and better medications, it is hoped that the course of the disease may be altered. More individuals in whom MS was diagnosed in young adulthood are living to see old age and achieve an average life span. It is important to note that those who have lived with MS for decades before experiencing the effects of old age will have adjusted and adapted to the disease, so aging may take place for them in a similar manner to an able-bodied person who experiences these changes. However, the implications that the aging process has on their overall physical and mental health may be more severe and more costly in terms of functional limitations and independence. Basic information about MS is presented here, and specific nursing implications are addressed.

Characteristics of Multiple Sclerosis

The etiology of MS is unknown, but several characteristics of the disease can be noted. MS is more prevalent in cooler northern climates, with some areas being designated "MS belts." This disorder affects women more often than men and whites more than blacks or Orientals. The onset generally occurs between 20 and 40 years of age. MS is the third most common debilitating disease and is called the crippler of young adults (Namey & Schwetz, 1993). Some familial tendency is observed inasmuch as those with immediate relatives having MS are 15 times more likely to acquire it, although MS is not contagious. Theories related to MS suggest that it may be due to viral infection or an autoimmune response.

Currently, the clinical course of MS is divided into five classifications: benign, primary progressive, progressive relapsing, secondary progressive, and relapsing-remitting. The three main clinical patterns are thus benign, progressive, and relapsing. Those with benign MS may experience one or two episodes that result in neurologic dysfunction, but recovery is complete and does not lead to disability over time (Halper & Costello, 1997; Rosebrough, 1997). Primary progressive MS results in increased disability over time, with or without exacerbations and sometimes with plateaus or a steady increase in disability. Progressive relapsing MS is characterized by remissions and exacerbations that result in increased levels of disability over time, with a type of cumulative effect. The secondary progressive type may be characterized by one or two events with complete recovery, followed by progressive disability over time. Relapsing-remitting MS is generally characterized by more frequent periods of exacerbations that result in either healing during the remission phase or progressive, cumulative disability with partial healing during remission in which a person may experience temporary recovery from the neurological effects. According to Halper and Costello (1997), the majority of relapsing patients change to secondary progressive patterns. Although the clinical course of MS is highly variable and unpredictable, most patients progress from initial symptoms to measurable disabilities.

The signs and symptoms seen in those with MS (Table 11–11) result from destruction of the myelin sheath, which acts as a conductor for nerve impulses in the CNS. The symptoms may last from minutes to hours. As the myelin is destroyed, acute inflammation and swelling around the nerve take place. Although these areas may heal, scarring results and patches of sclerotic tissue are left that interrupt and slow transmission of impulses along nerve fibers. This process affects the white matter of the brain and spinal cord, including the optic nerve, and results in scat-

Table 11–11 SIGNS AND SYMPTOMS OF MULTIPLE SCLEROSIS

Fatigue
Impaired mobility
Weakness
Paresthesia
Uncoordination
Balance problems
Visual deficits
Bowel and bladder difficulties
Spasticity
Dizziness
Impaired cognitive function

tered areas of sclerosis (thus the term "multiple sclerosis"). The pattern of scattering varies from patient to patient.

One major indicator of the disease is that it is characterized by periods of remission and exacerbation. Impaired mobility is the most common sign, along with fatigue. Other early indicators of the disease may be visual problems (such as blurred vision, blind spots, or diplopia). Sensory changes seen include numbness, paresthesia, a heightened sensitivity to extremes in temperature, and ataxia. Alterations in mobility eventually occur and include paresis, spasticity, incoordination, and loss of balance (Brar, Smith, Nelson, Franklin, & Cobble, 1991). Nystagmus (rapid involuntary movement of the eyeball) is common. Bladder incontinence may occur, as well as bowel and sexual dysfunction (Dupont, 1995; Norbendo, 1996).

The diagnosis of MS is made primarily through clinical findings, with laboratory tests and magnetic resonance imaging (MRI) used to support the diagnosis. Although no one single test is reliable in detecting MS, MRI provides the most useful information in that physicians can visualize areas of sclerosis. Current guidelines suggest that the diagnosis is made after at least two remissions and exacerbations of MS symptoms, as well as noting separate areas of demyelination in the brain and/or spinal cord on MRI. In adults over 50 years of age, false-positive results are common. Additionally, cerebrospinal fluid may show elevated protein levels (in about 50% of cases), but more likely elevated IgG levels, and oligoclonal IgG bands are present in 90% of cases (Halper & Costello, 1997).

Nursing Implications

Nursing goals include maximizing and maintaining independence, preventing complica-

tions, and providing support and education to the family and patient. Table 11–12 presents common nursing diagnoses associated with care of a patient with MS. An older person who has lived with MS may have difficulty distinguishing between the effects of disease progression and traits associated with normal aging. Buchanan and Lewis (1997) found that younger adults with MS who resided in nursing facilities were more dependent in ADLs than were elderly residents in those facilities. However, younger adults with MS who are living in long-term care facilities most likely do so because their functional limitations are greater (or their resources are smaller) than those in the community. Yet, if at a young age many patients with MS require constant nursing care, how much more so as they get older? One could expect a person who has lived with progressive functional limitations to perhaps have aged more quickly. That is, a person's biological age may not be equal to the chronological age when disabilities are present earlier in life. Disabilities may have a cumulative effect as one ages. For a symptom such as fatigue, a person with MS is likely to experience additional decreases in endurance as a result of the aging process. Yet those changes happen slowly, so the person has

Table 11–12 COMMON NURSING DIAGNOSES ASSOCIATED WITH CARE OF PERSONS WITH MULTIPLE SCLEROSIS

Impaired physical mobility
Fatigue
Activity intolerance
Self-care deficit
Alteration in sensory-perceptual function
Impaired swallowing
Potential for injury: falls
Anxiety
Alteration in bowel elimination: constipation or incontinence
Alteration in bladder elimination: retention, incontinence, or combined
Altered body temperature
Self-concept disturbance
Sexual dysfunction
Impaired communication
Attention deficit
Grief
Knowledge deficit
Home health maintenance
Powerlessness
Sleep pattern disturbance
Depression
Pain (from spasticity)

time to adjust. It remains to be researched what effect aging has on persons who have lived many years with the disease.

Improving Physical Endurance

Several nursing indications are related to maximizing a person's endurance. First, fatigue is a major symptom in MS and results in decreased endurance during physical activity. Fatigue in MS can be caused by minimal effort. It is a chronic problem and one that a person with MS takes longer to recover from than the average elder (Hubsky & Sears, 1992; Svensson, Gerdle, & Elert, 1994). Fatigue may be a primary symptom of MS and result from a decrease in nerve conduction impulses, or it may appear secondary to sleep disturbance, depression, medications, deconditioning, or other factors.

One way for the GRN to help a person with MS to combat fatigue is to alternate rest and activity. Planning for frequent rest periods during days of therapy or at home will allow longer periods of function. Rest should include both physical and mental aspects. Types of interventions that could be used and taught to the patient and family include watching television during rest periods, taking a nap, meditation, listening to music, or reading. Other strategies for decreasing fatigue include conserving energy, setting priorities for what should be accomplished that day, reassigning tasks as needed, and getting at least 8 to 9 uninterrupted hours of sleep per day (Hubsky & Sears, 1992).

Another key intervention to increase endurance and strength is an exercise program. Of course, planned rest periods should be included in any such regimen. Svensson, Gerdle, and Elert's case study (1994) of five individuals with MS suggested that exercise improved endurance and decreased fatigue. Being involved in an exercise program takes additional planning for the MS patient.

Fatigue is often related to an alteration in regulation of body temperature. Although the mechanism of this phenomenon is unclear, heat has been shown to exacerbate symptoms whereas cool provides temporary relief. Cool baths or cooling vests have been associated with short-term improvement when done several times per day, but these measures provide only temporary relief (Namey & Schwetz, 1993). The principle of using coolness within the environment can, however, be useful in several ways to decrease fatigue. A person with MS should wear lightweight clothes during physical activity. The room should be cool, and air conditioning should be used during warm weather. Activities should be planned for the cooler parts of the day. So an exercise program might best be done early in the morning or after sunset in the evening. Additionally, aquatic activities are recommended as therapeutic for persons with MS, but long-term care facilities rarely provide such services (Buchanan & Lewis, 1997). However, for those living in the community, an exercise program that includes swimming might be ideal if adequate supervision is available. Other water sports such as snorkeling or scuba diving are also done by some elders, although location and expense prohibit many from engaging in these activities (Peterson & Bell, 1995). Persons with MS may feel a new freedom in the water. Water activities provide exercise by giving resistance to movements. The coolness of the water helps decrease fatigue, and fewer problems in the sense of balance are noted, without a fear of falling as one would have when ambulating.

Endurance should be built gradually. Activity should be increased slowly, but maintenance of function emphasized. Exercise programs may need to be modified as time progresses to account for aging changes and further functional limitations.

Promoting Self-Care

For a person with MS, continuing self-care may become a daily challenge. Not only does promotion of self-care as a nursing goal assist the individual toward independence, it can also help manage health care costs for long-term care. "Improving self-care and avoiding preventable hospitalizations might lower the considerable health costs of MS" (Bourdette et al., 1993). Table 11–13 suggests some key areas for teaching persons with MS, as well as some expected outcomes.

Several strategies may assist in maintaining self-care for an older adult with MS. A regular, daily exercise program is one of the most important ways to maintain the strength needed for independent ambulation and ADLs. Fostering social support and linking the person and family with appropriate resources are equally important. Further interventions related to providing psychosocial support are discussed later. Stress management skills should be taught, as well as how to make the environment optimal for function by controlling temperature and the physical

Table 11–13 CLIENT/FAMILY TEACHING: KEY AREAS IN MULTIPLE SCLEROSIS

Essential teaching areas

Promoting activity tolerance/managing fatigue: alternating rest and activity, following exercise regimens, planning activities for the cooler part of the day, avoiding hot temperatures, building endurance gradually, using relaxation techniques

Medication therapy: side effects of all medications; use of pain medications; may need to teach subcutaneous injection technique, site rotation, mixing of medication for injection

Safety promotion: prevention of falls and injury

Disease progression: expectations, current treatments

Bowel and bladder management: balancing intake and output, effects of fluids/diet/activity on bowel and bladder patterns, prevention of constipation/UTI, management of incontinence; may need to teach self-catheterization

Psychosocial needs: identifying and using community resources, strengthening social support systems, managing role changes and sexual dysfunction, combating depression, dealing with feelings of grief and loss, managing pain

Outcomes: Client (and/or family/caregiver) will be able to

Identify events/activities that precipitate incontinence

State the signs/symptoms of UTI

List ways to reduce the risk of falls at home and in the community

Engage in strengthening exercises

Build endurance level through participation in exercise programs and structuring activities to minimize/manage fatigue

Identify relaxing activities to decrease anxiety, manage stress, and promote sleep

Prepare a proper diet with adequate protein and fiber

Identify own strengths and weaknesses

Use community resources and support groups as needed

State medication effects and side effects

Adjust to changes in roles/relationships

Develop an individualized plan that promotes self-care in ADLs while maximizing functional capacity

---

UTI, urinary tract infection; ADLs, activities of daily living.

---

layout. Therapies of various kinds should be considered, including aquatics, art, music, pets, horticulture, mobility, or massage. These activities can be done as hobbies or through more formalized programs. The home should be set up to minimize energy expenditure while maximizing performance and safety. Balance problems can lead to falls, so strategies discussed in Chapter 7 should be implemented.

Other factors may be related to self-care. Wassem (1991) found that persons with an internal locus of control had better knowledge of the disease, increased self-care, a more benign MS course, and a lower divorce rate overall than those with external loci of control. Using Wassem's suggestions, GRNs could base the care plan on the person's locus of control. A person with an internal locus would wish to be involved and participate in setting up a long-term home maintenance program. A person with an external locus of control might rather be told what a good plan would be. Gulick (1987) developed a 15-item self-administered scale to measure self-care in

ADLs among persons with MS. The major factors used in Gulick's model included intimacy, sensory and communication, and recreation and socializing. The model achieved a good fit, with the 15 items on the scale explaining 71% of the variance. These results suggest that the aforementioned areas are key factors in maintaining self-care among persons with MS (Gulick, 1991, 1992).

Managing Bladder Dysfunction

Bladder problems are common in patients with MS, even those with minimal other symptoms, and are a frequent cause of hospitalization. Urinary incontinence is often a contributing factor to institutionalization of older adults with MS. Neurogenic bladder dysfunction may be manifested in a variety of ways, including difficulties with storage, emptying, spastic sphincters, or detrusor-sphincter dyssynergia (Beneton, De Parisot, Granjon, & Millet, 1996). More detailed discussion of the management of neurogenic bladder problems is found in Chapter 8.

GRNs should observe laboratory results to rule out the presence of UTI as a causative factor in incontinence. A detailed bowel and bladder history should be taken. Adequate hydration is essential. A postvoiding bladder scan or postvoiding residual obtained through catheterization will assist the GRN in determining whether the patient is completely emptying the bladder. The combination of the amount voided in addition to what is obtained from the postvoiding residual will assist in calculating bladder capacity in the absence of more extensive urodynamic and cystometric testing.

Anticholinergics are often used when urine storage is the problem. When the patient is unable to empty the bladder completely, intermittent catheterization may be necessary. A postvoiding residual of greater than 150 ml is an acceptable guideline for determining incomplete bladder emptying in a geriatric client. A combination of therapies may be indicated if several compounding problems exist. Some patients may eventually need to rely on intermittent catheterization as the primary means of bladder emptying. Self-catheterization may need to be taught. The GRN can also assist the patient in identifying what activities precipitate incontinence or leakage. Balancing intake and output may also need to be taught.

Providing Psychosocial Support

The psychosocial and emotional needs of patients with MS may be many. Cognitive changes occur in 55% to 65% of people with the disease and affect memory, learning, reasoning, and attention (Jansen & Cimprich, 1994). Psychological changes vary greatly and are not necessarily related to the degree of physical disability (Wineman, 1990), so even those with mild functional limitations may have cognitive deficits. A wide range of emotions may also be experienced. Persons with MS may experience chronic sorrow periodically over time when events remind them of the chronicity of their situation (Hainsworth, 1994). Other common feelings may include sadness, anger, frustration, helplessness, fear, anxiety, depression, and uncertainty.

Wineman (1990) found that those with more severe disability expressed less purpose in life and increased depression. Psychosocial adaptation was significantly influenced by perceived social supports, perceived unsupportiveness, and perceived uncertainty. Gulick (1994) found that women perceived lower social support than men did, thus suggesting that nurses need to aware of losses that females, in particular, have experienced. Being a good resource means that nurses must be knowledgeable about what services are offered within the communities in which they practice.

Caregivers of those with MS express feelings common to others who provide assistance in the home of the chronically ill. Fatigue and isolation, anxiety, and depression are commonly reported (Gregory, 1995; O'Brien, 1993). A majority of caregivers in a study by Gregory, Disler, and Firth (1996) were over 50 years of age, with 32% being elderly themselves. This circumstance caused concerns about the caregiver's health and worry about the responsibility of caring for a person with MS over an extended period. A reduction in quality of life was found among caregivers, and significant changes were found to occur within the household.

Clearly, emotional support is needed for the entire family trying to cope with the impact of MS (Case Study 11.3). GRNs should provide information about the disease process and be available to answer questions. Time should be taken to allow the person and family to reflect on the implications of the disease process. It is likely that because of the characteristics of MS, the person may achieve rapport with the rehabilitation team after consecutive admissions related to exacerbations. However, good discharge planning is essential. Support groups for both the patient and family should be identified. Social support networks and family ties should be strengthened, and community resources and other means of assistance should be investigated.

CASE STUDY 11.3
Aging with Multiple Sclerosis

About 17 years ago, having lived with MS for many years, Mrs. Case (68 years) lived in a modest home with her husband as caregiver. Significantly fewer resources and adaptive equipment were available at that time than at the present, which forced the family to rely on their own resources. Mrs. Case had, within the last 2 years, experienced a gradual deterioration in function to the point of being wheelchair- and home-bound. Mr. Case was in his 70s and lovingly cared for his wife in their home. The local visiting nurse association made regular visits to their residence but found that Mr. Case had invented his own ways of caring for his wife out of necessity. The couple had one son who helped create some of the tools and equipment that Mr. Case had devised to make life easier for him and his wife. A collaborative effort between the health care system and the family had enabled Mr. Case to keep his wife at home, although she required many hours of care each day. It had been suggested that he place her in a nursing home, but Mr. Case refused, saying, "She took care of me and our child all these years. Now it's my turn." Mrs. Case was essentially totally dependent on her husband for the necessities of life such as bathing, food, and toileting. She was light and of slight build, and he was large and strong, which made transferring easier for him. She had an indwelling Foley catheter that was monitored and changed monthly by the home care nurse. Mr. Case made sure that his wife took in plenty of fluids and fiber to prevent constipation, and he got her up into her wheelchair or a special reclining chair daily. Her clothes were comfortable, loose fitting, and easy to wash. A hospital bed in their room made her positioning at night more comfortable.

Mrs. Case had a soft, weak, thin voice and often seemed to struggle with her respirations, although her lungs were clear. Mr. Case could understand her and could often read her facial expressions. The home environment was clean, safe, and warm. Mrs. Case had a small amount of gross upper extremity movement. Her husband and son had rearranged the house so that she could look out the back sliding glass door into the peaceful woods during the day from the kitchen. The telephone had a large plastic frame with giant buttons connected, which allowed Mrs. Case to sit next to it and push a button to ring each of several different numbers she might need in an emergency. This phone was how she was able to get help if her husband went out for groceries or was working in the yard. They had a schedule planned for each day that they tried to adhere to. This schedule seemed to provide a sense of stability and security. Mr. Case was a good cook and helped feed his wife at meals, which they ate together. He seemed to have adjusted extremely well to his wife's condition, although her care was a full-time job. When the home health nurses made their scheduled visits, they found that Mrs. Case's condition was stable. Her skin was in beautiful condition, with no breakdown, and her nutritional sta-

tus was sufficient, although she had difficulty swallowing at times. The nurse gave instructions to Mr. Case on how to assist with swallowing and how to identify the signs and symptoms of aspiration. She also reminded the patient and her husband of the importance of range-of-motion exercises to avoid contractures. The couple stated that she did her exercises with his help every morning. Mr. Case provided the nurse with records of intake and output, medications given, and any problems he had encountered. The nurse also gave Mr. Case the name and number of a newly formed support group in his area. Mrs. Case praised her husband in front of the nurse for his good care of her. This mutual sharing and regular interaction demonstrate the team concept at a time when fewer resources were available for older caregivers and their spouses.

Medication Management

Treatment of MS has traditionally involved medical management of exacerbations. Such management has been accomplished through intravenous or oral steroids, including methylprednisolone and prednisone, or immunosuppressants such as azathioprine or cyclophosphamide. Immunomodulation treatments (such as copolymer 1) are used for relapsing MS to reduce the rate of exacerbations (Costello & Conway, 1997). Interferons of different types have been studied in drug trials for MS patients with varying results.

One of the most promising treatments, however, is interferon beta-1b (Betaseron), which was approved for public use in 1993. Betaseron was studied extensively before its approval and has been shown to significantly alter the course of MS. Fewer new CNS lesions were found in those receiving 8 million IU through subcutaneous injection of the drug when compared with a group that received placebo (Costello & Conway, 1997). This result represented the closest to a cure for MS (although it is not a cure) discovered until recently. Betaseron thus acts to decrease the overall number and severity of MS exacerbations, as well as the number of plaques resulting from scarring of the myelin sheath. With the development and widespread use of Betaseron, it may be anticipated that persons with MS will be able to live a longer life with fewer complications and lessening degrees of disability over time.

An interesting phenomenon occurred when Betaseron first came on the market. Because the initial demand for the drug was so great, not enough of the medication was immediately available from the supplier. Radio stations in the Chicago area then advertised a lottery that was held to determine who would receive the first available treatments. Persons with MS were told to talk to their doctor about whether they would be a candidate for this new drug. The physicians were then to write a letter recommending which of their patients should receive it as soon as possible, and a "lottery" based on those names was subsequently held. Once the supply caught up with the demand, this shortage was no longer a problem. Between 30,000 and 50,000 people currently use Betaseron for the management of MS (Costello & Conway, 1997).

A few implications with the use of Betaseron are of note. "Effective long-term management begins with selecting patients who are highly motivated and who understand the realistic potential outcomes of treatment" (Conway & Costello, 1997, p. 63). Not all patients will be able to successfully engage in the requirements necessitated by Betaseron therapy. A reliable support system is necessary, and the patient must be self-motivated. Subcutaneous injection (given every other day) techniques must be mastered, as well as the ability to correctly reconstitute the powder with diluent. This process requires knowledge of several ordered steps and the physical ability to carry out these tasks or the presence of a caregiver who can accomplish these tasks. Injection sites are the same as for insulin, but sites should be rotated.

Management of side effects is another area of concern. The common side effects of Betaseron therapy that pertain to older adults are skin reactions, flu-like symptoms, abnormal laboratory results, dyspnea and palpitations, mental disorders (including depression, anxiety, and confusion), and temporary worsening of MS symptoms. Side effects most often occur in the early stages of treatment. Patients and families should be advised that the use of Betaseron therapy requires a long-term commitment and the ability to learn and perform several key skills.

The most recent medication on the market is Copaxone (glatiramer acetate for injection), a noninterferon, nonsteroidal agent. Copaxone moderates the course of MS on a long-term basis by blocking myelin-specific autoimmune responses and thereby reducing the frequency of relapses. This new class of medication, particularly for those with relapsing-remitting MS, seems to be better tolerated (with fewer side effects) than forms of interferon-β. It should be noted, however, that Copaxone use in patients over the age of 68 has not been studied (Teva Marion Partners, 1997). Several other new medications are currently being researched and offer new hope for those with MS.

GUILLAIN-BARRÉ SYNDROME

Guillain-Barré syndrome is a postinfectious illness of unknown origin, also referred to as acute idiopathic polyneuritis, a subcategory of acute idiopathic demyelinating polyneuropathy. GBS was first recognized as a clinical entity in 1976 with introduction of the swine flu vaccine (Steinberg, 1993). At that time, unusual symptoms developed in an increased number of persons who received the vaccine, some resulting in unexplained death, particularly among the frail elderly in nursing homes. Even older adults are at risk for this rare illness, which may occur without warning and presents a particular challenge to the nurse (Parobeck, Burnham, & Laukhuf, 1992).

Characteristics of Guillain-Barré Syndrome

Although the cause is unknown, theories include those related to an autoimmune response, a viral infection, allergies, or other hypersensitivity reactions. This disease affects persons of all ages and ethnic backgrounds, both males and females, with an incidence of 1.7 in 100,000. The mortality rate is presently 5% (Steinberg, 1993), although some earlier sources stated a mortality rate of 10% to 20% when the illness was first recognized as a disease.

The effects seen in GBS are attributed to widespread inflammation resulting in demyelination of peripheral nerve fibers (Table 11–14). The onset of the disorder is often preceded by an infection and mild fever, usually respiratory or gastrointestinal, 1 to 3 weeks previously. GBS has also been associated with vaccinations, including flu shots and immunizations. The symptoms are thought to have an abrupt onset, although in some cases vague, nonspecific complaints related to paresthesias, fatigue, and "not feeling right" may be voiced shortly before. GBS is characterized by a flaccid paralysis that begins in the lower extremities and moves upward symmetri-

Table 11–14   SIGNS AND SYMPTOMS OF GUILLAIN-BARRÉ SYNDROME

Rapid onset of symptoms
Complaints of abnormal sensations in the extremities or face
Fatigue
Weakness progressing to paralysis
Ataxia
Paralysis that moves from the lower extremities upward
Decrease or absence of deep tendon reflexes
Elevated protein level in spinal fluid
Feelings of fear and anxiety
Possible history of febrile illness 1–3 wk before onset
Possible history of immunization or vaccine

cally. When paralysis reaches the thoracic region, the person must often be managed by mechanical ventilation because of paralysis of the respiratory muscles, which can occur within even 48 hours of onset (Borgman-Gainer, 1996). In many cases facial paralysis may ensue, even without respiratory paralysis, although this variation is less common (Easton, 1995).

The diagnosis is sometimes difficult to make, although the person's symptoms generally present a typical picture. The physician will also check for loss of reflexes, even though this loss may not occur until symptoms have significantly progressed. Confirmation of the diagnosis can be made, however, through a lumbar puncture, which will show elevated protein levels in spinal fluid. Electrical nerve and muscles tests such as an electromyogram may also assist with the diagnosis. On occasion, GBS and MS are confused because of similar symptoms. However, the GRN should remember that MS is characterized by remissions and exacerbations but a person with GBS should not have recurrences once the disease has run its course.

The clinical progress of the disease covers three stages. In the first stage the onset seems abrupt, with the person rapidly experiencing ataxia, progressive weakness, and paralysis. A plateau then occurs in the second stage, which can last from several days to weeks. The third phase, or recovery, can take from weeks to months or as long as a couple of years for maximal function to be obtained. Because the myelin can regenerate, recovery can be complete. However, in many cases, permanent functional and sensory deficits may result. Bakker-Hatten, Lankhorst, Kriek,

and Slootman (1995) found that in a follow-up study of persons with GBS, most with serious paralysis during the illness had some degree of disability 7 to 12 years later, although only about one fourth were seriously disabled. Many physicians believe that the earlier the diagnosis is made and treatment begins, the better the chance for complete recovery without residual deficits.

In the acute phase, the person may complain of burning sensations of the skin and great pain when touched. This change in sensation is thought to be due to the effects of destruction of the myelin sheath, which protects and facilitates nerve impulse conduction. The GRN will need to be particularly aware of this occurrence, although this phase may have passed by the time the person is ready to enter rehabilitation therapy.

Nursing Implications

Medical management of a person with GBS includes medications such as immunosuppressants, prednisone, adrenocorticotropic hormone, and methotrexate. Intravenous gamma-globulin is preferred by some physicians for the treatment of GBS. Plasmapheresis is a treatment of choice for other individuals. This therapy involves a type of "washing" of the blood to rid it of antibodies that may have built up in response to the disease. Such plasma exchange is aimed at shortening progression of the illness and may include several treatments. The procedure may temporarily exacerbate symptoms and result in uncomfortable sensations, even feelings of near death (Easton, 1995), which is a risk of the treatment. However, after each treatment, patients may gain strength and eventually be able to move on to intensive rehabilitation and experience fewer permanent functional deficits. It is generally believed that the sooner this treatment is instituted, the more likely the person will recover with less loss of function. Rehabilitative nursing management of a person with GBS is supportive-educative. Table 11–15 lists common nursing diagnoses associated with care of a person with GBS. Penrose (1993), with reference to the treatment of patients with GBS, reminded nurses that the goal of rehabilitation "is to help the patient pace recovery to obtain the maximum use of muscles as the nerve supply returns and aid the patient in adjusting to persistent limitations" (p. 89). Monitoring respiratory status is crucial for persons with GBS. The physician should be

Table 11–15 COMMON NURSING DIAGNOSES ASSOCIATED WITH CARE OF PERSONS WITH GUILLAIN-BARRÉ SYNDROME

Ineffective breathing pattern
Ineffective airway clearance
Impaired physical mobility
Fatigue
Activity intolerance
Self-care deficit
Alteration in sensory-perceptual function
Impaired swallowing
Impaired verbal communication
Anxiety
Alteration in bowel elimination
Alteration in bladder elimination
High risk for injury/high risk for falls
Altered body temperature
Self-concept disturbance
Grief
Knowledge deficit
Alteration in home health maintenance
Powerlessness
Depression
Pain (in acute phase)
Alteration in family process

notified of any change in respiratory function. There is also a chance of a second onslaught shortly after the initial onset, so GRNs should be alert to the possibility of further impairment throughout the course of the illness. Because no "cure" is known and the symptoms are treated medically, the GRN will need to engage in teaching the patient and family. A strong social and emotional support network will be needed for those with GBS to combat the effects of this disorder. Feelings of isolation, helplessness, hopelessness, and loneliness are common (Baier & Schomaker, 1986). Support groups may assist the person and family in feeling that they are not alone. The GBS Foundation International provides assistance to patients and families through support, education, and research. More than 130 chapters exist in the United States, Canada, Europe, Australia, and South Africa (Steinberg, 1993).

The patient will gain strength and rebuild endurance through participation in therapies and encouragement of the interdisciplinary team. GRNs should emphasize gradually increasing endurance, alternating rest and activity, and improving activity tolerance (Case Study 11.4). Bowel and bladder retraining may be necessary, and it can be expected that most patients will regain these functions

through scheduled voiding and previously discussed toileting techniques. It should be emphasized to the patient and family that return to one's former state of strength and abilities is not always possible and may take a period of months or longer. Sensitivity to light is sometimes a problem, and wearing sunglasses can provide some relief. Fatigue may be an ongoing problem that prohibits some persons from returning to their former jobs. The GRN may need to assist the individual in identifying new or alternative means of employment or income if return to the former work setting is not a viable option.

CASE STUDY 11.4
Guillain-Barré Syndrome

Mrs. Jones, an 84 year old African-American woman, was admitted to the acute rehabilitation unit with a diagnosis of GBS. Minimal upper extremity movement was noted, but both lower extremities were essentially paralyzed upon admission. She required the maximum assistance of three to four people to transfer with a sliding board. She also had a broken left wrist, arthritis, and cataracts. Mrs. Jones had an indwelling Foley catheter, with intake and output being monitored. Two pressure ulcers, both stage I–II, were noted on her coccyx and required daily dressing changes. She was in isolation for enteric precautions because of suspected *Clostridium difficile* in the stool. A peripherally inserted catheter was being used to administer intravenous antibiotics. Mrs. Jones also received immunosuppressants. Bilateral footdrop was noted. Mrs. Jones had some complicating factors that puzzled the physician. She had gross generalized edema and possibly some renal impairment as evidenced by a blood urea nitrogen value of 32, although no prior renal problems. The abnormally dry condition of her skin and constant flaking in large amounts required that she take a daily bath (because of exfoliation) and that special creams be applied.

Because of her great amount of edema in addition to the weakness from GBS, Mrs. Jones was not able to participate well in therapy, although she was highly motivated. Her main social supports were her family, especially an 80 year old sister who was a retired nurse. Although her strength was slowly increasing with therapy and immunosuppressive medications, she remained weak. Plasmapheresis was not a treatment of choice because of her age and other health problems. Because the overall swelling of her entire body hindered her progress, the physician started her on a regimen of furosemide (Lasix), and within a week her swelling was gone and her skin condition relieved. Her intake and output were within normal limits, and use of the Foley catheter was discontinued. Bladder training followed, and she was continent by discharge. Her stools were negative for *Clostridium*. The pressure ulcers on her coccyx healed before discharge. Mrs. Jones surprised the staff by being able to return home (requiring only minimal assistance with ADLs) with her sister as primary caregiver. Home health services would monitor within the home.

LUPUS

Systemic lupus erythematosus (SLE) is a connective tissue disorder thought to be caused by antigen-antibody complexes that affect many bodily organs. SLE is now believed to be genetically driven based on studies of identical twins who showed antibody patterns identical to each other (Michigan Lupus Foundation, 1993; Shaw & Bertino, 1994) Lupus affects 1 in 700 people per year, which makes it a relatively frequently occurring disease. SLE is more common in females than males (4:1 ratio), especially striking those between 15 and 45 years of age with an average onset at age 30. SLE affects blacks, Asians, Hispanics, and Native Americans more than whites. A summary of risk factors is given in Table 11–16.

Because no cure is known but better treatment is available, it is likely that GRNs will be seeing increasing numbers of older patients with lupus in long-term care and rehabilitation (Bertino & Lu, 1993). The illness

Table 11–16 POSSIBLE RISK FACTORS FOR LUPUS

Family history/genetic predisposition
Extreme stress
Infections
Other environmental factors
Adult females
African-American, Hispanic, Native American, or Asian background

Table 11–17 SOME SIGNS AND SYMPTOMS OF LUPUS

Fatigue
Low-grade fever
Joint and muscle pain similar to arthritis
A butterfly rash (fixed erythema) over the nose and cheekbones (aggravated by sunlight)
Other rashes on the face or chest
Alopecia
Seizures
Abnormal antinuclear antibody titer
Pleurisy
Decreased appetite
Sores in the nose or mouth
Painful sensitivity of the fingers to the cold

can result in functional disabilities, especially problems related to the joints. Renal failure is the leading cause of death.

Characteristics of Systemic Lupus Erythematosus

The disease is characterized by triggering of an inflammatory response that results in tissue damage to the skin, joints, and internal organs through an autoimmune reaction. The symptoms vary widely among patients, so medical management is individualized. Some common signs and symptoms are presented in Table 11–17. SLE is an unpredictable disease characterized by remissions and exacerbations (Ferrante & Derivan, 1995).

Arthritis results in 90% of cases, so care is often overseen by a rheumatologist. The GRN will need to assist the person in maintaining a balance between managing the symptoms and preventing adverse reactions to medications. Individuals may be taking nonsteroidal anti-inflammatory drugs for arthritis and fever or corticosteroids if major organs are involved. One of the most distressing side effects of steroid therapy for the patient is the "moon" face, which can significantly alter their physical appearance, even to the point that they are unrecognizable to some who knew them previously.

The diagnosis is made through observation of symptoms, history, and an antinuclear antibody test, which is positive in 95% of cases. Acute pericarditis may be the first sign of SLE (Spiera & Rothschild, 1995), although cardiac involvement varies from patient to patient. A red butterfly rash across the nose and cheeks is characteristic, as well as the presence of fever, fatigue, and pain.

Nursing Implications

Nursing management of an older person with SLE will be complex. Common nursing diagnoses appear in Table 11–18. GRNs will need to assist persons in dealing with a variety of symptoms, including fatigue, chronic pain, and disturbances in self-concept (Bertino & Lu, 1993). Mutual goals should be set, including goals related to activity. Pain management will be essential, particularly if physical rehabilitation is being undertaken and involves joint motion and muscle strengthening. The GRN should teach energy conservation techniques and the importance of alternating rest and activity. A person with SLE should avoid sun exposure inasmuch as sunlight can exacerbate symptoms. Adequate sunscreen, wide-brimmed hats, and layered clothing can be helpful. Good oral hygiene and adequate nutrition can help prevent ulcerations of the mouth and nose, as well as promote overall health. The nurse should teach the person about the side effects of medications, such as the need to take steroids with food to avoid stomach upset. Signs and symptoms of exacerbation, as well as precipitating factors, should be explored and understood by the patient (Ferrante & Derivan, 1995). The GRN may need to remind physical therapists to be in constant communication with nurses and the physician to help monitor the effects, both positive and negative, of medication therapy on functional outcomes (Moncur & Williams, 1995).

Emotional support for patients with SLE and their families is essential for this chronic disorder (Case Study 11.5). Many SLE support groups can help provide socialization, understanding, camaraderie, and emotional support to those struggling with SLE. GRNs should be aware of local chapters in their area. Some key resources for those with common neurological disorders are noted in Table 11–19.

CASE STUDY 11.5
Living with Lupus

Although many persons who age with chronic health problems require frequent use of rehabilitative services, many learn to rehabilitate themselves. This case study provides one such example. Lupus was diagnosed in Mira when she was in her 20s, and she had lived with the disease for several decades. Although she experienced numerous complications requiring hospitalization as a result of lupus, she was able to live rather independently in her parent's home. Mira never married, and at the age of 60 she still lived with her elderly mother, who was widowed and in poor health. Together, they formed a strong support system and used their church community as a mainstay. Mira had been forced to retire early from teaching because of her inability to keep up the demanding pace, but working was one of her major coping strategies. A recurring problem for Mira was her tendency to sustain fractures relatively easily. Pain from arthritic changes contributed to her feelings of frustration. She was no longer able to drive a car, which made her feel more isolated. Mira solved her problems by volunteering to work in her church by coordinating a children's ministry. The church leaders worked out a system of exchange that helped provide transportation and housekeeping assistance for Mira and her mother in return for her services in organizing the children's programs, a job that demanded more intellectual, delegatory, organizational, and communication skills than physical demands. Her job at the church was flexible and provided the satisfaction and diversion she needed to cope, as well as helping to meet her family's needs.

Table 11–18   COMMON NURSING DIAGNOSES FOR PERSONS WITH LUPUS

Pain
Potential for infection
Alteration in nutrition: less than
   body requirements
Impaired gas exchange
Fatigue
Activity intolerance
Alteration in sensory perception
Decreased endurance
Alteration in body temperature
Self-concept disturbance
Powerlessness
Impaired physical mobility
Knowledge deficit

TRAUMATIC BRAIN INJURY

Although TBI occurs more frequently in the young than the old, trauma to the head can occur at any age and often necessitates reha-

Table 11–19 RESOURCES FOR THOSE WITH NEUROLOGICAL DEFICITS AND THEIR FAMILIES

American Spinal Injury Association
  250 E. Superior, Room 619
  Chicago, IL 60611
  312-908-3425
  312-908-6207
National Spinal Cord Injury Association
  600 W. Cummings Park, Suite 2000
  Woburn, MA 01801
Paralyzed Veterans of America
  801 18th Street NW
  Washington, DC 20006
  202-872-1300
  1-800-424-8200
Guillain-Barré Syndrome (GBS) Foundation
  International
  P.O. Box 262
  Wynnewood, PA 19606
  610-667-0131
National Multiple Sclerosis Society
  733 3rd Avenue, 6th Floor
  New York, NY 10017
  1-800-Fight MS (1-800-344-4867)
  E-mail: nat@nmss.org
Multiple Sclerosis Society
  Indiana Chapter
  615 North Alabama #318
  Indianapolis, IN 46204
  1-800-762-1209
Lupus Foundation of America
  1300 Piccard Drive, Suite 200
  Rockville, MD 20850
  301-670-9292
  1-800-558-0121
  Website: www.lupus.org/lupus
Lupus Foundation of America
  Northwest Indiana Chapter
  3819 W. 40th Avenue
  Gary, IN 46408
  219-659-1611

The American Parkinson Disease Association, Inc.
  1250 Hyland Blvd., Suite 4B
  Staten Island, NY 10305
  1-800-223-APDA (2732)
National Parkinson Foundation
  1501 N. W. Ninth Avenue
  Miami, FL 33136
  1-800-327-4545
  E-mail: @:NTS.MED.MIAMI.EDU
  Website: http://www.Parkinson.org
Parkinson's Disease Foundation
  William Black Medical Research Building
  Columbia Presbyterian Medical Center
  710 West 168th Street
  New York, NY 10032
  1-800-457-6676
  E-mail: PDSCPMCAOL.com
  Website: http://www.Parkinson-Foundation.org
United Parkinson Foundation
  833 W. Washington Blvd.
  Chicago, IL 60607
  312-733-1893
National Head Injury Foundation
  1776 Massachusetts Avenue NW, Suite 100
  Washington, DC 20036
  202-296-6443
  1-800-444-6443
  Website: www.biausa.org
National Stroke Association
  300 E. Hampden Avenue, Suite 240
  Englewood, CO 80110-2654
  1-800-strokes (1-800-787-6537)
  E-mail: info@stroke.org
  Website: http://www.stroke.org
National Institute of Neurological and
  Communicative Disorders and Stroke
  Building 31, Room 8A52
  9000 Rockville Pike
  Bethesda, MD 20892
  301-496-9746

bilitation. Little research has been published on the results of head injury in older adults. Most of the research done in this area has of course used samples of younger patients because head injuries most often occur in those aged 35 and under. However, head injury from falls, motor vehicle accidents, or other trauma is not uncommon and is likely to increase among the growing elderly population as persons are enjoying more active lifestyles into the later years. A major difference between head injury in younger and older adults is that the elderly have much less reserve in all body systems; as a result, they have less chance of survival after such an insult and poorer rehabilitation outcomes.

This discussion will review the effects of brain injury and general principles to guide care.

Characteristics of Brain-Injured Persons

The deficits seen in brain injury may result from impact or rebound damage or even a twisting motion of the brain stem. Tearing, bleeding, and swelling within the brain cause damage to the delicate cranial tissues. The extent of brain injury, just as the amount of recovery possible, depends on several factors, but mainly which areas of the brain have been damaged and the severity of the trauma. Table 11–20 reviews some common structures

Table 11-20 MAJOR AREAS OF THE BRAIN AND CORRESPONDING FUNCTIONS

Area	Function	Results of Impairment/Damage
Frontal lobe	Voluntary movements (for opposite side) Motor speech Attention, concentration, judgment, emotions, personality, problem solving Autonomic functions	Hemiplegia/hemiparesis Broca's aphasia Inability to concentrate, poor judgment, lack of safety awareness Inappropriate social behavior, flat affect, personality changes Autonomic dysfunctions Focal seizures
Temporal lobe	Primary auditory area Auditory memory, complex perceptual organization, sequencing of incoming stimuli	Receptive aphasia Auditory hallucinations Difficulty with sequencing Irritability, psychomotor seizures
Occipital lobe	Primary visual area Integration of visual input	Hemianopia Visual hallucinations Seizures
Parietal lobe	Primary sensory area (for opposite side) Association of sensory input	Impaired sensation Inability to discriminate left/right Agnosias, neglect, apraxia, seizures
Basal ganglia	Control of fine motor movements Muscle tone, movement integration	Rigidity, bradykinesia, tremors (parkinsonism)
Thalamus	Major sensory integration center Focusing attention/concentration Memory retrieval	Impaired sensations related to touch, pain, temperature Impaired intellectual ability, difficulty initiating tasks Prolonged disorientation
Hypothalamus	Regulates ANS: controls appetite, sexual arousal, thirst, temperature Neuroendocrine control, emotions	ANS disturbances Inappropriate behavior Mood swings
Limbic system	Mediates memory and emotional behavior Directs attention, stores information	Short-term memory loss Changes in motivation or attitude, emotional changes
Mesencephalon	Relay station for impulses Auditory and visual reflexes Cranial nerves I–IV	Impaired auditory/visual reflexes Cranial nerve dysfunction
Pons	Relay center, cranial nerves V–VIII	Cerebellar disorders Cranial nerve alterations
Medulla	Basic CNS function control: blood pressure, heart rate, respiration Cranial nerves IX–XII	Severe damage is fatal Alteration in vital signs Cranial nerve dysfunction
Reticular activating system	Connections with all major parts of brain Controls sleep/wake cycle	Alterations in levels of consciousness Sleep pattern disturbance Coma
Cerebellum	Balance, coordination Regulates most motor impulses	Ataxia, incoordination Balance problems, tremors

ANS, autonomic nervous system; CNS, central nervous system.

and functions of the brain, along with deficits seen when damage to that area occurs.

Some people with mild head injury will recover without residual effects, but many will have permanent losses associated with the injury. When a person first experiences a head injury, massive swelling in the tissues, changes in level of consciousness, and coma may result. Severe injuries will cause the person to assume a fetal position or decorticate or decerebrate posturing. Generally, the longer the coma, the less chance of recovery, especially without residual impairment.

Nursing Implications

In the acute phase of treatment, interventions will be aimed at preserving life. Some patients survive but remain comatose. Coma stimulation programs that focus on providing consistent sensory stimulation to all senses with various modalities (often accompanied by hyperbaric oxygenation treatments) are a method used for those with coma (Helwick, 1994). Recovery from coma may be long but is possible in some cases and requires subsequent intensive participation in therapy. Rehabilitation will focus on returning the person to a maximal level of functioning in view of the extent of damage to the brain.

Many scales can be used to assess function in a brain-injured person. However, two scales may be particularly useful to the GRN. The Glasgow Coma Scale, used to measure lower levels of function and most often in acute care settings, is considered a standard and reliable tool for characterizing TBI. The scale provides a score for the best responses related to eye opening, motor function, and verbal ability. A score from 3 to 15 is possible, with 3 being essentially no response and 15 indicating spontaneous eye opening, the ability to obey motor commands, and full orientation. A score of 3 to 8 indicates severe brain injury, a score of 9 to 12 indicates moderate brain injury, and a score of 13 to 15 indicates mild brain injury.

The Rancho Los Amigos Levels of Cognitive Function Scale is a general assessment tool frequently used in rehabilitation. The scale delineates eight stages or phases through which many persons with brain injury progress (Rancho Los Amigos Medical Center, 1979). Level I indicates no response to pain, touch, sound, or sight. At levels II and III the person progresses from a generalized reflex response to stimulation or pain to a localized response such as blinking to strong light and responding to physical discomfort but gives inconsistent responses to commands. In level IV the person is confused and agitated, alert, active, and aggressive and performs motor activities, but the behavior is nonpurposeful. From levels V to VIII, the person moves from confusion (nonagitated) and being highly distractible, to being appropriate and automatic, and finally to being purposeful and appropriate. By the last level, the person is able to engage in goal-directed activities more consistently and has an increased attention span.

Using this tool to generally categorize the patient's behavior and responses can help guide care. For example, a person in stage IV on the Rancho scale may be aggressive and prone to agitation. This type of behavior is often thought to be a natural occurrence for some types of patients as they move toward greater levels of alertness. The GRN should take particular care to avoid sensory overload for this person, keep teaching periods short, and emphasize safety and protection of the patient, who at this time will have an especially high risk for falls. Likewise, the GRN would expect persons at stages VII and VIII to be preparing for discharge and community reentry. Persons at this stage of recovery should be better able to engage in discharge planning and be more receptive to teaching.

Recent studies have suggested that health care professionals can identify risk factors for aggressive behavior, including disorientation to time and place, use of antiseizure medications, and a number of comorbidities such as cardiovascular disorders, particularly hypertension (Brooke, Questad, Patterson, & Bashak, 1992; Galski, Palasz, Bruno, & Walker, 1994). If these results hold true, GRNs might expect certain elders to exhibit signs of aggressive physical and verbal behavior because of the increased incidence of hypertension in this population combined with the effects of aging, in addition to the head injury, which could cause disorientation or confusion in unfamiliar surroundings.

Patterson (1993) classifies brain injury into three main categories: minor, moderate, and severe. Minor TBIs are most common and result in a loss of consciousness that lasts 20 minutes or less, supposedly leaving no residual disability. However, a classic study by Rimel, Giordani, Barth, Boll, and Jane (1981) showed that of a group of 424 patients (mean age of 27 years) meeting the criteria of minor head injury, 79% complained of headaches at a 3-month follow-up evaluation and

59% had memory problems. Some may classify these symptoms as postconcussion syndrome. The results of this study appear to be contrary to general guidelines and expected outcomes. Most significantly, the researchers concluded that "the most striking observations of these studies are the high rates of morbidity and unemployment in patients 3 months after a seemingly insignificant head injury and the evidence that many of these patients may have, in fact, suffered organic brain damage" (p. 221). GRNs should advocate the use of formal rehabilitative facilities and programs for older adults with head injuries.

Moderate TBI usually necessitates rehabilitative treatment and may leave the person with problems of headaches, dizziness, and other persistent neurological signs, although return to pre-injury lifestyle patterns is generally possible. Supervision and lifestyle modifications are probably necessary, however. Those with severe TBI have extensive, diffuse effects and a loss of consciousness that lasts more than 6 hours. Scores on the Glasgow Coma Scale will be 8 or less. A person with severe TBI will be left with some degree of permanent disability if recovery is even possible.

If intervention is initiated early, patients with severe head injury who participate in a formal rehabilitation program have been shown to have shorter lengths of hospital stay and higher cognitive levels at discharge and were more likely to be discharged home than to an extended care facility when compared with patients who did not participate in a formal program (Frost & Barone, 1996; Mackey, Bernstein, Chapman, Morgan, & Milazzo, 1992). Rehabilitation of brain-injured persons, although possibly costly in the short term, is cost-effective when considering cost/benefit ratios and long-term outcomes (DiDonato & Schaffer, 1994), including improved quality of life and the ability to be discharged home.

Several common effects of brain injury should be noted by the GRN. Functional deficits, both sensory and motor, may be seen. Hemiplegia or generalized motor deficits may ensue. Spasticity and rigidity may interfere with progress in therapy. The person may be disoriented to time, place, and people. Memory problems are often seen. Seizure disorders, headaches, and altered sleep patterns may also result from head trauma. Patients who awaken after unconsciousness might recall the past but be unable to remember recent events such as how the accident occurred or what happened immediately afterward. Social behavior is often inappropriate because inhibitions are lost, and the person may make suggestive or lewd conversation or engage in overt sexual behavior without restraint (McLean, Dikmen, & Temkin, 1993) (Case Study 11.6). Visual-perceptual disturbances and communication deficits are common. Alterations in cranial nerve function (Table 11–21) may result in a decrease or loss of the ability to smell or taste. Changes in intellectual function and capacity often occur. Such persons may or may not remember their former state. Other possible complications of brain injury include neurogenic bowel and/or bladder function (Grinspun, 1993), risk of infection, respiratory compromise requiring mechanical support or tracheotomy, decreased endurance and activity intolerance, potential for deep vein thrombosis, potential for injury related to poor safety awareness, and impaired swallowing because of dysphagia.

CASE STUDY 11.6
Traumatic Brain Injury

Terry Judd was a 64 year old man in excellent health. He retired at the age of 60 from a career in business administration. His hobbies included high-risk activities such as sky-diving, water and snow skiing, boating, and motorcycling. He had five grown children and lived with his second wife, who was 10 years younger than him. When riding his motorcycle one winter he hit a patch of ice and skidded into a tree. Although he was wearing a helmet, he sustained a head injury affecting the frontal lobe and a broken right arm. Mr. Judd was admitted to the rehabilitation unit for intensive therapy, with the goal of continuing in an outpatient head injury program with the assistance of his wife. His functional limitations included motor dysfunction causing incoordination, unsteadiness with ambulation, and spasticity. His safety awareness was poor. He displayed inappropriate social behavior, often taking off his clothes, making suggestive comments to the nursing staff, and swearing loudly in front of other patients. This behavior greatly disturbed his wife, who stated that he had been a relatively well mannered person before his injury. She believed that he was no longer the same person she had married. The GRN and

Table 11–21 CRANIAL NERVE FUNCTION AND TESTING

Cranial Nerve	Chief Function/Indications for Assessment
I. Olfactory	Sense of smell (sensory); test each nostril separately
II. Optic	Visual sense (sensory); check acuity to newsprint or use Snellen chart; test both eyes separately and together for field of vision; test along with cranial nerves III, IV, and VI
III. Oculomotor	Eye movement, pupil constriction/dilation (motor); test upward, downward, and lateral movement of eye; assess for PERRLA
IV. Trochlear	Downward eye movement, eyelids (motor); test with cranial nerves II, III, and VI
V. Trigeminal	Chewing (motor), sensations of head/face (sensory); check blink reflex, ability to clench teeth, temporal musculature
VI. Abducens	Lateral eye movement (motor); test with cranial nerves II, III, and IV
VII. Facial	Movement of facial muscles (motor); saliva secretion, taste on anterior two thirds of tongue (sensory); assess forehead wrinkling, smiling to show teeth, saliva production, taste ability; observe for symmetry, drooping, weakness
VIII. Acoustic	Hearing and equilibrium (sensory); test each ear separately to whisper/spoken voice; assess gait and balance
IX. Glossopharyngeal	Saliva secretion, movement of swallowing (motor), taste on posterior third of tongue (sensory), reflexes of breathing and blood pressure; test with cranial nerve X; evaluate swallowing, cough, and gag reflexes; have person say "ah" and observe uvula and pharyngeal walls for symmetry/deviation
X. Vagus	Motor and sensory function of heart, larynx, digestive organs; test with cranial nerve XI; monitor vital signs, gastric motility, vocal quality
XI. Spinal accessory	Movement of head, shoulders, and parts of larynx related to vocal production (motor); check shoulder shrug, sternocleidomastoid muscle strength, vocal quality
XII. Hypoglossal	Tongue movements (motor); assess speech ability, ability to stick out tongue and move side to side

PERRLA, pupils equal, round, react to light and accommodation.

the social worker engaged in a large amount of teaching with the wife to increase her knowledge about the effects of brain injury. She continued to participate in therapy, although she seemed distant from her husband. As Terry made progress with therapy, he was able to learn to control some of the behavior that upset his wife. His attention to tasks improved, but he no longer had the adventurous personality he had before. The staff psychologist also met with the couple several times throughout the rehabilitation stay but noted that the wife seemed to lack sufficient coping abilities to manage this situation in the long term. Although the rehabilitation team helped identify support groups and attempted to help the wife enhance her coping strategies, Mrs. Judd announced just before Terry's discharge that she was divorcing him to be with someone else she had met before the accident. None of his children were will-ing to assume his care, even on a temporary basis, and Terry was unable to live alone without supervision because of his impaired judgment and poor safety habits. Mr. Judd then had to be transferred to a long-term care facility until other arrangements could be determined.

■

An older person with TBI may encounter additional problems besides the immediate effects of brain injury. For example, finding a family member who will help care for the elder with permanent brain injury is a significant problem. Brain-injured persons often require a long period of observation or care, which may even be needed 24 hours per day. The severity of the head injury and secondary complications help define the limits of rehabilitation and expected outcomes, with more severely injured and disabled adults having a poorer prognosis (Sargent & Patterson, 1993). Additional nursing interventions for a cognitively impaired elder include providing a safe environment and reducing the risk of injury, promoting self-care and independence, frequently orienting the person, and monitoring mental status (Dellasega & Shellenbarger, 1992).

Nursing care, as well as all rehabilitative therapy, should help persons with TBI realize what their problems or deficits are and learn techniques to compensate for them (Williams, 1990). GRNs should make sure that the person has an adequate level of alertness or arousal and attention before attempting any teaching. The person's major problem may be a decreased level of alertness, which must be addressed before attentional deficits. The nurse will need to help maintain a general level of arousal to assist the person to focus on a specific stimulus or task. This goal is especially difficult when distracting stimuli are present. Therefore, it is necessary to minimize noise and distractions to enhance learning. Once the person's attention is gained, processes of recognition and interpretation can begin. Finally, combining and processing information into meaningful input and making decisions for action can be addressed.

An elderly caregiver may be unable or ill equipped to cope with the demands required by a person with brain injury. Such patients may be highly unsafe and be unaware of their disabilities. Persons with trauma to the brain often experience personality changes and become egocentric. They may fail to realize the sacrifices made by the caregiver. Such behavior can contribute to caregiver frustration and feelings of helplessness and anger. The caregiver may feel unappreciated and dissatisfied if the patient does not offer thanks or appreciation for the care provided. This situation can in turn contribute to placement of a person with brain injury into a long-term care facility because the caregiver burden becomes overwhelming.

Informal caregivers have identified many needs, including time for themselves, need for support groups, help with housekeeping tasks, respite care, financial support, day care programs, and transportation. Many of these needs were reported as not being met (Grant & Bean, 1992). GRNs should pay particular attention to family dynamics and role functions. Linking the family/caregiver to community resources and support groups is essential to meet the needs of the caregiver.

REFERENCES

American Parkinson Disease Association (1993). *Be independent: A guide for people with Parkinson's disease.* Staten Island, NY: Author.

Athlin, E., Norberg, A., Axelsson, K., Moller, A., & Nordstrom, G. (1989). Aberrant eating behavior in elderly parkinsonian patients with and without dementia: Analysis of video-recorded meals. *Research in Nursing & Health, 12,* 41–51.

Bach, C. A., & McDaniel, R. W. (1993). Quality of life in quadriplegic adults: A focus group study. *Rehabilitation Nursing, 18*(6), 364–367, 374.

Baier, S., & Schomaker, M. Z. (1986). *Bed number ten.* Boca Raton, FL: CRC Press.

Bakker-Hatten, B. S., Lankhorst, G. J., Kriek, L., & Slootman, J. R. (1995). Functional outcome of Guillain-Barré syndrome. *Journal of Rehabilitation Sciences, 8*(3), 82–86.

Beneton, C., De Parisot, O., Granjon, M., & Millet, M. F. (1996). Management of bladder disorders in multiple sclerosis. *Sexuality and Disability, 14*(1), 21–31.

Bertino, L. S., & Lu, L. (1993). The bite of a wolf: Systemic lupus erythematosus. *Rehabilitation Nursing, 18*(3), 173–178.

Blake, K. (1995). The social isolation of young men with quadriplegia. *Rehabilitation Nursing, 20*(1), 17–22.

Borgman-Gainer, M. F. (1996). Independent function: Movement and mobility. In S. P. Hoeman (Ed.), *Rehabilitation nursing: Process and application* (pp. 225–272). St. Louis, MO: C. V. Mosby.

Bourdette, D. N., Prochazka, A. V., Mitchell, W., Licari, P., & Burks, J. (1993). Health care costs of veterans with multiple sclerosis: Implications for the rehabilitation of MS. VA Multiple Sclerosis Rehabilitation Study Group. *Archives of Physical Medicine and Rehabilitation, 74,* 26–31.

Bozzacco, V. (1993). Long-term psychosocial effects of spinal cord injury. *Rehabilitation Nursing, 18*(2), 82–87.

Brar, S. P., Smith, M. B., Nelson, L. M., Franklin, G. M., & Cobble, N. D. (1991). Evaluation of treatment protocols on minimal to moderate spasticity in multiple sclerosis. *Archives of Physical Medicine and Rehabilitation, 72,* 186–189.

Brooke, M. M., Questad, K A., Patterson, D. R., & Bashak, K. J. (1992). Agitation and restlessness after closed head injury: A prospective study of 100 consecutive admissions. *Archives of Physical Medicine and Rehabilitation, 73,* 320–323.

Buchanan, R. J., & Lewis, K. (1997). Services that nursing facilities should provide to residents with MS: A survey of health professionals. *Rehabilitation Nursing, 22*(2), 67–72.

Calne, D. B. (1995). Diagnosis and treatment of Parkinson's disease. *Hospital Practice, 30*(1), 83–89.

Campbell, J., & Humphreys, J. (1993). *Nursing care*

of survivors of family violence. St. Louis: C. V. Mosby.

Charbonneau-Smith, R. (1993). No-touch catheterization and infection rates in a select spinal cord injured population. *Rehabilitation Nursing, 18*(5), 292–299.

Chase, T. N., Engber, T. M., & Mouradian, M. M. (1994). Palliative and prophylactic benefits of continuously administered dopaminomimetics in Parkinson's disease. *Neurology 44*(Suppl 6), 15–18.

Chisholm, A. H. (1996). Fetal tissue transplantation for the treatment of Parkinson's disease: A review of the literature. *Journal of Neuroscience Nursing, 28*(5), 329–338.

Clayton, K. S., & Chubon, R. A. (1994). Factors associated with the quality of life and long-term spinal cord injured persons. *Archives of Physical Medicine and Rehabilitation, 75*, 633–638.

Costello, K., & Conway, K. (1997). Nursing management of MS patients receiving interferon beta-1b therapy. *Rehabilitation Nursing, 22*(2), 62–66.

Craig, A. R., Hancock, K., Dickson, H., & Chang, E. (1997). Long-term psychological outcomes in spinal cord injured persons: Results of a controlled trial using cognitive behavior therapy. *Archives of Physical Medicine and Rehabilitation, 78*, 33–38.

Decalmer, P., & Glendenning, F. (Eds.) (1993). *The mistreatment of the elderly people.* London: Sage.

Dellasega, C., & Shellenbarger, T. (1992). Discharge planning for cognitively impaired elderly adults. *Nursing & Health Care, 13*(10), 526–531.

DeVivo, M. J., Hawkins, L. N., Richards, J. S., & Go, B. K. (1995). Outcomes of post–spinal cord injury marriages. *Archives of Physical Medicine and Rehabilitation, 76*, 130–138.

DeVivo, M. J., Stover, S. L., & Black, K. (1992). Prognostic factors for 12-year survival after spinal cord injury. *Archives of Physical Medicine and Rehabilitation, 73*, 156–162.

DiDonato, B. A., & Schaffer, V. L. (1994). The importance of outcome data in brain injury rehabilitation. *Rehabilitation Nursing, 19*(4), 219–227.

Dupont, S. (1995). Multiple sclerosis and sexual functioning—a review. *Clinical Rehabilitation, 9*(2), 135–141.

Easton, K. (1995). When a serious illness hits home. *Rehabilitation Nursing, 20*(5), 283–284.

Emick-Herring, B. (1993). Stroke. In A. E. McCourt (Ed.), *The specialty practice of rehabilitation nursing: A core curriculum* (pp. 35–40). Skokie, IL: Rehabilitation Nursing Foundation.

Ferrante, C., & Derivan, M. C. (1995). Caring for patients with systemic lupus erythematosus. *Nursing 1995, 25*(11), 66–67.

Fitzsimmons, B., & Bunting, L. K. (1993). Parkinson's disease: Quality of life issues. *Nursing Clinics of North America, 28*(4), 807–818.

French, J. K., & Phillips, J. A. (1991). Shattered images: Recovery for the SCI client. *Rehabilitation Nursing, 16*(3), 134–136.

Fried, K. (1993). Spinal cord injury. In A. E.

McCourt (Ed.), *The specialty practice of rehabilitation nursing: A core curriculum* (pp. 58–61). Skokie, IL: Rehabiltation Nursing Foundation.

Frost, D., & Barone, S. H. (1996). Functional outcome in elderly patients with traumatic brain injuries. *Rehabilitation Nursing Research, 5*(1), 9–15.

Galski, R., Palasz, J., Bruno, R. L., & Walker, J. R. (1994). Predicting physical and verbal aggression on a brain trauma unit. *Archives of Physical Medicine and Rehabilitation, 75*, 380–383.

Gausch, A., Linder, S. H., Williams, T., & Ryan, G. (1991). Functional classification of respiratory compromise in spinal cord injury. *SCI Nursing, 8*(1), 4–10.

Gauthier, L., Dalziel, S., & Gauthier, S. (1987). The benefits of group occupational therapy for patients with Parkinson's disease. *The American Journal of Occupational Therapy, 41*(6), 360–365.

Gilbert, M., Counsell, C. M., & Snively, C. (1996). Pallidotomy: A surgical intervention for control of Parkinson's disease. *Journal of Neuroscience Nursing, 28*(4), 215–216.

Gokbudak, H. J. (1985). Maximizing rehabilitation for the elderly patient with spinal cord injury. *Rehabilitation Nursing, 10*(1), 16–20.

Grant, J. S., & Bean, C. A. (1992). Self-identified needs of informal caregivers of head-injured adults. *Family Community Health, 15*(2), 49–58.

Gray, M., Rayone, R., & Anson, C. (1995). Incontinence and clean intermittent catheterization following spinal cord injury. *Clinical Nursing Research, 4*(1), 6–21.

Greco, S. B. (1996). Sexuality education and counseling. In S. P. Hoeman (Ed.), *Rehabilitation nursing: Process and application* (pp. 594–627). St. Louis, MO: C. V. Mosby.

Gregory, R. J. (1995). Understanding and coping with neurological impairment. *Rehabilitation Nursing, 29*(2), 74–78.

Gregory, R. J., Disler, P., & Firth, S. (1996). Caregivers of people with multiple sclerosis: A survey in New Zealand. *Rehabilitation Nursing, 21*(1), 31–37.

Grinspun, D. (1993). Bladder management for adults following head injury. *Rehabilitation Nursing, 18*(5), 300–305.

Gulick, E. E. (1987). Parsimony and model confirmation of the ADL self-care scale for multiple sclerosis persons. *Nursing Research, 36*(5), 278–283.

Gulick, E. E. (1991). Reliability and validity of the work assessment scale for persons with multiple sclerosis. *Nursing Research, 40*(2), 107–112.

Gulick, E. E. (1992). Model for predicting work performance among persons with multiple sclerosis. *Nursing Research, 41*(5), 266–272.

Gulick, E. E. (1994). Social support among persons with multiple sclerosis. *Research in Nursing & Health, 17*(3), 195–206.

Habermann, B. (1996). Day-to-day demands of Parkinson's disease. *Western Journal of Nursing Research, 18*(4), 397–413.

Hainsworth, M. A. (1994). Living with multiple

sclerosis: The experience of chronic sorrow. *Journal of Neuroscience Nursing, 26*(4), 237–240.

Halper, J., & Costello, K. M. (1997, October). *Multiple sclerosis: Current therapies, future hope.* Paper presented at the meeting of the Association of Rehabilitation Nurses, Baltimore.

Helwick, L. D. (1994). Stimulation programs for coma patients. *Critical Care Nurse, 8,* 47–52.

Hely, M. A., & Morris, J. G. L. (1996). Controversies in the treatment of Parkinson's disease. *Current Opinion in Neurology, 9*(4), 308–313.

Holicky, R. (1996). Caring for the caregivers: The hidden victims of illness and disability. *Rehabilitation Nursing, 21*(5), 247–252.

Hubsky, E. P., & Sears, J. H. (1992). Fatigue in multiple sclerosis: Guidelines for nursing care. *Rehabilitation Nursing, 17*(4), 176–180.

Hurwitz, A. (1986). Home visiting by nursing students to patients with Parkinson's disease. *Journal of Neuroscience Nursing, 18*(6), 344–348.

Ivie, C. S., & DeVivo, M. J. (1994). Predicting unplanned hospitalizations in persons with spinal cord injury. *Archives of Physical Medicine and Rehabilitation, 75,* 1182–1188.

Jaeger, R. J., Turba, R. M., Yarkony, G. M., & Roth, E. J. (1993). Cough in spinal cord injured patients: Comparison of three methods to produce cough. *Archives of Physical Medicine and Rehabilitation, 74,* 1358–1361.

Jansen, D. A., & Cimprich, B. (1994). Attentional impairment in persons with multiple sclerosis. *Journal of Neuroscience Nursing, 26*(2), 95–102.

Kitamura, J., Nakagawa, H., Iiuma, K., Kobayashi, M., Okauchi, A., Oonaka, K., & Kondo, T. (1993). Visual influence on center of contact pressure in advanced Parkinson's Disease. *Archives of Physical Medicine and Rehabilitation, 74,* 1107–1112.

Krames Communications. (1996). *Parkinson's disease: Living with a chronic illness.* San Bruno, CA: Author.

Krause, J. S. (1992). Employment after spinal cord injury. *Archives of Physical Medicine and Rehabilitation, 73,* 163–169.

Krause, J. S., & Crewe, N. M. (1991). Chronologic age, time since injury, and time of measurement: Effect on adjustment after spinal cord injury. *Archives of Physical Medicine and Rehabilitation, 72*(2), 91–100.

Lannon, M. C., Thomas, C. A., Bratton, M., Jost, M. G., & Lockhart-Pretti, P. (1986). Comprehensive care of the patient with Parkinson's disease. *Journal of Neuroscience Nursing, 18*(3), 121–131.

Larson, J. L., Johnson, J. H., & Angst, D. B. (1996). Respiratory function and pulmonary rehabilitation. In S. P. Hoeman (Ed.), *Rehabilitation nursing: Process and application* (pp. 361–400). St. Louis, MO: C. V. Mosby.

Latham, L. (1994). When spinal cord injury complicates med/surg care. *RN, 57*(8), 26–29.

Lieberman, A. (1994, February). Protein distribution diets in the management of fluctuations in levodopa response. *Drugs & Nutrients in Neurology, 5.*

Lieberman, A. N., Gopinathan, G., Neophytides, A., & Goldstein, M. (1996). *Parkinson's disease handbook: A guide for patients and their families.* Staten Island, NY: The American Parkinson Disease Association, Inc.

Luis, S. A. (1997). Pathophysiology and management of idiopathic Parkinson's disease. *The Journal of Neuroscience Nursing, 29*(1), 24–31.

Mackay, L. E., Bernstein, B. A., Chapman, P. E., Morgan, A. S., & Milazzo, L. S. (1992). Early intervention in severe head injury: Long-term benefits of a formalized program. *Archives of Physical Medicine and Rehabilitation, 73,* 635–641.

Maness, J. E. (1995). The impact of spinal cord injury on older adults' growth and development: A case study. *Rehabilitation Nursing, 20*(1), 29–31.

Matthews, P., & Carlson, C. (Eds.) (1987). *Spinal cord injury: Rehabilitation Institute of Chicago procedure manual.* Rockville, MD: Aspen Publishers.

McGlinchey-Berroth, R., Morrow, L., Ahlquist, M., Sarkarati, M., & Minaker, K. L. (1995). Late-life spinal cord injury and aging with a long term injury: Characteristics of two emerging populations. *Journal of Spinal Cord Medicine, 18*(3), 183–193.

McLean, A., Dikmen, S. S., & Temkin, N. R. (1993). Psychosocial recovery after head injury. *Archives of Physical Medicine and Rehabilitation, 74,* 1041–1046.

Michigan Lupus Foundation. (1993). *Lupus fact sheet.* St. Clair Shores, MI: Lupus Foundation of America.

Miller, C. M., & Hens, M. (1993). Multiple sclerosis: A literature review. *Journal of Neuroscience Nursing, 25*(3), 174–179.

Mitchell, P. H., Mertz, M. A., & Catanzaro, M. L. (1987). Group exercise: A nursing therapy in Parkinson's disease. *Rehabilitation Nursing, 12*(5), 242–245.

Moncur, C., & Williams, H. J. (1995). Rheumatoid arthritis: Status of drug therapies. *Physical Therapy, 75*(6), 511–525.

Namey, M., & Schwetz, K. (1993). What's new in multiple sclerosis management? Paper presented at the 1993 Association of Rehabilitation Nurses annual conference, Denver, CO.

National Parkinson Foundation. (1994). *Parkinson report, XV*(II), 2–10.

Nijhof, G. (1995). Parkinson's disease as a problem of shame in public appearance. *Sociology of Health and Illness, 17*(2), 193–205.

Norbendo, A. M. (1996). Bowel dysfunction in multiple sclerosis. *Sexuality and Disability, 14*(1), 33–39.

Nutt, J. G. (1994, February). The pharmacokinetics and pharmacodynamics of levodopa. *Drugs & Nutrients in Neurology,* 8–15.

O'Brien, M. T. (1993). Multiple sclerosis: Stressors and coping strategies in spousal caregivers. *Journal of Community Health Nursing, 19*(3), 123–135.

Palmer, S. S., Mortimer, J. A., Webster, D. D., Bistevins, R., & Dickinson, G. L. (1986). Exercise therapy for Parkinson's disease. *Archives of Physical Medicine and Rehabilitation, 67*, 741–745.

Parobeck, V., Burnheim, S., & Laukhuf, G. A. (1992). An unusual nursing challenge: Guillain-Barré syndrome following cranial surgery. *Journal of Neuroscience Nursing, 24*(5), 251–255.

Patterson, T. (1993). Traumatic brain injury. In A. E. McCourt (Ed.), *The specialty practice of rehabilitation nursing: A core curriculum* (pp. 52–57). Skokie, IL: Rehabilitation Nursing Foundation.

Payne, J. A. (1993). Contribution of group learning to SCI rehabilitation. *Rehabilitation Nursing, 18*(6), 375–379.

Penrose, N. J. (1993). Guillain-Barré syndrome: A case study. *Rehabilitation Nursing, 18*(2), 88–94.

Pentland, W., McColl, M. A., & Rosenthal, C. (1995). The effect of aging and duration of disability on long term health outcomes following spinal cord injury. *Paraplegia, 33*(7), 367–372.

Peterson, J. L., & Bell, G. W. (1995). Aquatic exercise for individuals with multiple sclerosis. *Clinical Kinesiology: Journal of the American Kinesiotherapy Association, 49*(3), 69–71.

Pires, M. (1996). Bladder elimination and continence. In S. P. Hoeman (Ed.), *Rehabilitation nursing: Process and application* (pp. 417–451). St. Louis, MO: C. V. Mosby.

Pritchard, J. (1995). *The abuse of older people: A training manual for detection and prevention.* London: Jessica Kingsley Publishers.

Rancho Los Amigos Medical Center, Adult Brain Injury Service. (1979). *Levels of cognitive function scale* (adapted version) (pp. 78–80). Downey, CA: Author.

Rimel, R. W., Giordani, B., Barth, J. T., Boll, T. J., & Jane, J. A. (1981). Disability caused by minor head injury. *Clinical and Scientific Communication, 9*(3), 221–228.

Rosebrough, A. (1997). Chronic neurological disorders: Multiple sclerosis, Parkinson's disease, myasthenia gravis, and Guillain-Barré syndrome. In P. A. Chin, D. Finocchiaro, & A. Rosebrough (Eds.), *Rehabilitation nursing practice* (pp. 443–473). New York: McGraw-Hill.

Sanchez-Ramos, J. (1994). The use of pergolide as an adjunct to Sinemet in Parkinson's disease. *Parkinson Report, XV*(II), 2–10.

Sargent, M., & Patterson, T. S. (1993). Postacute, home-based head injury rehabilitation: An outcome study. *Rehabilitation Nursing, 18*(6), 380–383.

Shaw, M. C., & Bertino, L. M. (1994). Shedding light on lupus. *Rehabilitation Nursing, 19*(2), 120.

Sie, I. H., Waters, R. L., Adkins, R. H., & Gellman, H. (1992). Upper extremity pain in the postrehabilitation spinal cord injured patient. *Archives of Physical Medicine and Rehabilitation, 73*, 44–48.

Spiera, H., & Rothschild, J. (1995). When systemic lupus erythematosus involves the heart. *Journal of Musculoskeletal Medicine, 12*(1), 54–56.

Sprinzeles, L. L. (1993). The effects of neurological impairment and rehabilitation on patients with Parkinson's disease (PD) and their families. Paper presented at the 1993 Association of Rehabilitation Nurses annual conference, Denver, CO.

Steinberg, J. (1993). *GBS—Guillain-Barre syndrome (acute idiopathic polyneuritis).* Wynnewood, PA: Guillain-Barré Syndrome Foundation International.

Stover, S. L., Hale, A. M., & Buell, A. B. (1994). Skin complications other than pressure ulcers following spinal cord injuries. *Archives of Physical Medicine and Rehabilitation, 75*, 987–993.

Svensson, B., Gerdle, B., & Elert, J. (1994). Endurance training in patients with multiple sclerosis: Five case studies. *Physical Therapy, 74*(11), 1017–1026.

Swonger, A. K., & Burbank, P. M. (1995). *Drug therapy and the elderly.* Boston: Jones & Bartlett.

Temple, R. (1987). Mobility and sensory alterations: Alternations in skin integrity: Potential and actual. In P. Matthews, C. Carlson, & N. Holte (Eds.), *Spinal cord injury: Rehabilitation Institute of Chicago procedure manual* (pp. 76–82). Rockville, MD, Aspen Publishers.

Teva Marion Partners (1997). *All About COPAXONE.* Kansas City, MO: Author.

The New Webster's Medical Dictionary. (1992). Hartford, CN: Lewtan Line.

Toth, L. L. (1983). Spasticity management in spinal cord injury. *Rehabilitation Nursing, 8*(1) 14–17.

Washington, H. (1993). Parkinson's disease, Part 1. *Harvard Health Letter, 18*(7), 1–4.

Wassem, R. (1991). A test of the relationship between health locus of control and the course of multiple sclerosis. *Rehabilitation Nursing, 16*(4), 189–193.

Weekly, N. J. (1995). Parkinsonism: An overview. *Geriatric Nursing, 16*(4), 169–172.

Werner, P. (1997). New medications for brain and spinal cord injury: Minimizing the "second" injury. *The Journal of Care Management, 3*(1), 46–56.

White, M. J., Rintala, D. H., Hart, K., & Fuhrer, M. J. (1994, Summer). A comparison of the sexual concerns of men and women with spinal cord injuries. *Rehabilitation Nursing Research*, 55–61.

Wichmann, R. (1990). *Be active: A suggested exercise program for people with Parkinson's disease.* Minneapolis, MN: American Parkinson Disease Association.

Williams, M. H. (1990). The self-help movement in head injury. *Rehabilitation Nursing, 15*(6), 311–315.

Wilson, D. M. (1992). Ethical concerns in a long-term tube feeding study. *IMAGE: Journal of Nursing Scholarship, 24*(3), 195–198.

Wineman, N. M. (1990). Adaptation to multiple sclerosis: The role of social support, functional disability, and perceived uncertainty. *Nursing Research, 39*(5), 294–299.

Wineman, N. M., Durand, E. J., & Steiner, R. P. (1994). A comparative analysis of coping behaviors in persons with multiple sclerosis or a spinal cord injury. *Research in Nursing & Health, 17*, 185–194.

Chapter 12

Orthopedic Problems

As persons age, many significant changes occur in the musculoskeletal system affecting movement, gait, and range of motion. Bones act as a lever system for the body and form the basis for all movement. With advanced age, bones generally become more porous, increasing the risk of fracture. The intervertebral spaces narrow, leading to a progressive decrease in height. The articulating joint surfaces also change as the body ages. Arthritis is the most commonly reported chronic problem among the aged (Matteson, 1997). Muscle mass also declines and may lead to decreased muscle strength. Orthopedic disorders in the elderly often necessitate rehabilitation to promote maximal functioning. This chapter discusses assessment, goals, interventions, and treatments for the orthopedic problems most commonly seen in rehabilitation.

The skeletal structure of the human body serves several functions. Bones act as a framework to provide shape and form, over and around which muscles, ligaments, tendons, soft tissues, and the rest of the bodily systems are entwined. Although bones are by nature porous, they are normally dense enough to provide protection from injury for the vital organs which lie beneath. For instance, the skull is hard and closely knit to shield the control center of the body, the brain. The ribs encase the lungs and heart, essential to life, as built-in armor. The pelvic bones protect the bladder, and so forth. Bones help to regulate the body by producing red blood cells within the bone marrow, and they also store essential minerals.

Bone formation begins at conception and

continues through life in a process cycle called *bone remodeling* (Kessenich, 1997). Bone-resorbing osteoclasts and bone-forming osteoblasts regulate this activity to manufacture new bone constantly. This cycle is relatively balanced until about age 30, when bone mass begins to decrease because of changes in factors affecting the remodeling process (Kessenich, 1997). Attention to factors related to promoting strong and healthy bone development is always important, but particularly in younger years, when bone remodeling is most stable. It is especially necessary for girls to have an adequate intake of calcium before the age of 16 years (Scura & Whipple, 1997) while bones are still developing, to prevent osteoporosis in later life.

Several factors affect the process of bone formation. These include the balance of hormones (particularly estrogen, testosterone, calcitonin, insulin, and parathyroid/thyroid hormones), weight bearing status and activity, and diet (particularly vitamin D and calcium-rich foods). The delicate balance of these factors can be seen by examining the interrelationships among them relating to bone physiology. Plasma calcium controls the production of parathyroid hormone, either by stimulating it and decreasing those secretions that result in bone resorption or by inhibiting it by adequate levels of calcium in the blood. Likewise, when the production of estrogen is decreased, as with menopause, calcium may be taken from the bone and released into the bloodstream to maintain the balance of multiple other hormones. Vitamin D aids in the absorption of calcium from the gut, so it is needed to process ingested calcium. Calcitonin, which is secreted by the thyroid gland, inhibits bone resorption and helps to keep calcium balanced. However, estrogen may affect calcitonin levels, which, in turn, influence calcium levels (Kessenich, 1997). Weight bearing stimulates bone-building cells, promoting resorption and bone formation. This is one reason why even passive weight bearing is preferable to none. Standing boxes are used for persons with tetraplegia for both physical and emotional benefits. Exercise throughout the life span is important for many reasons, including the maintenance of musculoskeletal integrity. Early ambulation after a surgical procedure is now the norm, to prevent the hazards of immobility and disuse syndrome.

To summarize, when the balance among any of these factors is disrupted, changes in bone formation and density are likely to occur over time. Problems with the cycle of bone remodeling can lead to osteoporosis and pathological fractures, which may result in functional limitations and a decreased capacity for independence.

OSTEOPOROSIS

Osteoporosis is a common, yet preventable disease. According to the National Osteoporosis Foundation (1997), more than 25 million people are affected, incurring a national cost of more than $10 billion per year. Osteoporosis is not an inevitable part of aging, but its effects can be devastating. Current efforts are focused on developing a national prevention education campaign to halt the disease before it starts. Many health care centers across the United States have developed screening and teaching programs with this goal of primary prevention in mind.

Women are affected by osteoporosis more often than men. After menopause, the lack of protective effect from estrogen is decreased, and women are at increased risk to develop more porous bones. Thus, osteoporosis is often considered an endocrine disorder (Kessenich, 1997). Fifty percent of women in the United States older than the age of 45 years have some degree of osteoporosis, as do 90% of those older than age 75 (McMahon, Peterson, & Schlike, 1992).

Men, however, are not immune to this disease. Men experience a significant number of hip fractures (1.7 million per year as of 1990) related to osteoporosis, and those older than age 70 are more likely to die than women as a result of this type of injury (Galsworthy &

Wilson, 1997; Kessenich & Rosen, 1996b). Thus, osteoporosis prevention should be taught to both men and women, and at an early age.

Assessing Risk Factors

The risk factors associated with osteoporosis are many. Some are controllable, whereas others are not. The risk factors listed in Table 12–1 can be logically related to the previous discussion about the mechanism of bone development.

Although osteoporosis can affect both men and women, women, especially those who are white, are at a higher risk. Postmenopausal women experience an increased incidence of osteoporosis because of the lack of the protective effects of estrogen. Elderly women in northern climates may be especially susceptible to osteoporosis because of a decrease in exposure to sunlight, which can lead to vitamin D deficiency. For example, a study of women living in New England found that they demonstrated decreased bone density in fall and early winter even with vitamin D supplements (Kessenich & Rosen, 1996a).

When assessing the elderly individual for risk factors of osteoporosis, a detailed history

Table 12–1 RISK FACTORS FOR OSTEOPOROSIS

Controllable
Sedentary lifestyle, inactivity
Insufficient dietary calcium intake
Insufficient vitamin D intake
Hormonal imbalances
Cigarette smoking
Alcohol consumption
Excessive caffeine intake
Lack of exposure to sunlight

Uncontrollable
History of diseases that affect the thyroid, liver, reproductive organs, hormones
Surgery affecting reproductive organs (such as hysterectomy, salpingo-oophorectomy, orchidectomy)
Disorders that prohibit or affect full weight bearing (such as tetraplegia or amputation)
Menopause
Advanced age
Thin, small-boned frame
European or Asian descent
Fair skinned, blonde
History of use of corticosteroids or thyroid replacement medications
History of anorexia or bulimia

is needed. Controllable and uncontrollable factors should be identified. Direct questions about the person's diet may be needed. For example, "How many glasses of milk do you drink each day?" may elicit more specific information than "Do you get enough calcium in your diet?". The knowledge level of the patient in relation to dietary requirements must also be assessed.

Many women do not have an adequate calcium intake (Ali & Twibell, 1994). This may be related to several factors. Women may have a lack of knowledge about the effects of insufficient calcium on bone density, as well as the long-term consequences associated with this problem. Although the importance of diet in prevention of illness has recently received much greater emphasis within the school curricula of most educational institutions, the significance of one's present actions on one's future health state is not always acknowledged. Teenagers in the United States have particularly notorious eating habits including fast foods, frequent snacks, irregular meal patterns, and dieting. Many females on weight reducing diets do not consume enough calories to equal the amount of calcium required for healthy bones. Gerontological rehabilitation nurses (GRNs) need to advocate osteoporosis prevention teaching for young people, even at the grade school level. Economic barriers such as lack of money to purchase necessary food items may also present a problem. Many of the foods that contain calcium are dairy products, or perishables, and thus are not generally stocked by food pantries or other community service organizations that provide relief for those in need. GRNs can offer a service within the community by providing lists of calcium-rich foods that could be included in food distributions.

Likewise, because of the increased attention given to women in relation to osteoporosis, men may be likely to believe that this disease does not affect males. Yet, one of every three men is likely to develop osteoporosis by age 75 (Galsworhy & Wilson, 1997). If a man's testosterone level is lower than normal, he is twice as likely to sustain a hip fracture (Kessenich & Rosen, 1996b).

Signs and Symptoms

The signs and symptoms of osteoporosis are often not noted until a fracture occurs. Fractures occur most often in the long bones such as the vertebral spine, hip, rib, and wrist (Kes-

senich, 1997). Kyphosis, decreased height, and back pain may be also signs of osteoporosis or associated fractures. Back pain related to vertebral fractures is common, and it can be a debilitating factor in the elderly. Densitometry is one method of detection wherein bone mass or density can be measured. Some progressive communities have initiated mobile health van projects that take this method of screening for osteoporosis directly into the community. This form of primary prevention allows physicians to track high-risk individuals and to refer them to appropriate care providers for follow-up as necessary.

Effects

Fractures are among the most serious and devastating effects of osteoporosis in the elderly. Osteoporosis contributes to nearly 1.5 million fractures of the bones each year. About 1 in 4 women in America will have had an osteoporotic vertebral fracture by age 60, and about half of all women will have had an osteoporotic fracture by the age of 75 (Paier, 1996). However, both men and women add to such fracture statistics. Of the 1.7 million hip fractures in 1990, 30% were among men (Kessenich & Rosen, 1996b). Men older than 70 years also have a higher mortality rate from hip fractures than women (Galsworthy & Wilson, 1997). Although one cannot ascertain how many hip fractures are directly related to osteoporosis, this condition is known to be a major contributing factor.

Broy (1996) stated that 50% of osteoporotic hip fractures and 90% of vertebral fractures could be prevented, but prevention must begin early. The incidence of hip fracture among the general population is expected to more than double by the year 2050 (Houldin & Hogen-Quigley, 1995). Galsworthy and Wilson (1997) stated that 500,000 vertebral fractures occur each year, leading to numerous self-care deficits. Osteoporotic fractures are often difficult to treat, particularly vertebral fractures. Back pain can be a very limiting factor for the elderly, and it can result in decreased independence and a poorer quality of life. Functional ability is negatively affected by vertebral fractures among the elderly (Galindo-Ciocon, Ciocon, & Galindo, 1995). Elderly women with vertebral fractures also report difficulty in functioning independently and in dealing with constant pain, changes in appearance, isolation, vulnerability, and uncertainty about the future (Paier, 1996). These trends and statistics have serious implications with regard to primary prevention and secondary interventions as well as rehabilitation.

Nursing Implications

Osteoporosis provides an excellent illustration of how GRNs function at all levels of prevention, not just at tertiary levels. The major aim of rehabilitative nursing interventions regarding osteoporosis should be primary prevention, defined as early prevention before the disease starts. If an individual already has osteoporosis, then secondary prevention (such as preventing fractures and fall risk education) would prevail. Tertiary prevention, usually considered the rehabilitation phase, would target those patients who have sustained an osteoporotic fracture and who require rehabilitation. However, one can see that true holistic gerontological nursing must incorporate all three levels into practice, particularly given the diverse nature and settings in which GRNs are employed today.

Nursing measures used by the GRN focus on assessment and modification of controllable risk factors. Osteoporosis education and screenings have been shown to be effective in increasing awareness of persons who are at risk (Cook, Noteloviz, Rector, & Krischer, 1991). Table 12–2 provides a list of some essential components of an osteoporosis prevention program. GRNs should be prepared to teach principles of proper nutrition, weight bearing exercises, avoidance of cigarette smoking and excessive alcohol use, strengthening exercises, and fall prevention to any elderly rehabilitation client. GRNs work with physical and occupational therapists to develop a team-oriented plan of care for each person.

The GRN should understand that a balance is needed among many factors to maintain bone health. Clients should be taught that both vitamin D and calcium are essential for strong bones. Both men and women should be taught before the onset of old age that osteoporosis is not just a women's disease. Osteoporosis is often a silent disease (Kessenich & Rosen, 1996b), so individuals must be made aware of how to reduce their risk before the onset of symptoms. GRNs encounter elderly patients who are admitted to long-term care for diagnoses other than osteoporotic-related problems. However, every older person has an increased risk, so this is an essential area for GRNs to note when completing any physical assessment or history.

For those persons already experiencing os-

Table 12–2 TEACHING COMPONENTS OF AN OSTEOPOROSIS PREVENTION PROGRAM

Proper diet: role of calcium, vitamin D
Choosing healthy foods
Reducing risk factors: role of smoking, alcohol, caffeine
Weight bearing activity (walking versus stationary bike riding)
Role of sunlight in assisting body to use vitamin D
Estrogen replacement therapy for postmenopausal women
Calcium supplementation
Exercise: warm-ups and stretching, low resistance, progressive resistance, back, and abdominal
Fall prevention: reducing controllable risk factors, making the home environment safe
Role of medications (if applicable): estrogen, calcitonin, alendronate
Examination and diagnosis: bone density imaging, physician examination
Dealing with psychosocial and emotional issues: fear, avoidance and isolation, depression, grief
Coping with losses: decreased mobility, self-esteem, roles, and relationships
Pain management: exercise, meditation, prayer, breathing, relaxation techniques, medications

teoporotic fractures, a modification of nursing interventions may be necessary. Paier (1996) suggested several components for an intervention program for women with vertebral fractures, based on a phenomenological study of women's experience. These included education, rehabilitation aimed at regaining or maintaining function, pain management, stress-reduction techniques, reducing social isolation, and promotion of self-care activities. Patients who enter rehabilitation, subacute care, or long-term care for other reasons, but who have a history or risk of osteoporosis, should receive particular attention with regard to prevention of falls and fractures. Even improper turning or positioning can result in fracture for the very frail elderly. The principles of mobility described in Chapter 7 should be reviewed.

Dietary Considerations: Clients should be instructed in identification of foods that provide rich sources of calcium and vitamin D. Women should be consuming between 200 and 400 mg of vitamin D per day (Scura & Whipple, 1997). Vitamin D assists calcium uptake from the gut to the bloodstream, and it is synthesized in the skin through exposure to sunlight. Again, this illustrates the necessity for a holistic approach to prevention that addresses the numerous components related to osteoporosis.

Recommended daily calcium intake for postmenopausal females is 1500 mg. This is the same for men older than 65 years (Broy, 1996). The recommended dosage for a calcium supplement should not be exceeded, because damage to the kidneys could result.

Several preferred selections in the diet can be found in Table 12–3. Some foods provide both these essential nutrients (calcium and vitamin D), so clients should be encouraged to make these part of a daily dietary regimen. If increased calcium in the diet is for some reason contraindicated (such as in persons who have problems with renal calculi), the dietitian and physician should be consulted.

Currently, several companies advertise formulations or antacids that are said to provide daily calcium in pill form. It is better that these vitamins and minerals come from food sources than from a bottle. Some such products are not absorbed from the intestines sufficiently well to result in any benefit. An idea of whether or not the body will dissolve and absorb such a supplement can be gained by dropping the pill into a small amount of vinegar, waiting 15 minutes, and observing whether or not it has begun to dissolve (Scura & Whipple, 1997). If the tablet has not begun to break up in this time, then it is unlikely that the body will derive much benefit from the supplement. However, this simple test does not take into account the variations in intestinal absorption among people, which are also dependent on many other factors, such as nutritional status.

Estrogen Replacement Therapy: A combination of calcium, vitamin D, and estrogen replacement can lessen postmenopausal bone loss (Allen, 1994; Broy, 1996). Estrogen replacement therapy helps to protect against hip fracture in those younger than 75 years. Estrogen has a bone-promoting influence, and to reduce the risk of postmenopausal bone loss and subsequent fractures, estrogen replacement is often recommended (Kessenich, 1997). For women who have had both ovaries removed before the age of menopause, hormone replacement therapy may have already been initiated. Estrogen is still the most effective medication for women who already have osteoporosis, and it is an option for most postmenopausal women (Broy, 1996).

There are side effects to hormone replacement therapy, so individuals should make informed decisions about this approach after discussing concerns with their primary health care provider. A recently approved medication, alendronate, has been well tolerated and has demonstrated an increase of 8% in spinal bone density while decreasing vertebral fractures by 48% in postmenopausal women who had osteoporosis (Broy, 1996). Gastrointestinal effects are the major adverse reaction. The recommended daily dose of 10 mg is enough to inhibit bone resorption and to improve bone mass density over time, but this drug is not yet approved for use in women who are taking hormone replacements (Scura & Whipple, 1997).

Exercise: Weight bearing and strengthening exercises should be an essential part of any osteoporosis prevention program. An exercise program should involve intensity, duration, frequency, and specific types of activity (Allen, 1994). As discussed in Chapter 7, increasing flexibility, balance, and strength can prevent falls in the elderly. Allen (1994) stated that, "the primary goal of an 'osteoporosis exercise program' in postmenopausal women is to retard bone loss and improve mobility and flexibility" (p. 210). A daily regimen of at least 30 minutes of exercise per day, at least three to four times per week, has been suggested as a preventive measure for osteoporosis (McMahon et al., 1992; Scura & Whipple, 1997). Kessenich (1997) recommended "exercises aimed at the extensor

Table 12–3 CLIENT/FAMILY TEACHING: FOODS TO INCLUDE IN AN OSTEOPOROSIS PREVENTION DIET

Foods Rich in Calcium	Serving Amount	Provides
*Low-fat or skim milk	1 cup	300 mg
*Low-fat yogurt	1 cup	300–400 mg
Broccoli	1 stalk	150 mg
Enriched farina cereal	1 cup	150 mg
Whole wheat bread	1 slice	88 mg
Fresh orange	1 medium	50 mg

Other vitamin-rich foods
*Low-fat cottage cheese
Canned salmon and sardines (including bones)
Foods fortified with calcium (such as orange
   juice, bread, cereal): become a label reader

*Also rich in vitamin D.
Based on information from the National Osteoporosis Foundation.

Table 12–4   ASSOCIATIONS THAT SUPPORT RESEARCH AND EDUCATION

National Osteoporosis Foundation
1150 17th Street, N.W., Suite 500
Washington, DC 20036
(202) 223–2226 or 1-800-223-9994
   (for educational information)

Older Women's League
666 11th Street, N.W., Suite 700
Washington, DC 20001
(202) 783–6686

National Institute on Aging
National Institutes of Health
Federal Building, Room 6C12
Bethesda, MD 20892
(301) 496–1752

---

muscles of the upper and lower back" (p. 194). Because vertebral fractures are common, and difficult to treat, back strengthening exercises are essential.

Screening: Bone mass measurement, or assessment of bone density, is the only method to determine the status of a person's bone health and to predict the potential for future fractures (National Osteoporosis Foundation, 1997). Yet, Medicare does not currently pay for this test, a situation that advocates for osteoporosis research are trying to change. Out-of-pocket expenses for a bone density measurement may currently run from $100 to $350 (Scura & Whipple, 1997).

Many persons think that osteoporosis is a normal part of aging and thus ignore signs and symptoms until serious health consequences have resulted. Persons on Medicare both may have the most need and may derive the greatest benefit from such screenings and diagnostic tools. GRNs can become involved through national foundations that petition legislators on behalf of osteoporosis prevention activities and research. Table 12–4 gives information on a few such organizations.

ARTHRITIS

Arthritis is a chronic disease that affects 12.1% of the population of the United States or 15.8 million people (Hirano, Laurent, & Lorig, 1994). There are more than 100 different types of arthritis. In most cases, the cause of arthritis is unknown (Liang, 1988). Osteoarthritis (OA) is the most common rheumatic disease (Fisher et al., 1993; "The Right Treat-

ment," 1995; Verbrugge, 1995). OA is also considered the most common chronic disease among the elderly (Hughes & Dunlop, 1995). Rheumatoid arthritis (RA) is another common classification of arthritis and one that often results in disability. Discussion here focuses on these two most common kinds of joint disorder that affect persons seen in rehabilitation.

Osteoarthritis

Quinet (1986) referred to OA as "joint failure syndrome" (p. 36). This type of degenerative joint disease is characterized by deterioration of the cartilage in the ends of the bones. Such chronic degeneration can lead to pain, disability, and loss of independence. Wear and tear, as well as trauma on the joint, may predispose an individual to OA.

Arthritis is more common among women than men. From mid-life on, arthritis is ranked as the number one chronic condition among women. Even in young adulthood, women have about 50% higher incidence of arthritic conditions than men (Verbrugge, 1995). As age increases, the gender difference in incidence of the disease narrows. There also appears to be more disability among women experiencing arthritis than among men.

Signs and Symptoms

Several signs and symptoms of OA appear in Table 12–5. In addition to pain, aching, and stiffness in the joints that can lead to difficulty in performing activities of daily living (ADLs) and instrumental ADLs (IADLs), defined as household management tasks, some common physical conditions may be of note. Heberden's nodes are bony enlargements at the end joints of the fingers that indicate arthritis. Bouchard's nodes occur at the middle joints

Table 12–5   SIGNS AND SYMPTOMS OF OSTEOARTHRITIS

Heberden's nodes (bony enlargements at end
   joints of fingers)
Bouchard's nodes (bony enlargements at middle
   joints of fingers)
Degeneration in joints
Pain, stiffness, aching in joints
Limited range of motion
Crepitus of the joints
Frequent fractures

of the fingers, appearing as bony enlargements. OA can be distinguished from RA in that the degeneration occurring in the joint does not involve chronic swelling and inflammation, and it does not generally result in severe deformities as with RA (Dunbar & Seegall, 1990).

Effects

With joint degeneration come pain and difficulty with such activities as walking, bending, and other ADLs. This is particularly true when the lower extremities, such as the knees and hip joints, are involved. OA of the knees is especially disabling, resulting in pain and stiffness, as well as trouble with kneeling, walking, rising from a chair, and climbing stairs (Fisher et al., 1993). With hand involvement, the ability to perform such activities as self-feeding, fastening buttons, opening jars, and other grasping tasks may be impaired.

Household management tasks are also affected, particularly if arthritic conditions affect the hands. Persons with arthritis often have *comorbidity*, or other concurrent conditions. Some of the most common arthritis comorbidities include hypertension, hearing impairments, visual disturbances, heart disease, and diabetes (Verbrugge, 1995). This list should not be entirely surprising, however, because these conditions are considered among the most frequently occurring chronic diseases in the elderly (Eliopoulos, 1997).

Arthritis not only results in physical limitations, but also leads to more physician visits, hospital stays, and social limitations (Verbrugge, 1995). Hirano et al. (1994), in a review of arthritis patient education studies from 1987 to 1991, found several common effects of arthritis. These included pain, fatigue, uncertainty about the future, depression, lifestyle changes, and adjustments to the future. One national survey among persons older than 65 years (based on self-reports) demonstrated that life-threatening conditions such as cancer or heart disease did not account for a significant proportion of disability (Hughes & Dunlop, 1995). However, the combination of arthritis and other comorbidity of almost any type seemed to perpetuate disability. Additionally, a strong relationship has been shown to exist between advanced age and arthritis-specific disability (Hughes & Dunlop, 1995; Verbrugge, 1995).

Rheumatoid Arthritis

This chronic, progressive, painful condition related to inflammation of the joint affects 1% of the world's population and has an increased incidence with age (Miller-Blair & Robbins, 1993). Autoimmunity is one proposed cause of RA (Liang, 1988). Thought to occur first between the ages of 20 and 40 years, RA is most often diagnosed before the age of 60 (Elioupolos, 1997; Mirabelli, 1990; Nesher & Moore, 1994). The incidence of RA actually decreases after the age of 65, although its effects continue into old age (Eliopoulos, 1997). Three to five times as many women as men experience RA (Shaul, 1994).

Signs and Symptoms

RA is characterized by flare-ups and remissions of inflammation within the joints. The joints particularly affected include the fingers, wrists, knees, and spine. Pain, stiffness, swelling, and decreased range of motion are hallmark signs (Table 12–6). Other symptoms include fatigue, malaise, weight loss, decreased appetite, anemia, and weakness (Eliopoulos, 1997).

There are three classifications of RA according to level or type of inflammation (Mirabelli, 1990): (1) acute, (2) subacute, and (3) chronic. The acute phase involves swollen, painful joints, which may be reddened and warm to the touch, as well as elevated sedimentation rates. A subacute classification is characterized by still painful and swollen joints that are no longer inflamed. Laboratory results return to more normal limits. The chronic phase has no active inflammation. Pain and fatigue may be present, even in the post-acute phases.

Effects

RA is one of the most debilitating types of arthritis. Table 12–7 lists some of the compli-

Table 12–6 SIGNS AND SYMPTOMS OF RHEUMATOID ARTHRITIS

Malaise
Fatigue
Symmetrical pattern of joint inflammation
Pain and stiffness in involved joints
Gelling (joints stiff after rest)
Morning stiffness
Swelling, warmth, and tenderness with joint movement
Elevated sedimentation rate
Presence of serum rheumatoid factor
Elevated white blood cell counts in synovial fluid (of inflamed joint)
Erosions of bone on radiographs

Table 12–7   COMPLICATIONS OF RHEUMATOID ARTHRITIS

Physical
Contractures, joint deformities
Vasculitis
Cardiac involvement (especially pericarditis)
Interstitial fibrosis
Pneumonitis
Visual disturbances
Periarticular osteopenia
Osteoporosis
Fractures
Unstable gait

Psychosocial
Threats to self-image and self-esteem
Decreased ability for self-care
Depression
Decreased ability for independence with activities of daily living and household chores
Fear of being labeled
Lifestyle changes (of role, job, physical abilities)
Possible social isolation
Changes in sexual role with partner

cations associated with RA. This disease has a systemic effect, affecting multiple joints, with increased fatigue during flare-ups. Such fatigue can, however, be constant and may affect the person's ability to walk and to perform ADLs or household chores. Even activities considered relatively simple, such as holding eating utensils, may become difficult. In one study, the following variables explained a significant amount of variance in reported fatigue: pain rating, functional status, sleep quality, female gender, comorbid conditions, and disease duration (Belza, Heinke, Yelin, Epstein, & Gilliss, 1993).

Other effects of RA are far reaching and costly. Medical costs may be three times as great, hospital costs may double, and doctor visits are more frequent among those with RA than in the general population (Shaul, 1994). The chronic inflammation and joint deterioration caused by RA can lead to joint deformities, particularly in the hands, knees, hips, and vertebrae. Pain management associated with these conditions presents a constant challenge.

The effects of RA reach far beyond the physical, affecting every area of the person's life, including socially and emotionally. In a qualitative study by Shaul (1997), women with RA reported four stages of living with RA: (1) becoming aware, (2) receiving care, (3) learning to live with it, and (4) mastery.

The sample of 30 women described feelings of disconnectedness, uncertainty, withdrawal, and the struggle for control. Because women incur 40% more chronic illness than men do, and because women tend to live longer, they require, and will continue to require, more health services and care (Shaul, 1994). The direct and indirect costs are high, and this situation is worse for women who live longer with chronic illness yet have an income generally less than that of men. Most research in RA has been done with white women, so further studies need to include a more diverse sample, including those of other ethnic groups.

Bradbury and Catanzaro (1989) found that men in a sample with an average age of 60 years reported the greatest difficulty in coping with those activities that affected joints and physical strength, such as sports, bending, and lifting. Women reported more concern with activities such as ADLs. A positive attitude and an internal locus of control were found to result in a better perceived quality of life.

Nursing Implications

Elderly persons with arthritis may have numerous needs. Several common nursing diagnoses associated with arthritis are presented in Table 12–8.

The desired outcomes related to these nursing diagnoses focus on patients' independence within the limitations of their abilities. Goals include management of pain, use of alternative therapies, prevention of secondary complications such as contractures, establish-

Table 12–8   NURSING DIAGNOSES COMMONLY ASSOCIATED WITH ARTHRITIS

Pain
Impaired physical mobility
Fatigue
Decreased endurance
Powerlessness
Self-care deficits
Sleep pattern disturbance
Depression
Alteration in self home maintenance
Impaired coping
Social isolation
Fear
Anxiety
Body-image disturbance

ment of an appropriate exercise regimen, management of medications, and promoting independence. Many of the nursing interventions discussed here work best in conjunction with each other. For example, low-dose steroid medications can promote participation in an exercise program, which, in turn, can decrease pain (Lyngberg, Harreby, Bentzen, Frost, & Danneskiold-Samsoe, 1994).

Pain Management: One of the most significant effects of arthritis from the person's point of view is controlling the pain associated with flare-ups. Pain management has traditionally focused on medications, including the use of acetaminophen, nonsteroidal anti-inflammatory drugs (NSAIDs), and steroids.

Treatments for pain in OA are presented in Table 12–9. Exercise has also shown promise

Table 12–9 TREATMENTS FOR PAIN ASSOCIATED WITH OSTEOARTHRITIS

Medications
Acetaminophen
Aspirin
Nonsteroidal anti-inflammatory drugs such as ibuprofen, naproxen, sulindac
Capsaicin (topically, with other therapies)
Nabumetone

Nonpharmacological Pain-Management Strategies
Moist heat (as with warm water soaks)
Warm paraffin wraps (can be followed by range of motion)
Stretch gloves or stockings
Gentle range of motion (can be done in warm water)
Exercises: range of motion, stretching, strengthening, functional (as instructed by the physical and occupational therapists)
Specific activities that provide active exercise to joints (such as playing the piano or typing for upper extremities; walking or swimming for lower extremities and overall conditioning)
Splints/braces (for resting the joints, joint protection with use of a walker or cane, and preventing contractures)
Adaptive equipment (such as utensils with built-up handles)
Heat/cold applications (cold for numbing and pain relief; hot for relaxing muscles)
Warm bath (limit to 20 minutes)
Good posture
Special supportive orthotic shoes
Well-balanced diet (those with gout should avoid foods high in purine)
Maintenance of proper weight

with regard to decreasing pain, especially in OA of the knees (Fisher et al., 1993; Orr & Bratton, 1992).

Rehabilitation: The purpose of rehabilitation is to maintain function and to prevent secondary complications while assisting the person to achieve his or her maximal independence level. "The common goal of rehabilitation for all persons with arthritis is to raise and maintain physical capabilities, emotional stability, social integration, and economic independence" (Krutzen, 1984, p. 634). Persons with OA and RA are frequent users of assistive technology devices. Most of these adaptive devices are helpful for toileting, bathing, and lower extremity dressing (Rogers & Holm, 1992).

Prevention of complications is part of rehabilitation. Splints or braces are often used to prevent contractures and deformity from arthritis. Gilbert-Lenef (1994) suggested a way to splint the arthritic hand with a lightweight homemade device using Velcro, to straighten arthritic fingers, thus preventing contractures. Such splints are used to prevent secondary complications such as deformities that can result from flexion of muscles and joints without full range of active motion.

Exercise: GRNs need to encourage patients to begin exercise programs that will help to minimize the effects of arthritis. Common types of activities for persons with arthritis include walking, cycling, swimming, and stretching (Keefe et al., 1996). Active hand exercises reduce stiffness and pain, resulting in increased range of motion (Dellhag, Wollersjo, & Bjelle, 1992). Although in the past, exercise for the treatment of OA of the knees was not recommended, several studies have confirmed that exercise programs resulted in improved outcomes for persons with arthritis, including a decrease in pain (Fisher et al., 1993; La Mantia & Marks, 1995; Orr & Bratton, 1992). In a study involving persons with OA of the knees, "improvements in muscle function resulted in improvements in functional capacity" (Fisher et al., 1993, p. 846). A 3-month physical therapy program studied by Fisher et al. (1993) was successful in increasing strength and decreasing pain without exacerbating symptoms. La Mantia and Marks (1995) summarized findings as follows: "beneficial effects have been demonstrated to improve aerobic capacity, exercise endurance, physical activity, six-minute test of walking distance, 50-foot walking time, gait velocity due to gain in stride length and not increases in cadence, pain, depression, and anxiety without apparent worsening of disease-related symptoms" (p. 27).

Medications: Medical treatment of arthritis takes several common forms. The most commonly used medications to relieve arthritis symptoms are NSAIDs. Examples of those used most often are aspirin, ibuprofen, and naproxen. NSAIDs relieve pain and decrease inflammation, but they often result in side effects, particularly gastrointestinal disturbances (Moncur & Williams, 1995) (Table 12–10). Another potential side effect of NSAID use is the elevation of blood pressure by an average of 5 mmHg. This increase could be significant for elderly adults with pre-existing hypertension. Elderly patients who are taking NSAIDs or higher doses of aspirin need to be monitored with regard to hematological status. This includes complete blood count, urinalysis, blood urea nitrogen, creatinine, potassium, and serum transaminase several times per year (Quinet, 1986).

Acetaminophen (Tylenol) is still the number one choice of many physicians and primary health care providers for the treatment of arthritis. Acetaminophen is recommended as a first drug of choice over NSAIDs for OA because it has fewer side effects. However, the long-term use of acetaminophen (more than two pills per day) may result in chronic renal failure ("The Right Treatment," 1995). Capsaicin (trans-8-methyl-N-vanillyl-6-nonenamide), an active ingredient in chili peppers, used topically, has caused a decrease in pain for those with OA and RA in certain studies, but it is not generally effective as a sole therapy for arthritis (Watson, 1994).

Nabumetone is a newly approved NSAID for treatment of RA and OA. This medication has fewer gastrointestinal side effects and is safer for those with impaired renal function (Roth, 1992).

All elderly persons on medication regimens should be instructed to take prescribed drugs regularly, not just as needed. In addition to drug therapy, persons with arthritis may benefit from alternative therapies, as discussed in the next section.

Alternative Therapies: Several types of alternative therapies have shown promise in the treatment of arthritis (see Table 12–9). Some of these are used alone, but most are used in combination with other treatments. For example, transcutaneous electrical nerve stimulation units can provide pain relief in OA, particularly in conjunction with capsaicin (Nicholas, 1994). Warm paraffin wax treatment followed by active hand exercises has been shown to improve range of motion and grip function significantly in persons with RA (Dellhag et al., 1992). However, wax baths alone may not be of significant benefit. Acupuncture has been used for treatment of pain among persons with OA of the knees. Takeda and Wessel (1994) found that acupuncture significantly reduced pain, stiffness, and physical disability in the osteoarthritic knee. An interesting aspect of this study, however, was that those receiving real acupuncture and those receiving placebo acupuncture showed similar results, with no difference between groups. This finding suggests either a significant psychological component to pain treatment among these patients or physiological effects in both groups. Additionally, men showed greater effects than women.

Additional aspects of pain management are worth mentioning. Interferential therapy is a bipolar technique in which electrodes are placed on either side of the knee for delivery of electrical currents. This technique has been shown to decrease pain in OA. Persons with certain personality traits or disorders (such as depression or hysteria) were previously thought to respond poorly to pain therapy. Shafshak, El-Sheshai, and Soltan (1991) found that personality traits had no significant effect on pain response.

Surgery

When pain and joint dysfunction limit range of motion enough to interfere with the per-

Table 12–10 SOME SIDE EFFECTS OF NONSTEROIDAL ANTI-INFLAMMATORY DRUGS

Indigestion
Peptic ulcers, complications of ulcers
Vomiting
Chronic renal failure
Hematological changes
Urticaria
Rashes
Bronchospasm
Headache
Dizziness
Tinnitus
Confusion

Data from Moncur, C., & Williams, H. J. (1995). Rheumatoid arthritis: Status of drug therapies. *Physical Therapy, 75,* 511–525.

son's perceived quality of life, surgery can be a viable option. Hip and knee replacements are common and successful in the elderly. These are discussed later in this chapter. The best benefit of surgery (for the person) is decreased pain.

Educational Programs

Several types of educational programs have been developed and researched in patients with arthritis. Orr and Bratton (1992) measured the effect of an inpatient arthritis rehabilitation program on self-assessed functional ability. A volunteer sample of 97 persons participated in a 6-day intensive program with exercise and mobility, education, counseling, and individual physical and occupational therapy, with the focus of promotion of independence in ADLs with self-care. Nursing care was provided 24 hours a day. Measures of outcomes were determined on admission and discharge. The results indicated that, after the program, participants experienced a significant decrease in disability, pain, and the need for assistance. The interdisciplinary approach used seemed to be effective in promoting positive outcomes.

Education is not only useful for improving functional outcomes. Based on a meta-analysis by Superio-Cabuslay, Ward, and Lorig (1996), patient education interventions provided additional benefits (beyond the effects of NSAID treatment) of pain relief, functional ability, and reduction in tenderness of the joint. The effects of education were greater for persons with RA than for those with OA.

Many patients with arthritis benefit from emotional, social, and financial support (Reisine, 1995). Chaney et al. (1996) found that shorter illness duration, greater perceived pain, and increased functional disability led to greater levels of depression. Illness duration was found to have a modifying effect between function and depression. These findings should cause the nurse to be alert to the patient's emotional status and to realize that many persons, especially those newly diagnosed with RA, may experience significant distress related to their condition.

Pain coping and exercise training have also been shown to enhance pain control. Although patients vary in coping ability, pain is generally a major concern. Coping skills to deal with pain can be learned. In a study by Keefe et al. (1996), a 10-week program was run in which participants met for 90 minutes per week with a nurse educator and a psychologist. Topics discussed included progressive relaxation, exercise and activity, distraction techniques such as imagery, cognitive restructuring, and problem solving. Results showed that patients expressed enhanced pain control. Another study by Keefe et al. (1996) also showed that spouse-assisted pain-coping skills training resulted in better outcomes. These included significantly lower levels of pain, less psychological disability, improved pain behavior, and higher self-efficacy and marital adjustment.

Joint protection programs typically consist of education on a variety of concepts including pain management, rest, exercise, energy conservation, use of adaptive equipment, and prevention of deformity. Hammond (1994) found that a joint protection education program for patients with RA did not result in a behavioral change. The sample Hammond used had only 11 subjects and lasted just 6 weeks. Yet, the participants did report a change in attitude toward management of their arthritis. Hammond's pilot study suggests that behavioral change may require more time and more specific target outcomes to be effective.

Research

Many published studies deal with RA. More studies are needed for OA. The less common forms of arthritis also warrant further examination. Research should focus on fatigue and dealing with life changes. Staff members need to be further educated about the effects and nursing interventions related to care of the elderly person experiencing arthritis. Cost-effectiveness of treatments and evaluation of arthritis education groups are also areas for further study (Hirano et al., 1994).

The effect of combinations of therapies such as pain coping and exercise training needs to be researched. Variables should be identified that predict a person's response to biopsychosocial treatment (Keefe et al., 1996).

JOINT REPLACEMENT SURGERY

Total Hip Arthroplasty

Many conditions necessitate total replacement of the hip. Arthritis, osteoporosis, traumatic fractures, and degeneration of the joints can make ambulation painful and difficult, resulting in decreased range of motion, impaired physical mobility, and decreased independence. In one study (Levy, Levy, Snyder, & Digiovanni, 1995) with patients aged an average of 85.2 years, OA was the most common diagnosis among those admitted for total hip arthroplasty (THA).

Hip fractures are the most common orthopedic condition among the elderly, especially the frail old (Rush, 1996). Ninety-seven percent of hip fractures occur in persons older than 65 years, with a cost of $7 billion to $34 billion each year in the United States for surgery and rehabilitation (Thomas, 1996). The typical patient with a hip fracture is a woman more than 65 years of age. One third of all women who survive to age 90 have had a hip fracture (Perez, 1994). The primary risk factor for hip fracture is trabecular bone loss and decreased bone strength from postmenopausal osteoporosis (Perez, 1994).

Surgery, including THA, often gives the best results, by decreasing pain, stabilizing the joint, and providing increased mobility. Four types of hip repair are noted: pinning, nailing, fixation, and arthroplasty. Persons who have undergone uncomplicated hip surgery may return directly home postoperatively. Those with complications or additional factors, particularly after THA, may go to rehabilitation or subacute care. Persons with severe impairments who are poor surgical risks may benefit more from non-surgical treatment, resulting in lower levels of morbidity. This is assuming that quality care will be provided in the extended care facility to which they are discharged. For the purposes of this text, discussion focuses on THA, because this is more commonly seen in rehabilitation.

Expected Outcomes

Outcomes after THA are varied because of the interaction of several factors including age, functional status on admission, existing comorbidities, and psychosocial issues. Older persons generally have lower functional scores on admission than younger adults. Often, the older the person is on admission, the worse the functional status (Oberg & Oberg, 1996). Many patients never regain full function after THA, and they may be discharged to a nursing home or extended care facility (Thomas, 1996). Pre-fracture mobility is often the best predictor of post-fracture outcome (Perez, 1994).

About 15% of patients with hip fractures require long-term care (Perez, 1994). Up to 70% of nursing home residents, and 30% of those in the community, die within a year of complications of hip fracture (Resnick, 1994). Increased mortality after hip fracture has been associated with male gender, increased age, residence in a nursing home before the fracture, and the presence of comorbidities (Lu-Yao, Baron, Barrett, & Fisher, 1994).

THA significantly improved outcomes in most studies. Outcomes were also improved through exercise programs emphasizing strength and mobility training (Sherrington & Lord, 1997). Berman, Quinn, and Zarro (1991) found that THA improved gait characteristics in persons with degenerative arthritis, especially in those with unilateral hip disease. Levy et al. (1995) found that 88% of persons (n = 76, average age = 85.2 years) remained able to walk after THA. Sixty percent used a cane. A total of 96% remained independent, and most were satisfied with their health outcome. This research demonstrated strong positive results for those undergoing THA for OA.

Complications of THA abound among older adults. These include blood clots (deep vein thrombosis, pulmonary emboli), pressure ulcers, delirium (often from unfamiliar surroundings of the hospital and especially in those older than 85 years), urinary tract infections (from indwelling catheters), and infection at the operative site (Perez, 1994).

Nursing Implications

Two general areas to assess are injury factors and patient factors. Injury factors include assessment of bone and soft tissue quality, extent of trauma, presence of degenerative joint disease, and the possibility of comorbidities such as cancer with metastasis. Patient factors include psychological issues as well as the person's pre-injury status including the presence of other unrelated diseases such as congestive heart failure, chronic obstructive pulmonary disease, or diabetes (Zuckerman, Zetterberg, & Frankel, 1995). Also important to consider are family support, history of falls, and independence level at home.

Assessment: The GRN should consider several key components when examining a person after THA. First, circulation and sensation should be noted. The surgical site should be assessed. The wound edges should be well approximated. Staples will probably still be present and should be intact. Slight redness is common, but the surgical site should not be warm or edematous, although some edema at the site is also common. The GRN should note any drainage when changing the dressing (if applicable). A scant amount of serosanguineous drainage is common soon after surgery. A sterile dressing is often applied over the incision to protect it during activity and mobility training. The site should be kept clean and dry. Some physicians order the incisional site to be cleansed with povidone-iodine (Betadine) or iodine daily. Sterile swabs are used for this cleansing, taking care not to snag the cotton tip on the staples. The physician may order half of the staples to be removed one day, and half later. Sterile adhesive strips can be applied as needed, particularly to any areas where the wound edges are not well approximated.

Some edema is common to the lower extremities among elderly patients after THA and should be documented in terms of amount and whether it is pitting or non-pitting. The GRN should ask the patient whether or not swelling was present in the extremities before surgery, because edema may be related to other causes or to less activity postoperatively. The operative leg should be examined for signs and symptoms of deep venous thrombosis. Any such factors should be promptly reported to the physician. The pedal pulses should be palpable. It may be necessary to mark the area in which the pulse is palpated if pulses were premorbidly weak, so that other nurses will be assisted in locating the pulse. Additionally, a Doppler examination may be needed if pulses cannot be palpated.

Goals/Outcomes/Nursing Diagnoses: Early ambulation and prevention of complications such as skin breakdown, deep venous thromboses, pneumonia, and delirium are keys to successful rehabilitation after THA. The goal of treatment is to restore the pre-injury level of functioning, but this is not always possible or probable. As previously stated, outcomes depend on a variety of factors, all of which should be considered when setting realistic goals and planning interventions. Mutual goal setting should be incorporated into the interdisciplinary plan of care.

Specific nursing goals may include that the patient will remain free from injury (safety), regain independent bladder functioning (after Foley catheter removal, if applicable), be free from skin breakdown, have adequate peripheral tissue perfusion, and remain alert and oriented. Additionally, the GRN would expect to see stable vital signs, willing participation in teaching/learning and preparation for discharge, and participation in therapeutic activities to promote self-care. Nursing diagnoses related to hip fracture and THA are presented in Table 12–11.

Interventions: One initial yet essential nursing intervention falls under the role of the nurse as patient advocate. GRNs can assist persons undergoing THA by advocating placement in a formal rehabilitation program soon after surgery. Although rehabilitation does begin immediately postoperatively, therapy in the acute care setting lacks the intensity and focus of the acute rehabilitation unit. Patients with THA benefit from rehabilitation measures if they are admitted within 6 months after surgery (Kolarz, Maager, Scherak, El Shohoumi, & Wottawa, 1995). Failure in rehabilitation of the elderly could be due to poor conditions on admission. However, all types of patients benefit from rehabilitation, but the sooner they enter the program, the better.

Physical Indications: Proper posture is important in maintaining mobility and range of motion. A backrest support should help to maintain proper posture and "either correct or accommodate lumbar spinal and thoracic spinal postural deviants such as lateral flexion, scoliosis, and kyphosis" (Stinnett, 1996, p. 25).

Hip precautions must be maintained to prevent dislocation, a relatively common occurrence after surgery. An abductor wedge or pillow may be used to keep the knees apart, either in a chair or in bed. Pillows should be kept between the patient's legs when turning on the side in bed at home until the physician

---

Table 12–11 COMMON NURSING DIAGNOSES RELATED TO HIP FRACTURE AND REPLACEMENT

Pain
Alteration in peripheral tissue perfusion
Alteration in physical mobility
Impaired skin integrity
Potential for injury (high risk for falls)
Potential for infection (related to surgical wound)
Alteration in home maintenance
Self-care deficit (related to bathing, activities of daily living)
Alteration in urinary elimination (related to indwelling catheter or removal of catheter)
Alteration in bowel elimination (related to constipation from inactivity)

Table 12–12 PATIENT/FAMILY TEACHING: POSTOPERATIVE HIP CARE

Do Not:	Rationale
Cross legs	Can dislocate hip by pushing out joint
Bend past 90 degrees at the waist	Puts undue stress on prosthesis; can fall out of chair
Bear full weight on the operative side until the physician gives permission	Time is required for bone to heal and strengthen around prosthesis; full weight bearing too soon may cause fracture

Do:	Rationale
Sit with legs 3–6 inches apart	Prevents dislocation
Keep 2 pillows between legs when turning/side lying	
Inform dentist and other physicians before treatment that you have a prosthesis	Antibiotics may be needed to prevent possible infection
Inform security officials of prosthetic device before going through metal detectors	Prosthesis may trigger metal detectors in government buildings or airports
Report signs and symptoms of infection	So that prompt treatment may be initiated
Continue leg strengthening, range of motion, and other activities as prescribed by physical therapist	Promotes bone and wound healing
Continue to wear elastic stockings at home as directed by physician	Prevents blood clots and swelling; promotes circulation

permits otherwise. Routine hip precautions and postoperative care to be taught to the patient and family appear in Table 12–12.

Education: Teaching by the GRN can significantly influence the outcome for persons after joint replacement. Education has been shown to increase feelings of control from increased knowledge (Orr, 1990) and to result in more active participation in the recovery process. Favorable outcomes were obtained when persons were given preoperative education. This

included being allowed to discuss fears and options (Lichtenstein, Semann, & Marmar, 1993). A postoperative support group also can assist with addressing the concerns of older adults.

An educational program for older adults should include pre-surgical discussion of joint replacement, arthritis and medication management, exercises, pain management, stress and coping skills, joint protection (including hip precautions and energy conservation), and discharge planning (Orr, 1990). Although many units that emphasize rehabilitation do not have standard THA protocol, certain activities need to be included in discharge planning. These include a home exercise program, maintenance of hip precautions, recognition of complications (Table 12–13), and the ability to demonstrate the skills to negotiate stairs properly and safely and to ambulate (Enloe, Shields, Smith, Leo, & Miller, 1996). Written instructions should be provided for the patient and caregiver.

No teaching program should neglect the psychosocial and emotional aspects related to recovery after THA. Houldin and Hogen-Quigley (1995) found that visits by a psychiatric clinical nurse specialist decreased trait anxiety scores. Patients in this study also expressed gratitude at having their emotional needs attended to by the nursing staff. Persons should receive counseling and should be allowed to discuss coping strategies with the GRN before discharge.

The GRN may also need to assist the patient with follow-through in the use of adaptive equipment. This is particularly important on the off-shifts if no therapist is present, when supervising persons in a long-term care setting, as a review before discharge, or when

Table 12–13 PATIENT/FAMILY TEACHING: SIGNS AND SYMPTOMS OF WOUND INFECTION

Wound Observations
Increased pain at the surgical site
Drainage (not present at discharge), especially foul smelling, bloody, and yellowish or green
Redness or swelling at the incision site
Wound edges that are gaping

General Observations
Fever
Chills, sweating
Nausea or vomiting
Loss of appetite
Malaise

instructing the family. Important aspects of instruction to remember will be related to the use of crutches, canes, and walkers.

For example, the patient should hold the cane in the hand opposite to the affected hip. This relieves 20% to 25% of the body weight (Perez, 1994). Crutches are more stable than a cane, but they are rarely used by elderly patients because more energy is required, and most elderly persons feel less steady, perhaps increasing the risk of falls. Crutches also place an increased demand on the heart. A person using a cane or crutches should be reminded to move the device with the affected leg, then move the unaffected leg.

For stairs, the person should be reminded that the un-operative leg steps up first, followed by the operative leg. When going down stairs, the operative leg goes first, followed by the un-operative leg. Because the use of the terms "good" and "bad" is contraindicated in rehabilitation, it may help the person to remember the saying, "up with the strong, down with the weak," when negotiating stairs.

A walker is more steady and easy to use, but it requires increased time and patience. Many persons use walkers successfully as their primary assistive device for walking after discharge. However, some reminders should be given. The person using a walker should be reminded not to hold onto it when rising from a chair. It is used to steady the person once he or she is standing. The walker should not be placed too far in front of the person before stepping through. This can throw the user off-balance. Nor should the walker be carried. If this is the case, it may not be needed, except perhaps for psychological comfort. Some elderly persons have found that pushing a wheelchair from behind provides added support, as does pushing the grocery cart at the store. However, these devices can also be hazards if a wheelchair or cart cannot be controlled and causes the person to become off-balance.

Research

More research is needed on the specific outcomes related to persons of different ethnic groups who undergo THA. Additional studies could focus on measuring outcomes after THA, particularly variations in mobility over extended periods of time. Length of time related to wearing down of the prosthesis also warrants further study.

Total Knee Arthroplasty

Pain and immobility related to arthritis or other degenerative joint disease are major reasons leading to total knee arthroplasty (TKA). This surgical procedure involves replacement of the worn joint with prosthetics that allow more freedom of movement. TKA for persons with arthritis has resulted in decreased pain, increased mobility, a better emotional state, and improved perceived quality of life (Pitson, Bhaskaran, Bond, Yarnold, & Drewett, 1994).

Physicians try to postpone this operation in older persons until it is absolutely necessary, so that the likelihood of having to replace the parts from the first surgical procedure is lessened. At present, the life expectancy of the prosthetics used in TKA is approximately 10 to 12 years. However, TKA is highly successful, even in persons of advanced age. Research by Bohannon and Cooper (1993) showed that 96% of the 146 subjects in the study having TKA were discharged home. Functional improvements were significant with rehabilitation. Gains were noted especially in the areas of transfers, ambulation, and the ability to negotiate stairs. The mean stay in acute rehabilitation for a unilateral TKA was 9.9 days at a cost of $16,149. A cost of $23,594 was associated with an 11.9-day stay. However, as with THA, elderly patients admitted with lower functional scores will probably have less positive outcomes than those with previously higher scores (Oberg & Oberg, 1996).

TKA is considered so effective that even persons who were not considered good candidates in the past have had successful outcomes. For example, persons with Parkinson's disease were deemed poor candidates for TKA, but a case study by Fast, Mendelsohn, and Sosner (1994) suggested that a person with mild Parkinson's disease may still benefit from surgery. These authors found that rehabilitation of a person with Parkinson's disease who underwent TKA was prolonged, but it was found to be effective if the person was able to ambulate before surgery and demonstrated the ability to learn.

A common preference of physicians at this time is to perform bilateral TKA when needed. Previously, two separate operations were done, allowing time in between for the first knee to heal. This method was thought to be more beneficial to the patient than having both knees operated on at the same time. However, physicians now believe, particu-

larly in the older patient, that replacement of both knees at the same time is preferable. Not only does it lengthen recovery only slightly (over unilateral operations), but also the person does not have to undergo two anesthetics or incur the cost of separate surgical procedures. The entire procedure for bilateral TKA takes roughly 2 to 3 hours and can even be done using spinal anesthesia. Blood lost during the operation may be filtered via the use of specialized and highly technical equipment and given directly back to the person during the surgery. However, postoperative pain may be significant and will need to be addressed by GRNs.

Goals/Outcomes/Nursing Diagnoses

As with hip replacement, education of the person and family can play a key role in promoting positive outcomes. The GRN should emphasize the importance of exercise, the role of medications, joint protection, ambulation skills, positive coping strategies, and discharge preparation. Increased knowledge related to these topics leads to feelings of more control as well as more active participation in the rehabilitation process (Enloe et al., 1996; Orr, 1990).

The major goal of TKA is to return the person to a maximal independent level of functioning and mobility with decreased pain. Expected outcomes include a well-healed surgical wound, good peripheral circulation, improved ambulation and the ability to climb stairs, the ability to perform ADLs and IADLs, joint protection skills, and pain management. Nursing diagnoses are similar to those for THA (see Table 12–11).

Nursing Implications

One of the ways in which early mobility is enhanced is through the use of continuous passive motion (CPM). The benefit of CPM to improve the rate of change in flexion occurs early postoperatively, yet the benefit of CPM machines has been questioned by some. At present, the physician's preference determines whether or not a CPM machine is used. The theory behind CPM is that early movement enhances healing of the cartilage, promotes wound healing, and increases mobility of the joint, particularly with regard to flexion. One study showed no difference in improving flexion or extension in patients with degenerative joint disease when CPM was used and when it was not, but CPM did enhance the rate of return of active knee

flexion (Chiarello, Gundersen, & O'Halloran, 1997).

Nursing responsibilities related to caring for a person rehabilitating after TKA include assessment of the wound, education (see Table 12–13), and monitoring the use of the CPM. As with THA, the surgical incision site should be examined each shift at minimum. Hemovacs may have been inserted during surgery to assist in relieving drainage from the operative site, but such devices are generally removed before admission to the rehabilitation unit. The person will probably wear elastic stockings to promote blood flow and to deter clotting. Antiembolism stockings are often effective in helping to promote circulation and in preventing edema. These stockings need to be removed to assess the lower extremities properly, then reapplied. The wound edges should be well approximated. It is common for the staples to remain in place until shortly before discharge. Sterile adhesive strips may be applied to the incision site after removal of the staples. Dressings are rarely necessary. There should be no (or scant) drainage from the incision site. Pedal and posterior tibial pulses should be palpated. The legs should be inspected for any signs of deep venous thrombosis. The patient should be questioned about sensations such as coolness of the extremities.

The GRN also monitors the use of the CPM machine. The person with bilateral TKA may have two machines. Typically, the physician orders degrees of flexion and extension postoperatively, with gradual increases daily. A dial or digital buttons on the machine will be set for the specified degrees. The GRN needs to assist the person in complying with the prescribed number of hours on the machine, as well as placing the person's leg appropriately in the device. Some beds have machines attached to them that elevate and lower. Other units have portable CPM machines that need to placed on the bed when ready to use. The minimal goal of range of motion for the person with TKA is 0 degrees of extension (fully extended) and 90 degrees of flexion. This right angle of flexion is needed to rise from a chair or bed, and full extension is needed for walking with proper balance.

Ambulation and exercising should be encouraged, particularly on the off-shifts when physical therapy and occupational therapy are no longer in session. Exercises prescribed by the physical therapist generally work all the major muscle groups. Leg raising, ankle/foot flexion and extension, sitting knee flexion with resistive bands, supine hip abduction/adduction, and other exercises aid in strengthening.

AMPUTATION

More than 100,000 amputations are performed each year in the United States. Of those, 85% involve the lower extremity, particularly below-knee and above-knee amputations (Heafey, Golden-Baker, & Mahoney, 1994). Persons admitted to rehabilitation, subacute care, or long-term care after an amputation have undergone surgery for a variety of reasons. The most common cause is peripheral vascular disease, with diabetes as an underlying pathologic process about 50% of the time (Heafey et al., 1994). Sometimes, a small foot injury or wound in the elderly diabetic patient can lead to major complications and amputation.

Lower extremity amputations may simply be classified into two broad categories: above-knee and below-knee amputations, also called transfemoral and transtibial amputations. However, amputations can occur at many levels. The type of amputation performed depends largely on the cause of injury and the extent of damaged tissue. In the case of diabetes-related amputations, it is not uncommon for persons to undergo multiple surgical procedures beginning with the toes and progressing upward, as the physician attempts to spare as much of the lower extremity as possible. All diseased tissue is removed with each amputation to prevent further infection, gangrene, and sepsis.

Goals/Outcomes/Nursing Diagnoses

Nursing care of the elderly person who has undergone an amputation is crucial in promoting positive outcomes. These include helping to protect and preserve the residuum (regardless of the location of the amputation), preparing the stump for a prosthesis, and addressing psychosocial and emotional issues. The goals of an amputee program are "to provide the knowledge, skills, and attitude necessary for physical and emotional adjustment and to help the patient achieve self-care at home and in the community" (Yetzer, Kauffman, Sopp, & Talley, 1994, p. 358). Table 12–14 provides a list of common nursing diagnoses associated with care of the person who has undergone an amputation. For the purposes of this text, the discussion focuses on special indications for care of older persons with lower extremity amputations.

Table 12–14 NURSING DIAGNOSES RELATED TO AMPUTATION

Alteration in peripheral tissue perfusion
Impaired physical mobility
Impaired skin integrity
Alteration in bowel elimination
Potential for deconditioning
Body image disturbance
Altered body image
Pain
Fear
Anxiety
Powerlessness
Self-care deficits
Decreased endurance
Potential for injury
Knowledge deficit
Alteration in home maintenance
Grief
Impaired social interaction
Alterations in family process
Ineffective individual coping
Disuse syndrome

Nursing Implications

Rehabilitation for the person with an amputation must begin immediately after surgery. GRNs may need to educate nurses in acute settings about appropriate care of the stump. This is particularly true with regard to positioning the stump after surgery. The physician may order stump elevation postoperatively to reduce edema, and if the nurse is not careful, the pillow may be placed in a way that actually contributes to contractures and can even prevent the later use of a prosthesis. The pillow should never be placed under the knee, because this can lead to contracture of the knee joint. Complete extension is required for optimal walking and for prosthesis use, so decreased range of motion must be prevented. The prone position is excellent for promoting stump extension, but few elderly persons can tolerate lying on their stomach for a variety of reasons, not the least of which is restricted air flow caused by increased pressure on the chest.

Conditioning a stump has six main objectives (Table 12–15). Generally, the stump must have minimal swelling and tenderness and maximal shrinkage. A stump is conditioned and shaped for prosthesis fitting in several ways. The person may be fitted with a rigid removable dressing, elastic (Ace) bandage wraps after surgery, or a shrinker sock. Rigid removable dressings decrease swelling and

Table 12–15 OBJECTIVES FOR STUMP CONDITIONING

Conical shape, maximal shrinkage
Absence of tenderness, ability to tolerate contact
  with prosthetic cup and to bear weight
Freely movable scar
Decreased swelling, minimal edema
Firm, nonfragile skin
Normal muscle power and range of motion in
  preserved structures and joints
Decreased phantom limb pain

pain and may help to prepare the stump more quickly for the fitting of a prosthetic limb. When elastic bandage wraps are used, the GRN must have proficiency at stump wrapping to promote proper stump conditioning.

The stump should be inspected at each wrapping. It is common for a dressing to be needed at first. Initially, the stump may be squarish and will need to be more conical for prosthetic use. A black eschar forms at the incision line and should be examined for any open areas or drainage. Clips should never be used to secure bandages, because they can cause skin damage to the already compromised limb. Instead, one should use tape to hold the elastic wrap in place and to secure it to itself, thus avoiding tape contact with the person's skin.

When wrapping the stump, the nurse may use a pelvic anchor (around the waist) or may start the wrap *perpendicular* to the stump, covering the end of it first, instead of beginning *around* the stump. Diagonal wraps (figure eight) are used with more tension applied at the bottom than the middle or the top. No creases should be permitted. The goal is a conical shape that will fit the prosthetic limb. This technique may also help to reduce the risk of phantom limb pain later.

Persons with an amputation need to have normal range of motion and power in the rest of the joints. Arm strengthening exercises are needed, and balance is especially important when learning to walk with a prosthesis. Additionally, three main goals related to prosthesis use after an amputation are the person's accepting the amputation, integrating the prosthesis into the person's body image, and using the prosthesis to attain the maximal level of functional independence (Theuerkauf, 1996). Additionally, the GRN should be alert to improperly fitting prostheses and should be in close communication with the physical and occupational therapists and the

prosthetist as the person adjusts to the prosthesis. When the person is first wearing the prosthesis, the device should be removed at 15- to 20-minute intervals to check the skin condition. Weight loss or gain can also affect the fit of the prosthesis.

Most persons believe that the work related to wearing a prosthesis is worth it. Age was not found to be a major factor in successful use of a prosthesis, and 73% of persons in one study used their prosthetic limb full time as a main method of locomotion (Steinberg, Sunwoo, & Roettger, 1985).

Emotional issues surrounding amputation can be many. Phantom limb pain, or awareness of a sensation in the amputated limb as if it were still present, presents a nursing challenge. Such sensations may last up to 6 months postoperatively. This is a physiological disorder unrelated to psychological problems. The GRN should explore with the patient the sensations experienced and whether or not any type of stimulus acts as a trigger. Tactile sensations such as touching or lightly tapping the stump (or a desensitization program as provided by the therapists), or using heat or electrical stimulation, may help to alleviate these distressing sensations (Davis, 1993).

The person with an amputation should begin to deal with this change in body image. The GRN should help the person to identify positive coping strategies and should assist him or her in engaging in self-care. The family should be included in care. Visits with the unit psychologist may be of help. Support groups may also provide needed emotional support for the person and family. Although aged persons may be able to adjust to an altered body image, additional complications such as regaining mobility may present other problems. However, the presence of disease is more of a determining factor of prosthesis use than age (Steinberg et al., 1985). Technological advances in the development of adaptive equipment, including prosthetics and orthotics, give new hope for those with amputations to regain and maintain independence. Case Study 12.1 provides an excellent example of a well-adjusted man who has lived with an amputation and chronic disabilities for more than 50 years.

CASE STUDY 12.1
Aging with an Amputation and Chronic Disabilities

Mr. George was a medic in World War II at the age of 17. He was on the front lines, providing life-saving care to wounded soldiers and caring for the dying. At age 19, while performing his duties, he was hit by a mortar, resulting in multiple, near-fatal injuries including the loss of his right leg. Mr. George spent many months recovering in the hospital and in rehabilitation, but he lived the rest of his life with an above-knee amputation and severely impaired circulation in the other leg. Army physicians told Mr. George that he was lucky to be alive, but that his injuries would cause him to age about 12 to 15 years faster physically than his chronological age.

Mr. George's medical history is complex, including hypertension, heart disease, diabetes, arterial insufficiency, a fractured left hip, a left knee replacement, and cancer of the kidney, bladder, and prostate. His left kidney was removed several years ago, and he was recently diagnosed with an inoperable malignant tumor on his remaining kidney, which was already degenerating. Mr. George was not a candidate for dialysis because of his history of blood clots and other medical problems. He is aware that his condition is terminal, but he maintains an optimistic attitude, relying on his strong faith in God and the support of his family to cope with his uncertain future. The doctors have told him that because his kidney tumor is slow-growing, kidney failure or heart problems will most likely take his life before the cancer does.

As of this writing, Mr. George is 70 years old. He has experienced several major problems in aging with an amputation and multiple chronic illnesses including decreased mobility, skin impairment, circulatory changes, pain, and nutritional concerns. These include problems with lifting, standing, and sitting. Arthritis in his shoulders, arms, and elbows limits his mobility. Pain in the neck, vertebra, and arms makes even sleeping on his side difficult. Lying on his left side sometimes causes him to pass out. Tilting his head forward or back causes great pain. He is unable to lie in a prone position. Greater stress was placed on his left leg from wheeling around in the wheelchair, as well as from standing. Mr. George has had pressure sores on the buttocks and must do frequent weight shifts, because he is now mainly confined to a wheelchair. Because of injuries to his left leg suffered during the war, he has no arterial blood flow past the knee, so he must keep it elevated to prevent venous stasis. Although he often wears his prosthesis to church, Mr. George is unable to stand for any period of time, because he loses feeling in his other leg

and is prone to falls. He also must maintain a balanced diet with no sodium, no sugar, no caffeine, low protein, and low potassium. These dietary restrictions have caused major lifestyle adjustments.

Psychosocially, Mr. George has battled the stigma of disability, adjustment of lifestyle, lack of accessibility to community resources, lack of social acceptance, role changes, personal depression, fatigue, decreased energy reserve with increased age, and constant pain since the age of 19. Mr. George estimates that about 60% of his present condition is due to disabilities and "extra wear and tear," and 40% is due to increased age.

Mr. George has many strengths that allow him to cope remarkably well with these multiple issues and problems. He has a very supportive wife who believes in "teamwork," and they have recently celebrated their 50th wedding anniversary. He has two grown children and seven grandchildren, all of whom live close by and provide a strong support mechanism. Mr. George credits his strong faith in God and the loving support of his wife for his longevity. He focuses on personal hygiene each morning, promoting a healthy self-image. He carefully follows dietary restrictions. He strives to make himself participate in some activity or to go outside every day. He accomplishes many projects by adapting his environment and carefully planning ways to do things himself. He also spends about 2 hours per day in devotions, reading, and prayer together with his wife. In addition to these coping mechanisms, Mr. George received help from the federal government throughout the time after his service-related disability. The Veterans Affairs service provided for his medical needs, including building a "handicapped home" for him that is at ground level and has larger doorways and halls to accommodate a wheelchair. Mr. George reports that this accessibility and architectural changes in the community, as well as the more relaxed attitudes of others to those with disabilities, have increased his quality of life.

Despite his terminal diagnosis, Mr. George continues to encourage others and willingly shares his story. He has learned to accept his limitations and is grateful for each day of life. He states, "I won't go one day sooner than God wants me to. Nor will I stay one day longer." Mr. George offers the following advice to rehabilitation nurses: Be more attentive. Be informed about resources for those with disabilities. Be a great listener. Take time to hear what the person is saying. Listen to the whole person. Taking time to assess and evaluate the entire person properly has resulted, for him, in taking fewer prescription medications, better coping, and more correct diagnoses of his situation and unique needs.

REFERENCES

Allen, S. H. (1994). Exercise considerations for postmenopausal women with osteoporosis. *Arthritis Care and Research, 7*(4), 205–212.

Ali, N. S., & Twibell, R. (1994). Barriers to osteoporosis prevention in perimenopausal and elderly women. *Geriatric Nursing, 15*(4), 201–205.

Belza, B. L., Heinke, C. J., Yelin, E. H., Epstein, W. V., & Gilliss, C. L. (1993). Correlates of fatigue in older adults with rheumatoid arthritis. *Nursing Research, 42*(2), 93–99.

Berman, A. T., Quinn, R. H., & Zarro, V. J. (1991). Quantitative gait analysis in unilateral and bilateral total hip replacements. *Archives of Physical Medicine and Rehabilitation, 72,* 190–194.

Bohannon, R. W., & Cooper, J. (1993). Total knee arthroplasty: Evaluation of an acute care rehabilitation program. *Archives of Physical Medicine and Rehabilitation, 74,* 1091–1094.

Bradbury, V. L., Catanzaro, M. L. (1989). The quality of life in a male population suffering from arthritis. *Rehabilitation Nursing, 14*(4), 187–190.

Broy, S. B. (1996, February). A "whole patient" approach to managing osteoporosis. *Journal of Musculoskeletal Medicine,* 15–29.

Chaney, J. M., Uretsky, D. L., Mullins, L. L., Doppler, M. J., Palmer, W. R., Wees, S. J., Klein, H. S., Doud, D. K., & Reiss, M. J. (1996). Differential effects of age and illness duration on pain-depression and disability-depression relationships in rheumatoid arthritis. *International Journal of Rehabilitation and Health, 2*(2), 101–112.

Chiarello, C. M., Gundersen, L, & O'Halloran, T. (1997). The effect of continuous passive motion duration and increment on range of motion in total knee arthroplasty patients. *Journal of Orthopedic and Sports Physical Therapy, 25*(2), 119–127.

Cook, B., Noteloviz, M., Rector, C., & Krischer, J. P. (1991). An osteoporosis patient education and screening program: Results and implications. *Patient Education and Counseling, 17,* 135–145.

Davis, R. W. (1993). Phantom sensation, phantom pain, and stump pain. *Archives of Physical Medicine and Rehabilitation, 74,* 79–85.

Dellhag, B., Wollersjo, I., & Bjelle, A. (1992). Effect of active hand exercise and wax bath treatment in rheumatoid arthritis patients. *Arthritis Care and Research, 5*(2), 87–92.

Dunbar, R. E., & Seegall, H. F. (1990). *Arthritis: Rheumatism and gout.* Chicago: Budlong Press.

Eliopoulos, C. (1997). *Gerontological nursing* (4th ed.). Philadelphia: J. B. Lippincott.

Eliopoulos, C. (1993). *Gerontological nursing.* Philadelphia: J. B. Lippincott.

Enloe, L. J., Shields, R. K., Smith, K., Leo, K., & Miller, B. (1996). Total hip and knee replacement treatment programs: A report using consensus. *Journal of Orthopedic and Sports Physical Therapy, 23*(1), 3–11.

Fast, A., Mendelsohn, E., & Sosner, J. (1994). Total knee arthroplasty in Parkinson's disease. *Archives of Physical Medicine and Rehabilitation, 75,* 1269–1270.

Fisher, N. M., Gresham, G. E., Abrams, M., Hicks, J., Horrigan, D., & Pendergast, D. R. (1993). Quantitative effects of physical therapy on muscular and functional performance in subjects with osteoarthritis of the knees. *Archives of Physical Medicine and Rehabilitation, 74,* 840–847.

Galindo-Ciocon, D., Ciocon, J. O., & Galindo, D. (1995). Functional impairment among elderly women with osteoporotic vertebral fractures. *Rehabilitation Nursing, 20*(2), 79–83.

Galsworthy, T. D., & Wilson, P. L. (1996). It steals more than bone. *American Journal of Nursing, 96*(6), 27–34.

Gilbert-Lenef, L. (1994, January–March). Splinting the arthritic hand. *Journal of Hand Therapy,* 29–30.

Hammond, A. (1994). Joint protection behavior in patients with rheumatoid arthritis following an education program. *Arthritis Care and Research, 7*(1), 5–9.

Heafey, M. L., Golden-Baker, S. B., & Mahoney, D. W. (1994). Using nursing diagnoses and interventions in an inpatient amputee program. *Rehabilitation Nursing, 19*(3), 163–168.

Hirano, P. C., Laurent, D. D., & Lorig, K. (1994). Arthritis patient education studies, 1987–1991: A review of the literature. *Patient Education and Counseling, 24,* 9–54.

Houldin, A. D., & Hogen-Quigley, B. (1995). Psychological intervention for older hip fracture patients. *Journal of Gerontological Nursing, 21*(1), 20–26.

Hughes, S. L. & Dunlop, D. (1995). The prevalence and impact of arthritis in older persons. *Arthritis Care and Research, 8*(4), 257–264.

Keefe, F. J., Kashikar-Zuck, S., Opiteck, J., Hage, E., Dalrymple, L., & Blumenthal, J. A. (1996). Pain in arthritis and musculoskeletal disorders: The role of coping skills training and exercise interventions. *Journal of Orthopedic and Sports Physical Therapy, 24*(4), 279–290.

Kessenich, C. R. (1997). The pathophysiology of osteoporotic vertebral fractures. *Rehabilitation Nursing, 22*(4), 192–195.

Kessenich, C. R., & Rosen, C. J. (1996a). Vitamin D and bone status in elderly women. *Orthopaedic Nursing, 15*(3), 67–71.

Kessenich, C. R., & Rosen, C. J. (1996b). Osteoporosis: Implications for elderly men. *Geriatric Nursing, 17*(4), 171–174.

Kolarz, G., Maager, M., Scherak, O., El Shohoumi, M., & Wottawa, A. (1995). Rehabilitation after total hip replacement. *International Journal of Rehabilitation Research, 18,* 266–269.

Krutzen, P. (1984). Living with and adjusting to

arthritis. *Nursing Clinics of North America, 19,* 629–636.

La Mantia, K., & Marks, R. (1995, August). The efficacy of aerobic exercises for treating osteoarthritis of the knee. *New Zealand Journal of Physiotherapy,* 23–30.

Levy, R. N., Levy, C. M., Snyder, J., & Digiovanni, J. (1995). Outcome and long-term results following total hip replacement in elderly patients. *Clinical Orthopaedics and Related Research, 316,* 25–30.

Liang, M. H. (1988, December). Living with arthritis. *Medical Forum,* 5–6.

Lichtenstein, R., Semann, S., & Marmar, E. C. (1993). Development and impact of a hospital-based perioperative patient education program in a joint replacement center. *Orthopaedic Nursing, 12*(6), 17–23.

Lu-Yao, G. L., Baron, J. A., Barrett, J. A., & Fisher, E. S. (1994). Treatment and survival among elderly Americans with hip fractures: A population-based study. *American Journal of Public Health, 84,* 1287–1291.

Lyngberg, K. K., Harreby, M., Bentzen, H., Frost, B., & Danneskiold-Samsoe, B. (1994). Elderly rheumatoid arthritis patients on steroid treatment tolerate physical training without an increase in disease activity. *Archives of Physical Medicine and Rehabilitation, 75,* 1189–1195.

Matteson, M. A. (1997). Age-related changes in the musculoskeletal system. In M. A. Matteson & E. S. McConnell (Eds.), *Gerontological nursing: Concepts and practice* (pp. 197–221). Philadelphia: W. B. Saunders.

McMahon, M., Peterson, C., & Schlike, J. (1992). Osteoporosis: Identifying high-risk persons. *Journal of Gerontological Nursing, 18*(10), 19–26.

Miller-Blair, D. J., & Robbins, D. L. (1993, June). Rheumatoid arthritis: New science, new treatment. *Geriatrics, 48,* 28–38.

Mirabelli, L. (1990, September). Caring for patients with rheumatoid arthritis. *Nursing90,* 67–72.

Moncur, C., & Williams, H. J. (1995). Rheumatoid arthritis: Status of drug therapies. *Physical Therapy, 75,* 511–525.

National Osteoporosis Foundation (1997). *Osteoporosis Alert Petition Drive.* Washington, DC: Author.

Nesher, G., & Moore, T. L. (1994). Clinical presentation and treatment of arthritis in the aged. *Clinics in Geriatric Medicine, 10,* 659–675.

Nicholas, J. J. (1994). Physical modalities in rheumatological rehabilitation. *Archives of Physical Medicine and Rehabilitation, 75,* 994–1001.

Oberg, U., & Oberg, T. (1996). Worse functional status among old people when admitted for arthroplasty. *Scandinavian Journal of Caring Sciences, 10,* 96–102.

Orr, P. M. (1990). An educational program for total hip and knee replacement patients as part of a total arthritis center program. *Orthopaedic Nursing, 9*(5), 61–86.

Orr, P. M., & Bratton, G. N. (1992). The effect of an inpatient arthritis rehabilitation program on self-assessed functional ability. *Rehabilitation Nursing, 17,* 306–310.

Paier, G. S. (1996). Specter of the crone: The experience of vertebral fracture. *Advances in Nursing Science, 18*(3), 27–36.

Perez, D. E. (1994). Hip fracture: Physicians take more active role in patient care. *Geriatrics, 49*(4), 31–37.

Pitson, D., Bhaskaran, V., Bond, H., Yarnold, R., & Drewett, R. (1994). Effectiveness of knee replacement surgery in arthritis. *International Journal of Nursing Studies, 31*(1), 49–56.

Quinet, R. J. (1986). Osteoarthritis: Increasing mobility and reducing disability. *Geriatrics, 41*(2), 36–50.

Reisine, S. T. (1995). Arthritis and the family. *Arthritis Care and Research, 8*(4), 265–271.

Resnick, B. (1994, July). Die from a broken hip? *RN,* 22–26.

Rogers, J. C., & Holm, M. B. (1992, February). Assistive technology device use in patients with rheumatic disease: A literature review. *American Journal of Occupational Therapy, 46,* 120–126.

Roth, S. H. (1992, May). Nabumetone: A new NSAID for rheumatoid arthritis and osteoarthritis. *Physician Assistant,* 59–66.

Rush, S. (1996). Rehabilitation following ORIF of the hip. *Topics in Geriatric Rehabilitation, 12*(1), 38–45.

Scura, K. W., & Whipple, B. (1997). How to provide better care for the postmenopausal woman. *American Journal of Nursing, 97*(4), 36–44.

Shafshak, T. S., El-Sheshai, A. M., & Soltan, H. E. (1991). Personality traits in the mechanisms of interferential therapy for osteoarthritic knee pain. *Archives of Physical Medicine and Rehabilitation, 72,* 579–581.

Shaul, M. P. (1997). Transitions in chronic illness: Rheumatoid arthritis in women. *Rehabilitation Nursing, 22*(4), 199–205.

Shaul, M. P. (1994). Rheumatoid arthritis and older women: Economics tell only part of the story. *Health Care for Women International, 15,* 377–383.

Sherrington, C., & Lord, S. (1997). Home exercise to improve strength and walking velocity after hip fractures: A randomized controlled trial. *Archives of Physical Medicine and Rehabilitation, 78,* 208–212.

Steinberg, F. U., Sunwoo, I., & Roettger, R. F. (1985). Prosthetic rehabilitation of geriatric amputee patients: A follow-up study. *Archives of Physical Medicine and Rehabilitation, 66,* 742–745.

Stinnett, K. A. (1996). Occupational therapy intervention for the geriatric client receiving acute and subacute services following total hip replacement and femoral fracture repair. *Topics in Geriatric Rehabilitation, 12*(1), 23–31.

Superio-Cabuslay, E., Ward, M. M., & Lorig, K. R. (1996). Patient education interventions in osteoarthritis and rheumatoid arthritis: A meta-analytic comparison with nonsteroidal antiinflammatory drug treatment. *Arthritis Care and Research, 9*(4), 292–301.

Takeda, W., & Wessel, J. (1994). Acupuncture for

the treatment of pain of osteoarthritic knees. *Arthritis Care and Research, 7*(3), 118–122.

The right treatment for arthritis (1995, March). *Johns Hopkins Medical Letter,* 3.

Theuerkauf, A. (1996). Self-care and activities of daily living. In S. Hoeman (Ed.), *Rehabilitation Nursing: Concepts and Application* (pp. 156–187). St. Louis, MO: C. V. Mosby.

Thomas, R. L. (1996). Management of hips fracture in the geriatric patient: A team approach in the institutional setting. *Topics in Geriatric Rehabilitation, 12*(1), 59–69.

Watson, C. P. N. (1994). Topical capsaicin as an adjuvant analgesic. *Journal of Pain and Symptom Management, 9*(7), 425–432.

Verbrugge, L. M. (1995). Women, men, and osteoarthritis. *Arthritis Care and Research, 8*(4), 212–220.

Yetzer, E. A., Kauffman, G., Sopp, F., & Talley, L. (1994). Development of a patient education program of new amputees. *Rehabilitation Nursing, 19*(6), 355–358.

Zuckerman, J. D., Zetterberg, C., & Frankel, V. H. (1995). Principles of treatment of orthopedic injuries in the elderly. *Topics in Emergency Medicine, 17*(2), 47–62.

Part IV

Issues in Gerontological Rehabilitation Nursing

■

Chapter 13

Cultural Competence in Gerontological Rehabilitation Nursing

■

At present, the majority of the 12.7% of the United States population (32.8 million individuals) older than 65 years of age is white or Anglo-American (Fowles, 1994). However, the ethnic elderly is the fastest growing subgroup of the elderly (Espino, 1995). Various ethnic groups use social and health-related resources differently. This has enormous implications for nursing, because minority elders have been shown to be at increased risk of morbidity and mortality resulting from socioeconomic and health status factors. Yet, these groups may use health services less than those in a white majority group (Angel, Angel, & Himes, 1992; Ries, 1990).

Despite ethnic differences among groups, most elderly persons across cultures have some common problems. More women tend to be widowed than men. Women have a longer life span than men. Females tend to be a somewhat disadvantaged group, at least socioeconomically, regardless of ethnic or racial background. The major health problems experienced by the general elderly population are chronic. These include arthritis, hearing impairments, hypertension, heart conditions, and orthopedic problems. The leading causes of death include heart disease, cancer, and cerebrovascular disease. A few variations in these statistics are seen among the elderly ethnic minority groups discussed in this chapter.

African-Americans and Hispanic Americans constitute the two largest ethnic minority groups in this country, and their numbers are growing faster than those of the white majority. It is estimated that by the year 2025,

5% of the nation's aged will be minorities (Espino, 1995). Because most research has been done on an Anglo-American population, it makes generalizations to other groups incongruent with culture-competent care goals. Some general comparisons are made among the major ethnic groups commonly recognized. However, these are mere generalities to assist the gerontological rehabilitation nurse (GRN) in exploring possible differences in health belief or practices and are not meant to be a substitute for further study about the specific groups or subgroups with which the nurse may work.

Some generalities may be noted. Persons of ethnic minority groups have an increased need for health services resulting from more functional limitations, increased medical problems, poorer health, and more work-related disabilities (Damron-Rodriguez, Wallace, & Kington, 1994; Gibson & Burns, 1992). They are less likely to use the hospital and may rely on more informal services. However, minority groups seem to have less access to the health care system. Utilization of important services for the elderly is decreased among these groups (Damron-Rodriguez et al., 1994).

Latinos and African-Americans use nursing homes less than Anglo-Americans. Some research has demonstrated that nursing staff within long-term care facilities communicate less frequently with ethnic elders than with white Canadians or Anglo-Americans, but all elders had only minimal verbal interaction with staff (Jones & Van Amelsvoort Jones, 1986).

Psychometric instruments have largely been developed with a white population in mind and often do not consider cultural factors in measurement. These include assessments of vocational aptitudes of African-Americans in rehabilitation settings (Alston & McCowan, 1994a) and mental status examinations such as those that measure depression (Baker, Espino, Robinson, & Stewart, 1993). The development of culturally sensitive tools is an area now being addressed in research.

The GRN should realize the importance of assessing the generation of family members. The length of time spent in the United States can affect behavior (Gelfand & Barresi, 1987; Gelfand & Kutzik, 1979). First-generation families tend to be more traditional than those who have experienced American culture for a longer period of time.

Two dynamics should be considered when discussing aging in minorities: culture and the aging process. These issues are interrelated yet distinct. As age increases, so does the incidence of chronic illness and disability, often more so among ethnic minorities. Yet, all elderly groups have many commonalities. Those older than age 65, regardless of race or ethnic group, experience universal changes associated with aging. Compared with younger persons, elders suffer more from chronic illnesses than from acute diseases. The human body shows effects of wear and tear such as wrinkles, changing hair color, slower reflexes, decreased muscle strength, and a general slowing of bodily functions. Yet, this, too, is an individualized phenomenon in that each person ages differently, and some show fewer effects of normal aging than others. For several reasons, nurses and other health care professionals should be concerned with differences among elderly ethnic groups, particularly minorities. "Aging is a cultural as well as a biological process" (Clark & Anderson, 1967, p. 3). All people experience physical aging, but the process of becoming older, or aged, is greatly influenced by one's culture. Yet, the way in which various cultural groups define aging is generally unknown. In one study, nearly two fifths of representatives of cultures surveyed failed to provide information on what "old" meant for them, and in those members of a culture who could specify definitions used by people for aging, there was great variation (Cowgill, 1986). Some African cultures do not keep calendars, or time, and thus members of these cultures have no notion of their ages (Van den Berghe, 1987). Because of the scarcity of cultural definitions of aging, this chapter focuses on similarities and differences among the major ethnic groups, particularly those in the United States, on whom more research is available. Additionally, suggestions of what constitutes culturally competent nursing care are addressed.

BACKGROUND ON AGING OF MINORITIES

Anthropologists suggest that the value placed on later life depends on the ideals of the culture. This belief causes many elderly persons to be devalued because they are unable to perpetuate their society's cultural ideals (Clark & Anderson, 1967). When this is true, then how much greater is the plight of the disabled elderly? The status of the elderly in different societies may be reflected by historical beliefs and traditions, as in the older black population (Coke & Twaite, 1995). Blakemore and Boneham (1994), in discussing differences among Asian and Afro-Caribbean elders, state that "it is this changing experience of what it is to age as a member of a minority community which ensures that ethnicity, race and culture are not static entities"(p. x). The ways in which ethnic groups mourn a loved one's death, participate in burial activities, or commemorate a lost one also reveal distinctive differences (Irish, Lundquist, & Nelsen, 1993; Kastenbaum, 1991).

The concept of double jeopardy has been used to characterize minority aging (Salmon, 1994). This term reflects the notion that "negative effects of aging are compounded among minority group members" (Kart, 1994, p. 401). Research generally supports this concept among African-American and Mexican-American elderly persons. If culture helps to define or characterize aging, then certainly it warrants further examination.

DEFINITIONS

Many variations of the terms discussed here can be found in the literature. For the purposes of this text, some common definitions are used. The reader is advised to consider carefully the specific meanings set forth by other authors within the context of each work.

Culture is defined as those attitudes, thoughts, feelings, values, and beliefs that influence behavior. The component of behavior is particularly important, in that behaviors can be observed and are thought to be a reflection of one's inner feelings and beliefs. Culture is related to actions. Elderly persons belonging to ethnic minority groups may express their strengths through cultural values, creating alternative solutions to problems they may face (Fry, 1981).

The term *race* is often used in a broad sense as a way of "collectivizing people in our minds" (Sowell, 1994, p. xiii). *Race* refers to "one distinct type of group whose ethnic identity is based on their physical characteristics" (Gelfand, 1994, p. 5). Sowell (1994) stated that race was an illusory dichotomy applied to observable differences in people's skin color and the like and was used to distinguish among broad categories of people such as whites and blacks, whereas ethnicity denoted variations among subgroups within the races. Manuel (1982) argued that "racially labeled groups are ultimately socially defined" (p. 15). For the purposes of this text, the term *ethnic* as defined later is used to encompass all such differences.

The concept of ethnicity is broader. Holzberg (1982) defined ethnicity as "social differentiation based on such cultural criteria as a sense of peoplehood, shared history, a commonplace of origin, language, dress and free preferences, and participation in particular clubs or voluntary associations" (p. 252). According to this definition, the concept of culture can be subsumed under the term *ethnicity*. This word is more generic than *race*, but it incorporates the racial dimensions (Manuel, 1982).

The major ethnic and racial minority groups in the United States are generally considered to be: African-American (or black), Asian or Pacific Islander, Hispanic American (or Latino), and Native American. The term black is used interchangeably with African-American, and the term Latino is used interchangeably with Hispanic American (Gelfand, 1994).

Within each major ethnic group are subgroups. Hispanic/Latino refers to persons of Spanish descent whose primary language is Spanish, but it includes Cubans, Puerto Ricans, and Mexican-Americans, for example, all of whom have distinct cultural beliefs and ethnic traits. Likewise, there are 300 recognized tribes of Native Americans in the United States (Gelfand, 1994), each with differences as well as similarities. Additionally, all people with dark or "black" skin do not consider themselves "black" or African-American unless their roots were in slavery.

This is to be distinguished from those Caribbean natives whose origins are in the islands.

The groups known as Anglo-Americans or whites fall under what was formerly termed Caucasian, but they have many subgroups as well, each with distinct characteristics and origins. Examples include those who are Jewish, Irish, Italian, or Polish. Each of these groups may view itself as separate, yet members of these groups consider themselves white (a racial distinction based on physical appearances). Some experts consider European American elderly persons a majority among minority groups of the elderly in American society (Hayes, Kalish, & Guttman, 1986), yet ethnic groups from European backgrounds are not recognized with minority status (Gelfand, 1994).

A minority is "a group that has experienced discrimination, oppression, and subordination in America" (Browne & Broderick, 1991, p. 2). An ethnic minority is a "group that shares a common heritage and past and has suffered from discrimination and subordination within society" (Markides & Mindel, 1987, p. 13).

The distinction between terms such as those previously defined can be confusing. The reader is encouraged to approach the literature with the definition used by each particular author, because many terms can be used loosely or interchangeably. *Ethnic*, or *ethnic group*, is used here in a general sense to include culture, race, religious preferences, nationality, and other commonalities shared by groups of people. Of prime importance is that within all racial and ethnic groups are subgroups as well as individuals. No person should be stereotyped based on race or culture. Yet, it is helpful for nurses to understand the historical roots and similarities among those with cultural backgrounds different from their own, because these cultural factors can be an integral part of a person's health and illness experience. Cultural competence begins with an awareness of one's own culture.

RESEARCH ON ELDERLY ETHNIC MINORITY GROUPS

Although the elderly have been a population increasingly scrutinized for several decades now, research on the influence of race, culture, or ethnicity on aging and health behaviors has been much more recent. Most studies have been conducted on samples of white males, so they may have limited applicability to other subgroups. Kart (1994) stated that "recognition of the ethnic (and racial) diversity present in the U. S. experience has only recently begun to rub off on the field of social gerontology" (p. 376). Published medical research on specific minority elderly groups only began to flourish within the last decade. One collection of articles on ethnogeriatrics appearing in *Clinics of Geriatric Medicine* attests to the finding that physicians are becoming more sensitive to the difference among ethnic groups within the older population, yet it acknowledges that the available literature on ethnic subgroups is scant and limited in generalizability (Espino, 1995).

Nursing research on elderly minority groups has received increased attention with the development and testing of Leininger's model for transcultural nursing. Ethnonursing was established by Leininger (1985) as a way to help nurse researchers within the qualitative paradigm discover phenomena about health care and well-being among those of different cultures. Leininger (1995) proposed that "the goal of transcultural nursing . . . is ultimately to provide *nursing care that fits with or has beneficial meanings* and health outcomes to people of different or similar cultural backgrounds" (p. 12).

ANGLO-AMERICANS OR EUROPEAN-AMERICANS

Anglo-American is a general term used for white, non-Hispanic individuals. Most research among the aged has been done with this group. However, according to more recent trends, the white majority will "soon become one of several 'minority' groups in several states" (Stanford & Yee, 1992, p. 15). Although those age 65 years and older are the fastest growing age group in the country, even faster growth is occurring in the non-white populations.

Anglo-Americans are considered overall to have more formal education, have higher income levels, better health, and longer life spans than Hispanic Americans or African-Americans (Aiken, 1995). In 1988, only 10% of elderly white persons had incomes below the poverty level, versus 32% of blacks and 22% of Hispanic Americans (Eliopoulos, 1993). White persons have a higher rate of physician contacts and tend to utilize the health care system more frequently than African-Americans (Ries, 1990).

Anglo-Americans typically value youth, beauty, and achievement. Competition and rewards are common themes. Anglo-Americans tend to be more materialistic than persons of other cultures and value high-technology goods. Equal gender rights as well as independence and freedom are also recurring themes in this culture. Anglo-Americans also tend to be generous and helpful to others during crises (Leininger, 1995).

European-Americans are considered another ethnic group with many subgroups. More research has been done with those of Jewish or Italian descent. Other subgroups of European-Americans come from German, Irish, English, French, and Polish backgrounds. More recently, most of those with European-American heritage are likely born in the United States. Traditionally, in most of these cultures, the woman was subservient to the man, and a commitment to the family was paramount for the success and preservation of the family.

Much research has been done with the Jewish ethnic group, in part because of their interesting history. Having long been a persecuted group in many countries, Jews developed a self-sustaining social structure. Jews have immigrated to the United States from all over the world. Yet, some constants such as religious heritage, dedication to the family unit, and value of education and medical care remain relatively stable. However, there is a vast difference in religious practices within Judaism, from the strict Hassidic Jews, who observe the biblical laws and maintain a kosher diet, to the liberal or Reform Jews, who do not practice such stringent rules and lean more toward gender equality. Observance of religious ceremonies such as Passover traditionally have great significance in the lives of almost all Jewish people. Being Jewish is more than the practice of a religion or a heritage. It is considered a way of life. Some researchers, however, believe that the American-Jewish community may be disintegrating, largely because of a decline in religious observance as well as changing gender roles between younger and older individuals (Kart, 1987).

In Judaism, folk remedies such as chicken soup are common to treat simple ailments, but medical care is highly valued. Jews are highly represented in prestigious professions such as law and medicine, reflecting the emphasis placed on education (Gelfand, 1994; Leininger, 1995). Guttman (1986) found that elderly Jews used more formal support services than any of the other white ethnic groups, and a large percentage also used community centers.

Italian elders pass their values on through family ties. Johnson (1985) named three factors that distinguish Italians from other European subgroups. These include interdependence, authority and power, and affect and emotions. Elders maintain authority within the family unit that helps to perpetuate the norms of the culture. The Roman Catholic church helped to influence beliefs concerning marriage and family within Italian culture.

The scope of this book does not permit discussion of the many other ethnic subgroups within the European-American tradition. The reader is encouraged to search the literature for research and information on the health practices and beliefs of those to whom care is being provided. An insider's perspective is necessary to provide culture-specific care to any group of people.

AFRICAN-AMERICANS

Within the total African-American population, 8% are older adults (Browne & Broderick, 1991). African-Americans account for about 8.3% of the elderly population (Kart, 1994).

The historical roots of these persons are important in understanding common traits. African-Americans were dislocated from Africa through slavery and suffered many years of discrimination and hardship in the United States. Besides the numerous psychosocial implications inherent in an oppressed people, slavery caused family ties to be destroyed and resulted in lower educational levels and less than average income among black persons (Clavon, 1986). About one third of African-Americans are poor (Kart, 1994), the highest poverty rate among ethnic minorities.

Elderly African-Americans are at an even greater disadvantage than the rest of the black population. They are the least healthy, suffer from more chronic conditions, and are most likely to lose physical function compared with other groups. About 59% of males and 50% of females experience hypertension, and usually at a younger age than among other groups (Brangman, 1995; Gillies, 1991). Black women are more likely to suffer a stroke than white women (Cameron, Badger, & Evers, 1989), a finding that could largely be due to the incidence of hypertension, the number one risk factor for stroke. Mortality from stroke is two to three times greater for blacks than whites of either gender between the ages

of 55 and 64 (Gelfand, 1994). This difference gradually narrows until after the age of 85 and is referred to as a crossover effect. Similar patterns are seen for coronary artery disease and death from acute myocardial infarction.

The leading causes of death are the same as in other elderly groups: coronary heart disease, cerebrovascular disease, and cancer (Brangman, 1995). However, the incidence of types of cancer varies. For example, cancers of the esophagus, pancreas, stomach, prostate, and larynx are more common among blacks than among whites in the same age group (Gelfand, 1994).

The cultural beliefs of African-Americans greatly affect their use of the health care system. Strong family and religious ties make it more likely that they will be involved in intergenerational care. Elders are respected, and extended family living arrangements are common. Elders often care for younger family members such as grandchildren (Lockery, 1992). They may have strong beliefs against the use of nursing homes, and they may need special counseling to resolve value conflict if placement of a loved one in long-term care becomes necessary (Clavon, 1986).

Social supports are extremely important in maintaining health and in providing for those with disabilities. Alston and McCowan (1994) stated, "If an African American woman with a disability loses (or perceives to lose) her support network, she may feel alienated from her culture and experience difficulty functioning in her multiple roles" (p. 39). GRNs should be alert to the possibility that clients may need assistance in establishing new social support systems. Those clients who have successfully adapted after a disability or impairment may be willing to act as role models or mentors for new patients. More of an effort to meet the unique needs of this population is needed.

Church and religious involvement is particularly integral to many African-Americans. Religious training begins at an early age, and the role of leaders within the church is highly esteemed. A strong religious heritage can easily be seen in the words and music of many Negro spirituals that have survived to the present day. The early religious origins in Africa were more than just ceremonial; they were a way of life.

The history of African-Americans is significant in their use of health care. African-Americans often prefer to seek advice of family members, friends, neighbors, or spiritual healers before that of health care professionals. There is a sense of greater trust in the familiar folk remedies and healers than today's health care system, which may be perceived as slow, unfriendly, or incongruent with their values (Morgan, 1995). Older blacks may be less inclined to trust a white physician's diagnosis and may rely on family members and friends to guide their care. They may be more comfortable with a caregiver of the same ethnic/racial background. This should not be cause for alarm, but can be used to the patient's advantage. More ethnic minority nurses are needed and can be excellent teachers to those of different backgrounds.

Although African-American elders tend to have less access to needed health care services, they use the emergency room as a primary care source more often than their white counterparts. When utilizing doctors, they may shop around, visiting several physicians for similar problems. Hospital length of stays may be slightly longer (Ries, 1990). Folk medicine and home remedies may be preferred to more formal health care.

Nurses who are not African-American should be aware of cultural differences between themselves and African-American clients or patients, yet without stereotyping, because each person is unique. A study by Cameron et al. (1989) demonstrated that white nurses and disabled black patients had limited knowledge about each other. These nurses did not know about their patients' history, family structures, or customs. Black patients were also less informed about the role of the nurses in the community setting. Lack of communication among those of different cultures seems to be a recurring theme within the health care literature. Table 13–1 gives some suggestions for nurses in providing culture-sensitive care. Strong family bonds should be supported by nursing staff, realizing that these socialization ties can prevent isolation and depression in the elderly. Time should be taken to ask pertinent questions and to ascertain family relationships and social support structures. In these changing times, one cannot assume that traditional familial values will continue to the next generation. As with all patients, each one should be treated as unique.

HISPANIC AMERICANS

Hispanic Americans are the fastest growing minority group in the United States, although only 5% of the Hispanic population is elderly.

Table 13–1 SUGGESTIONS FOR PROVIDING CULTURALLY SENSITIVE NURSING CARE TO OLDER ADULTS

Ask culturally pertinent questions and listen carefully to responses.
Make expectations and roles clear within the health care setting.
Recognize differences between ethnic groups, but avoid stereotyping.
Gear informational material to the appropriate level of the learner, taking into account age and educational level.
Recognize the importance of family and kinship ties.
Do not assume that the family structure is intact or that elders will automatically be cared for at home.
Realize that institutionalization may not be an acceptable option in some cultures.
Assess generations of family members and how long they have lived in the present country, realizing that first-generation families may have more traditional values.
Ascertain the use of informal services (folk medicine, home remedies, and the like).
Be an advocate for the patient, knowing that the elderly have unique needs that may be influenced by culture, yet misunderstood by others.
Acknowledge that although patterns of behavior exist, each individual is unique.
Remember that traditional values may be changing, and support structures may not be intact.
Encourage cultural and ethnic expressions within the nursing care plan as able, such as food from home, more lenient visiting privileges, allowing smaller children to visit, or communicating with religious leaders as an integral part of the health care team.
Be familiar with ethnographic interviewing techniques.
Encourage ethnic minorities to become involved in health related occupations.
Utilize appropriate resources such as translators and consultants from the patient's ethnic group.
Become involved in attempts to bring health care to communities in need instead of expecting them to use services that may be inaccessible.
Support the patient's autonomy and rights.
Consciously increase communication with older adults and promote socialization activities.

Half of the present elderly group was foreign born. About 60% of the total Hispanic population is of Mexican origin (Gelfand, 1994). The rest have Puerto Rican, Cuban, Central American, or South American backgrounds. This diverse population is not easily categorized, so the available research is less than systematic. Most research on Hispanic Americans considers them as a whole group, further complicating issues, because there is diversity among the subgroups. More studies have examined Mexican-Americans, yet this is a smaller group in the older population than Cubans or Puerto Ricans (Kart, 1994). Thus, this section deals with some generalities suggested by the available literature.

Some socioeconomic issues distinguish this group from black persons. Hispanic Americans average a higher income, yet about 20% of the elderly lived below the poverty level in 1989 (Kart, 1994). Fewer Hispanic elders have college educations than do black elders. Perhaps in part because of these disadvantages, many Hispanic Americans report a poor health status and more disabilities than whites (McKenna, 1989). Those who reside in urban areas are at higher risk of chronic conditions, yet they may be unable to use or access the care needed, often because they do not speak English.

Kinship ties are of great significance in the Hispanic community. Family pride is greatly valued, and old age is respected. The man is the head of the household, which has a patriarchal structure (Bassford, 1995). Women are traditionally submissive, and men are dominant. The family is supportive and flexible. The extended family and family caregiving are very important. There is a deep sense of family obligation and loyalty, with respect being a key concept. The rights of elders are considered of prime importance.

Inherent in the value of respect is politeness. This concept may be misunderstood by health care workers. Hispanics may perceive the health care staff as their "hosts," in that they are "guests" in the facility (Bedolla, 1995). This perception can lead to different expectations and conflicts between staff and families. Patients may be hesitant to voice complaints out of sense of respect for the staff. Nurses should use care when determining what the patient would like to be called while receiving care. One should not assume that the patient would be most comfortable on a first-name basis. Additionally, female patients may be uncomfortable receiving intimate bodily care from a male caregiver. Privacy and modesty are equally important.

Independence and control may be important issues, especially for Hispanic American men. They are less likely to admit to health problems than women. Having been socialized to independence, men may benefit from feeling like active contributors (Seabrooks, Kahn, & Gero, 1987), an essential component of rehabilitation. An individualized self-care framework for planning interventions could be of more use than traditional nursing plans for this population as well as for black persons (Butler, 1987).

Traditional cultural foods are an important aspect of healthy living. Alcohol may be considered a food staple in this culture (Pousada, 1995). It is important for health care professionals to be aware of this because of potential interactions with medications that may be prescribed during illness.

Many Hispanic Americans use herbs and teas for minor problems but more formal health services for major difficulties. Older Hispanic immigrants define health most often as feeling well (Ailinger & Causey, 1995). There is a holistic nature to their perception of health, a balance of the physical, mental, and spiritual. Many believe in good and evil spirits, folk healing, and rituals (Gillies, 1991; Pousada, 1995). The concept of *curanderismo* refers to a holistic cultural system based on knowledge of herbal remedies, prayers, and healing rituals. The *curandera*, or folk practitioner, combines her knowledge and skills with healing powers and abilities from God to provide care to Hispanic Americans (Villarruel & Leininger, 1995). Health and illness are seen as reflections of one's favor or disfavor with God.

Spanish is spoken as the primary language. This fact alone may decrease elders' use of available resources and may isolate them socially. They may be hesitant to share feelings with Anglo-Americans, although they visit physicians more often than white persons according to some reports (Damron-Rodriguez et al., 1994). Hispanic Americans have more chronic illnesses, yet they utilize fewer medical, dental, and hospital services (Johnson et al., 1988). They are more likely to use these services if they are accessible and non-threatening (McKenna, 1989).

Hispanic Americans report lower life satisfaction scores and poorer mental health than blacks or Anglo-Americans (Ailinger, 1989; Johnson et al., 1988). A greater percentage of Hispanic Americans are functionally impaired when compared with whites (Ailinger, Dear, & Holley-Wilcox, 1993). More members of this group report their health as poor, and self-assessed health seems to be related to educational level (Ailinger, 1989; McKenna, 1989).

The principal health problems of Hispanic Americans are common to the aged population, but they are unique in other ways. The major health alterations reported include arthritis, hypertension, circulatory difficulties, and diabetes (Gillies, 1991). Diabetes (non-insulin-dependent) affects nearly 25% of Puerto Rican–Americans and Mexican-Americans (Bassford, 1995). The top causes of death in this group are heart disease and cancer, much like the general elderly population.

The nurse needs to develop a rapport with the patient and family. Good interviewing skills are essential and can provide better information than static forms and documentation. Ascertaining the patient's role within the family is important in planning care, but direct questions may not yield the desired results. Ethnographic methodology can be used with greater success than quantitative methods in research situations (Garfinkel, 1967; Gitlin, Corcoran, & Leinmiller-Eckhardt, 1995), and basic tenets of ethnographic interviewing should be taught to health care professionals working with people of different cultures. If a language barrier exists, an interpreter would be a great asset.

Although extended family ties are important to Hispanic Americans, tradition changes with each generation, so it may be incorrect to assume that this network is intact. The nurse's demeanor should be informal, yet respectful. Family members and patients may view themselves as guests of the hospital, so nurses working in this setting should be careful to ascertain expectations. In summary, the need for more minority health care workers, nurses who are culturally sensitive, translation services, and socialization clubs for older adults cannot be overemphasized.

ASIANS AND PACIFIC ISLANDERS

This ethnic group is large and of diverse backgrounds. Many Asians came to the United States and Canada as refugees. Asian-Americans in the United States (accounting for 2.9% of the total population in 1990) include Chinese, Koreans, Vietnamese, Indians, Pakistanis, Filipinos, Afghans, Hmong, Montagnards, Cambodians, Laotians, Thais, and Japanese (Gelfand, 1994).

Islanders, such as those from the Caribbean or Virgin Islands, may rely heavily on folk cures tied to beliefs about spirits. Little traditional professional medical or health care may be available or utilized. Although from outward appearances they may be labeled by others as black, most Islanders do not refer to themselves that way. They may prefer to be known as Caribbean Islanders or the like, depending on their heritage.

In many ways, Asian-Americans are similar to whites. They generally enjoy more financial success and stability than African-Americans, Latinos, or Native Americans. Asian-Americans experience about the same, if not slightly better, health as older white groups. The largest numbers of elderly in the Asian ethnic group are Chinese and Japanese. They experience less incidence of hip fractures and coronary artery disease, but they have a higher incidence of liver, stomach, esophageal, and pancreatic cancers than their white counterparts (Gelfand, 1994). However, differences in health status among all subgroups of this type are beyond the scope of discussion for this text. Although little information is available on many of the subgroups, mortality rates indicate a good level of overall health (Markides & Mindel, 1987). Despite usually strong family ties, many Asian elders have serious barriers to health care. Stereotypes suggest that Asian Americans are cared for by their families, yet this assumption may be in error. Many elders are unable to speak fluent English and may have difficulty accessing the health care system. Some literature suggests that many Asian-Americans experience functional limitations and disabilities, yet they are unable to access needed services or do not recognize what services are available (Markides & Mindel, 1987).

With the family unit as the dominant social structure, being single has had severe emotional and spiritual implications for the Chinese. One of the worst things that can happen to a Chinese elder is to be left living without relatives. Some elders who live alone have learned to adapt without traditional supports. Others have become part of non-traditional social networks, such as "sisterhoods," that allow them to survive and have social support apart from the traditional organization of the family (Sankar, 1981).

The Japanese utilize professional health services regularly. However, they also practice folk medicine and home remedies. Such traditions may involve the use of acupuncture, herbal tonics, and spiritual exercises. Kinship ties are important, as is children's education, which is highly valued. Elders are honored and esteemed. Self-control and pride in work are other cultural norms. The importance of "saving face," or avoiding shame and disrespect, is learned through this culture. Thus, a Japanese elder within the hospital setting may be reluctant to voice complaints about care because this could be seen as disrespectful to the staff. He or she may endure pain rather than request medication.

Chinese and Japanese cultures are steeped in the religious practices of Confucianism, Taoism, and Buddhism. Illness may be viewed as an imbalance between good and evil forces. Some Asians may refer to the yin and the yang, or the positive and negative forces that affect the universe. These forces must be in balance for health to be maintained. Other subgroups use the term "chi" to describe the life force that keeps the body in a state of balance and health. When the flow of the chi is disrupted, illness can occur. Treatment may be aimed, through physicians who practice folk cures, at removing barriers to the flow of chi, to return the body to a state of harmony.

The GRN must take care to avoid disrespect to Asian elders if trust is to be established. Calling a man by his first name, using sustained direct eye contact, or using physical contact may be seen as disrespectful. Gestures may have different meanings in this culture than they do for Anglo-Americans. What is natural in one culture may be considered hostile or insulting in another (Leininger, 1995).

Harmony between good and bad forces is believed to be related to health. The body and the mind are inseparable. Rest and quietness are thought to help restore the body's natural balances. The GRN can foster a calm environment and can promote the presence and support of family to encourage the healing process.

NATIVE AMERICANS

Aged American Indians are among the most deprived groups of people in the United States, with many living in absolute poverty (Gelfand & Kutzik, 1979). There is a lack of information and research on this group, more than on any other minority. Part of this difficulty lies in the number and diversity of tribal groups and in a lifestyle that may cause them to relocate frequently on reservations. Tribal differences influence the status of the elderly.

Although old age is generally respected, some nomadic tribes traditionally abandoned their aged members in times of hardship, or the elder would go away from the tribe to die in a sort of suicide. The Navajos have a matriarchal system that places more value on the females of the tribe. Old age is highly esteemed, and a sense of individualism is maintained despite close familial ties (Phillips & Lobar, 1995).

For those Native Americans living in urban areas away from reservation lands, fewer governmental programs are accessible to assist with health care. About one fourth of Native Americans live on reservations, and the rest are nearly equally split between rural and urban areas (Gelfand, 1994). Those trying to integrate into the rest of American society apart from the reservation do not have access to the same funding or services as those on the reservations, thus complicating an already difficult situation.

The stress of relocation and forced assimilation put on American Indians by governmental administrators may have contributed to the higher rates of certain health problems found in this group. Native American elders suffer more from tuberculosis, diabetes, liver disease, kidney disease, hearing impairments, and visual impairments than the general aged population. More than 25% have diabetes. Major causes of death include alcoholism (459% higher than the general population), tuberculosis, accidents, diabetes, pneumonia and influenza, and homicide (Gelfand, 1994).

More health care and nursing services are needed in accessible areas for Native Americans. Although clinics may be set up to provide such care, it is more likely that Indians will rely on tribal folk cures for treatment. Rapport must be established, particularly on the reservation where time takes on a different dimension and persons tend to move around, to conduct needed research to meet the health care needs of these people.

Additionally, nurses should be advocates for Native Americans who are trying to work and raise families off the reservation and improve their quality of life, by encouraging the government to provide equitable funding for those choosing to live in the city.

DEVELOPING CULTURAL SENSITIVITY

The first step toward developing cultural sensitivity or competence is to know oneself. GRNs must understand their own values, beliefs, and attitudes. One's upbringing and conditioning affect the way things are perceived. Ethnocentrism, or an attitude that one's own culture is the right way, must be avoided if two-way communication is to take place. Other barriers to cultural competence include prejudices such as ageism, sexism, and racism. Nurses may have cultural blind spots that cause them to assume that a client is like themselves based on physical appearance. The variation among cultures can also pose a problem. Nurses may assume that persons from similar backgrounds share the same language and beliefs, but this is not always true. Case Studies 13.1 and 13.2 describe such instances.

CASE STUDY 13.1

An elderly gentleman was admitted to the emergency room of a large hospital. He reported himself to be Yugoslavian, but spoke little English. The nursing administrator attempted to find a nurse who would be able to translate so the man's medical complaint could be determined. She located a nurse of Serbian descent working on a medical floor of the hospital at the time and requested her translation services. The floor nurse came to the emergency room only to discover that the patient was Macedonian and they did not share a common language. The medical staff insisted that the staff nurse should have been able to translate for the patient because they were from the same part of the world. The staff nurse became extremely frustrated that the emergency room personnel had unrealistic expectations and very little understanding of the vast number of languages spoken by this minority group.

CASE STUDY 13.2

A nurse of Hispanic origin was asked to assist her elderly relatives who were going to the physician for a check-up. They spoke little English. However, as the young nurse was translating the medical instructions to the elders, she used her Americanized Spanish dialect, which contained some slang, and the elders became offended. Their dialect was different, although the language was the same,

and what was appropriate in one dialect was insulting in the other.

Culturally competent nursing care involves integration of the knowledge of a person's culture into their care. Leininger (1995) stated that "in the twenty-first century all nurses will need to be prepared in transcultural nursing with substantive knowledge and skills to function in an intense multicultural world" (p. 4). Whether it is labeled transcultural nursing, cultural sensitivity, cultural awareness, cultural competence, or ethnorelativity, there is no doubt that effective nursing care must incorporate cultural knowledge. Quality nursing care should strive to be culturally congruent.

As seen in the previous discussion, culture influences how people view health and illness, as well as whether or not they seek treatment and from whom they seek it. The GRN with knowledge of the culture of the person for whom care is being given stands a much better chance of providing what the *patient* needs. Sex and gender differences should be considered. For example, a male nurse may need to refer care of a woman of Middle Eastern background to a female nurse. A female nurse may prefer that her male colleague teach a diabetes management class to a group of Arab Muslims in her care.

Nonverbal communication should be done with care. Touching the head in some cultures means that something has been taken from the other person. Eye contact is culturally determined, because for some this is insulting, but for others, lack of eye contact may indicate feelings of guilt. The "evil eye" in many cultures is what makes a person ill. Silence may show respect in the Native American culture, but it could show disagreement for an African-American.

Campinha-Bacote (1995) stated that "conducting a culturally sensitive cultural assessment is a critical factor in rendering culturally relevant service to our growing ethnically diverse patient population" (p. 19). In assessing for cultural differences, the nurse should ask questions of the patient or family that elicit information about self-care practices. Table 13–2 lists several non-threatening questions that the nurse could ask to show sensitivity and to obtain useful information.

The use of folk medicines or remedies, and alternative healers, should be explored with-

Table 13-2 EXAMPLES OF CULTURALLY SENSITIVE QUESTIONS

What do you think caused these problems?
Has this happened before? If so, what kind of things helped you feel better?
Who do you turn to most often when you have a problem?
What would you like me to call you? (By Mr., Mrs., a nickname?)
Are there any special things that you need that would make you feel more comfortable while you are here?
Would you like a family member to be with you during your treatment?
What type of routine are you used to at home?
Are there any special foods from home that you would like to have during your stay here?
Who will be helping you at home after you are discharged?
How do you see your role in the family? (breadwinner, homemaker, boss, etc.)
What activities do you enjoy? What is your favorite pastime?

out being judgmental. The GRN should generally support the patient's cultural beliefs unless they are in direct contradiction with known medical and nursing research showing a hazard to health. In this case, the GRN should provide needed information in a non-threatening manner. Folk practices such as wrapping an inflamed toe in raw bacon to draw out infection (Case Study 13.3), or taking small amounts of olive oil to prevent or control hypertension, do not need to be discouraged. Other practices, such as making a cross on the door to ward off evil spirits or opening scissors under the mattress of the bed to cut pain, may be important parts of a person's culture. The GRN should remain aware that such practices have long family and social traditions attached to them and are likely used before seeking, or at least in conjunction with, more professional health services.

Additionally, the use of long-term care facilities may be culturally incongruent within many groups. Alternative arrangements should always be explored, and if long-term care is necessary, then appropriate interventions to assist the family with coping should be examined (Case Study 13.4).

dies instead. The GRN spent a great deal of time educating P.T. and his wife on foot care, particularly related to slower healing due to age and the higher risk of infection related to his diabetes. One day, on a visit to the home, the GRN inspected the foot that the wife had complained was showing redness and swelling from a gouty flare-up. The GRN noted what appeared to be an unusual dressing on the foot and began to unwrap it. Thin, whitish strips with a greasy texture first appeared to the nurse to be peeling skin, and she became alarmed. Just then, the wife exclaimed, "Oh, I meant to take that off before you got here!" The wife removed the "dressing" and explained that it was raw bacon, a folk cure for inflamed toes. The saltiness was thought to draw out infection and to decrease redness and swelling. As the GRN observed the toe, it had indeed improved since the last observation. The GRN then used the opportunity to explore the cultural norms and folk remedies used by the couple and discussed ways in which they would prefer to receive care. In particular, P.T. wished to avoid hospitalization, so a plan of care was established to incorporate mutual goals.

■■■

CASE STUDY 13.3

P.T. was an elderly man of Polish-American descent. He experienced diabetes and flare-ups of gouty arthritis in his left great toe. The home care GRN was making daily visits to perform wound care on an ulcerated area on his right foot, where he had tried to treat a callus by removing it with a razor blade. P.T. voiced strong objections to going to physicians for any problem, preferring home reme-

CASE STUDY 13.4

Mrs. L. was an 84 year old, widowed, African-American woman who had 7 children, 14 grandchildren, and 10 great-grandchildren. All but 1 of her children lived within an hour's drive of their mother's house. Mrs. L. lived with her 82 year old sister in a large 2-story home, where both were visited daily by family members. Both sisters had been active in their local church until Mrs. L. fractured her hip in a fall. After recovery from a total hip arthroplasty in an acute care hospital, Mrs. L. was deconditioned and sent to a rehabilitation unit for continued therapy, hoping to be discharged home to her previous living arrangements. Her children and grandchildren visited regularly. While in rehabilitation, Mrs. L.'s sister, with whom she lived, had a stroke and experienced right hemiplegia and aphasia, necessitating a change in the discharge arrangements for Mrs. L. The GRN and the social worker discussed possible discharge destinations for Mrs. L., one of which was placement in a long-term care facility until she became strong enough to return home alone. Mrs. L.'s children strongly objected to the idea of their mother or aunt being placed in a nursing home. They considered that alternative unacceptable. The GRN and other members of the interdisciplinary team then worked with the extended family to establish a culturally congruent discharge plan. This included one of the daughter's leaving her job to become a full-time caregiver for both the mother and aunt in the home, until Mrs. L. was strong enough to provide care for her sister, who would require some assistance with activities of daily living. The other family members set up a schedule to provide respite for the caregiver daughter and contributed monetarily to the care costs not covered by insurance. Church friends also helped with transporting Mrs. L.'s sister to outpatient speech therapy. With the combined efforts of the family, church, and health care system, Mrs. L. and her sister were able to return home after discharge.

IMPLICATIONS FOR RESEARCH

Although aging is universal, little is known about the diversity of the aged in different cultures. Much more research is needed among ethnic minority groups. Of particular interest is the diversity within major ethnic and racial groups and subgroups. Questions must be raised such as: How does culture influence the aging process? How is an "elderly person" defined or perceived among groups and subgroups? What is considered "old" in various cultures? How can nurses be trained to become more culturally sensitive to the needs of elders?

Nurses can begin to move in the right direction by being informed of basic ethnic and cultural differences. Colleges of nursing are attempting to include education on multiculturalism, but more formal coursework needs to be available. Additionally, focus on diversity within the elderly population needs more emphasis.

Recruitment of ethnic minorities into health care professions should be a priority. Likewise, services need to be more community-based and accessible to all. The unique needs of the disabled and chronically ill elderly make this an essential concern of the future. Nurses can take a leadership role by staying abreast of and being actively involved in multicultural research.

REFERENCES

Aiken, L. R. (1995). *Aging: An introduction to gerontology*. Thousand Oaks, CA: Sage.

Ailinger, R. (1989). Self-assessed health of Hispanic elderly persons. *Journal of Community Health Nursing, 6*(2), 113–118.

Ailinger, R. L., & Causey, M. E. (1995). Health concept of older Hispanic immigrants. *Western Journal of Nursing Research, 17*, 605–613.

Ailinger, R. L., Dear, M. R., & Holley-Wilcox, P. (1993). Predictors of function among older Hispanic immigrants: A five-year follow-up. *Nursing Research, 42*(4), 240–244.

Alston, R. J., & McCowan, C. J. (1994, January, February, March). African American women with disabilities: Rehabilitation issues and concerns. *Journal of Rehabilitation*, 36–40.

Angel, R., Angel, J., & Himes, C. (1992). Minority group status, health transitions, and community living arrangements among the elderly. *Research on Aging, 14*, 496–521.

Baker, F. M., Espino, D. V., Robinson, B. J., & Stewart, B. (1993). Assessing depressive symptoms in African American and Mexican American elders. *Clinical Gerontologist, 14*(1), 15–29.

Bassford, T. (1995). Health status of Hispanic elders. In D. V. Espino (Volume Ed.), *Clinics in Geriatric Medicine: Ethnogeriatrics, 11*(1), 25–38.

Bedolla, M. A. (1995). The principles of medical ethics and their application to Mexican-American elderly patients. In D. V. Espino (Volume Ed.), *Clinics in Geriatric Medicine: Ethnogeriatrics, 11*(1), 131–138.

Blakemore, K., & Boneham, M. (1994). *Age, race, and ethnicity: A comparative approach*. Buckingham, United Kingdom: Open University Press.

Brangman, S. A. (1995). African American elders: Implications for health care providers. In D. V. Espino (Volume Ed.), *Clinics in Geriatric Medicine: Ethnogeriatrics, 11*(1), 15–24.

Browne, C., & Broderick, A. (1991). *Aging and ethnicity: A replication handbook for social work education for practice with Asian and Pacific Island elders*. Manoa, HI: Pacific Gerontology Social

Work Education Curriculum Replication Project, University of Hawai'i.

Butler, F. R. (1987). Minority wellness promotion: A behavioral self-management approach. *Journal of Gerontological Nursing, 13*(8), 23–28.

Cameron, E., Badger, F., & Evers, H. (1989). District nursing the disabled and the elderly: Who are the black patients? *Journal of Advanced Nursing, 14*(5), 376–382.

Campinha-Bacote, J. (1995). The quest for cultural competence in nursing care. *Nursing Forum, 30*(4), 19–25.

Clark, M., & Anderson, B. G. (1967). *Culture and aging: An anthropological study of older Americans.* Springfield, IL: Charles C Thomas.

Clavon, A. (1986). The black elderly. *Journal of Gerontological Nursing, 12*(5), 6–12.

Coke, M. M., & Twaite, J. A. (1995). *The black elderly: Satisfaction and quality of later life.* Binghamton, NY: Haworth Press.

Cowgill, D. O. (1986). *Aging around the world.* Blemont, CA: Wadsworth Publishing Company.

Damron-Rodriguez, J., Wallace, S., & Kington, R. (1994). Service utilization and minority elderly: Appropriateness, accessibility and acceptability. *Gerontology and Geriatrics Education, 15*(1), 45–62.

Eliopoulos, C. (1993). *Gerontological nursing.* Philadelphia: J. B. Lippincott.

Espino, D. V. (Volume Ed.). (1995). *Clinics in Geriatric Medicine: Ethnogeriatrics, 11*(1), xi.

Fowles, D. G. (1994). *A profile of older Americans.* Washington, DC: American Association of Retired Persons and Administration on Aging, U.S. Department of Health and Human Services.

Fry, C. L. (1981). *Dimensions: Aging, culture, and health.* New York: J. F. Bergin Publishers.

Garfinkel, H. (1967). *Studies in ethnomethodology.* Englewood Cliffs, NJ: Prentice-Hall.

Gelfand, D. (1994). *Aging and ethnicity.* New York: Springer Publishing.

Gelfand, D., & Barresi, C. M. (1987). *Ethnic dimensions of aging.* New York: Springer Publishing.

Gelfand, D. E., & Kutzik, A. J. (Eds.) (1979). *Ethnicity and aging.* New York: Springer Publishing.

Gibson, R. C., & Burns, C. J. (1992). The health, labor force, and retirement experiences of aging minorities. In E. P. Stanford & F. M. Torres-Gil (Eds.), *Diversity: New approaches to minority aging* (pp. 53–63). Amityville, NY: Baywood Publishing Company.

Gillies, D. A. (1991). Content and significance of minority aging curriculum guide. *MAIN Dimensions, 2*(9), 1–4.

Gitlin, L. N., Corcoran, M., & Leinmiller-Eckhardt, S. (1995). Understanding the family perspective: An ethnographic framework for providing occupational therapy in the home. *American Journal of Occupational Therapy, 49*, 802–808.

Guttman, D. (1979). A perspective on Euro-American elderly. In C. L. Hayes, R. A. Kalish, & D. Guttman (Eds.), *European-American elderly: A guide for practice.* New York: Springer Publishing.

Hayes, C. L., Kalish, R. A., & Guttman, D. (Eds.) (1986). *European-American elderly: A guide for practice.* New York: Springer Publishing.

Holzberg, C. (1982). Ethnicity and aging: Anthropological perspectives on more than just the minority elderly. *Gerontologist, 22*, 249–257.

Irish, D. P., Lundquist, K. F., & Nelsen, V. J. (1993). *Ethnic variations in dying, death, and grief.* Washington, DC: Taylor & Francis.

Johnson, C. (1985). *Growing up and growing old in Italian-American families.* New Brunswick, NJ: Rutgers University Press.

Johnson, F., Foxall, M. J., Kelleher, E., Kentopp, E., Mannlein, E. A., & Cook, E. (1988). Comparison of mental health and life satisfaction of five elderly ethnic groups. *Western Journal of Nursing Research, 10*, 613–628.

Jones, D. C., & Van Amelsvoort Jones, G. M. M. (1986). Communication patterns between nursing staff and the ethnic elderly in a long-term care facility. *Journal of Advanced Nursing, 11*, 265–272.

Kart, C. S. (1987). Age and religious commitment in the American-Jewish Community. In D. Gelfand & C. Barresi (Eds.), *Ethnic dimensions of aging* (pp. 96–105). New York: Springer Publishing.

Kart, C. S. (1994). *The realities of aging.* Boston: Allyn and Bacon.

Kastenbaum, R. J. (1991). *Death, society, and human experience.* New York: Macmillan Publishing Company.

Leininger, M. (1985). Ethnonursing: A research method to generate nursing knowledge [In *Summer research conference monograph*]. Detroit, MI: Wayne State University.

Leininger, M. (1995). Jewish Americans and culture. In M. Leininger (Ed.), *Transcultural nursing: Concepts, theories, research and practices* (pp. 471–484). New York: McGraw-Hill.

Lockery, S. A. (1992). Caregiving among racial and ethnic minority elders: Family and social supports. In E. P. Stanford & F. M. Torres-Gil (Eds.), *Diversity: New approaches to minority aging* (pp. 113–122). Amityville, NY: Baywood Publishing Company.

Manuel, R. C. (1982). *Minority aging: Sociological and social psychological issues.* Westport, CT: Greenwood Press.

Markides, K. S., & Mindel, C. H. (1987). *Aging and ethnicity.* Newbury Park, CA: Age.

McKenna, M. (1989). Twice in need of care: A transcultural nursing analysis of elderly Mexican Americans. *Journal of Transcultural Nursing, 1*(1), 46–52.

Morgan, M. (1995). African Americans and cultural care. In M. Leininger (Ed.), *Transcultural nursing: Concepts, theories, research and practices* (pp. 383–400). New York: McGraw-Hill.

Phillips, S., & Lobar, S. (1995). Navajo child health beliefs and rearing practices within a transcultural nursing framework: Literature review. In

M. Leininger (Ed.), *Transcultural nursing: Concepts, theories, research and practices* (pp. 485–500). New York: McGraw-Hill.

Pousada, L. (1995). Hispanic-American elders: Implications for health-care providers. In D. V. Espino (Volume Ed.), *Clinics in Geriatric Medicine: Ethnogeriatrics, 11*(1), 39–52.

Ries, P. (1990). Vital and health statistics: Health of black and white Americans, 1985–1987. National Center for Health Statistics. *Vital Health Statistics, 10*(171).

Salmon, M. A. (1994). *Double jeopardy: Resources and minority elders.* New York: Garland Publishing.

Sankar, A. (1981). The conquest of solitude: Singlehood and old age in traditional Chinese society. In C. Fry (Ed.), *Dimensions: Aging, culture, and health* (pp. 65–83). New York: J. F. Bergin Publishers.

Seabrooks, P. A., Kahn, R., & Gero, G. (1987). Cross-cultural observations. *Journal of Gerontological Nursing, 13*(1), 18–22.

Sowell, T. (1994). *Race and culture: A world view.* New York: Basic Books.

Stanford, E. P., & Yee, D. L. (1992). Gerontology and the relevance of diversity. In E. P. Stanford & F. M. Torres-Gil (Eds.), *Diversity: New approaches to minority aging* (pp. 15–23). Amityville, NY: Baywood Publishing Company.

Van den Berghe, P. (1987). Age differentiation in human societies. In J. Sokolovsky (Ed.), *Growing old in different societies: Cross-cultural perspectives.* Littleton, MA: Copley Publishing Group.

Villarruel, A., & Leininger, M. (1995). Culture care of Mexican Americans. In M. Leininger (Ed.), *Transcultural nursing: Concepts, theories, research and practices* (pp. 365–382). New York: McGraw-Hill.

Chapter 14

Psychosocial Concepts and Issues

■

The elderly person experiencing functional limitations deals with more than physical problems. Many persons with disabling or limiting conditions express feelings of anxiety, sorrow, depression, anger, and frustration. Chronic conditions challenge the person's and the family's abilities to cope and adapt to a long-term situation involving uncertainty and fear. This chapter presents some of the psychosocial concerns associated with, and factors influencing, gerontological rehabilitation nursing. The use of coping strategies and the concepts of quality of life, social support, loss and grief, spiritual well-being, and sexuality are discussed. Negative outcomes such as abuse of elders and suicide among the elderly are also addressed.

FACTORS INFLUENCING GERIATRIC REHABILITATION

The literature contains suggestions of many factors that can influence outcomes in rehabilitation of the elderly. Many such *physical* factors have been discussed in the preceding chapters. However, additional factors related to other aspects of care must be noted. These include but are not limited to: the use of coping strategies, social support, motivation, and spiritual well-being.

Coping Strategies

More than 31.5 million people in the United States have a chronic illness (Martin, 1995). Long-term illness may require the mobilization and integration of new coping mecha-

nisms in order to attain positive outcomes. Several ways in which persons cope with limiting physical conditions have been studied. The coping strategies of patients with chronic health problems, as well as their caregivers, have been shown to be positively influenced by the rehabilitation process (White, Richter, & Fry, 1992). The use of appropriate coping mechanisms results in decreased psychological distress, including less anger, depression, guilt, and anxiety (Roberto et al., 1995).

One common theme that emerges across the research is the desire to be in control (Easton, Rawl, Zemen, Kwiatkowski, & Burczyk, 1995; Gallagher, Wagenfeld, Baro, & Haepers, 1994; Martin, 1995). This seems to apply to both patients and family caregivers. Feelings of stress, fear, and anxiety can lead to helplessness, or a sense of having no control over one's situation. In a sample of 297 healthy elderly volunteers, Speake, Cowart, and Pellet (1989) found that perceived health status and health locus of control were significant predictors of healthy lifestyles. This suggests that control, or even perception of it, can assist in maintaining health in the absence of illness, not just promoting health in the presence of illness. Gass (1987) studied the relationships between bereavement, coping, resources, and health among 100 elderly widows. The results of that study indicated that "social support, strong religious beliefs, practice of rituals, belief in control over bereavements, and good prior mental health were related to less psychosocial and/or physical dysfunction" (Gass, 1987, p. 39). Additionally, the more resources a person had, the less psychosocial and/or physical dysfunction was likely to occur, regardless of the number of coping strategies used. Again, control (in addition to resources) emerged as an important factor.

Returning control to the person, in whatever form is possible or needed, is one of the foundations of promoting self-care. Rehabilitating older adults are at particular risk for feeling loss of control over their situation. Gerontological rehabilitation nurses (GRNs) should make a concerted effort to allow the person to retain as much control as possible in the rehabilitation setting from the time of admission. GRNs should also take every opportunity to return each aspect of control, whether that be control of bodily functions or a sense of control over one's future, in order to promote wellness among the elderly.

In addition to control, other factors such as humor, activity, and developing relationships have been identified as common means of coping with stress and chronic sorrow (Hainsworth, 1996; Hainsworth, Eakes, & Burke, 1994; Reinhardt, 1996). Chronic sorrow is to be distinguished from depression, in that it is a pervasive sadness that is permanent, periodic, and progressive (Hainsworth, 1996). This type of sorrow is related to a normal mourning that commonly occurs in those with cancer, Parkinson's disease, infertility, multiple sclerosis, or other chronic disorders. Hainsworth's work in chronic sorrow showed that caregivers with a mean age of 61.2 years reported feelings of depression, frustration, and mental exhaustion. Again, these findings emphasize that chronicity affects the entire family, not just the patient. Thus, GRNs need to remain aware that family members and caregivers will grieve also and may require additional interventions to promote positive coping and adjustment.

Talking to persons in similar situations and therapeutic venting of feelings are ways in which a feeling of control is maintained. Developing relationships can occur with a sharing of feelings of sorrow and suffering. Such relationships may then form the basis of new, or strengthened, social support networks.

Other coping strategies that have been used by rehabilitation patients include positive thinking, keeping a sense of normalcy, and taking things one step at a time (Easton et al., 1995). Hope also emerges as an important coping mechanism among those with chronic illness (Miller, 1992). This may be related to the hope that the situation will improve, that

a cure will be found, or that things will get better. Hope is a coping strategy that GRNs should consistently support, because an absence of hope leads to hopelessness, feelings of loss of control, and poor (or negative) outcomes.

Social Support

Thomas and Hooper summarized the thoughts of many researchers by stating, "although it is not possible to conclude that adequate social bonds and an internal locus of control 'cause' good health, this indeed may be the case" (1983, p. 15). Numerous studies have reported the benefits of social support for patients. Social support can be defined in a variety of ways, but it is essentially the resources that provide the person with a sense of stability, security, social interaction, and social connectedness. Differences in perceived social support varied between studies and are influenced by age, type of disability, and sometimes degree of functional limitations.

Turner (1996), in a study of physically disabled elders in Ontario, Canada, demonstrated that factors influencing family support and conflict change across the life span. Elders perceived greater support and lesser conflict from family members when compared with younger adults (between ages 18 and 64). Elders with more severe functional limitations expressed less negative and conflictive interactions with the family.

One study examined social support among 241 elders with age-related visual impairment (Reinhardt, 1996). The majority of older adults had both a close friend and a close family member, suggesting that perhaps elders have developed social skills that promote the maintenance of social support structures. Reinhardt stated that "close relationships were perceived as providing greater attachment in females and greater instrumental assistance and social integration with males" (1996, p. 268). Cummings et al. (1988) reported that older patients with hip fracture who had a greater number of social supports had significantly better functional outcomes.

Similarly, involvement of a spouse has been shown to promote positive functional outcomes among stroke patients (Baker, 1993). Generally, increased support from family and friends is associated with greater life satisfaction and less depression.

Social class differences in support were discussed in one study. Krause and Borawski-

Clark (1995) found that those elders with a high school diploma had more contact with friends than those with lesser education. Those having higher education (beyond high school) had more well-developed social support networks later in life.

Other differences in the use of social support can be seen. Logan and Spitze (1994) found that family support sometimes substituted for formal services. The greater the functional disability, the more use of formal services took place. Likewise, Miner (1995) found that African-American families may combine formal and informal services, and advanced age was associated with greater use of formal services. The black elderly are willing to use formal services but value both types of resources, desiring to maintain the close family links that help decrease caregiver burden. Social support quality and perceived rewards and costs were more important than caregiving demand or income among African-American caregivers (Picot, 1995).

Social support can also have a negative impact on the person. For example, family members who form the person's main support network may not provide the needed emotional or physical support for the person and may even impair rehabilitative progress by conveying negative attitudes toward the person's goals. GRNs should assist persons and their caregivers in exploring their social support networks, to determine whether they are positive or negative. Accessibility continues to be a major issue in the use of services among elderly of minority groups. The coping skills used often depend on a person's resources, so knowledge of these must be gained before interventions can be planned. Efforts should be made to assist the person in identifying strong, positive support persons who will be an asset to the person's self-care activities and goals.

Differences in social support among elders may also be related to medical diagnosis. For example, Heidrich (1996) found that women with arthritis had more functional health problems and more symptoms and perceived their illness as worse, more chronic, and less controllable than elderly women with breast cancer. However, when the social networks of both groups were examined, those with better social support matrixes had increased psychological well-being regardless of their health problems. Similarly, Kemp, Adams, and Campbell (1997) found that elderly polio survivors reported no overall significant differences in depression when compared with a nondisabled control group. Although older polio survivors often experienced depression, it was related to attitude and family function more than physical disability.

Although nursing care influences a variety of outcomes, it is of note that follow-up after discharge seems particularly important for elderly persons with long-term health alterations. Nursing care that continues after discharge seems to act as a social support mechanism. Roberts et al. (1995) found that persons receiving telephone call support from a nurse experienced less psychological distress than those who did not. Persons generally report a high degree of satisfaction with care provided by discharge follow-up nurses, as well as decreased anxiety (Easton et al., 1995). Cognitive behavioral interventions can also help patients achieve rehabilitation goals and decrease distress, while promoting the use of positive coping mechanisms (Lopez & Mermelstein, 1995). Nurses can assist those who are having difficulty adjusting through matching coping and support strategies used by the patient, fostering the use of positive coping mechanisms (Martin, 1995). GRNs should also remember that family members may be hidden victims of aging and disability, and that long-term health alterations affect the entire family. Thus, family dynamics, resources, and coping strategies used by family members should also be examined.

Motivational Factors

Resnick (1996) used critical ethnography to explore factors related to motivation on a geriatric rehabilitation unit. Key informants (five white women) with an average age of 87 provided information about factors that improved motivation. These included goals, humor, caring, beliefs, encouragement, motive disposition, and power resulting from relationships. Within the same study, domination, or the sense of being ruled or controlled by others, resulted in reported feelings of valuelessness and hopelessness. Empowerment was found to be much more effective than forced compliance or domination in motivating women toward rehabilitation. These findings are consistent with previous studies that showed that an internal locus of control resulted in more positive rehabilitation outcomes.

Additionally, the use of therapeutic humor in health and healing has long been established. Easton et al. (1995) also demonstrated that humor was an often used, and highly effective, coping mechanism among rehabilitation patients.

Spiritual Well-being

Spiritual well-being is an often overlooked aspect of holistic health care. Landis (1996) found that spiritual well-being was an internal coping resource for persons adjusting to the uncertainty of life with long-term health alterations. A strong relationship was found between spiritual well-being and psychosocial adjustment. Persons reporting feelings of increased spiritual well-being showed less uncertainty and fewer problems related to living with chronic illness. In a study of 100 rehabilitation patients, other researchers found that the response "prayed or put your trust in God" was given as a top coping strategy by more than 90% of respondents both at discharge and at 4 months after discharge (Easton et al., 1995). This strategy was also rated as highly effective. A study of coping in African-American caregivers (Picot, 1995) showed that prayer and faith in God was a more frequently used coping strategy than problem-solving and information seeking.

Nurses working with elderly clients or residents can strengthen the benefits the person may gain from spiritual resources through several interventions. First, GRNs should acknowledge that each person is a spiritual being. All people have a component that represents this holistic aspect of the self. Much as nurses have been educated to provide culturally competent care, so GRNs should strive to plan care that is also spiritually sensitive and congruent. Acknowledging persons' religious beliefs and facilitating their ability to worship or pray as they desire give permission for a person to be a spiritual being. Spirituality includes religious beliefs but also encompasses one's sense of life's meaning and significance. The GRN should include spiritual assessment as part of the admission procedure and may need to be sure that the appropriate person from the person's church, parish, or temple is notified when a person is admitted to the health care facility.

Even persons who do not consider themselves particularly religious may in a time of crisis request the services of a pastor, priest, rabbi, or other spiritual leader. This suggests that many persons derive comfort from the presence of a spiritual leader. For many individuals, the pastor represents a source of inner strength and encouragement. Pastors may be lifelong friends of the family and provide insightful information into the person's thoughts, feelings, and social situation that can help the GRN provide spiritually sensitive care. Incorporating the spiritual leader into the health care team promotes care of the entire person. Pastors often act as counselors, providing health care for the soul, and may be the sole professional source of follow-up for the person after discharge. GRNs should make every effort to bolster communication with members of the clergy in the community, so that appropriate resources may be identified and utilized to the fullest.

QUALITY OF LIFE

Quality of life is often related to the use of coping patterns, or the person's ability to deal with stressful situations. Quality of life is always perceived from the emic (or insider's) perspective and is nearly impossible to measure with any objectivity from an outsider's viewpoint. Thus, when speaking of quality of life, GRNs should note that this is a subjective term and should be interpreted as such. For example, an older person who has lived with a disability for many years may report a higher quality of life than a younger person with lesser limitations. From an observer's point of view, the older person may have a poorer quality of life, yet reports the opposite. Indeed, Mold, Looney, Viviani, and Quiggins found that "sociodemographic and functional status variables are relatively weak predictors of personal values and directives" (1994, p. 461).

Elderly patients seem to value quality of life over quantity of life. In a study of 178 cognitively intact elders, those persons with better social and family support were more likely to express advance directives (see Chapter 15 for further discussion) indicating a desire for cardiopulmonary resuscitation (Mold et al., 1994). The ability to think clearly was highly valued (64% of respondents), and most did not wish to live in a vegetative state.

Being married has been positively correlated to a higher perceived quality of life (Rickelman, Gallman, & Parra, 1994). Marital adjustment and income were found to be the best predictors of quality of life for spouses of continuous ambulatory peritoneal dialysis (CAPD) patients (Dunn, Lewis, Bonner, & Meize-Grochowski, 1994). Economic factors may also play a role in the perception of quality of life. Visually impaired elders who maintained supportive friendships in later life in addition to family relationships also reported a higher life satisfaction (Reinhardt, 1996).

LOSS AND GRIEF

Older adults experience a great many losses throughout their life span. The longer one lives, the more likely one is to encounter multiple losses. This may include the death of loved ones, divorce, loss of a job, or loss of health. With advanced age, the incidence of chronic illness rises, necessitating assistance with daily activities for many older adults, which contributes to a feeling of loss of independence or control. Many elderly in rehabilitation or long-term care settings have lost the ability to ambulate or lost control of bowel and bladder function. For others, the losses are more obvious, as with the loss of a limb through amputation.

With any type of loss comes a process of grieving. "Adaptation to losses is believed to occur gradually through a process of grief resolution" (Harden, 1997, p. 691). Kubler-Ross' (1969) theory can provide a framework for GRNs to view the grieving process through which older adults may work in order to cope with loss. The five stages of grief are (1) denial, (2) anger, (3) bargaining, (4) depression, and (5) acceptance. GRNs may use this model to ascertain at which stage patients are in the grieving process. Patients may move between the stages at various rates, and this is highly individualized.

It has been this author's clinical experience that patients in rehabilitation are more likely to have positive outcomes if they are in the acceptance phase. Persons who are in denial, exhibit persistent anger, or those with clinical depression are often not ready to participate in an intense rehabilitation program and do not generally display readiness to learn. However, although patients may exhibit signs of anger or depression, this is more often seen from family members, while the patients themselves often move through the process more quickly. GRNs should recall that family members will also experience grief but may need assistance in moving toward acceptance, sometimes more so than the patient. GRNs can help persons and families move toward acceptance of and adjustment to losses by enhancing a person's positive social support systems, helping him or her access community resources, and promoting the use of positive coping mechanisms.

SEXUALITY

Sexuality is a general term used to describe the behaviors associated with expressing one's sexual identity (McConnell & Murphy, 1997). It encompasses, but is not limited to, sexual activity or relationships. The frequency of sexual intercourse declines with advanced age, but interest in and capacity for sexual relations does not decline (in the absence of disease). Surveys of the elderly report that the median age for cessation of intercourse for men was 68 years and for women it was 60 years (Aiken, 1995). Of course, these figures may be largely dependent on social circumstances and other factors.

Several changes in the reproductive system occur with aging. For women, atrophy of the reproductive organs, thinning of the vaginal wall, and decreased vaginal lubrication can result in pain during intercourse. Additional lubrication with a water-soluble substance such as K-Y jelly can assist with this problem. GRNs should caution women against the use of petroleum jelly (such as Vaseline), because it is not as effective as a lubricant and can predispose the woman to infection. Vaginal irritation and urinary tract infections may be common, especially after intercourse, as a result of thinning of the vaginal wall. GRNs should instruct older women on the importance of good feminine hygiene and the importance of emptying the bladder after intercourse to decrease the risk of infection.

Men also experience some changes with aging with regard to sexual functioning. Degenerative changes occur in the reproductive organs, but men remain fertile through late life (Patrick, 1993). Erections may take longer to occur and may be less firm. Periodic difficulties with erection and ejaculation are common and do not necessarily indicate impotence. The refractory period lengthens with advanced age, and it may be 1 to 2 days before the man is able to achieve full orgasm again (Miller, 1995).

Miller (1995) summarizes the results of studies on sexuality and aging in six major points: (1) older adults continue to have a capacity for and interest in sexual relations although the frequency of sexual activity gradually declines with age; (2) a decrease in sexual activity with advancing age is due to social circumstances, risk factors, or pathophysiology; (3) a decrease in sexual activity is more often due to social circumstances such as the death or illness of a spouse, particularly in the case of older women; (4) lifelong sexual patterns, interest, and activity continue into old age, not changing significantly; (5) men are more sexually active than women throughout the life span; and (6) masturbation is not an uncommon practice among the elderly, being most common among healthy 80 to 102 year old men.

It is particularly important for GRNs to acknowledge each person as a sexual being, because this is an essential aspect of providing holistic care. Providing privacy, realizing the need for intimacy, and opening up the topic of sexuality for discussion are especially important for persons with chronic illness or functional limitations. In addition to normal aging changes, older adults with rehabilitative problems may require special consideration in this area. Changes in body image, physical functioning, or perception of self are common issues that older adults must face when chronic illness or disability is experienced. Fears of rejection or pain may need to be addressed. For example, the man who has experienced a myocardial infarction may be afraid to resume sexual activity for fear of another heart attack. Persons experiencing a stroke with residual hemiparesis may need to learn new positions for intercourse with their partner in order to feel comfortable both physically and emotionally. Those with a colostomy may feel embarrassment because of odor or scars and may fear rejection by their sexual partner. Persons with spinal cord injury require special instructions on their physical ability to engage in sexual activities.

Most important is that GRNs should emphasize the many ways in which sexuality may be expressed, including holding hands, caressing, talking, kissing, and other mutual expressions of affection, not just sexual intercourse. Allowing patients and spouses to discuss their concerns before discharge is an important intervention. Booklets and instructional videos may be suggested. Cultural norms may preclude or influence discussion of sexuality, but GRNs should be aware that most elderly persons are interested in information about how their disease or disability affects this aspect of their lives (Staab & Hodges, 1996).

POLYPHARMACY

The use of multiple medications is common among the elderly. Some patients require multiple medications to manage a number of chronic illnesses. Between 20% and 32% of all drugs are prescribed for the elderly, and they use 40% of all over-the-counter medications, resulting in a cost of several billion dollars per year (Grossberg & Grossberg, 1998; Stone, 1991). Most elderly take two or more medications, with the most commonly prescribed medications being analgesics, cardiovascular agents, antihypertensives, and antibiotics, although there is some variation in types of drugs taken depending on the health care setting (whether long-term facility or the community) (Swonger & Burbank, 1995). Sedatives, laxatives, and antacids are also commonly used. Glickstein cited these facts: "the average elderly person receives 13 prescription drugs per year for multiple disease conditions," and "estimates indicate that half of all medications prescribed for those over age 65 are not taken correctly" (1989, p. 1). Drug-related illnesses are associated with a significant number of hospital admissions each year, and also deaths among the aged. Table 14–1 shows the most commonly prescribed medications for the elderly.

Because of polypharmacy, or the prescription of multiple medications, elders are at risk for negative drug effects. Several factors contribute to this. First, physiological changes in the aging body can alter the way medications are absorbed and processed. Medications are absorbed more slowly and less efficiently in the older person because of changes in the gastrointestinal system, such as decreased motility and enzymes. The liver may be less efficient at detoxification than in a younger individual, and the kidneys are slower to excrete waste products, largely as a result of the loss of a number of functional nephrons with age and decreased cardiac output leading to diminished glomerular filtration rate. A slower metabolic system, as well as the lack of available protein for medication to bind with, allows the drugs to remain in the body longer and may produce a cumulative effect. Thus, although an elderly person shows no adverse effects to a medication, this could change rapidly, and constant awareness is required on the part of the GRN to assess for side effects. Additionally, the more medications a person is taking the more likely that an adverse reaction will occur. However, signs and symptoms may be different in an older adult, and side effects may be slower to appear. Thus, special dosage requirements are often indicated in the management of medications for the elderly. Those with kidney and liver problems are particularly at risk for toxicity, even with very low drug dosages (Glickstein, 1989). Even commonly used non-

Table 14-1 MOST COMMONLY PRESCRIBED MEDICATIONS FOR THE ELDERLY

Type	Side Effects
Heart Medications	
Lanoxin (digoxin)	Loss of appetite, nausea, vomiting, weakness, blurred vision, yellow or spots before the eyes
Blood Pressure Medications	
Dyazide (triamterene; hydrochlorothiazide)	Drowsiness, lethargy, gastrointestinal upset, cramping diarrhea, tingling in toes and fingers
Lasix (furosemide)	Dermatitis, tingling in extremities, nausea and vomiting
HydroDIURIL (hydrochlorothiazide)	Thirst, weakness, lethargy, muscular tiredness, low potassium, upset stomach
Tenormin (atenolol)	Coldness in feet, dizziness, tiredness, decreased heart rate, tingling in extremities, nausea, vomiting, low pulse
Aldomet (methyldopate HCl)	Sedation, weakness
Minipress (prazosin HCl)	Dizziness, headache, drowsiness, take first dose at bedtime
Capoten (captopril)	Rash, fever, loss of taste perception, protein in urine, very low blood pressure, weakness, dizziness
Vasotec (enalapril maleate)	Low blood pressure, weakness, dizziness
Cardizem (diltiazem HCl)	Abnormal heart rhythms, fluid accumulation in hands, feet, dizziness
Procardia (nifedipine)	Dizziness, flushing, weakness, swelling of arms and legs
Arthritis Medications	
Feldene (piroxicam)	Upset stomach, nausea, darkening of stools
Naprosyn (naproxen)	Upset stomach, nausea, stomach pain, heartburn, dark stools
Clinoril (sulindac)	Upset stomach, stomach irritation, nausea, vomiting, swelling of legs and feet, dark stools
Indocin (indomethacin)	Stomach irritation, stomach cramps, dizziness, mental confusion, ringing in the ears, dark stools
Aspirin	Nausea, stomach irritation, ringing in the ears, dark stools
Antianxiety Medications	
Xanax (alprazolam)	Mild drowsiness, confusion, depression, lethargy, sleepiness
Ativan (lorazepam)	Mild drowsiness, confusion, depression, lethargy, disorientation, slurred speech, dry mouth
Sleeping Medications	
Restoril (temazepam)	Drowsiness, confusion, lethargy
Halcion (triazolam)	Drowsiness, dizziness, lightheadedness, disorientation
Other Medications	
Zantac (ranitidine HCl)	Headache, dizziness, stomach discomfort, rash
Tagamet (cimetidine)	Mental confusion, diarrhea, muscle pains, dizziness, hallucinations, breast enlargement

From Glickstein, J. K. (1989). Polypharmacy: Drug-induced illness in the elderly. *Focus on Geriatric Care & Rehabilitation*, 2(8), 4. © 1989, Aspen Publishers, Inc.

prescription medications can cause adverse reactions (Table 14–2).

Having several physicians can lead to miscommunication or overprescription of medications. The nurse cannot assume that all physicians on the patient's case are equally knowledgeable or informed about the drug interactions among multiple medications that can have a damaging effect on the patient (Case Study 14.1). There are several ways the GRN can facilitate communication between health care professionals. First, it is essential that an accurate picture of the person's medication regimen is obtained on admission to the facility. In addition to requesting a written list of medications, including over-the-counter drugs, that the patient has been taking, it is wise to ask the family to bring all the medications to the GRN in a paper bag to be checked. Most family members will gladly oblige. The GRN should check the bottles, labels, and appearance of the pills against

Table 14–2 NONPRESCRIPTION MEDICATIONS COMMONLY USED BY THE ELDERLY

Medication	Adverse Effects	Precautions
1. Pain Relievers		
Aspirin 　Ecotrin 　Ascriptin 　Bufferin	Nausea, vomiting, GI irritation, ulceration, bleeding, prolongation of bleeding time, sodium and water retention, ringing in ears.	Do not use with history of peptic ulcer, GI bleeding, or gout (will increase uric acid levels).
Ibuprofen 　Advil 　Nuprin 　Haltran 　Medipren	Nausea, vomiting, GI irritation, ulceration, bleeding, sodium and water retention.	Do not use with history of peptic ulcer, GI bleeding, hepatic/renal disease. Do not mix with alcohol.
Acetaminophen 　Tylenol 　Anacin-3	Hepatic necrosis after acute ingestion of 15 g or more.	Use with caution in client with history of liver or kidney disease. Do not exceed the maximum daily dose because of potential hepatic toxicity with overdose. Do not use with alcohol because of increased risk of hepatotoxicity.
2. Antacids	Antacids with primarily aluminum tend to be constipating. Those with magnesium may cause diarrhea. Those containing primarily calcium carbonate will tend to be constipating.	Do not use if taking a prescription antibiotic containing tetracycline. The sodium content of the antacid should be considered in elderly with high blood pressure or congestive heart disease.
3. Laxatives Metamucil Colace Doxidan Perdiem Correctol Dulcolax Ex-Lax Peri-Colace Effer-Syllium	Use with moderation because routine use can lead to dehydration and loss of electrolytes such as sodium and potassium. Can also lead to dependency.	Depending on the type, can cause interference with absorption of medications if taken together.
4. Cold Medications Actifed Benadryl Contac Comtrex Dimetapp Drixoral NyQuil Ornex	Those that contain phenylpropanolamine should not be taken with antihypertensive medications except under supervision of a doctor. May cause drowsiness. Avoid alcoholic beverages (alcohol may increase drowsiness). Avoid operating a motor vehicle while taking these medications.	If client has high blood pressure, heart disease, diabetes, thyroid glaucoma, or difficulty in urination, take only under the advice of a doctor.

From Glickstein, J. K. (1989). Polypharmacy: Drug-induced illness in the elderly. *Focus on Geriatric Care & Rehabilitation*, 2(8), 5. © 1989, Aspen Publishers, Inc.

the list provided by the family. Elders often become confused when reading multiple prescription labels and may interchange dosages or times. For example, the physician may have ordered three tablets twice per day, but the person may be taking two pills three times per day. Elders are often frugal with medications, causing them to save old prescriptions, use antibiotics for conditions other than those for which they were ordered, or put pills into different containers to save for a later illness. Most of these types of errors are not done intentionally but can be caused by lack of knowledge about the effects and purposes of prescription drugs. Additionally, when asked what medications the person takes at home, many people will not include over-the-counter items such as antacids, analgesics, or laxatives. The GRN should specifically inquire about these medications to ensure accurate documentation. Once a precise history of medication regimen has been obtained, the GRN should make sure that all physicians, including consultants, are informed about the patient's prescriptions. The pharmacist is an invaluable resource to the GRN when drug interactions are questioned. Nurses must also take responsibility for being informed about potential adverse reactions and drug interactions, because they are most likely going to administer the drugs and teach the patient and family.

CASE STUDY 14.1
Polypharmacy

Nora Collins, age 71, came to the rehabilitation unit because of a complicated hospital stay following a surgical operation to remove her appendix. Her family (a husband of nearly 50 years, several children and grandchildren) had become distraught over Nora's deterioration during her hospital stay. Previously active and in good health, she was confused and disoriented, even combative at times after the surgery. The physician had ordered medication to help her relax, including Haldol and Xanax. Before long, Nora became totally dependent, incontinent, lethargic, and dysphagic. Her hospital stay lengthened to over a month and she experienced functional debility. Her family feared she had given up and would die, so she was referred for rehabilitative services. Feeling she could benefit from intensive therapy to regain ambulatory ability, speech, and continence,

she was accepted to the rehabilitation program for a 10-day trial period. She had a nasogastric tube and catheter on admission. When admitted to rehabilitation, she was also taking at least 14 medications, not including medications given on an as-needed basis, prescribed by more than five different physicians. After performing a thorough physical and neurological examination, the physiatrist, suspecting that polypharmacy might be contributing to the patient's difficulties, discontinued all but the necessary medications Nora took for cardiac problems and hypertension. Within one full week, Nora was alert and oriented, able to feed herself and carry on a conversation. The family said that a miracle had occurred. Nora was discharged home to her husband and family after intensive rehabilitation and was able to return to her former abilities and activities.

A more common source of medication problems is related to the patient's and family's lack of knowledge about the effects produced. This is an area in which GRNs can positively influence the health of the person through the teaching role. Basic medication teaching should be part of every discharge plan. General rules that should be reinforced with the patient and family are presented in Table 14–3. More specific instructions should include the major effects and adverse reactions of each medication the person will take home. The person or caregiver should be able to identify the drug by its appearance, state the time it should be taken, its purpose, and the major side effects. A plan of action if side effects occur should be made. For example, if the person taking Lanoxin has a heart rate below 60 beats per minute, the medication should not be taken, and the physician should be called; or if anginal pain is unrelieved by nitroglycerin tablets sublingually as ordered, the physician should be called or the person should go to the emergency room. Whatever the individualized plan, it should be written down on the discharge papers and understood by the patient and caregivers. A medication box can be used to help organize the patient's pills. Mistakes are less likely to occur if medications are given around mealtimes and bedtime. The drug list should be scrutinized by both nurse and physicians before discharge to eliminate any unnecessary medications for use at home. A general rule of

Table 14-3 CLIENT/FAMILY TEACHING: MEDICATION MANAGEMENT

- Have one place at home where all medications are kept.
- Organize pills by times of day they are taken. If using a medication box, medications for the entire day can be prepared in the morning but should still be checked again before taking them.
- Take your pills at the same time each day. Work with your nurse to develop a schedule that fits your lifestyle. Taking pills with meals helps many people to better manage several medications.
- Do not keep pills in the bathroom. The humidity can damage them. The kitchen cupboard may be a safer place.
- Keep all medicines out of the reach of grandchildren. Many pills taken by older people can be lethal to small children.
- Keep a list of your daily medications in a conspicuous place, such as taped to the refrigerator, so it is easy to see and refer to.
- If you have memory problems, keep a book or journal to cross off pills when you take them. A medication box can help with this also. Don't hesitate to ask family members to help.
- If you miss a dose and it is not too long after the scheduled time, take the missed dose. If it is close to the time for the next dose, do not double up, but get back on schedule as soon as possible.
- Diuretics should be taken in the morning so they don't make you have to get up to urinate at night.
- Take all of your antibiotics as the doctor ordered. Although you may feel better after a few days, if you don't continue taking the pills the entire length of time, the most resistant germs will still be in your body, and could cause you to have a worse infection later. Although you may be tempted to save some antibiotics for a subsequent infection to save money, there is also no guarantee that your next infection will be susceptible to the same medicine.
- Refill your prescriptions on time. Do not wait until it is gone; you may be unable to get it filled immediately. This is particularly important for your heart and blood pressure medicines. Skipping doses or days can lead to heart problems, elevated blood pressure, and even stroke.
- Do not cut pills in half to save money. Your doctor or nurse practitioner bases the care they plan for you on the expectation that you are following their recommendations. You only hurt your own health and make it more difficult to treat you by making changes of which the doctor is not informed.
- Do not use alcohol when taking your medications unless you have discussed this with your doctor. Some drugs are made stronger when mixed with alcohol in your system and can cause an overdose or even death.
- Make sure your doctor knows about any over the counter cold medicine you may need to take when ill, because some drugs can inactivate your medicine or cause it to be extra powerful and hurt you. Be a label reader and an informed consumer.
- Even if your blood pressure is "normal" or "good" when you check it or it is checked in the office, this does not mean you no longer have a problem and can stop taking your medicine. Remember, your blood pressure medication is what is helping it to be normal. There are often no signs of high blood pressure until it is so high that it can cause a stroke.
- Your best defense against having negative reactions to your medications is to know about them and work with your health care provider to keep you safe and healthy.

thumb is to start low and go slow; medications should be reduced to the essentials. A schedule to normalize pill taking with the daily routine can help improve compliance when multiple medications are required.

Polypharmacy can be avoided in some cases. However, it is highly likely that older rehabilitation clients will have multiple chronic health problems that are treated by a medication regimen. This requires GRNs to be knowledgeable about the possible negative effects of polypharmacy, many of which can be avoided through carefully planned nursing care.

ABUSE OF ELDERS

GRNs work with older adults in a variety of settings and situations. Because the majority

of patients seen in acute rehabilitation are discharged home, numbers of disabled older adults living in the community are likely to increase. Likewise, as the population ages, so will the number of elderly requiring assistance with activities of daily living, placing strains on family caregivers and taxing the already overburdened staff of long-term health care facilities. Trends such as these, as well as cuts in Medicare and Medicaid funding, suggest that additional stressors will be introduced into these care situations, perhaps putting many older adults at higher risk for mistreatment or abuse.

The National Center on Elder Abuse estimated that 818,000 older Americans were victims of some type of domestic abuse in 1994 (Thobaben, 1996). Others estimated that 1.5

million elders are victims of abuse or mistreatment each year (Frost & Willette, 1994). Pritchard (1995) stated that 5% to 10% of elders experience some kind of abuse. The vast majority of cases are hidden or unreported, yet abuse of elders is likely to be an increasing problem as the number of aged in this country grows. The use of the term *abuse of elders* is preferred to *elder abuse* (by some) as more concise and avoiding possible offense to the aged. However, the majority of the literature, as well as recent texts on family violence, still refers to "elder abuse" when discussing mistreatment of the elderly. Both terms are used here to refer to violence against older adults.

Types of Abuse

There are several types of elder abuse that are discussed in the literature. Those types most frequently cited include physical abuse (including sexual), psychological or emotional abuse, material or financial abuse, and neglect. Some authors also include violation of constitutional rights as another category. Pritchard (1995) named four categories of abuse: physical, psychological, sociological, and legal. Sengstock and Barrett (1992) distinguished six types of abuse or neglect: psychological or emotional neglect, psychological or emotional abuse, violation of personal rights, financial abuse, physical neglect, and direct physical abuse. Using this system, degrees of abuse or neglect can be specified. Abuse can also be divided into categories of active and passive. Active abuse would include such things as assault, battery, and other forms of aggressive violence. Passive abuse involves the presence of threats of bodily harm and instilling fear in the victim. Whatever the categories used, abuse of elders can range from physical beating or gross neglect to financial abuse as in stealing money and property. Several kinds of abuse are often present at once, and abuse or neglect tends to be recurring (Quinn & Tomita, 1986). Case Study 14.2 provides an example.

CASE STUDY 14.2
Abuse of Elder by an Adult Child

Fred Orston was a widowed 83 year old man who had progressive osteoarthritis and chronic respiratory disease. His only daughter, Ellen, age 49, had come to live with him when it became difficult for him to care for himself in such activities as shopping, paying bills, and preparing meals. Ellen worked evenings and nights full-time as a waitress at a restaurant 20 minutes away. She had three grown children, none of whom lived at home, and was single. Fred was well known in the community, because he had been a resident in the small town most of his life. Many of the neighbors knew him, because he often walked around the block before the degeneration of his joints due to arthritis and further respiratory problems from emphysema. After Ellen moved in to care for him, Fred was seen less and less in the neighborhood. Concerned friends and neighbors asked the daughter about Fred's health, but she told them that he was bedfast, and she was evasive of further questions. Telephone calls and visits to the home by friends were unanswered. A woman who lived next door finally called the police when she heard yelling coming from inside the house, fearing for "Fred's welfare." On entering the home, the house was found to be neatly kept except for one back bedroom. Fred was found sitting in a chair in that room, door closed, appearing emaciated and despondent. His surroundings were filthy, and he was dressed in dirty clothes that smelled of dried urine and feces. He told the police, "I never wanted to be a burden." Fred suffered from malnutrition and neglect. He was taken to the hospital, then discharged in satisfactory condition with daily home health aide care. When Ellen was questioned, she expressed anger and resentment at being an only child and having to "give up my life" to take care of her ailing father "after I raised three kids of my own by myself." She had promised her mother that she would not put her dad in a nursing home. It was also discovered that she had cashed his pension and Social Security checks and spent them on clothes and entertainment for herself. Ellen was guilty of neglect as well as psychological and financial abuse.

It is important to note, however, that elders may also exhibit abusive behavior toward their caregivers, and this is not uncommon. This might include hitting, slapping, throwing things, and yelling. Caregivers also cite other behaviors used by elders to control the situation: crying, pouting, manipulating, invading privacy, calling the police, and physical violence (Steinmetz, 1988). Reasons for this behavior in the elder should be explored but are likely related to frustration, feelings of hopelessness or loss of control, or to psychiatric disorders. Adverse effects of medications, electrolyte imbalances, or other pathophysiological conditions should be ruled out.

The major category of abuse against elders is thought to be neglect of a dependent elder (Campbell & Humphreys, 1993). Neglect may take the form of ignoring the person's normal physical needs, such as food, drink, and elimination, or withholding nutrition or medication. Emotional isolation and verbal abuse often accompany neglect. It would seem, then, that older adults in long-term care or in need of rehabilitation are a high-risk group for several types of abuse.

Characteristics of Abusers

One of the most popular theories to explain elder abuse is the stress model, which states that elders who become abused have created extreme levels of stress for their caregiver, resulting in an intolerable burden that leads to mistreatment. Wilson summarized caregiver stress theory by stating that the hypothesis is that "elder's physical, emotional, and financial dependency needs create an unfair and inescapable relationship with the caregiver" (1992, p. 69), which leads to abuse. More recent research, however, suggests that "the dependency of the victim may simply be a catalyst for abuse in a caretaker who cannot cope effectively" (Barnett, Miller-Perrin, & Perrin, 1997, p. 26). Buckwalter, Campbell, Gerdner, and Garand (1996) supported this view with four case studies of rural caregivers of persons with dementia. These researchers found that several factors were associated with abuse in caregiving situations. These included "denial and maladaptive personality characteristics in the caregiver, and anxiety and lack of knowledge" (Buckwalter et al., 1996, p. 249). Similarly, Saveman, Hallberg, and Norberg (1996) found in a study of 44 cases of elder abuse within families that this was a complex problem and was related to the inability of the caregiver to meet the care demands of the elder. A history of violence on the part of the caregiver was found to be a recurring theme. Thus, current research supports the notion that abusers are more likely to have social, psychological, or emotional problems, which when combined with a high life stress, can create an abusive situation. This would suggest that elder abuse is more highly related to characteristics of the perpetrator than the victim. In either case, however, the role of the nurse may be crucial in preventing mistreatment of elders in the long-term care setting or the home. Nurses must assess the entire family dynamics and social support system and take appropriate actions in high-risk cases.

Sense of coherence (developed by Antonovsky) is an orientation to life that can help prevent breakdown related to stress through the use of appropriate coping strategies. Gallagher et al. (1994) found that caregivers of sick elders needed to be able to cope by redefining the relationship with the dependent. This research suggested that there was a threshhold effect of the nature of patient disability on the protective effects of the sense of coherence. Sense of coherence protected against role overload and could be used to predict role overload. Additionally, care of a patient with functional impairments and dementia was positively associated with role overload.

Given current findings, care for the caregiver is particularly important if potential abusive situations are to be avoided. Pritchard (1995) lists five main factors that caregivers said pushed them over the edge into abuse: (1) behavior traits of the person (patient), (2) tasks that they had to perform on the person's behalf, (3) frustration, (4) the carer's sense of isolation, and (5) lack of services or other support. Stressors such as burnout, lack of knowledge or training, and increased care demands are likely contributing factors (Wierucka & Goodridge, 1996). The nurse is in an ideal position to connect the caregiver with support services that can buffer against the effects of the stress of caregiving. This is especially important for those who care for elders with Alzheimer's-type dementia, because this is associated with abuse (Barnett et al., 1997). Caregiver support is available in many areas for those caring for the cognitively impaired. The nurse should know about resources in the community and initiate appropriate referrals.

Nurses need to be aware of the risk factors and typical characteristics of those involved with elder abuse. A study by Trevitt and Gallagher (1996) showed that nurses in Canada and Australia were not knowledgeable about types of elder abuse, nor comfortable in dealing with these situations. It is important for nurses to remember that mistreatment of the elderly crosses cultural and socioeconomic barriers. There is no one "type" of victim or perpetrator. There is conflicting evidence for arguments on all sides of the concern, such as the characteristics of socioeconomic class or gender of abusers or victims. However, contributing factors to abuse include increased dependency, the presence of psychological problems, a history of abuse or poor family relations, poor living conditions, financial difficulties, and behavioral problems of the person or caregiver (Pritchard, 1995).

The abuser is often a family member or relative and often lives with the victim (Decalmer & Glendenning, 1993). The perpetrator is more likely to be a man who has a history of abuse or violence or has been abused himself (Pritchard, 1996). Spouse abuse is probably more common than previously thought, and includes men as victims as well. Abusers are more likely to have social, emotional, or psychological problems or be users of drugs or alcohol. High life stress and care demands as well as poor coping abilities, lack of resources, and knowledge deficits are also common characteristics of abusers (Buckwalter et al., 1996).

Loneliness can contribute to financial abuse of the elderly. Elders who feel isolated and have no significant social support system or family members are easy victims for opportunists. One particular scenario that seems to recur is the younger couple living in the neighborhood who befriend the lonely widow with ailing health. The woman feels a need to acknowledge the favors they do for her such as mowing the lawn, providing transportation to the doctor's office, and generally "looking after" her. She may leave them her home or other money in her will or even legally "adopt" them so they become heirs to what she owns when she dies. In extreme cases, the "caretakers" who prey on such isolated individuals will steal from them while they are living, handle their finances, abuse or neglect them, and try to keep others away, feeling threatened if they perceive that neighbors or others may be moving in on their territory. This is one reason why it is essential that GRNs who act as advocates for the elderly in their communities be knowledgeable about resources and support groups available. GRNs should take a proactive approach to preventing abuse of older adults by promoting access to community resources, activities, and educational opportunities. Such interventions can help older adults cope with isolation and feelings of loneliness, strengthening their support systems and de-creasing the likelihood of their becoming victims of abuse.

Characteristics of the Victim

Several early studies and texts characterized "typical" victims of elder abuse as being female, older than 80, vulnerable, having dementia, and being functionally impaired and lonely (Hocking, 1988; Tomlin, 1989). The majority of literature in the 1980s supported this idea. Conflicting information was provided by Pillemer and Finkelhor (1988), suggesting that spouse abuse was higher than previously thought, and that men were often victimized. Their research also contradicted other stereotypes, finding that the victims of abuse did not appear more ill or disabled than others. Pritchard (1996) maintains, however, that most victims are women, and most abusers are men, although agreeing that research does not support the stereotype of the victim as being a woman older than 75 and dependent and the abuser as a middle-aged woman (often the daughter acting as caregiver).

Despite conflicting research and new evidence that may suggest a changing pattern in the 1990s, there are several factors that emerge as common in the literature (Table 14–4). Many of those who are abused are confused or demented. There are likely to be more female than male victims, and women may be more severely injured than men when comparing extent of abuse (Pritchard, 1995, 1996). Decalmer and Glendenning (1993) summarized the characteristics of most research done on elder abuse before 1990. The profile of the abused person they suggested included the following traits: elderly female, physically or mentally impaired, socially isolated and depressed, an abusing parent in

Table 14–4 RISK FACTORS FOR ELDER ABUSE (VICTIM)

- Lives alone or with another person (shared living arrangement)
- Elderly
- Poor or of limited means
- Poor health
- Widowed
- Significant functional or cognitive limitations
- Female (more than male, proportionately)
- Socially isolated
- Dependent on others
- History of family violence

the past, lower socioeconomic class, stubborn, willing to adopt the sick role, and unable to live independently. The presence of such factors should alert the nurse to the potential for victimization.

Detection and Prevention

A thorough physical assessment is necessary to detect possible abuse. GRNs working in home care, clinic settings, long-term care facilities, or acute rehabilitation may encounter older adults who have been physically abused or neglected. Detection is extremely difficult in many elders, because many of the signs and symptoms are not only normal parts of aging (Decalmer & Glendenning, 1993) but could be present in a person who is trying to maintain self-care and may experience falls, bruises, and emotional lability (as a result of stroke or other related pathophysiology). However, some specific interventions merit mention. The nurse should note the size, color, and location of bruising, especially on the upper arms and thighs. Clustering of bruises of different colors (yellow, green, blue, faded) may indicate that an individual has been repeatedly hit or slapped. The shoulders and inner arms can also be checked for fingerprint type bruises indicating grabbing, shaking, or squeezing. Unexplained burns should be suspect. For the fragile aged, skin tears or pressure sores may be present. Of particular suspicion should be those cases in which the elder presents with poor hygiene, malnutrition, dehydration, and withdrawal.

Sexual abuse is an additional area to which

Table 14–5 INDICATIONS OF POSSIBLE ELDER ABUSE

- Poor hygiene
- Unexplained bruises of different stages of healing
- Broken bones
- Malnutrition
- Dehydration
- Depressed mood
- Withdrawn, fearful
- Cowering
- History of treatment in a variety of facilities and by different physicians
- Person left alone in the home
- Person brought for treatment by someone other than the caregiver
- Elder expresses feelings of hopelessness, helplessness
- Elder expresses ambivalent feelings toward family

the nurse should be alert. Although this is a statistically rare occurrence among the elderly in comparison with the general population, it is not considered uncommon and is probably significantly underreported. There are several commonly seen situations in which sexual abuse of elders takes place. Pritchard (1996) cites three commonly seen types of cases: history of incest (usually between son and mother), marital situations, and the abuse of older gay men by younger men in the community. Assessment of the family situation is crucial in order to detect possible sexual mistreatment of vulnerable elders. The nurse should note any signs of discomfort when

Table 14–6 NURSING INDICATIONS IN THE PREVENTION OF ELDER ABUSE

- Establish a trusting relationship with the elder.
- Be able to refer families to resources available in the community.
- Strengthen social supports.
- Encourage regular respite for the caregiver.
- Identify caregivers at highest risk to be abusers, and target interventions to prevent stress from caregiver burden.
- Interview the patient and family or caregiver to find out normal patterns for stress management.
- Identify possible scenarios and facilitate strategies to cope with the situation.
- Observe family interactions, dynamics, and body language.
- Encourage single patients to stay involved and connected socially.
- Be aware of risk factors and contributing factors.
- Perform thorough physical assessments and carefully document findings, including appearance, nutritional state, skin condition, mental attitude and awareness, and need for aids to enhance sensory perception.
- If abuse is suspected, interview caregiver and other possible informants to confirm or refute suspicions.
- Know the laws governing reporting of abuse.
- Encourage the patient to let a trusted person know where valuable papers are stored.

Table 14–7 WAYS TO REDUCE THE POTENTIAL FOR ABUSE

- Stay active, keep involved in social activities.
- Have access to a telephone and use of it in private.
- Maintain contact with family and friends.
- Know your financial situation and when to expect deposits.
- Know where your important files are kept.
- Have a family member or friend visit regularly unannounced.
- Have an emergency safety plan if you are concerned about potential abuse.

the person walks or sits in a chair. Physical examinations may reveal vaginal or rectal tears, bleeding, bruising of the inner thighs, buttocks, or legs, or other indicators of forced sexual activity.

In addition to assessing for signs of abuse (Table 14–5), the nurse can use preventive techniques such as those noted in Table 14–6. Interviewing should be done on a one-on-one basis with the possible victim and the nurse. The nurse should ask direct, yet sensitive, questions if abuse is suspected (Appendices 14A, 14B, and 14C). Victims are often reluctant to discuss their situation if abuse is present, partly for fear of retaliation from the abuser. Opening the door to discussion of the elder's fears or worries is the beginning of treatment. The nurse's main concern should be for the victim's welfare and safety, but a non-judgmental attitude must be maintained for effective intervention.

GRNs should caution patients and their families to carefully check out any person they allow into their home to provide care. Several ways to reduce the potential for abuse appear in Table 14–7. Many so-called professional caregivers work independently but are substance abusers who are later found to be abusive to the client. The nurse should be able to provide names of reliable agencies who do extensive background checks on employees. This should not, however, take the place of educating patients on ways to protect themselves from those who might try to take advantage of them.

SUICIDE AMONG THE ELDERLY

Contrary to popular belief, the incidence of suicide among the elderly is the highest of any age group, even teenagers (Bowles, 1993; Sorenson, 1991). Suicide rates among the elderly declined between 1933 and 1981, in part because of the increasing proportion of older women present in the population (McIntosh, 1984; Strasburger & Welpton, 1991). The suicide rates for African-American men older than age 85 have tripled in the last few decades; however, white men older than the age of 85 have the highest suicide rate of all elderly groups (Matteson, Bearon, & McConnell, 1997). Persons age 65 years and older accounted for 20.9% of suicides (Courage, Godbey, Ingram, Schramm, & Hale, 1993; McIntosh, 1992). Adamek and Kaplan (1996) reported that in Western society, those older than 65 committed 30% of all suicides, 10% of suicides in the United States.

Some gender and ethnic differences in suicide are apparent. White men older than the age of 85 are particularly at risk, whereas elderly women less frequently commit suicide. Women historically tended to use pills or poisoning to commit suicide; men used more violent means. However, more recent research showed an increased rate of suicide among older women, and a larger proportion using firearms as lethal weapons (Adamek & Kaplan, 1996; Meehan, Saltzman, & Sattin, 1991). The increased use of firearms may indicate either a change in culture or, more likely, a more serious intent to succeed.

Suicide rates vary between countries, although patterns have emerged. Suicide has been strongly correlated with age in England, Wales, Germany, Austria, Switzerland, and Hungary and positively correlated (but less strongly) with age in Canada, Finland, and Australia for women (Osgood, 1986). Variations in suicide rates may have less to do with age and gender than with cultural and environmental conditions. Economic variables, such as poverty, are also thought to play a role.

Differences in the means used for suicide are also evident. Elders more often use firearms or other lethal means (such as hanging) to commit suicide, indicating a total intention of death (McIntosh & Santos, 1986). They may go to remote places where they are not easily found, in contrast to teenagers, for whom attempted suicide may be a cry for help. For the older adult, suicide is often carefully planned and more likely to be successful (Osgood, 1986). Additionally, elders may give fewer or no warning signs of a suicidal intent. Despite these statistics, less research or attention has been given to prevention of elderly suicide than in younger age groups. This is perhaps reflective of the value placed on older adults by society.

The presence of chronic illness and suicide rate appear to be linked. The suicide rate has been especially documented in the aged with cancer (Conwell, Caine, & Olsen, 1990) and chronic respiratory disease (Horton-Deutsch, Clark, & Farran, 1992). Courage et al. (1993) found that elders viewed suicide as a way of staying in control over the dying process. These researchers found that the primary cause of suicide among elders was intolerable life circumstances, but that they desired to talk about ending their lives, depression, and suicide. Linn and Lester studied 40 German suicide notes, revealing "suicide notes of older people had fewer feelings of inadequacy and more indications of illness and grief over widowhood" (1996, p. 370).

Risk factors associated with suicide are many. These include bereavement, stroke (especially left-sided), severe medical illness, history of depression, alcoholism, white and male, a visit to the physician within 1 month of the suicide attempt, and several specific medical diagnoses (Table 14–8). Of particular interest is the incidence of persons visiting a physician prior to the suicide attempt. In one study, 9% to 11% of 268 subjects in the sample had visited the doctor during the week preceding the suicide attempt, and 40% saw the physician during the month before the attempt (Michel, Runeson, Valach, & Wasserman, 1997). Many of these subjects expressed ideas of suicide to the physician, suggesting that health care professionals need to be more alert to risk factors and help-seeking behaviors exhibited prior to a person's attempting suicide. This study supported previous research. Forsell, Jorm, and Windblad (1997) researched suicidal thoughts in the elderly. Among 969 subjects in Sweden, 13.3% had recent suicidal thoughts, often associated with depression. Suicidal thoughts were also associated with an increase in physical dysfunction, institutionalization, visual problems, being single, use of psychotropic drugs, history of psychiatric disorders, and advanced age.

In today's society, GRNs need to be knowledgeable about depression, alcoholism, and suicide patterns in the elderly. These are often neglected components in nurses' education, so warning signs may go unnoticed (McIntosh, 1987). Suicide may be a negative outcome of depression or alcohol misuse. Knowledge of risk factors, as summarized in Table

Table 14–8 RISK FACTORS FOR ELDERLY SUICIDE

Cancer or fear of cancer
Chronic respiratory disease
Presence of other chronic disease (such as AIDS; degenerative illness; Parkinson's, Huntington's, or Alzheimer's disease; those on renal dialysis)
Intractable pain
Diagnosis of terminal illness
Feelings of isolation
Poor social support
Single, divorced, or widowed
Alcoholism
Depression
Drug abuse
Psychiatric disorders
Multiple losses, bereavement
White male older than 75
Desire to have control over the end of their life
Feelings of an intolerable life situation
Feelings of uselessness, hopelessness, or inadequacy
Chronic sleep problems
Strong need for independence
Inflexible personality type (need to be in control and avoid uncertainty)
History of suicide in family
Previous attempted suicide

14–8, is essential. Depression is highly correlated with suicide. Because the GRN works with individuals and families who are at high risk of depression, nursing interventions are indicated. Table 9–3 reviewed signs and symptoms of geriatric depression. Alcoholics have a significantly higher suicide rate than the general population (Strasburger & Welpton, 1991). Yet, late onset alcoholism is highly treatable (Osgood, 1986). "Early detection and treatment of depression, alcoholism, and suicidal ideation is one key to suicide prevention" (Osgood, 1986, p. 300).

Risk assessment is important when working with older adults in long-term care. A mental examination should become a routine part of assessment. Mental status screenings are convenient and efficient tools to assist the GRN with this evaluation. Questions about depression and alcohol or drug use should be asked. If suicidal tendencies or history is suspected, more direct questions should be asked. Contrary to previously held beliefs, direct questioning about suicidal intent does not encourage the person to follow through with suicide. Any verbal statement by an elder that suggests a desire to die, that life has no meaning, should be taken seriously and not simply as attention-seeking behavior (Strasburger & Welpton, 1991). In particular, the nurse should determine whether the person has an expressed suicide plan with the means and intention to carry it out (Badger, 1995).

For the person with suicidal ideations, the nurse must take definitive action. The physician and other team members should be consulted immediately, and a treatment plan implemented. Removal of all means of suicide, including sharp objects, nonessential medication, or items that could be used as weapons, is indicated. More frequent monitoring and supervision should be instituted while the person is at acute risk (Valente, 1993). Psychiatric interventions by trained medical professionals should be started. Psychotropic medications may be needed, but care should be taken that these are used appropriately and with discretion, because overdose of these types of pills is a common means of suicide. The person may need to be transferred out of the rehabilitation facility and into inpatient psychiatric care. The person's expectations about old age should be addressed. The person must also perceive that help is immediately available when needed. Social support systems should be identified, encouraged, and strengthened. Religious leaders previously acquainted with the person may be included as part of the team treatment to enhance spiritual ties that can buffer against stress.

The development, availability, and use of services that promote mental and physical health and increase socialization are imperative for preventing suicide among the elderly. Such outreach programs have been shown to improve case findings and potential for early intervention (Mellick, Buckwalter, & Stolley, 1992). Educational programs for staff working with the aged are also needed.

A significant area in which the GRN may have influence is that of social support. Promoting links to societal interactions and the development of significant relationships can prevent depression and isolation associated with increased suicide rates. Also, as discussed previously, elders having strong religious affiliations and involvement seem to cope better with chronic problems and losses, and report a higher level of satisfaction with life, than those who do not. However, one study demonstrated that the specific religious affiliation must be considered when assessing for risk of depression, because Pentecostals

were found to be at three times greater risk for major depression than those of other religions (Meador et al., 1992). Self-esteem and perceived quality of life may be related to suicide rates. Several studies have shown that satisfaction with life as one ages is associated with social ties. For example, successful aging has been linked to living with or having a spouse, and the strong level of attachment to a person (a spouse in particular) is positively correlated to a higher perceived quality of life (Rickelman et al., 1994). Additionally, the spouse has been shown to significantly influence positive functional outcomes of stroke patients (Baker, 1993). Likewise, persons with spinal cord injury (albeit of younger age) reported that contact with others who share common problems helped in adjustment to injury (Payne, 1993).

Self-esteem is closely related to a person's self-concept. In later life, many losses occur, such as the death of a spouse, retirement from a job, loss of friends, and decreased earning potential. Ageism can also undermine self-esteem in elders because self-esteem may be based, at least partially, on a reflection of the perceptions of others. Case Study 14.3 presents a situation related to elderly suicide.

CASE STUDY 14.3
Suicide

Mr. Jenkins was a 76 year old man with a suspected history of alcoholism, admitted to the inpatient rehabilitation unit after a stroke that left him with mild lower extremity weakness, moderate upper extremity paresis, and also some dysphagia. Mr. Jenkins was divorced and lived alone in a small apartment, having no contact with his ex-wife. He also had two grown daughters. He was estranged from the elder, but the younger daughter lived nearby and visited him occasionally on the rehabilitation unit, although their relationship seemed strained. He claimed no religious affiliation or church attendance. The friends he "hung out with" at the bar he frequented were his main support system. At the first team meeting, several concerns were voiced by the staff. Although the patient stated that his main goal was to return home and live independently as before, he displayed little motivation during therapy sessions, although his prognosis was good. The speech therapist felt that he was tolerating a mechanical soft diet well, but had a rather flat affect. The primary nurse shared that the patient had had some delirium tremens prior to admission and now seemed anxious, at times showing hand tremors. He had also made a statement on admission that his life was now worthless. The staff psychologist was consulted and Mr. Jenkins was diagnosed with clinical depression and scheduled for regular counseling sessions. In light of his suspected alcoholism, he was also referred to Alcoholics Anonymous, but the patient exhibited no interest in pursuing this. As treatment went on, Mr. Jenkins seemed to be making satisfactory progress. Before discharge, Mr. Jenkins was scheduled for a home pass. Mr. Jenkins had seemed more cheerful, although quiet, and by now could walk well with a walker and minimal assistance. One of his friends picked him up and dropped him off at home. When Mr. Jenkins did not return from his pass at the scheduled time, the nurses became concerned. The daughter telephoned shortly afterward to say that her father had killed himself at home by hanging. The staff was in shock. This was the first experience with a patient's suicide that this team had encountered. The unit psychologist held an inservice session to help team members deal with their feelings of anger, disbelief, and guilt. This experience helped heighten the awareness of the team to the issue of elderly suicide, an event that they had previously thought was unlikely to occur among their patients. New policies and procedures were implemented as a result, and risk factors brought to the forefront. The impact of this incident, however, had long-lasting effects on the staff.

GRNs can help older adults to strengthen social ties and promote a positive self-esteem through various techniques. One such strategy is group therapy that is designed to help meet the psychosocial needs of the aged while promoting social interaction. This is particularly important in long-term care facilities, where elders may be more confined, than for those dwelling in the community. Support programs have been linked with postponing death and nursing home placement, as well as decreasing length of hospital stay (Oktay & Volland, 1990).

Such groups can be based on any number of premises. Nurses may wish to form groups based on specific diagnoses, depending on the types of patients in the facility (e.g., stroke support group, chronic obstructive pulmonary disease support group, amputee group). Including the family or significant others may be preferred. Groups could center around a certain activity, such as upper extremity strengthening, ambulating, or personal care. The GRN could work with the facility's activity director to plan meaningful projects that promote social interaction as well as leisure, based on the needs of the residents. Pet therapy groups are often therapeutic. Crafts or cooking classes may appeal to many of the women residents. The formation of a bowling league may encourage men to become more socially active while promoting a healthy competitive spirit. Special parties based on holidays or events should include and encourage family participation, thus strengthening familial ties and promoting positive memories and interactions. For example, some senior housing centers have regular birthday brunches where the family can sponsor a party for their loved one right in the facility and invite the rest of the residents to join in the celebration. This gives residents events to look forward to and allows them to be honored in the presence of family and friends.

Long-term care facilities (LTCFs) in general need to examine the layout and furnishings of the building to allow for installation and maintenance of items that promote healthy leisure activity. Pool tables, exercise bikes, bowling alleys, grounds suitable for walking, and pleasant surroundings all are important. The environment in LTCFs should promote independence for those who make it their home.

SUMMARY

To summarize, GRNs should be knowledgeable about available resources within the community and local health care systems in order to advocate quality care for older adults. By examining psychosocial concerns that influence the rehabilitation process, GRNs can enhance the positive aspects of a person's support network. By identifying and enlisting the help of positive support persons, social support is strengthened. The person may need assistance in identifying and developing coping mechanisms to deal with an uncertain life situation. Spiritual well-being and the inclusion of the spiritual leader as part of the health care team should be explored. Quality of life issues should be considered, particularly within the context of the person's life situation. The person's ability to deal with loss and grief should also be examined in relation to coping with disability or disease. Sexuality and the need to express oneself as a sexual being throughout the life span should be addressed with each person. Lastly, the potential for negative outcomes related to patients' or families' inability to cope or adjust to changes in one's life situation should be considered, particularly the potential for mistreatment of the elderly or the potential for suicide.

REFERENCES

Adamek, M. E., & Kaplan, M. S. (1996). The growing use of firearms by suicidal older women, 1979–1992: A research note. *Suicide and Life-Threatening Behavior, 26*(1), 71–77.

Aiken, L. R. (1995). *Aging: An introduction to gerontology.* Thousand Oaks, CA: Sage.

Badger, J. (1995). Reaching out to the suicidal patient. *American Journal of Nursing, 95*(3), 24–32.

Baker, A. C. (1993). The spouse's positive effect on the stroke patient's recovery. *Rehabilitation Nursing, 18*(1), 30–33.

Barnett, O. W., Miller-Perrin, C. L., & Perrin, R. D. (1997). *Family violence across the lifespan.* Thousand Oaks, CA: Sage.

Bowles, L. (1993). Logical conclusion?: Mental health, older people. *Nursing Times, 89*(31), 32–34.

Buckwalter, S. C., Campbell, J., Gerdner, L. A., & Garand, L. (1996). Elder mistreatment among rural family caregivers of persons with Alzheimer's disease and related disorders. *Journal of Family Nursing, 2*(3), 249–265.

Campbell, J., & Humphreys, J. (1993). *Nursing care of survivors of family violence.* St. Louis: Mosby.

Conwell, Y., Caine, E., & Olsen, K. (1990). Suicide and cancer in late life. *Hospital and Community Psychiatry, 41,* 1334–1339.

Courage, M., Godbey, K., Ingram, D., Schramm, L., & Hale, W. (1993). Suicide in the elderly: Staying in control. *Journal of Psychosocial Nursing, 31*(7), 26–31.

Cummings, S. R., Phillips, S. L., Wheat, M. E., Black, D., Gossby, E., Wlodarczyk, D., Trafton, P., Jergesen, H., Hunter Winograd, C., & Hulley, S. B. (1988). Recovery of function after hip fractures: The role of social supports. *Journal of the American Geriatrics Society, 36,* 801–806.

Decalmer, P., & Glendenning, F. (Eds.). (1993). *The mistreatment of elderly people.* London: Sage.

Dunn, S. A., Lewis, S. L., Bonner, P. N., & Meize-Grochowski, R. (1994). Quality of life for spouses of CAPD patients. *ANNA Journal, 21,* 237–247, 257.

Easton, K. L., Rawl, S. M., Zemen, D., Kwiatkowski, S., & Burczyk, B. (1995). The effects of nursing follow-up on the coping strategies used by rehabilitation patients after discharge. *Rehabilitation Nursing Research, 4*(4), 119–127.

Forsell, Y., Jorm, A. F., & Windblad, B. (1997). Suicidal thoughts and associated factors in an elderly population. *Acta Psychiatrica Scandinavica, 95,* 108–111.

Frost, M. H., & Willette, K. (1994). Risk for abuse/neglect: Documentation of assessment data and diagnoses. *Journal of Gerontological Nursing, 29* (8), 37–45.

Gallagher, T. J., Wagenfeld, M. O., Baro, F., & Haepers, K. (1994). Sense of coherence, coping and caregiver role overload. *Social Science Medicine, 19,* 1615–1622.

Gass, K. A. (1987). The health of conjugally bereaved older widows: The role of appraisal, coping and resources. *Research in Nursing & Health, 10,* 39–47.

Glickstein, J. K. (1989). Polypharmacy: Drug-induced illness in the elderly. *Focus on Geriatric Care & Rehabilitation, 2*(8), 1–8.

Grossberg, G. T., & Grossberg, J. A. (1998). Epidemiology of psychotherapeutic drug use in older adults. *Clinics in Geriatric Medicine: Psychotherapeutic Agents in Older Adults, 14*(1), 1–5.

Hainsworth, M. A. (1996). Helping spouses with chronic sorrow related to multiple sclerosis. *Journal of Psychosocial Nursing, 34*(6), 36–40.

Hainsworth, M. A., Eakes, G. G., & Burke, M. L. (1994). Coping with chronic sorrow. *Issues in Mental Health Nursing, 15,* 59–66.

Harden, J. T. (1997). Nursing diagnoses related to psychosocial alterations. In M. A. Matteson, E. S. McConnell, & A. D. Linton (Eds.), *Gerontological nursing: Concepts and practice* (2nd ed., pp. 661–735). Philadelphia: W. B. Saunders.

Heidrich, S. M. (1996). Mechanisms related to psychological well-being in older women with chronic illnesses: Age and disease comparisons. *Research in Nursing and Health, 19,* 225–235.

Hocking, E. D. (1988). Miscare—A form of abuse in the elderly. *Update, 15,* 2411–2419.

Horton-Deutsch, S., Clark, D., & Farran, C. (1992). Chronic dyspnea and suicide in elderly men. *Hospital and Community Psychiatry, 43,* 1198–1204.

Kemp, B. J., Adams, B. M., & Campbell, M. L. (1997). Depression and life satisfaction in aging polio survivors versus age-matched controls: Relation to postpolio syndrome, family functioning, and attitude toward disability. *Archives of Physical Medicine and Rehabilitation, 78,* 187–192.

Krause, N., & Borawski-Clark, E. (1995). Social class differences in social support among older adults. *Gerontologist, 35,* 498–508.

Kubler-Ross, E. (1969). *On death and dying.* New York: Macmillan.

Landis, B. J. (1996). Uncertainty, spiritual well-being, and psychosocial adjustment to chronic illness. *Issues in Mental Health Nursing, 17,* 217–231.

Linn, M., & Lester, D. (1996). Content differences in suicide notes by gender and age: Serendipitous findings. *Psychological Reports, 78,* 370.

Logan, J. R., & Spitze, G. (1994). Informal support

and the use of formal services by older Americans. *Journal of Gerontology: Social Sciences, 49* (1), S25–S34.

Lopez, M. A., & Mermelstein, R. J. (1995). A cognitive-behavioral program to improve geriatric rehabilitation outcome. *Gerontologist, 35,* 696–700.

Martin, S. D. (1995). Coping with chronic illness. *Home Healthcare Nurse, 13*(4), 50–54.

Matteson, M. A., Bearon, L. B., & McConnell, E. S. (1997). Psychosocial problems associated with aging. In M. A. Matteson, E. S. McConnell, & A. D. Linton (Eds.), *Gerontological nursing: Concepts and practice* (2nd ed., pp. 603–659). Philadelphia: W. B. Saunders.

McConnell, E. S., & Murphy, A. T. (1997). Nursing diagnoses related to physiological alterations. In M. A. Matteson, E. S. McConnell, & A. D. Linton (Eds.), *Gerontological nursing: Concepts and practice* (2nd ed., pp. 407–551). Philadelphia: W. B. Saunders.

McIntosh, J. (1984). Components of the decline in elderly suicide: Suicide among the young-old and old-old by race and sex. *Death Education, 8,* 113–124.

McIntosh, J. (1987). Suicide: Training and education needs with an emphasis on the elderly. *Gerontology and Geriatric Education, 7,* 125–139.

McIntosh, J. L. (1992). Epidemiology of suicide in the elderly. *Suicide and Life-Threatening Behavior, 22* (1), 15–35.

McIntosh, J., & Santos, J. (1986). Methods of suicide by age: Sex differences among the young and old. *International Journal of Aging and Human Development, 22,* 123–139.

Meador, K. G., Koenig, H. G., Hughes, D. C., Blazer, D. G., Turnbull, J., & George, L. K. (1992). Religious affiliation and major depression. *Hospital and Community Psychiatry, 43,* 1204–1205.

Meehan, P., Saltzman, L., & Sattin, R. (1991). Suicides among the older United States residents: Epidemiologic characteristics and trends. *American Journal of Public Health, 81,* 1198–1200.

Mellick, E., Buckwalter, K., & Stolley, J. (1992). Suicide among elderly white men: Development of a profile. *Journal of Psychosocial Nursing, 30*(2), 29–34.

Michel, K., Runeson, B., Valach, L., & Wasserman, D. (1997). Contacts of suicide attempters with GPs prior to the event: A comparison between Stockholm and Bern. *Acta Psychiatrica Scandinavica, 95,* 94–99.

Miller, C. A. (1995). *Nursing care of older adults: Theory and practice.* Philadelphia: J. B. Lippincott.

Miller, J. F. (1992). *Coping with chronic illness: Overcoming powerlessness.* Philadelphia: F. A. Davis.

Miner, S. (1995). Racial differences in family support and formal service utilization among older persons: A nonrecursive model. *Journal of Gerontology: Social Sciences, 50B*(3), S143–S153.

Mold, J. W., Looney, S. W., Viviani, N. J., & Quiggins, P. A. (1994). Predicting the health-related

values and preferences of geriatric patients. *The Journal of Family Practice, 39,* 461–467.

Oktay, J. S., & Volland, P. J. (1990). Post-hospital support program for the frail elderly and their caregivers: A quasi-experimental evaluation. *American Journal of Public Health, 80*(1), 39–46.

Osgood, N. (1986). *Suicide and the elderly.* Rockville, MD: Aspen.

Osgood, N., & McIntosh, J. (1986). *Suicide and the elderly: An annotated bibliography and review.* Westwood, CT: Greenwood Press.

Patrick, M. (1993). Characteristics of older people and introduction to theories of aging. In D. L. Carnevali & M. Patrick (Eds.), *Nursing management for the elderly* (pp. 87–98). Philadelphia: J. B. Lippincott.

Payne, J. A. (1993). The contribution of group learning to the rehabilitation of spinal cord injury adults. *Rehabilitation Nursing, 18,* 375–379.

Picot, S. J. (1995). Rewards, costs, and coping of African American caregivers. *Nursing Research, 44*(3), 147–152.

Pillemer, K., & Finkelhor, D. (1988). The prevalence of elder abuse: A random sample survey. *Gerontologist, 28*(1), 51–57.

Pritchard, J. (1995). *The abuse of older people: A training manual for detection and prevention.* London: Jessica Kingsley Publishers.

Pritchard, J. (1996). Darkness visible . . . elder abuse. *Nursing Times, 92*(42), 26–31.

Quinn, M. J., & Tomita, S. K. (1986). *Elder abuse and neglect.* New York: Springer Publishing.

Reinhardt, J. P. (1996). The importance of friendship and family support in adaptation to chronic vision impairment. *Journal of Gerontology: Psychological Sciences, 51B,* P268–P278.

Resnick, B. (1996). Motivation in geriatric rehabilitation. *Image: Journal of Nursing Scholarship, 28* (1), 41–45.

Rickelman, B. L., Gallman, L., & Parra, H. (1994). Attachment and quality of life in older, community residing men. *Nursing Research, 43*(2), 68–72.

Roberts, J., Browne, G. B., Streiner, D., Gafni, A., Pallister, R., Hoxby, H., Drummond-Young, M., LeGris, J., & Meichenbaum, D. (1995). Problem-solving counselling or phone-call support for outpatients with chronic illness: Effective for whom? *Canadian Journal of Nursing Research, 27* (3), 111–137.

Saveman, B., Hallberg, I. R., & Norberg, A. (1996). Narratives by district nurses about elder abuse within families. *Clinical Nursing Research, 5,* 220–236.

Sengstock, M. C., & Barrett, S. A. (1992). Abuse and neglect of the elderly in family settings. In J. Campbell & J. Humphreys (Eds.), *Nursing care of survivors of family violence* (pp. 173–208). St. Louis: Mosby.

Siegel, K. (1986). Psychosocial aspects of rational suicide. *American Journal of Psychotherapy, 40,* 405–418.

Sorenson, S. (1991). Suicide among the elderly: Issues facing public health. *American Journal of Public Health, 18,* 1109–1110.

Speake, D. L., Cowart, M. E., & Pellet, K. (1989). Health perceptions and lifestyles of the elderly. *Research in Nursing and Health, 12,* 93–100.

Staab, A. S., & Hodges, L. C. (1996). *Essentials of gerontological nursing: Adaptation to the aging process.* Philadelphia: J. B. Lippincott.

Steinmetz, S. K. (1988). *Duty bound: Elder abuse and family care.* Newbury Park, CA: Sage.

Stone, J. T. (1991). Preventing physical iatrogenic problems. In W. C. Chenitz, J. T. Stone, & S. A. Salisbury (Eds.), *Clinical gerontological nursing* (pp. 359–375). Philadelphia: W. B. Saunders.

Strasburger, L., & Welpton, S. (1991). Elderly suicide: Minimizing risk for patient and professional. *Journal of Geriatric Psychiatry, 22,* 235–259.

Swonger, A. K., & Burbank, P. M. (1995). *Drug therapy and the elderly.* Boston: Jones and Bartlett.

Thobaben, M. (1996). Beyond physical care. Elder abuse and neglect. *Home Care Provider, 1*(5), 267–269.

Thomas, P. D., & Hooper, E. M. (1983). Healthy elderly: Social bonds and locus of control. *Research in Nursing and Health, 6,* 11–16.

Tomlin, S. K. (1989). *Abuse of elderly people: An unnecessary and preventable problem.* London: British Geriatrics Society.

Trevitt, C., & Gallagher, E. (1996). Elder abuse in Canada and Australia: Implications for nurses. *International Journal of Nursing Studies, 33,* 651–659.

Turner, H. A. (1996). Determinants of perceived family support and conflict: Life-course variations among the physically disabled. *International Journal of Aging and Human Development, 42*(1), 21–41.

Valente, S. (1993). Evaluating suicide risk in the medically ill patient. *Nurse Practitioner, 18*(9), 41–50.

White, N. W., Richter, J. M., & Fry, C. (1992). Coping, social support, and adaptation to chronic illness. *Western Journal of Nursing Research, 14*(2), 211–224.

Wierucka, C., & Goodridge, D. (1996). Vulnerable in a safe place: Institutional elder abuse. *Canadian Journal of Nursing Administration, 9*(3), 82–104.

Wilson, J. S. (1992). Granny dumping: A case of caregiver stress or a problem relative? *Home Healthcare Nurse, 10*(3), 69–70.

Appendix 14A

The Hwalek-Sengstock Elder Abuse Screening Test

Violation of Personal Rights or Direct Abuse

4. *Who makes decisions about your life—like how you should live or where you should live?

9. Does someone in your family make you stay in bed or tell you you're sick when you know you're not?

10. Has anyone forced you to do things you didn't want to do?

11. Has anyone taken things that belong to you without your O.K.?

15. Has anyone close to you tried to hurt you or harm you recently?

Characteristics of Vulnerability

1. Do you have anyone who spends time with you, taking you shopping or to the doctor?

3. Are you sad or lonely often?

6. Can you take your own medication and get around by yourself?

Potentially Abusive Situation

2. Are you helping to support someone?

5. Do you feel uncomfortable with anyone in your family?

7. Do you feel that nobody wants you around?

8. Does anyone in your family drink a lot?

12. Do you trust most of the people in your family?

13. Does anyone tell you that you give them too much trouble?

14. Do you have enough privacy at home?

---

*Numbers refer to the order in which items appeared on the questionnaire.
Used with permission of Melanie Hwalek and Mary G. Sengstock.

Appendix 14B

Elder Abuse Assessment Protocol

■

See figure on opposite page

General Assessment

Clothing:	Hygiene:	Grooming:	Nutrition:	Skin:
Torn _____	Body odour _____	Unkempt nails _____	Pallor _____	PAs: _____
Soiled _____	Unclean _____	Uncut nails _____	Lips _____	Sites _____
Disarrayed _____		Finger _____	Mouth _____	
		Feet _____	Hydration _____	Ulcers:
				Sites _____

Physical assessment: Evidence of:

1. Bruising:

Site: Colour of bruises/size

Shoulders	_____	_____
Buttocks	_____	_____
Thighs	_____	_____
Forearm	_____	_____
Lips	_____	_____
Mouth	_____	_____
Face	_____	_____
Eyes	_____	_____
Other	_____	_____

Colour of bruises: Please indicate black/purple/yellow
(this may give some indication of age of bruises)

Urine burns:
Sites _____

Excoriation:
Sites _____

2. Abrasion/Laceration:

Site: Colour/state

Mouth	_____	_____
Lips	_____	_____
Gums	_____	_____
Genitalia	_____	_____
Buttocks	_____	_____
Others	_____	_____

Please state colour/state: e.g. red/pink/open/
closed/scarred/scabbed/tenderness etc.

Please indicate site of bruising/abrasion/laceration on torso
Colour code: bruise (black)
Abrasion/laceration. (red)

3. Alopecia/hemorrhaging:
Comment:

6. Cognitive/emotional assessment:
- (a) Worried/anxious _____
- (b) Aggressive
- (c) Depression:
  - Sad _____
  - Loss of interest _____
  - Feeling hopeless _____
  - Withdrawn _____
  - Tearful _____
- (d) Slurred speech _____
- (e) Drowsiness _____
- (f) Reduced responsiveness _____
- (g) Cowering _____
- (h) Irritable, easily upset _____
- (i) Defensive _____
- (j) Evasive _____
- (k) Guarded _____
- (l) Suspicious _____
- (m) Confused _____
- (n) Disoriented _____
- (o) Sleep disturbances _____
- (p) Evidence of infantilization _____

Comment:

Assessor's summary and general opinion:

4. Obvious deformities: _____
Comment/site:

Contractions _____
Comment/site:

	Site
Pain	_____ _____
Tenderness	_____ _____
Swelling	_____ _____

7. Relationship with carer:
- (a) Defensive _____
- (b) Guarded _____
- (c) Hostile _____
- (d) Passive _____
- (e) Afraid _____

Any change after carer has left?

Comment:

5. Sexual abuse (by observation not examination)
Genitalia: vaginal and anal area
- Bruising
- Bleeding
- Pain _____
- Redness _____
- Itching _____
- Scratch marks _____
- Discharge _____
- Marked embarrassment evident _____
- Comments:

8. Personal possessions:
- Petty cash _____
- Toiletries _____
- Tissues
- Newspaper _____
- Writing material _____
- Stamps _____
- Confectionery _____
- Cordials _____
- Personal clothing _____

Signed: ....
Date(s): ....

From Davies, M. (1993). Recognizing abuse: An assessment tool for nurses. In P. Decalmer & F. Glendenning (Eds.), *The mistreatment of elderly people* (p. 116). London: Sage. Reprinted by permission of Sage Publications Ltd.

Appendix 14C

Carr Abuse Assessment Protocol

■

1. Relationship to patient:
   Relative _____
   Other _____

2. Age range:
   Under 21 _____
   21–39 _____
   40–59 _____
   60–75 _____
   75+ _____

3. Gender
   Male/Female

4. Marital status:
   Married _____
   Single _____
   Separated _____
   Divorced _____
   Widowed _____
   Other _____

5. Domestic arrangements:
   Alone _____
   With patient _____
   With spouse _____
   With children _____
   With others _____

6. Evidence of:
   Alcohol dependence _____
   Drug dependence _____
   Physical illness _____
   Mental illness _____
   Mental retardation _____
   Financial dependence _____
   History of family
   violence _____
   Other _____

7. Evidence of stress:
   Frustration _____
   Exhaustion _____
   Anxiety _____
   Low self-esteem _____
   Lack of leisure time _____
   Problems with
   children/marriage _____

8. Knowledge of patient's situation:

	Good	Poor
(a) Physical/emotional health		
(b) Assistance with ADLs:		
Bathing		
Dressing		
Eating		
Mobility		
Toiletting		
(c) Any treatment regime:		
Medication		
Nutrition		
Exercise		
Treatments		
Others		

9. Attitude towards patient:
   (a) Angry _____
   (b) Blaming _____
   (c) Critical _____
   (d) Over-concerned _____
   (e) Resentful _____
   (f) Non-concerned _____

10. Attitude toward staff:
    (a) Defensive _____
    (b) Aggressive _____
    (c) Irritable _____
    (d) Suspicious _____

11. Behaviour with patient during
    visiting:
    Demonstrates lack of:
    Physical contact _____
    Facial contact _____
    Eye contact _____
    Verbal contact _____

Assessor's summary and
general opinion:

Signed: ....
Date(s): ....

From Davies, M. (1993). Recognizing abuse: An assessment tool for nurses. In P. Decalmer & F. Glendenning (Eds.), *The mistreatment of elderly people* (p. 116). London: Sage. Reprinted by permission of Sage Publications Ltd.

Chapter 15

Ethical, Legal, and Moral Issues

■

Inherent in gerontological rehabilitation nursing are many ethical, legal, and moral dilemmas that the gerontological rehabilitation nurse (GRN) might face. Working with an older population brings difficult situations that will require nurses to examine their own feelings, values, and beliefs. Examples of common issues that arise include the patient's right to die, withholding and withdrawing treatment, assisted suicide, rehabilitation of the older terminally ill patient, and the use of restraints or safety devices. These are but a few of the topics that GRNs may be called on to discuss as they arise in the clinical setting. The time to examine one's feelings is before the situation occurs, not while it is occurring. This requires careful thought and discussion among GRNs and knowledge of appropriate alternatives available to patients and families. Some of these issues are discussed in this chapter in the hope that nurses will give prior thought to how they would handle certain situations. Case studies are provided for several issues to stimulate critical thinking about possible scenarios.

ETHICAL PRINCIPLES

Although making ethically correct choices is a complex process, decision-making can be thought of as generally guided by four basic principles: autonomy, beneficence, nonmaleficence, and paternalism. As these values come into conflict, an ethical or moral dilemma can result.

Each principle is discussed here briefly as a point of reference.

Autonomy refers to the person's right to make an independent decision. Nurses are taught that part of being a patient advocate is to uphold the person's autonomy. This is thought to apply to competent adults who are cognitively intact. So, exceptions to the "rule" of autonomy are people who may not be "of sound mind." This notion allows for liberal interpretation. For example, is a depressed elderly person who wishes to end his life shortly after suffering a complete and debilitating spinal cord injury truly able to make such a decision, given that these feelings may be considered common immediately after such an incident? Physicians do not order ventilators to be turned off at the immediate demand of each person. Traditional values cause most people to prize life, and mourn the loss of it. The grieving process experienced after a physical loss such as occurs with chronic illness and disability can cause emotional upheaval that may cloud the person's judgment. So autonomy must be viewed in light of each person's situation. The age factor is also considered. If the patient is a teenager, there is likely to be more resistance to upholding the wish to terminate his or her life than if the person is considered old. Although this might be considered ageism, arguments can be made that the younger patient has not "lived his life" but the older person has. GRNs must explore their own feelings and beliefs about patient autonomy, yet consider each situation and person as unique.

One of the most common situations GRNs encounter involves the conflict between autonomy and paternalism. This occurs when the person's right to decide is in direct conflict with the nurse's beliefs. *Paternalism* refers to the caregiver's (whether health care professional or family member) tendency or desire to make decisions for the person based on his or her own set of values and beliefs. A paternalistic decision in health care must always be justified. That is, health care professionals should strive to uphold the person's autonomy and not support his or her decisions only if there is ample and sufficient cause (such as questionable mental capabilities). In some instances, the nurse or physician may take away a person's right to choose and make the decision for him or her. This is paternalism. Family members often also exercise paternalism. For example, a patient living at home could have clear advance directives that specify that no life-supporting measures be initiated in the event of cardiac arrest, yet if such a situation arises, the family can still call emergency personnel to try to revive the person. Once called, the paramedics are obligated to perform life-saving procedures. Such an example is described in Case Study 15.1. Likewise, there is the case of a terminally ill person who has specified advance directives to avoid life-prolonging procedures and then becomes unable to speak for himself or herself. If the family insists that all measures be taken to preserve life, the person's living will may not be honored. In this case, paternalism has overruled autonomy, partly because health care professionals must still deal with the family long after the person has died.

CASE STUDY 15.1
Withholding Treatment

Mrs. Low was an elderly woman caring for her terminally ill husband at home. He was in his eighties and had been hospitalized many times. His health had continued to deteriorate with no hope of recovery. They had decided together, and with the full cooperation of his doctor, that no life-saving measures would be taken, and he would be allowed to die peacefully if a crisis should arise. Home health care aides and nurses visited regularly during daytime hours. Mrs. Low had no family support, but she had several close church members who provided emotional and social support. One couple, Dr. and Mrs. Gibbs, who helped care for the woman and her husband, were a physician and nurse from their church. Mrs. Gibbs encouraged Mrs. Low to maintain as high a level of self-care and independence as possible but assisted her with instrumental activities of daily living (IADLs) such as driving to doctor appointments, doing laundry, and helping bathe Mr. Low regularly. When Mrs. Low told the couple of their decision to allow Mr. Low to die peacefully, Dr. and Mrs. Gibbs were supportive. They told Mrs. Low that if a crisis arose, she could call them and they would come right over to be with her and her husband at the end, although his condition at the time did not indicate imminent death. Mrs. Low agreed and such was the plan. However, Mr. Low took a turn for the worse one day, and Mrs. Low called the Gibbses to be with her. Yet, in her upset state, Mrs. Low had also called the ambulance. The Gibbses arrived at the same time as the paramedics, who began to start intravenous fluids and intubated Mr. Low. Despite the fact that Dr. Gibbs was a medical doctor and attested to the fact that Mr. and Mrs. Low did not wish life-saving measures to be taken, the paramedics stated that they were legally bound to do all they could to resuscitate Mr. Low. The end result was that extensive measures were taken to revive Mr. Low, a hospital stay with large medical bills followed, and frustration was experienced by all involved. Mr. Low died shortly thereafter.

DISCUSSION QUESTIONS: From a rehabilitation perspective, what interventions could the home care GRN devise to support the patient's autonomy? What ethical principles are present in this situation? Whose autonomy is at risk? Is paternalism a factor? If so, which people in the situation acted in a paternalistic manner? If one were operating according to the principle of distributive justice, would the outcome have been different? Which person would be the focus of the GRN's interventions and ethical decision-making in this case? What legal documents needed to be in place for Mr. and Mrs. Low to have their decision about a peaceful death without life support upheld? What questions might the physician friend (Dr. Gibbs) have asked Mrs. Low in order to avoid the situation that occurred when the paramedics arrived? What could Mrs. Low have done differently to prevent the extensive measures taken to prolong her husband's life after she called the ambulance? What might she have done prior to calling the ambulance? Why do you think she called for emergency help instead of calling her friends as they had agreed? If anyone had produced the appropriate advance directive document stating that no life-supporting measures were to be instituted, what should the paramedics have done?

Beneficence implies actively doing good. This is in contrast to the more passive principle of *nonmaleficence,* which means to do no harm. Both concepts should be applied to situations of concern. Nursing care should not be aimed only at preventing harm but also at actively promoting what is beneficial to the person and family.

For example, in Case Study 15.2, the nurse was informed by the patient that he felt he was going to die, was preparing to, and wished to. Given the information provided by the patient, the nurse could have actively done good (beneficence) by making certain that the patient had the opportunity to exercise his autonomy through legal documents that would express his wishes for no life support. The nurse did not have time to do so in this particular case. However, she was in conflict when the patient became unresponsive because she wanted to do no harm (nonmaleficence) and uphold his autonomy, yet she actively tried to save his life, feeling this was doing good (beneficence). Was this also paternalism on the nurse's part, or a legal obligation? The appropriate paperwork was not in the chart, and she felt a legal obligation to call a code and begin rescue measures. She later learned that the physician had had a similar discussion as she with the patient a day before and had also not completed the appropriate documentation to support the patient's wishes. Several ethical principles are involved in Case Study 15.3. The reader is encouraged to read and discuss them.

CASE STUDY 15.2
Decision-Making

Casey, a GRN with 2 years of experience in nursing, was working on the skilled nursing floor of a large hospital before the mandatory laws regarding advance directives were insti-

tuted. One of her patients, Mr. Lloyd, age 87, had been admitted for a short stay to regain strength after minor hernia surgery. As Casey made her evening rounds, Mr. Lloyd calmly announced to her that he was going to die. He revealed that his wife had dementia and was in a nursing home, no longer able to recognize him. Mr. Lloyd stated that he was ready to die and that it was going to happen soon. He had called his lawyer, pastor, and doctor in the past 3 days to settle his affairs. Mr. Lloyd was up independently in the room, had progressed well, and was scheduled for discharge the next day. Casey listened to him verbalize, asked appropriate questions about suicidal ideations (Mr. Lloyd exhibited none), and then reassured him that he was doing well and that there was no physical reason to think that his condition was terminal. Casey returned 20 minutes later to give Mr. Lloyd his bedtime medications and found him unresponsive in a sitting position with the head of the bed up. Because there were no advance directives on the chart, and Mr. Lloyd was considered to be full code status, Casey called the code and began cardiopulmonary resuscitation (CPR). The code team arrived and worked to revive Mr. Lloyd while Casey tried to contact the physician. The physician arrived at Mr. Lloyd's room and stated that the patient had told him the same thing as he had told Casey. The code was stopped per the physician's order after 45 minutes of resuscitative measures, and Mr. Lloyd was pronounced dead.

DISCUSSION QUESTIONS: What are the ethical principles involved in this situation? Is there an ethical dilemma here? Which team members does it involve? Did the nurse and the physician fulfill their ethical and legal obligations? Was a moral obligation involved? From the perspective of distributive justice, what would be of major concern? How have situations like this been altered since the institution of advance directives? What could the GRN have done differently? What could the physician have done differently? In your experience, is a situation such as this one rare?

CASE STUDY 15.3
Withdrawing Treatment

Mr. Smith, age 68, was a patient on the skilled nursing unit of a small county hospital in the

1980s. He had been diagnosed with terminal cancer of the liver from years of alcoholism. Mr. Smith, a widower, had not specified any advance directives. His daughter and son-in-law, who lived in another state, were called when his condition deteriorated. Intravenous fluids and enteral feedings had been initiated by the physician. Upon visiting with her comatose father, the daughter expressed fear that he was "suffering" in being incapacitated, so termination of life-sustaining procedures was discussed with the physician and GRN. The daughter informed the physician that she did not wish her father to "linger" when there was no chance of recovery or improvement. Because it was apparent that the patient was no longer able to make competent decisions, the daughter, being the next of kin, stated she wished all treatments to be stopped. She said that her father would never have wanted to be kept alive like this. The physician agreed to this and wrote the appropriate orders. The GRN discontinued the tube feeding and intravenous line, leaving the Foley catheter in place as directed by the physician to monitor urinary output and keep the patient clean and dry. It was not until after the treatments were discontinued and Mr. Smith did not die immediately that the daughter began to express doubts about her decision. Although she and her husband had undergone lengthy discussions about the impact of her decision, she was not prepared for the emotional conflict that ensued. Mr. Smith was kept comfortable and repositioned regularly, but no hydration or nutrition was given. Urinary output slowly diminished over days as the family waited and watched. The daughter approached the GRN with many questions as they waited for Mr. Smith's death. "How long will it take?" "Is he in pain?" "Is this the right thing to do?" The most difficult question for the GRN to address was "Isn't this really like starving him to death?" The GRN spent a great deal of time with the family reinforcing that Mr. Smith had no chance of recovery, that he was not suffering being in a comatose state, and that he would be kept comfortable in a peaceful environment. A cot was placed in the room for the daughter to stay around the clock if she desired. As the days passed and Mr. Smith lingered in an unconscious state, the daughter became more distraught that he had not died immediately. Through counseling and arranging for a pastor to visit, the GRN was able to reinforce to the family that

they had upheld their father's wishes, even though it was difficult for them. Had legislation regarding advance directives been in place at the time, the daughter might not have had to bear the burden of this decision. The guilt and emotional conflict experienced by the family escalated during the long 6 days before Mr. Smith's death. Although such crises cannot always be avoided, advance directives provide support, both legal and emotional, for families faced with such decisions.

DISCUSSION QUESTIONS: Once the daughter expressed doubts about her decision to terminate life support, can she reverse that decision at any time? What interventions on the part of the staff might have made the daughter's decision to terminate life support less difficult? How might the GRN respond to the comment "Isn't this really like starving him to death"? How should the GRN explain end-of-life care to the family? What other team members might assist with comforting the family in a situation such as this? What nursing diagnoses are likely to have precedence in this situation?

Distributive justice deals with "allocation and equitable distribution of scarce resources" (Henderson & McConnell, 1997, p. 133). Some maintain that distributive justice has a built-in bias against the elderly in that they may be viewed as less productive than younger members of society. It must be remembered, however, that older persons have contributed to society for a much longer period of time and still have experiences, expertise, and wisdom to share with others. Additionally, many older adults continue to stay in the workforce or volunteer in hospitals, churches, and the like. An extreme example of distributive justice is the "lifeboat" scenario in which decisions about life and death are based on the greatest good for the greatest number or who is sacrificed for the greatest good. With the expectation that health care resources will continue to decline, or at least be limited, GRNs may need to examine their feelings about this ethical principle and how it relates to the rehabilitation process. Case Study 15.4 presents a situation for consideration.

CASE STUDY 15.4
Rehabilitation of the Terminally Ill Elder

Mrs. Linden, age 62, came to the inpatient rehabilitation unit for strengthening following an extended hospital admission in acute care. She had a history of a recent brain tumor with metastasis to the lymph nodes and was told by her oncologist that she probably had only weeks to months to live at the most. Mrs. Linden had been through radiation and chemotherapy, as well as surgery to remove the tumor. Her head was shaved and she had a large scar on the right temporal area. She wore a turban-type scarf during therapy to cover her head. Mrs. Linden wanted to be in rehabilitation. Her goal was to be strong enough to go home and live the days she had left at home, as strong as possible. She was a cheerful participant and was well liked by the entire staff. Her family, a supportive husband and three children, participated in her care and visited daily. The nurses on the unit, however, questioned the ethics of the decision to have her admitted to the rehabilitation unit. One of the doctors said she would be "lucky to last 3 more weeks at home" with her advanced stage of brain cancer. Yet, she was fully alert and oriented and seemed able to make rational decisions. In order to build endurance and increase her strength for home discharge, the nurses encouraged her to sit up a little longer each evening. However, they felt guilty about "pushing" her endurance because of Mrs. Linden's condition, which left her drained and exhausted by the end of a day in therapy. The nurse clinician met with the nursing staff and allowed them to discuss their feelings. The nurses supported each other by making Mrs. Linden and her family's desire to return home their primary goal. The staff chose to take the position that they were supporting the patient's autonomy and right to choose how she would spend her final days, even though several of them expressed reservations saying, "This sure isn't how I would want to spend my last weeks on earth." Mrs. Linden was able to return home, where she died under hospice care 3 weeks later.

DISCUSSION QUESTIONS: What is the ethical dilemma in this situation? What are the major ethical principles involved? How would one argue the perspective of distributive justice in this case?

ADVANCE DIRECTIVES

The Patient Self-Determination Act (PSDA) (1990) gives patients the legal right to formulate choices about the withholding or withdrawal of treatment under specific conditions. It is the nurse's responsibility to make certain that patients and their families are informed of these rights, to provide information about advance directives, and to help ensure that the person is competent when such decisions are made. *Advance planning* involves a process of communication, reflection, and discussion about the person's treatment preference for end-of-life care (Miles, Koepp, & Weber, 1996). Each agency or facility must have specific and detailed policies and procedures that uphold this patient right (Weber, 1993).

Elderly persons in rehabilitation may have more cause than most to specify their wishes about treatment because of advanced age and diagnoses of chronic conditions. It is then essential for the GRN to be informed about the documentation required to legalize the person's wishes. The purpose of advance directives is to support a person's autonomy by allowing him or her to make decisions about end-of-life treatment. These directives are only effective in the case that the person has an incurable injury, disease, or illness that has been certified as terminal by a physician. Such declarations make it legal for the person to die naturally instead of artificially prolonging life.

Several types of advance directives have been recognized in various states. These may include a living will, a life-prolonging procedures declaration, a health care representative appointment, and a durable power of attorney. Individuals older than the age of 18 who are admitted to a health care facility will be asked whether they have formulated, or wish to formulate, an advance directive. It is generally the role of the nurse to see that this is done.

The *living will* is a written document, made when the person is competent, that directs caregivers to allow natural death to occur in the event of terminal illness. This directive becomes operative only when two conditions are met: (1) the attending physician has certified that the person has a terminal illness, and (2) death is imminent from that terminal condition within a short period of time if artificial life-sustaining procedures are not implemented.

A *life-prolonging procedures declaration* is also made in advance by a competent individual to state that life-prolonging procedures *should* be instituted in the event of a terminal illness that would cause death if not for artificial procedures. This is in contrast to the advance directive expressing no life support in the event of inevitable death due to terminal illness. The person would be stating that all possible measures should be instituted to sustain or prolong life.

An *appointment of a health care representative document* allows a person to specify another individual to make health care decisions in his or her behalf if the individual becomes incapacitated or unable to make his or her own decisions. The health care representative is authorized to act in good faith for the other person. Individuals may also list persons who are disqualified from making decisions about their health care. This must be done in writing.

A *durable power of attorney* for health care is a more broad document than that of health care representative, although the latter may be subsumed by the former. This legal document permits the person to designate another individual to make decisions for him or her in the event that he or she becomes incapable of doing so. This can include authority in financial matters, personal and family business, as well as health care decisions. For the purposes of withholding and initiating treatment for the terminal patient, the power of attorney document should be combined with another signed declaration such as the living will or the others previously mentioned.

Studies have shown that rehabilitation programs may be valuable sites for educating persons about advance directives. Although only 9% of 845 cardiac rehabilitation sites in one study provided educational sessions on advance directives, more than 50% stated that they were in favor of including such information (Heffner & Barbieri, 1996). Cardiac rehabilitation programs provide an excellent site to educate patients about advance directives, but they are not widely used for this purpose. Similarly, most pulmonary rehabilitation programs did not educate patients about advance directives but are potential sites for improving dialogue and disseminating information about this topic (Heffner, Fahy, & Barbieri, 1996). Such studies suggest that GRNs may facilitate communication about advance directives in a variety of settings.

THE "RIGHT TO DIE"

The right to die, or a person's right to choose death over life, is a subject of much debate in health care. The living will declaration supports the patient's right to choose. Nurses are taught to uphold the patient's autonomy, but this is often in conflict with their own values and beliefs. In the area of gerontological rehabilitation nursing, the issue can be compounded by the person's age, the presence of chronic illnesses, and whether or not the person is deemed mentally competent. As a person ages, some memory loss is common, and cognitive deficits may result. A judgment as to a person's capacity to choose to end his or her life may be difficult. Depression and other emotional processes could be the result of disease or injury. All factors should be weighed before an evaluation can be made.

If a decision is made to support the right to die, then the issue becomes even more complex. There is a fine legal line between withholding and withdrawing treatment. Withholding treatment could be the result of advance directives or living wills that specify that no treatment is to be initiated. However, in many cases, the issue is withdrawing treatment, or removing treatment that may be life-saving or life-sustaining. Although family members may wish to uphold their loved one's wishes, the effects of withdrawal of feeding tubes or a ventilator may not be clearly understood by them.

The issue of tube feeding as a life-sustaining measure is controversial and unclear, yet a common dilemma among the elderly in long-term care facilities. Wilson's study demonstrated that "respect for the patient's autonomy does not guide tube feeding decisions" (1992, p. 198). Instead, most decisions to begin or end tube feedings are made by the physician and with the input of someone other than the patient.

Life support legislation varies from state to state in the United States. Krynski, Tymchuk, and Ouslander (1994) found that the elderly in long-term care facilities lacked understanding of various medical practices such as tube feeding. This would suggest that even among those elders who have living wills, specific directives about tube feeding may not be given. This study also indicated that elders showed improvement in knowledge with directed teaching, suggesting that nursing interventions for the elderly should include explanation of such procedures. Because tube feeding can sustain life for a long period of time, the decision to withdraw it often rests with the family.

Some states exclude provision of nutrition such as food and water as life-prolonging events. However, according to 1994 amendments to the Living Will Act, individuals can now specify in the living will whether or not they wish tube feeding or hydration to be given or that they wish this decision to be left to health care professionals or another designated person (Costas, 1994). GRNs should make certain that the patient's wishes are explicitly and accurately documented to the last detail.

Even though in the case of the terminally ill, there is no hope of recovery, the family may not realize until after the decision is made what the result of withdrawal of intravenous fluids or feeding tubes may be. Wilson (1992) stated, "the right to die legislation arising from Nancy Cruzan's case would indicate that tube feeding can be withdrawn in some instances" (p. 198). Withdrawing treatment is usually much more emotionally difficult for the family than withholding it. Case Study 15.3 describes the questions that arose when one family made the decision to terminate treatment.

An individual's right to die may be more in question in cases of a competent younger person who has sustained a high-level spinal cord injury and is ventilator-dependent. For an alert person placed on a ventilator permanently necessary to sustain life, legal actions must be taken to discontinue treatment because death is not imminent and the condition is not terminal. Such instances are less common with older adults, who are more likely to deal with issues surrounding life-prolonging procedures such as tube feedings or intravenous fluids.

Also embroiled in the right to die controversy are the issues of assisted suicide and euthanasia. The media coverage surrounding Dr. Jack Kevorkian's "death machine" attests to this fact. Only about half of Kevorkian's "patients" were terminally ill. Helping or causing these people to die constituted euthanasia, sometimes referred to as rational suicide. This has serious implications for those with disabilities or chronic illness, who may fear that legalization of euthanasia will cause those with various kinds of limitations to be seen as undesirable, even expendable. Individuals may desire to terminate their life when chronic illness or pain causes them to perceive no quality of life. Yet, because of personal or religious beliefs, or the inability

to carry out a plan, the idea of suicide is unacceptable. Assisted suicide occurs when another individual helps a person to end his or her life. Thus, assisted suicide may allow persons to believe that they have escaped the implications of suicide if it was assisted by another, particularly a doctor. To some, this validates the process and yet achieves the desired end.

GRNs should explore their own feelings about assisted suicide and euthanasia, because these are likely to continue to be issues in gerontology and rehabilitation. Two opposing views are given as representative examples here. Pohlmeier stated that "every physician is familiar with the situation in which he stops medication so that his patient may die peacefully and quietly—an act of passive euthanasia" (1985, p. 121). He continued to question why we should prevent suicide when "suicide and euthanasia do not represent opposites, because efforts toward choosing one's death do not contradict efforts of suicide prevention" (p. 121). Pohlmeier believed that laws and regulation could not help doctors to decide the right strategy for suicide prevention, but that it was a matter of conscience and a special type of relationship between individuals. Yet, as Siegel (1986) pointed out, only a small percentage of those who commit suicide fall under the category of the incurably ill seeking self-determination. She stated that potential abuses of laws giving individuals the right to suicide include tragic deaths "among individuals for whom the suicidal urge was transitory and irrational" (Siegel, 1986, p. 411). Siegel goes on to argue that by making euthanasia legal, it would become easier for people to decide that suicide is a reasonable alternative and hinder the possibility of treatment interventions and professional help.

The possibility of future legalization of euthanasia and rational suicide exists and would have serious implications for health care professionals working with older adults. The nurse who focuses on rehabilitation of the older adult will likely have grave concerns about the statements that euthanasia makes about the value of life among the elderly and disabled. GRNs should be informed of both sides of these issues and be prepared to offer guidance and alternatives to family members and patients seeking answers. Being active on hospital ethics committees and in community or political organizations is one way for GRNs to protect the rights of the elderly with functional limitations through the roles of advocate, mediator, and educator (see Case Study 15.4).

USE OF PHYSICAL RESTRAINTS

The use of physical restraints is a highly controversial issue, and one which has undergone significant changes in the health setting since the late 1980s. The Omnibus Budget Reconciliation Act (OBRA) of 1987 set stricter criteria for the use of physical restraints in nursing homes in order to protect the rights of patients. It declared that nursing home residents have the right to be free from physical or chemical restraints that are not needed to treat medical symptoms (Janelli, Kanski, & Neary, 1994). Prior to OBRA, restraints were thought to be often used for the convenience of long-term care staff with limited personnel and resources. The Nursing Home Reform Act "now requires nursing homes to develop psychosocial rehabilitation programs and to follow guidelines for antipsychotic drug and restraint use" (Rovner, Steele, Shmuley, & Folstein, 1996, p. 12). Six basic categories for reasons of restraining residents were noted in one study: (1) ambulation (falling, balance), (2) behavioral (agitation, combativeness), (3) positioning (in wheelchair, bed, or chair), (4) wandering (outside or into others' rooms), (5) jeopardizing life support (such as pulling on tubes), and (6) new admission (such as wandering) (Cohen, Neufeld, Dunbar, Pflug, & Breuer, 1996). Guidelines for use of mechanical restraints state that they are to be used only when (1) the patient is unable to walk without falling as a result of a neurological or medical disorder, or (2) the patient poses an immediate risk to harming himself or herself or others because of combativeness (Rovner et al., 1996).

The use of restraints has been associated with both an increase (Case Study 15.5) and a decrease in falls and resulting injury. Restraints can cause increased agitation and thus heighten the risk of injury to the patient or others. New federal guidelines have greatly reduced the number of restrained nursing home residents, but nurses often express conflicting feelings about wishing to keep the person safe. As Werner, Cohen-Mansfield, Koroknay, and Braun stated, "although the use of physical restraints requires a physician's order, nurses have been the primary decision makers for the use of physical restraints. This decision, however, is accompanied by contradictory feelings" (1994, p. 19). Physicians agree that the nursing staff

generally "initiate, monitor, and discontinue restraint use independently" (Schleenbaker, McDowell, Moore, Costich, & Prater, 1994, p. 427). This issue then is certainly relevant to GRN practice.

CASE STUDY 15.5
Use of Physical Restraints

The acute care unit of a small county hospital had a large percentage of elderly patients. Nellie, a frail 80 year old awaiting discharge to an extended care facility, was confused and tended to wander. She had a history of falls, but without serious injury. The nursing assistant had restrained Nellie in a highback chair in her room, using a vest restraint tied in the back and bilateral wrist restraints that secured her arms to the arms of the chair. Upon passing the room, a student nurse and her instructor found the chair upside down, with Nellie still restrained to it, on her knees in urine, screaming for help. The pair called for help but were unable to undo any of the restraints because there were multiple knots tightly tied. The instructor cut the restraints away with her scissors as the student nurse reassured Nellie that they were there to help. Although Nellie was physically unharmed except for a bruise on her forehead, the emotional trauma of being hung upside down with a chair on top of her might have done immeasurable damage to her trust of the staff. In Nellie's case, alternatives to restraints should have been used, and restraints posed a greater threat to her safety than her wandering. Because this case happened some years ago, new OBRA regulations were not yet in effect. More recent laws should help prevent such occurrences in the future.

DISCUSSION QUESTIONS: What are some possible alternatives to the physical restraints in this case? What are the legal ramifications that may have resulted? What general guidelines should have been followed to prevent such an incident? What fall risk factors can be identified by the information given, and what nursing interventions are most appropriate?

Schleenbaker et al. (1994) examined the records of 323 inpatient rehabilitation patients to evaluate restraint use. Results showed that 78.3% of patients had restraints ordered, but they were used in only 32.2% of patients, with vest restraints as the most common type. These data support the notion that use of physical restraints in the rehabilitation setting continues to be high. Their findings led this interdisciplinary team of researchers to conclude that age was not associated with restraint use as much as diagnosis, decreased mental status, lower Functional Independence Measure (FIM) scores, and male gender, but that restraints may also not prevent falls, because falls occurred in 25% of restrained and 10.1% of the unrestrained patients in the sample.

Several interventions within nursing home settings can help reduce the use of restraints. Rovner et al. (1996) found that activities done with psychiatric supervision could decrease the use of antipsychotic drugs and restraints, as well as decrease behavior disorders. Another study demonstrated that when physical restraint use decreased and an educative/consultation intervention was implemented, the use of neuroleptic or benzodiazepine medication did not increase. This research suggested that a decrease in both medications and restraint use could occur together (Siegler et al., 1997).

Within the acute care setting, use of physical restraints is also strictly regulated. In rehabilitation, such devices are avoided when at all possible, yet the incidence of falls among rehabilitation patients is high and associated with injury. This undoubtedly contributes to the use of safety devices. The main reason for physical restraint use is to protect the person from harm. This includes preventing falls or pulling out tubes, which could injure or traumatize the individual. Conflicting reports add to the confusion regarding restraints. Fall prevention has been ingrained in nurses throughout their training, yet in rehabilitation the goal is independence and self-care, so physical restraints would seem contradictory.

Some nurse researchers contend that although restraint use has decreased significantly during the 1990s, the overall impact in the United States has been slight. The practice continues because of factors such as fear of reprimand or lawsuit if a patient falls, belief that there are not good alternatives to physical restraint, staff perceptions, or lack of knowledge on the part of nursing staff (Evans & Strumpf, 1990; Janelli et al., 1994). Ludwick and O'Toole's study (1996) demonstrated that restraint use was the major treatment for confusion in the acute care hospital, being used by 84% of the 100 nurses

in the study. Less frequently used were the interventions of orienting, monitoring, and protecting.

Part of this issue involves cultural norms. Restraint use is more prevalent in the United States and Canada than in the United Kingdom, although there are not discernible differences in the characteristics between elders in long-term care facilities (Strumpf, Evans, & Schwartz, 1991). Evans and Strumpf (1990) pointed out that in Scotland and England "falls and accidents are an expected occurrence in geriatric care settings, where active rehabilitation is the rule" (p. 124). In these countries, beds are used that are closer to the floor, more like beds at home. The authors go on to say that falls there are common, but do not often result in serious injury. American nurses also viewed restraints as more beneficial than did Scottish nurses.

GRNs should be aware that many good alternatives to physical and chemical restraints exist. However, "the provision of ongoing education to nursing staff members is a necessary step to decrease feelings of frustration and stress and to assist the staff in being aware of alternatives to restraints" (Werner et al., 1994, p. 24). Several alternatives are given in Table 15–1. Every effort must be made in the rehabilitation setting to ensure that GRNs not only know the facts about use of restraints but also practice other means of fall prevention. A balance must be struck between promoting independence and

Table 15–1 ALTERNATIVES TO RESTRAINTS

Wheelchair adaptations
Wedge seats
Cushions to prevent sliding
Alarm devices on bed or wheelchair and exits
Special beds that promote comfort and safety but allow increased activity
Reclining chairs
Call light in easy reach
Increased supervision and observation
Daily exercise and ambulation programs
Toileting schedules and frequent assistance to the bathroom
Increased social activities and interactions
Increased number of volunteers to assist residents
Promotion of staff and resident interactions
Change in medications
Environmental changes that promote activity in a controlled setting

ensuring safety. This transition requires a change in mindset for many nurses. There is a need for formal, continuing education programs and role modeling by expert clinicians to help staff make decisions and identify workable alternatives to restraint use.

GRNs should be at the forefront of creative and individualized nursing care that provides options to the use of physical restraints. Baldwin, Craven, and Dimond suggested that "there may be a range of acceptable risk" (1996, p. 20) with regard to physical restraints, because trying to remain free of risks can impede the goals of independence, autonomy, and achievement of maximal functional level (Fagier & Greenwood, 1993). All factors must be weighed before implementing any approach. The GRN should consider that a primary purpose of rehabilitation is to regain independent function, including ambulation. Strengthening exercises, proper nutrition, walking programs, and medication management all are important aspects in reducing restraint use while ensuring patient safety. Additionally, the GRN should work with other team members and medical staff to reduce the risk for injury. There is also a significant role for administrators to support the philosophy of least restraint. Other nursing interventions for preventing falls without the use of restraints are discussed in Chapter 7.

REFERENCES

Baldwin, R. L., Craven, R. G., & Dimond, M. (1996). Falls: Are rural elders at greater risk? *Journal of Gerontological Nursing, 22*(8), 14–21.

Cohen, C., Neufeld, R., Dunbar, J., Pflug, L., & Breuer, B. (1996). Old problem, different approach: Alternatives to physical restraints. *Journal of Gerontological Nursing, 22*(2), 23–29.

Costas, H. J. (1994). Indiana living will update. *Quality Times, 3*(3), 1–2.

Evans, L. K., & Strumpf, N. W. (1990). Myths about elder restraint. *IMAGE: The Journal of Nursing Scholarship, 22*(2), 124–127.

Fagier, J., & Greenwood, M. (1993). Outside risk. *Nursing Times, 89*(40), 56–58.

Heffner, J. E., & Barbieri, C. (1996). Involvement of cardiovascular rehabilitation programs in advance directive education. *Archives of Internal Medicine, 156,* 1746–1751.

Heffner, J. E., Fahy, B., & Barbieri, C. (1996). Advance directive education during pulmonary rehabilitation. *Chest, 109*(2), 299.

Henderson, M. L., & McConnell, E. S. (1997). Ethical considerations. In M. A. Matteson & E. S. McConnell (Eds.), *Gerontological nursing: Concepts and practice* (pp. 123–157). Philadelphia: W. B. Saunders.

Janelli, L. M., Kanski, G. W., & Neary, M. A. (1994). Physical restraints: Has OBRA made a difference? *Journal of Gerontological Nursing, 20*(6), 17–21.

Krynski, M. D., Tymchuk, A., & Ouslander, J. G. (1994). How informed can consent be? New light on comprehension among elderly people making decisions about enteral tube feeding. *Gerontologist, 34*(1), 36–43.

Ludwick, R., & O'Toole, A. W. (1996). The confused patient: Nurse's knowledge and interventions. *Journal of Gerontological Nursing, 22*(1), 44–49.

Miles, S. H., Koepp, R., & Weber, E. P. (1996). Advance end-of-life treatment planing. A research review. *Archives of Internal Medicine, 156,* 1062–1968.

Pohlmeier, H. (1985). Suicide and euthanasia—special types of partner relationships. *Suicide and Life Threatening Behavior, 15*(2), 117–123.

Rovner, B. W., Steele, C. D., Shmuley, Y., & Folstein, M. F. (1996). A randomized trial of dementia care in nursing homes. *Journal of the American Geriatrics Society, 44,* 7–13.

Schleenbaker, R. E., McDowell, S. M., Moore, R. W., Costich, J. F., & Prater, G. (1994). Restraint use in patient rehabilitation: Incidence, predictors, and implications. *Archives of Physical Medicine and Rehabilitation, 74,* 427–430.

Siegel, K. (1986). Psychosocial aspects of rational suicide. *American Journal of Psychotherapy, 40,* 405–418.

Siegler, E. L., Capezuti, E., Maislin, G., Baumgarten, M., Evan, L., & Strumpf, N. (1997). Effects of a restraint reduction intervention and OBRA '87 regulations on psychoactive drug use in nursing homes. *Journal of the American Geriatrics Society, 45,* 791–796.

Strumpf, N. W., Evans, L. K., & Schwartz, D. (1991). Physical restraint of the elderly. In W. C. Chenitz, J. T. Stone, & S. A. Salisbury (Eds.), *Clinical gerontological nursing* (pp. 329–344). Philadelphia: W. B. Saunders.

Weber, G. (1993). Tips on implementing the Patient Self-Determination Act. *Nursing and Health Care, 14*(2), 86–91.

Werner, P., Cohen-Mansfield, J., Koroknay, V., & Braun, J. (1994). Reducing restraints: Impact on staff attitudes. *Journal of Gerontological Nursing, 20*(12), 19–24.

Wilson, D. M. (1992). Ethical concerns in a long-term tube feeding study. *IMAGE: The Journal of Nursing Scholarship, 24*(3), 195–198.

Chapter 16

Trends in Gerontological Rehabilitation Nursing

■

The future of gerontological rehabilitation nursing is likely to be reflective of the progress within the separate specialties of gerontological and rehabilitation nursing. Gerontological rehabilitation nursing is in its infancy, with little nursing research specifically in this area. As such, few publications are available that help define the scope and standards of practice. This text represents a beginning attempt to provide some essential information within a single source to which gerontological rehabilitation nurses (GRNs) can refer. Nurses must continue to build the knowledge base and engage in research and practice relating to the rehabilitation of older adults. The emergence and acceptance of gerontological rehabilitation nursing as a new specialty will not be without its struggles. Yet the development of this field is necessary to prepare nurses to meet the needs and demands of the future population.

In the writing of this text, it became apparent that there is great diversity in the knowledge and basic preparation of nurses across the United States, as well as those in different countries (such as United States and Canada). The fact that bachelor's degree preparation is still not the minimum for entry level nursing positions in the United States, combined with the fact that nursing programs often do not include rehabilitation as a separate course in the curriculum, has caused debate over the level of practice for GRNs. Some assume that the knowledge of the average staff nurse (regardless of when he or she completed basic nursing education) includes the content presented in this book, although it has been this

author's experience—both as an educator and practitioner—that this is not so. Even if nurses do possess knowledge and education in this area, it is not always translated into practice, particularly in the long-term care setting. There are various levels of knowledge in these areas; in addition, resources and education available to promote minimal competence may be lacking. Many nursing programs gear teaching toward passing the state board examination for licensure. However, the examination's focus is not on the content needed to practice in gerontological rehabilitation nursing. The state board examination will likely be changing to reflect the changes in the population, but until the questions are representative of the population, materials written on the subject are less likely to take priority over more traditional texts that have an acute care focus. Additionally, nurses working in long-term care facilities may have completed their nursing education long before rehabilitative content received emphasis in the curriculum. These nurses may or may not return for continuing education and may be less likely to be required to do so than if they were employed in an acute care or academic setting. So, although the demographics of the population may be shifting toward a gerontological/rehabilitation focus, education of the nursing workforce may not be keeping pace with the changes. This idea is supported by the priorities delineated for geriatric rehabilitation: (1) education, (2) policy, and (3) research (Hoenig, Nusbaum, & Brummel-Smith, 1997).

DIRECTIONS FOR ACADEMIC CURRICULA

Some schools and colleges of nursing are beginning to offer courses that combine gerontology and rehabilitation, because these two areas fit well together if separate courses cannot be offered. From such combinations naturally emerges a focus on rehabilitative care of the elderly. Yet, few articles in the literature provide any direction for the development of these courses. Academia and nursing texts should reflect the current state of the knowledge within the discipline; however, a survey of texts in gerontology reveals that most include only a single chapter on rehabilitation. Likewise, rehabilitation texts have a broad focus, with a single chapter on gerontological issues.

Health care professionals are just beginning to realize the impact the aging population will have on nursing. In their position paper, *Nursing Education's Agenda for the 21st Century,* the American Association of Colleges of Nursing (1993) identified the importance of including health promotion and maintenance (in relation to chronic and acute conditions) in the curriculum. The federal government's report, *Healthy People 2000,* identified health promotion and disease prevention as essential goals (Office of Disease Prevention and Health Promotion, 1990). In addition, the National League for Nursing (NLN) published a book entitled *Determining the Future of Gerontological Nursing Education.* In it, Tagliareni states that members of the associate degree focus group "recognize that provision of safe and competent care to older adults requires a strong knowledge base in rehabilitation, maintenance of functional ability, and promotion of self-care" (1993, p. 63). Likewise, a 1994 report from the National Institute of Nursing (Research Priority Expert Panel of Long-term Care) discussed the increased visibility of long-term care issues for the older adult population. This document details many specific areas in which nursing research is needed along with the challenges and opportunities presented by an aging society. The clinical problems identified by the panel included behavior, confusion, mobility, skin integrity, restraints, infection, urinary incontinence, and sleep. The nursing community seems to be in agreement that rehabilitation is key to maintaining quality of life for older adults with chronic health alterations.

As previously stated, the texts available on a subject often provide the direction it may take and certainly reflect much of the current state of knowledge in the field. Prior to the 1990s, many "gerontological nursing texts" were basically medical-surgical texts with some bits and pieces of gerontology thrown in. However, there are many fine gerontological nursing textbooks and references on the market today. Each of them offers different strengths, and each is geared to particular levels of study. The more recently published gerontology nursing texts have obviously recognized the need for a more long-term care focus. The trend is toward more comprehensive care with a prevention and wellness focus in a holistic gerontology framework. This provides evidence that both the fields of gerontological nursing and rehabilitation nursing are attempting to clarify and distinguish their respective roles. References are needed for long-term caregivers that have an emphasis on post-acute care, separating them from more traditional works. Academicians can help influence the demand for more texts of this type if gerontological rehabilitation concepts are taught in the classroom.

Questions remain as to what needs to be included in the academic curriculum to prepare nurses for future care of the elderly. Many nursing programs do not have enough room for additional credits in the curriculum to add a course in rehabilitation or gerontology. Some feel these concepts are incorporated into the rest of the coursework; others offer a class in chronic illness, with a gerontology component.

One solution to the problem of integrating rehabilitation and gerontology into the curriculum is the development of a single course that specifically focuses on tertiary care or prevention. Such a class can be modified to fit the particular needs of students at each university. An example of a topical outline for a course on tertiary care of the adult and the long-lived adult is given in Table 16–1. This course was structured to focus on rehabilitation and gerontological nursing, emphasizing application of rehabilitation principles, while incorporating some "medical-surgical" information as well in order to achieve a better fit within the overall framework of the nursing program.

Although nursing students should be familiar with concepts of rehabilitation from beginning coursework, an in-depth exploration with clinical practice to reinforce learning seems to enhance comprehension of the rehabilitation process. General nursing diagnoses may be presented first, because students are

Table 16–1 EXAMPLE OF GENERAL TOPICS TO BE COVERED IN A COURSE IN REHABILITATION AND GERONTOLOGICAL NURSING

Introduction to rehabilitation
  Concepts, scope of practice
  Conceptual framework
  History
  Theories
  Holistic care
  Interdisciplinary rehabilitation team
    members (roles and functions)
Nursing process related to long-term care and
  rehabilitation
  Assessment (including functional scales)
  Nursing diagnoses and interventions
    Health perception
    Nutritional/metabolic
    Body temperature
    Skin integrity
    Bowel elimination
    Bladder elimination
    Activity/exercise
    Self-care
    Mobility (including falls)
    Tissue perfusion
    Sleep/rest, comfort
    Cognitive/perceptual
    Self-perception/role
    Sexuality
    Stress/coping
    Value/belief
    Communication
  Goal setting
  Evaluation
Specific rehabilitation diagnoses: Nursing
  management related to chronic health
  alterations
  Stroke
  Seizures
  Brain injury

Orthopedic problems:
  Arthritis
  Joint replacements
  Amputation
Neurological problems: Spinal cord injury
Neurological and endocrine problems:
  Myasthenia gravis
  Multiple sclerosis
  Parkinson's disease
  Guillain-Barré syndrome
  Muscular dystrophy
  Amyotrophic lateral sclerosis
  Lupus
  Huntington's chorea
  Diabetes
The aging population
  Aging theories
  Defining gerontological nursing
  Review of normal aging (by system)
  Abnormalities of aging (by system)
Geriatric and long-term care issues
  Support for the family/caregiver
    Social support and support groups
    Community resources
    Caregiver burden
  Ethical/legal issues
    Polypharmacy
    Abuse/neglect of elders
    Withholding/withdrawing treatment
    Pain management
    Assisted suicide
    Advance directives
  Death and dying
    Support for the person and family
    Postmortem care

familiar with these, but they are discussed in the context of tertiary care practice. The content then moves to more specific nursing care of persons with common diagnoses seen in rehabilitation and geriatrics. Gerontological nursing principles are covered, along with issues that relate specifically to the older adult with chronic health alterations. This course builds on previous classes in which students have studied the normal effects of aging and basic medical-surgical principles. It is offered toward the end of the program in the senior year (bachelor of science in nursing [BSN] level). Students participate in clinical practicums in acute rehabilitation facilities and long-term care units. The students' clinical experiences include care of an elderly adult with a rehabilitative problem and multi-

ple chronic health alterations. The required nursing care plan paper allows them to apply the nursing process in the total nursing care of a patient through the rehabilitation process. Following the same patient through the rehabilitation process allows them to get a better sense of the long-range implications that chronic illness and disability have on the patient and family, as well as the various roles of nurses within the interdisciplinary team. Students are treated as team members, giving them the added benefit of experience within a team framework. Additionally, students attend a field trip to a major, nationally renowned rehabilitation institute to gain exposure to the total range and diversity of those who require rehabilitation nursing care. This type of course, which incorporates rehabilitation and gerontological nursing principles, may better prepare nurses to meet the future demands of the population.

CERTIFICATION

Certification is a means of recognizing that an individual has demonstrated a certain level of expertise within a specialty. This is generally obtained by first meeting certain specific criteria and then achieving a passing score on a written examination. Certification is available in both gerontological nursing and rehabilitation nursing. The requirements are similar in either area for basic certification. To be able to sit for the certification examination, a person must possess a current registered nurse (RN) license, have at least 2 years of experience in the specialty, and obtain letters from professional colleagues that confirm eligibility to sit for the examination.

Rehabilitation

On successful completion of the written examination in rehabilitation, the nurse may use the title CRRN (Certified Rehabilitation Registered Nurse). The CRRN examination is given through the Association of Rehabilitation Nurses (ARN). According to the Rehabilitation Nursing Foundation (RNF), "the goal of ARN certification examination is to recognize nurses who, through an examination process, are able to demonstrate an agreed-upon level of expertise in rehabilitation nursing" (Habel, 1993, p. 17). The first certification examination was given in 1984. As of 1993 there were more than 7000 certified rehabilitation nurses. By the year 2000, a nurse will have to hold a bachelor's degree in nursing to be eligible to take the basic CRRN examination. This will provide additional distinction to this credential.

Gerontology

In gerontology, the nurse may add the credential "C" to the RN title, thus RNC (meaning registered nurse, certified). The examination was first given in 1975, through the American Nurses Association (ANA). By 1997, more than 8000 nurses were certified in gerontological nursing practice (Eliopoulos, 1997).

It is interesting to note that although the specialty of rehabilitation nursing is much younger (officially recognized in 1974), it has grown much more quickly as a specialty than gerontological nursing (officially recognized in the 1960s). Given the current progress, certifications within rehabilitation may become even more specialized. Texts such as this one on gerontological rehabilitation nursing as well as one for pediatric rehabilitation are firsts in the field. Perhaps examinations for pediatric, geriatric, cardiac, or other subspecialties may not be far off.

ADVANCED PRACTICE

The state of the art of nursing in rehabilitation and gerontological nursing is partially reflected in the area of advanced practice. Current trends indicate an increase in the number of nurses prepared at the graduate level and an availability of diverse jobs for them. There are several changes occurring within rehabilitation nursing at the time of this writing that support future projections.

Advanced practice nurses in rehabilitation have published a core curriculum, and the ARN had previously published a booklet defining roles, scope, settings, and standards for this level of expertise. The field of gerontological nursing has already accomplished these tasks, having established master's programs throughout the United States both for clinical nurse specialists (CNSs) and nurse practitioners (NPs) in care of the aged. The ANA, through the American Nurses Credentialing Center (ANCC), offers advanced certification in gerontological nursing as a clinical specialist or a nurse practitioner.

The ARN offered the first advanced certification in rehabilitation in December 1997 and January 1998. The examination is practice-based, and examinees must be minimally prepared at the master's level with a specified amount of experience in rehabilitation. Those passing the certification examination earn the credential CRRN-A (Certified Rehabilitation Registered Nurse–Advanced). Content areas on the advanced rehabilitation examination are also similar to the gerontological clinical nurse specialist examination. The content area includes core knowledge (pathophysiology, pharmacology, and theory), direct practice, research, and systems and policy (Association of Rehabilitation Nurses, 1997).

PRACTICE SETTINGS

As has been presented throughout this book, practice settings for the GRN are currently diverse and will continue to diversify. Gerontological rehabilitation nursing is practiced wherever there are elderly persons and nurses who use the principles of gerontological rehabilitation. These settings include acute care facilities, rehabilitation units of every level, subacute care, nursing homes, the person's home, and the community. More important than the settings, however, is the need for preparation in the field of gerontological rehabilitation nursing.

Quality of care in extended care facilities continues to be of concern. The staffing patterns within long-term care facilities vary widely throughout the nation and internationally, and the general public might be surprised to learn of the accepted lack of registered nurses managing residents' care within long-term care facilities. In many parts of the United States, licensed practical nurses (LPNs) and nursing assistants make up the majority of nursing staff. One LPN may be the only nurse on duty on the night shift, with nursing assistants providing the direct patient care. Such organizational structures require the LPN to supervise and manage many other staff members. A concern is that an LPN with 1 year of basic nursing education may lack the skills and preparation to do this. The quality and competence of nursing assistants within long-term care facilities are

also varied and depend largely on the skill and expertise of the person from whom their assistant training was taken. Teaching other direct caregivers such as LPNs and certified nursing assistants (CNAs) to provide safe, competent care, while providing it with a rehabilitative focus and cultural sensitivity, will be a major task for GRNs working in long-term care. Future research efforts may focus on the relationship between educational preparation of caregivers (LPNs and CNAs in particular) to quality of patient care. Given these trends, experts have recommended that Congress pass legislation requiring (by the year 2000) that a registered nurse be present around the clock in all nursing facilities. Family members should be taught to look at the level and ratio of trained staff to residents when considering placement in extended care facilities.

RESEARCH

Crane (1995) described research utilization by nurses at different levels of practice. Baccalaureate-prepared nurses should value science-based practice, whereas master's-prepared nurses should evaluate practice outcomes and engage in pilot testing but not conduct re-

---

Table 16–2 EXAMPLE OF AN ABSTRACT FOR A QUANTITATIVE NURSING RESEARCH PROPOSAL

The Effects of Advanced Practice Nurse Teaching on Fall Incidence in Elderly Stroke Patients in Rehabilitation

Falls are one of the most costly, yet preventable, health care problems affecting the elderly. Elderly stroke patients are particularly at risk for falls. The broad objectives of this study are to discover the effect of nursing teaching about fall prevention on elderly stroke survivors who are patients in rehabilitation, and what effect this teaching has on persons' self-care agency (using Orem's conceptual framework).

The specific aims of this research are (1) to explore the effectiveness of nursing teaching about fall prevention on the fall incidence of elderly stroke patients in a rehabilitation setting and after discharge, (2) to determine whether patients with left-sided or right-sided stroke benefit more from nursing teaching with regard to prevention of falls, and (3) to examine the effect of supportive-educative nursing interventions about fall prevention on the self-care agency of stroke survivors.

The proposed study is a pre-experimental, pilot nursing intervention study. A convenience sample of 128 volunteers from two comparable units will be used. Each unit (two different sites) will have a control group (who will receive usual care) and a treatment group (who will receive additional teaching and follow-up from the nurse regarding fall prevention). The independent variable (IV) is the fall prevention teaching provided by the nurse. The dependent variables (DVs) are the incidence of falls and self-care agency. A control variable is left-sided or right-sided stroke. Investigator-developed instruments will be used in addition to the Functional Independence Measure (FIM) scale and the Appraisal of Self-Care Agency Scale (ASA-A) to measure self-care agency. The ASA-A tool has high validity and reliability (alpha range .77 to .86) and has been used in at least seven different countries with equivalent consistency. Comparisons between groups will be made using chi-square for categorical data and t-tests and analysis of variance (ANOVA) for continuous data.

Table 16–3   EXAMPLE OF AN ABSTRACT FOR A QUALITATIVE NURSING RESEARCH PROPOSAL

The purpose of this study is to explore the adaptive behaviors used by elderly stroke patients of various cultural backgrounds, using an ethnographic design resulting in a cultural picture. Adaptive behaviors will be defined generally as those actions that reflect the attitudes, beliefs, values, and coping mechanisms used by individuals adjusting to life after a stroke. The experiences of post-stroke adults older than age 65 will be examined in order to observe both differences and similarities of the stroke experience within and between four cultural groups: African-American, Hispanic, Amish, and Anglo-American. Subjects will be recruited from stroke support groups, community centers, and local churches. Participation of subjects will be voluntary with informed consent obtained. There is no set number of subjects, but data collection will continue until no new themes or patterns emerge.

Methods of data collection will include using 3–5 focus groups, then ethnographic interviews with key informants, which will be tape recorded. The participants will be asked: How did you adjust to life after your stroke? How has your life changed since your stroke? Questions will be refined after the focus groups, and additional questions are likely to emerge. Field logs and a reflective journal will be kept, with ongoing data collection and analysis. The software program entitled Ethnograph will be used, and analysis of data will follow qualitative methods as the researcher identifies patterns and themes that emerge from the transcribed interviews.

Evaluation of the research will be done using guidelines for qualitative studies. The researcher will confirm results using techniques outlined by Lincoln and Guba (1985) on establishing trustworthiness. Evaluation of validity and reliability will also follow Leininger's (1994) six major evaluative criteria for qualitative research, which include examining results for credibility, confirmability, meaning-in-context, recurrent patterning, saturation, and transferability.

search. The advanced practice nurse with a master's level of education should be able to critique research and use the findings to improve practice. Doctorally prepared nurses should be learning skills and gaining experience to design and conduct research, as well as to direct others in this area. Crane further stated, "more than ever, there is a need for nursing to use in practice the findings and methods of research in order to show that the interventions used improve patient outcomes and that the care given is cost effective" (1995, p. 567). An example of research utilization is using research-based risk assessments to decrease hospital-acquired pressure ulcers. Research utilization should lead to more positive outcomes. Hoenig et al. (1997) listed seven research priorities for geriatric rehabilitation: (1) define rehabilitation interventions according to reliable criteria; (2) refine outcome measures; (3) examine the effects of well-defined rehabilitation interventions on outcomes; (4) explore the role of assistive technology in geriatric rehabilitation; (5) determine outcomes, costs, and access to rehabilitation for different methods of care (such as managed care, fee for service); (6) optimize cost effectiveness; and (7) determine the optimal timing for rehabilitation. These suggestions, although not nursing specific, provide some direction for study.

Nursing research is needed in both the qualitative and quantitative paradigms. The methods chosen depend on the question the researcher wishes to answer. Quantitative research focuses on the use of specific statistical measurements to analyze and evaluate results of data in an objective manner. Qualitative research is often used to explore problems about which little is known or written. Examples of abstracts using each different approach are given in Tables 16–2 and 16–3. The problems proposed represent areas in gerontological rehabilitation nursing where research is needed.

There continues to be a great debate about whether nurse researchers can conduct inquiries using a combination of both methods. Many experienced researchers do not favor mixing methods. However, triangulation, or the use of both quantitative and qualitative methods, may be a future trend for research in gerontological rehabilitation nursing. The most important thing to remember when designing a research study is that the method chosen must be the most appropriate one to answer the researcher's question. Often, nursing research studies generate other questions that are best answered within a different paradigm. GRNs must be open to research using whichever methods provide the most accurate and reliable answers.

Although research studies are often designed by a doctorally prepared nurse, GRNs at any level can participate in research through problem identification, information gathering, and utilization. One of the most significant contributions staff nurses can make to the research process is identifying questions and ideas from their own clinical practice that they would like to see answered. Many important nursing discoveries have been made in just this way. GRNs with advanced degrees should participate in mentoring other nurses with regard to the appropriate utilization of nursing science. All nurses, regardless of educational level, are expected to be discriminating consumers of research. This should translate into incorporating substantiated clinical findings into everyday practice.

Quantitative Research

As has been suggested, there is a lack of statistically sound quantitative nursing research in the elderly population with regard to the effects of rehabilitation. Some contributing factors to this include accessibility to adequate sample sizes, ethical and legal issues in performing clinical trials, availability of necessary research funds, and a lack of nurse researchers working in this area.

Quantitative methods are best used when numerical outcomes are being measured. For example, scores on the Functional Independence Measure (FIM) scale or ratings on a Likert scale would provide quantitative data. The level of the data (nominal, ordinal, interval, or ratio) depends on what is being measured and will help determine the type of statistical test used to analyze the results. Data are often collected through surveys, questionnaires, or other self-report measures. Investigators will need to develop instruments that are reliable and valid. Many tools already tested for reliability and validity are available. Proper design and sampling techniques provide reliable information and allow researchers to make inferences about the general population. This research method is considered more objective than the qualitative method and is often preferred by nurse researchers because of the measurable degree of reliability and validity that can be obtained.

Qualitative Research

What if the researcher wants to know about the experience of an older adult who is living with a spinal cord injury, what stroke survivors do to adapt and cope at home, or what it is like to grow older with an amputation? A questionnaire could be developed, but what if there is no published research on the subject? How does the researcher know what questions to ask or what items to include in a survey? Questions such as these would best be answered by using qualitative research methods. Methods for gathering qualitative data vary widely but are likely to include focus groups, personal interviews, discussion groups, participant observation, videotaped interviews, and photographs. The researcher is the instrument and must have a good understanding of qualitative methods and techniques. Data are recorded and transcripts of the data are analyzed through a continuous process by identifying commonalities and patterns, drawing conclusions about the information and revisiting information gained. Software programs are available to help with data analysis by making large amounts of data more manageable and allowing the researcher to explore different themes and patterns. Questions of validity and reliability of the study are particularly important to address, because the subjectivity of this type of research lends itself to criticism, especially secondary to the possibility of bias on the part of the researcher.

Because there are so many areas of gerontological rehabilitation in which little research exists, qualitative methods can provide beginning information and stimulate other questions that would best be answered using quantitative measurements. An example of a proposal for a qualitative research study using ethnography appears in Table 16–3. Ethnography involves examination of culture and is used to look at the influence of beliefs, values, and ideals on the topic of interest.

MANAGED CARE

A concern for those working in gerontological rehabilitation is the effect that managed care will have on this specialty. Capitation, or primary care physician managed care, could work for the good of the field, because managed care offers the potential to align the goals of cost containment with the goal of maximizing functional status for older adults (Lachs & Ruchlin, 1997). However, the current system provides little help in achieving these goals and may even provide an incentive for physicians to undertreat frail elders (Hoenig et al., 1997). Thus, fee-for-service payments or "by the head" reimbursement may have a negative effect on outcomes.

"For larger populations of older adults with frailty or incipient frailty, the aggregate cost of providing care is inversely proportional to functional status" (Lachs & Ruchlin, 1997, p. 1126). The prevention of functional decline is important because it leads to new and more costly care. As previously discussed, further research needs to be done on the effects of rehabilitation on the elderly in various settings. As some researchers stated, "one of the most important challenges for geriatric rehabilitation will be to develop a method for measuring outcomes across a continuum of care, but this will not be an easy task" (Hoenig et al., 1997, p. 1378).

CONCLUSIONS AND RECOMMENDATIONS

The field of gerontological nursing is continuing to expand. The knowledge suggested by texts and clinical reference books on the market will help determine the direction in which future nurses are educated. More texts are needed relating to the practical information required to provide quality care for older adults with multiple chronic health problems. Care of the older adult with long-term illnesses cannot be adequately given apart from the principles and concepts of rehabilitation. Nurses and nursing assistants are not sufficiently knowledgeable in the areas of prevention and rehabilitation. Future projections suggest that there will be an increased need for health care professionals who can adapt and care for the aged in a wide variety of settings outside of the hospital. A nurse educated in the principles of rehabilitation, with sufficient knowledge of the aging process, will be able to meet the future challenges of the complex elderly population. New roles for health professionals may emerge, and families will likely play a more crucial part in care of the aged than ever before. More aged adults will be cared for in the home. Nurses must then be prepared to teach family members to care for their older relatives with complex health care needs. Specific areas in which nurses caring for older adults should be further educated include changes related to the normal aging process, principles of promoting self-care, improving nutritional status, maintaining skin integrity, promoting functional mobility, establishing bowel and bladder patterns, and enhancing memory and cognition. Additionally, nurses need to know how to apply principles in these areas to care for those with long-term illnesses or functional limitations. Once nurses have developed expertise in these areas, they can teach family members these principles as well.

The home health industry is already bursting at the seams, and managers are just beginning to realize that something else is needed, that there is a missing link to long-term care. Nursing resources are needed to guide us into the future and provide direction for those seeking answers to the questions addressed in this text: What is the key to quality care for our elderly patients? How can the older adult maintain self-care as long as possible? What is the nurse's role in promoting continued independence for disabled older adults in the community? The answers to these questions are most likely to be found in the marriage between rehabilitation concepts and gerontological nursing, paving the way for a new nursing specialty in gerontological rehabilitation.

REFERENCES

Aiken, L. R. (1995). *Aging: An introduction to gerontology.* Thousand Oaks, CA: Sage.

American Association of Colleges of Nursing. (1993). *Nursing education's agenda for the 21st century.* New York: Author.

American Association of Retired Persons (AARP). (1994). *A profile of older Americans.* Washington, DC: Author.

Association of Rehabilitation Nurses. (1995). *The gerontological rehabilitation nurse: Role description* [Brochure]. Skokie, IL: Author.

Association of Rehabilitation Nurses. (1997). Certification update. *ARN Network, 13*(1), 5.

Crane, J. (1995). The future of research utilization. *Nursing Clinics of North America, 30,* 565–577.

Eliopoulos, C. (1993). *Gerontological nursing* (3rd ed.). Philadelphia: J. B. Lippincott.

Eliopoulos, C. (1997). *Gerontological nursing.* Philadelphia: Lippincott.

Habel, M. (1993). Rehabilitation nursing practice. In A. McCourt (Ed.), *The specialty practice of rehabilitation nursing: A core curriculum* (3rd ed.). Skokie, IL: Rehabilitation Nursing Foundation.

Hoenig, H., Nusbaum, N., & Brummel-Smith, K. (1997). Geriatric rehabilitation: State of the art. *Journal of the American Geriatrics Society, 45,* 1371–1381.

Kuhn, T. (1995). Scientific revolution. In R. Boyd, P. Gasper, & J. D. Trout (Eds.), *The philosophy of science* (pp. 139–158). Cambridge, MA: Massachusetts Institute of Technology.

Lachs, M. S., & Ruchlin, H. S. (1997). Is managed care good or bad for geriatric medicine? *Journal of the American Geriatrics Society, 45,* 1123–1127.

National Institute of Nursing Research, Priority Expert Panel of Long-term Care. (1994). *Long-term care for older adults.* Bethesda, MD: U.S. Department of Health and Human Services.

Office of Disease Prevention and Health Promotion. (1990). *Healthy people 2000: National health promotion and disease prevention objectives.* U.S. Public Health Service. Pub No. 017-001-00473. Washington, DC: U.S. Government Printing Office.

Staab, A. S., & Hodges, L. C. (1996). *Essentials of gerontological nursing: Adaptation to the aging process.* Philadelphia: J. B. Lippincott.

Tagliareni, E. (1993). Issues and recommendations for associate degree education in gerontological nursing. In C. Heine (Ed.), *Determining the future of gerontological nursing education* (pp. 60–63). New York: National League for Nursing.

U.S. Department of Commerce, Economics and Statistics Administration, Bureau of the Census. (1992). *Profiles of America's elderly: Growth of America's oldest-old population.* Washington, DC: U.S. Government Printing Office.

Appendix 16A

Philosophical Perspective on the Foundations of Gerontological Rehabilitation Nursing

■

There are several questions that arise when considering the foundations of gerontological rehabilitation nursing. These sorts of "puzzles" in the Kuhnian tradition are discussed here.

One may argue whether nursing as a whole can even be considered a science according to Kuhn, who makes distinctions between basic and applied science. Nursing, when called a science, is more often thought of as applied science. However, three evidences of basic science cited in Kuhn's writings include the goal of increasing understanding rather than control of nature, the existence of exemplars as part of the disciplinary matrix, and the characteristic repetitive problems of trying to bring existing theory and existing observation into agreement. Both the general discipline of nursing and the specialty of gerontological nursing exhibit these traits to some degree, as is expounded on in the following sections. But, for the purpose of this discussion, the following assumptions are presupposed: (1) there exists a metaparadigm for nursing theory; (2) there exists a paradigm for gerontological nursing, whether explicitly defined in the literature or not, which depends on various other paradigms such as those in biology and sociology; and (3) the field of nursing in general has characteristics of both basic and applied science in the Kuhnian view, so is loosely referred to as a science.

Three main factors currently propel the need for change in nursing care of the aged: (1) the essential tension inherent between the specialties of rehabilitation and gerontological nursing, (2) the projected needs of an elderly society, and (3) the cyclical nature of scientific discovery. These points also serve as a basis for discussion of resolutions of the observed anomalies.

The "Essential Tension"

Kuhn's theory of science illuminates some of the problems that have emerged in gerontological nursing. He stated that although the productive scientist must be a traditionalist, this very role is necessary to become a successful innovator. During gerontological nursing's many years of "normal science," GRNs have expanded knowledge about caring for the older adult, becoming clinicians, advanced practitioners, educators, and researchers. Gerontological nurses have certainly advanced in knowledge, so the objective of increased understanding of the paradigm is constantly being met. But what is the pinnacle of all this accumulation of wisdom? Kuhn answered this question rather well when he described the concept of "essential tension" implicit in scientific research. Just as the aging population is changing, nursing must also mature. As Kuhn said, "the old must be revalued and reordered when assimilating the new" (1995, p. 140). Traditional gerontic nursing is in need of change in order to progress as a specialty within the science of nursing.

One force propelling change is the growing "tension" between views of acute and chronic illness. Traditionally, these concepts have represented "opposing" sides of the range of nursing care. Although we can simplify these terms into working definitions, reality is quite different. There is no sharp dividing line between what is "acute" and what is "chronic" illness. The problems of reconciliation between these views, in light of the Kuhnian tradition, have led some to question the existing paradigm. It is possible that the gap in care that arises from traditional divisions between gerontology and rehabilitation nursing involves the sort of puzzles, problems, and anomalies that Kuhn sees as leading to revolution. One of the greatest anomalies in gerontological nursing is that it is not rehabilitation based. For example, most gerontological texts focus on acute care, without an emphasis on rehabilitation of those persons with chronic problems, especially those elderly living in the community. It could be said that the present "theory" of gerontological nursing, which does not focus on rehabilitation, has come under scrutiny because observations have told us that more people are aging with disabilities and chronic illnesses than our present system allows for or anticipated. As life span has increased, so has the number of elderly with long-term health alterations. While this knowledge must be reconciled, nursing as a science, whether basic or applied, or both, is inherently affected because the demands of the changing population warrant it. However, since the emergence of rehabilitation as a nursing specialty in 1974, the disciplines of gerontological and rehabilitation nursing have attempted to close the gap between acute and chronic health care for the elderly, trying to bring their ideas together for the sake of the prevailing paradigm and the good of the aged.

A second problem that arises from the essential tension between gerontological and rehabilitation nursing is that of education. Kuhn's position that the nature of natural science education is conducted primarily through textbooks is demonstrated here in nursing. There are only two comprehensive rehabilitation nursing books on the market today. Although care of the ill adult is discussed in virtually all nursing texts on the subject, the same books are reluctant to give even a scant chapter on long-term therapeutic care of the older adult. Is this to suggest that rehabilitation is not a part of gerontological nursing? Surely this could not be the case, given that more than half of the elderly suffer from at least one chronic illness, and more are likely to die from a long-term illness than an acute one (Eliopoulos, 1993). Are we also, then, educating nurses in the principles of rehabilitation as well as gerontological nursing? I think not. One need only survey the curricula of schools and colleges of nursing to see that this is true. Rarely do nursing programs offer a single course in rehabilitation. In fact, many still do not include intensive education in gerontology despite the projections that more than half of the total supply of registered nurses will be caring for persons in the older age category (U.S. Department of Commerce, 1992).

Now, I must again clarify what is meant by rehabilitation, for most nurses will probably exclaim that they practice these techniques already. Experience has shown that such is just not the case. Rehabilitation nurses are specially trained to care for individuals (and their families) who have experienced a long-term health alteration, such as stroke or amputation, helping them cope and adapt to a life-changing crisis. This care begins "day one" (in "acute" care) and is necessary to maintain function, promote independence and self-care, and prevent secondary complications. In fact, according to Kuhn's view, rehabilitation nursing could be considered an exemplar of the entire nursing field. Rehabilitation specialists have worked out problems with patients with the most complex medical conditions, applying principles of the paradigm to unique cases. Take, for example, a recent situation faced by one rehabilitation team: to teach a young woman with traumatic quadruple amputations to function again in her roles as a wife, mother, and member of society. Such a case represents the ultimate challenge for physicians, nurses, therapists, and technologists to expand the existing paradigm by necessary innovations.

Rehabilitation nurses work from a broad knowledge base and must cooperatively function as an interdisciplinary team member, because this approach to goal attainment is the lifeblood of this specialty. These concepts and principles are not typically taught in depth in nursing school and are unfamiliar to many nurses. Indeed, most nurse educators are themselves lacking in this crucial education and so are reluctant to teach these concepts to others.

Thus, there needs to be discussion between leaders, clinicians, and academicians in gerontology and rehabilitation to further define and clarify the roles of each, their differences and similarities. A joint agenda should be established to ensure continuity of care between specialty groups. Textbooks need to be written to expound new theories and ideas that emphasize rehabilitation. Additionally, nurses must be educated in both these areas at the basic level to be prepared to face the challenges ahead as our society ages.

Social Forces

Although Kuhn agrees that social forces alone are not sufficient to drive science, he acknowledges the powerful impact such changes have on promoting the development of new knowledge. According to the American Association of Retired Persons (AARP), persons older than age 65 represent more than 12.9% of the U.S. population, or about one in every eight Americans (1994). By 2030, when the "baby boomers" reach age 65, they will account for about 20% of the population. Life expectancy as of 1992 was 75.7 years (Aiken, 1995), so people are living longer than in years past. The group of those 85 and older is the fastest growing age group (U.S. Department of Commerce, 1992). However, approximately 29% of elders assessed their health as fair or poor (AARP, 1994), and more than 7 million reportedly needed help with activities of daily living (Staab & Hodges, 1996). In addition, elders accounted for 35% of all hospital stays in 1992, but the average length of stay was only 8.2 days (Staab & Hodges, 1996). With most hospitalized elders staying in the hospital a little more than a week, where should the focus of care be? Do these aged individuals recover so quickly, or are they being discharged quicker and sicker into a community that is ill prepared to handle their complex medical needs? I suggest that the latter is true. One of the foremost problems facing health care today is how to manage the needs of the growing aged population. More frail elderly are living in the community with multiple chronic problems and complex needs. Some still believe that such elderly provide no useful contribution to society. But what will happen when 20% of the population is old? If we do not focus on rehabilitation, teaching these individuals to perform self-care and maintain independence as long as possible, the supply of health care workers will not meet the demand for services. The family members will then become the primary caregivers. We already see this happening with increasing frequency in the community. Then who will teach the families to care for their loved ones? Most likely, nurses will be the instructors. But how can they teach what they themselves have not learned? These facts provide a compelling reason for gerontological nurses of the future to be educated in the rehabilitation process.

It is at this point that we may introduce a final solution to the anomaly present in gerontological nursing. This is the emergence of a new subspecialty, which, ideally, will eventually influence the way nursing care of the aged is practiced. This is the field of gerontological rehabilitation nursing, which represents an exemplar of gerontological nursing, much as rehabilitation is an exemplar of nursing in general. This "subspecialty" has been defined by the Association of Rehabilitation Nurses: "Gerontological rehabilitation nurses use a holistic approach in the assessment and provision of services to geriatric clients. Helping geriatric clients achieve their optimal level of physical, mental, and psychosocial well-being is the primary goal" (1995, p. 1).

However, as the Kuhnian theory suggests, new problems arise with the emergence of gerontological rehabilitation nursing. If this new branch of rehabilitation nursing is accepted, what does this say about gerontological nursing? That it is not holistic? That it has only an acute care focus? Are gerontological nurses prepared to give up the rehabilitative piece of their specialty? Are rehabilitation nurses ready to subsume that portion of care in its entirety? Under whose domain does care of the chronically ill elderly fall? One must also ask why gerontological rehabilitation nursing did not grow out of gerontological nursing, the more mature established tradition, rather than the "infant" field of rehabilitation nursing. If, as Kuhn suggests, the process of solving puzzles and anomalies precedes scientific revolution, then perhaps gerontological nursing will soon be on the horizon of such an event.

This growing dilemma can have but one satisfactory outcome. That is the change in our approach to holistic care of the elderly. Our methods and procedures must reflect the idea that rehabilitation is at the core of, and the prevailing framework for, all gerontological nursing. This can only occur as nurses become more educated about the process of rehabilitation. It could be that over time, as this idea is developed, that a shift will occur and a new paradigm will emerge.

The Cyclical Nature of Science

If, as Kuhn believes, science is cyclical in nature, consisting of periods of normal science and revolution, then we must consider gerontological nursing to be in a time of normal science. We have developed and continue to research the existing paradigm. Our thinking and studying has been quite convergent. One need only compare a few of the dozens of gerontological nursing texts recently published to observe how very similar each is in its approach and scope. We emphasize primary care and promoting wellness, as well as care of the ill adult. But where are the principles that lead us to new discoveries in the care of the elder with long-term health problems and improvement of their quality of life? Why is it that nursing professionals acknowledge a gap in the health care of the elderly but are so slow to diverge from the comfortable circle we have come to accept as gerontological nursing?

Although, as Kuhn states, there would be no normal science without commitment to a paradigm, instead of being content with the status quo of gerontological nursing science, we may need to seek those personalities who will lead nurses to expand their knowledge (pure), skills (applied), and creativity (inventor), to meet the future challenge of gerontic care. The concepts of gerontological rehabilitation nursing stand as an example of the beginning of new theories emerging from the old, teaching that the elderly are to be valued throughout their entire life span and that independence can and should be maintained as long as possible.

To summarize, Kuhn's theory of science can be used to illuminate the problems and solutions that have arisen within the field of gerontological nursing. By examining a few of the characteristics of Kuhnian science that apply to this specialty, questions about the prevailing paradigm are raised and patterns of struggle and growth become evident. Gerontological rehabilitation nursing represents a viable solution to the dilemma of continuity of care for the elderly, and it has emerged from factors such as the essential tension between views of acute and chronic illness, social forces, and the cyclical nature of scientific methods. Gerontological and rehabilitation nurses need to work together to refine the new ideas and concepts proposed by gerontological rehabilitation nursing, whose future may serve as an exemplar of the profession, even to the point of promoting a shift in the present paradigm. In Kuhn's view of science, the solving of puzzles and problems that are becoming more obvious in nursing with the changing elderly population, leads to the discovery of new ideas and eventually revolution.

Index

Note: Page numbers in *italics* indicate figures; those followed by t indicate tables.

ISBN 0-7216-6344-3

90038

9 780721 663449